Emergency Nursing Certification (CEN)

SELF-ASSESSMENT AND EXAM REVIEW

Emergency Nursing Certification (CEN)

SELF-ASSESSMENT AND EXAM REVIEW

Jayne McGrath, MS, RN, CEN, CCRN, CNS-BC
Clinical Nurse Specialist—Emergency Department
University of Wisconsin Hospital and Clinics
Faculty Associate—University of Wisconsin—Madison School of Nursing
Madison, Wisconsin

Andi Foley, DNP, RN, ACCNS-AG, CEN
Emergency Services Clinical Nurse Specialist
CHI Franciscan Health—St Francis Hospital
Federal Way, Washington

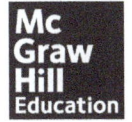

New York / Chicago / San Francisco / Lisbon / London /
Madrid / Mexico City / Milan / New Delhi/ San Juan / Seoul /
Singapore / Sydney / Toronto

Emergency Nursing Certification

ISBN 978-1-259-58714-6
MHID 1-259-58714-2

Copyright © 2017 by The McGraw-Hill Companies, Inc. All rights reserved. Printed in the United States of America. Except as permitted under the United States Copyright Act of 1976, no part of this publication may be reproduced or distributed in any form or by any means, or stored in a data base or retrieval system, without the prior written permission of the publisher.

1 2 3 4 5 6 7 8 9   LOV   21 20 19 18 17 16

Notice

Medicine is an ever-changing science. As new research and clinical experience broaden our knowledge, changes in treatment and drug therapy are required. The authors and the publisher of this work have checked with sources believed to be reliable in their efforts to provide information that is complete and generally in accord with the standards accepted at the time of publication. However, in view of the possibility of human error or changes in medical sciences, neither the authors nor the publisher nor any other party who has been involved in the preparation or publication of this work warrants that the information contained herein is in every respect accurate or complete, and they disclaim all responsibility for any errors or omissions or for the results obtained from use of the information contained in this work. Readers are encouraged to confirm the information contained herein with other sources. For example and in particular, readers are advised to check the product information sheet included in the package of each drug they plan to administer to be certain that the information contained in this work is accurate and that changes have not been made in the recommended dose or in the contraindications for administration. This recommendation is of particular importance in connection with new or infrequently used drugs.

This book was set in Minion Pro by Aptara, Inc.
The Editors were Susan Barnes and Brian Kearns.
The production supervisor was Richard Ruzycka.
Project Management was provided by Dinesh Pokhriyal, Aptara Inc.
The cover designer was Dreamit, Inc.
The index was prepared by Kathrin Unger.

Library of Congress Cataloging-in-Publication Data

Names: McGrath, Jayne, editor. | Foley, Andi, editor.
Title: Emergency nursing certification (CEN) : self-assessment and exam
   review / [edited by] Jayne McGrath, Andi Foley.
Description: New York : McGraw-Hill Education, [2017] | Includes
   bibliographical references and index.
Identifiers: LCCN 2016047951| ISBN 9781259587146 (pbk.) | ISBN 1259587142
Subjects: | MESH: Emergency Nursing–education | Certification | United
   States | Outlines | Examination Questions
Classification: LCC RC86.9 | NLM WY 18.2 | DDC 616.02/5076–dc23 LC record available at https://na01.safelinks.protection.outlook.com/?url=https%3A%2F%2Flccn.loc.gov%2F2016047951&data=01%7C01%7Cmidge.haramis%40mheducation.com%7Cbcc4cb5f528540ea6adf08d402679b57%7Cf919b1efc0c347358fca0928ec39d8d5%7C1&sdata=0Eafgkto1ty%2Bx9szRwNq48j%2Bx2JlF4D2nIAFjxqs7go%3D&reserved=0

McGraw-Hill Education books are available at special quantity discounts to use as premiums and sales promotions, or for use in corporate training programs. To contact a representative please visit the Contact Us page at www.mhprofessional.com.

To the emergency staff at University of Wisconsin Hospital: I am privileged to work alongside you and appreciate the interesting things we see and learn together. Thank you for your kindness and sense of humor.

To my mom, who taught me to set goals and work to attain them. To my husband, Ed, who continues to support and love me as we walk through the many seasons of life together; and to our four sons, who give me good reason to smile every day.

Everything on earth has its own time and its own season. Ecclesiastes 3:1,
(Contemporary English Version—American Bible Society)

Jayne McGrath

One of my favorite quotations is from Rumi: Be a Lamp, a Lifeboat, or a Ladder. In that spirit, I wanted to take this opportunity to especially thank those in my life who have embodied that quote.

To my family, and especially my mom, Ruth Greatens: Thank you for being my lamp and my guiding inspiration.

To my CNS mentors: Thank you for being there when I needed you. Marisa Gillaspie-Aziz, Patti Howard, Melissa Irwin, Terri Repasky, Darleen Williams—you have been and are my lifeboat. Thank you.

To all the ED and ICU teams I have worked with over the years: Thank you for lifting me up or forcing me to climb those ladders past my comfort zone. I have great friends in Wisconsin, Kansas, Utah, Florida, and Washington who make me a better nurse.

And finally—to my husband, Steve Foley. You are my lamp, my lifeboat, and my ladder, every day! Without your support and encouragement, I would not be the person I am today.

Andi Foley

Contents

Contributors .... *ix*
Reviewers .... *xi*
Preface .... *xiii*

1. Getting Ready for the CEN 1
Andi Foley, DNP, RN, ACCNS-AG, CEN

2. Cardiovascular Emergencies 5
Tammy Kasprovich, PhD, RN, CEN

3. Respiratory Emergencies 37
Jamie Vranak, MSN, RN, CEN

4. Neurologic Emergencies 63
Edward Hunt, BS, RN, CEN

5. Shock 91
Jayne McGrath, MS, RN, CEN, CCRN, CNS-BC

6. Gastrointestinal Emergencies 105
Jayne McGrath, MS, RN, CEN, CCRN, CNS-BC

7. Genitourinary, Gynecology, and Obstetrical Emergencies 131
Geraldine M. Maurer, DNP, CRNP, FNP-C, RNC-OB, MPM and
Lorna Woodhall, Ed.D(c), MSN, RN, CEN, EMT-P

    Genitourinary 131
    Gynecology 136
    Obstetrical 143

8. Psychosocial Emergencies 165
Nathan Whitman, DNP, RN, PMHNP-BC, PMHCNS-BC

9. Medical Emergencies and Communicable Diseases 179
Carla Brim, MN, RN, PHCNS-BC, CEN, FAEN and Tami Wheeldon, BSN, RN, CEN

    Medical Emergencies 179
    Communicable Diseases 193

10. Maxillofacial and Ocular Emergencies 211
Jayne McGrath, MS, RN, CEN, CCRN, CNS-BC and Andi Foley, DNP, RN, ACCNS-AG, CEN

    Maxillofacial 211
    Ocular 221

11. Orthopedic and Wound Emergencies 235
Jenna Hannity, MSN, RN, CEN

    Orthopedic 235

    Wound Emergencies 241

12. Environment and Toxicology Emergencies 253
Michael J. Chicarelli, DNP, RN, CEN

    Environmental Emergencies 253

    Toxicology 265

13. Professional Issues in Emergency Nursing 279
Dino Johnson, MHA, BSN, RN

Answer Page for 150 Question CEN Prep Quiz 297

150 Question CEN Prep Quiz 299

Index 341

Contributors

Carla Brim, MN, RN, PHCNS-BC, CEN, FAEN
Trauma Coordinator
Providence Health Care
Instructor
Washington State University College of Nursing
Spokane, Washington
Medical Emergencies and Communicable Diseases

Michael J. Chicarelli, DNP, RN, CEN
Administrator of Professional Services
University of New Mexico Hospitals
Albuquerque, New Mexico
Environment and Toxicology Emergencies

Andi Foley, DNP, RN, ACCNS-AG, CEN
Emergency Services Clinical Nurse Specialist
CHI Franciscan Health—St Francis Hospital
Federal Way, Washington
Getting Ready for CEN
Maxillofacial and Ocular Emergencies

Jenna Hannity, MSN, RN, CEN
Emergency Unit Based Educator
CHI Franciscan Health—St Clare Hospital
Lakewood, Washington
Orthopedic and Wound Emergencies

Edward Hunt, BS, RN, CEN
Emergency Room Nurse
Ocean Beach Hospital
Captain/Training Officer
Wahkiakum County Fire District #3
Rosburg, Washington
Neurologic Emergencies

Dino Johnson, MHA, BSN, RN
Vice President of Patient Services and Chief Nursing Officer
CHI Franciscan Health—St Francis Hospital
Federal Way, Washington
Professional Issues in Emergency Nursing

Tammy Kasprovich, PhD, RN, CEN
Clinical Professor
Columbia College of Nursing, Milwaukee, Wisconsin
Registered Nurse—Emergency Department
Wheaton Franciscan Healthcare Franklin, Franklin, Wisconsin
Cardiovascular Emergencies

Geraldine M. Maurer, DNP, CRNP, FNP-C, RNC-OB, MPM
Assistant Professor—University of Pittsburgh School of Nursing
Family Nurse Practitioner—University of Pittsburgh Medical Center Urgent Care Centers
Pittsburgh, Pennsylvania
Genitourinary, Gynecology, and Obstetrical Emergencies

Jayne McGrath, MS, RN, CEN, CCRN, CNS-BC
Clinical Nurse Specialist—Emergency Department
University of Wisconsin Hospital and Clinics
Faculty Associate—University of Wisconsin—Madison School of Nursing Madison, Wisconsin
Gastrointestinal Emergencies
Maxillofacial and Ocular Emergencies
Shock

Jamie Vranak, MSN, RN, CEN
Director of Ambulatory Services
Wheaton Franciscan Healthcare—Franklin
Franklin, Wisconsin
Respiratory Emergencies

Tami Wheeldon, BSN, RN, CEN
Longview, Washington
Medical Emergencies and Communicable Diseases

Nathan Whitman, DNP, RN, PMHNP-BC, PMHCNS-BC
Clinical Nurse Specialist Psychiatric Liaison
UW Health, University Hospital
Madison, Wisconsin
Psychosocial Emergencies

Lorna Woodhall, Ed.D(c), MSN, RN, CEN, EMT-P
Nursing Faculty
Pittsburgh Technical Institute
Oakdale, Pennsylvania
Genitourinary, Gynecology, and Obstetric Emergencies

Reviewers

Mark Blaney, BScN, RN, CEN
Regional Nurse Educator
CHI Franciscan Health
Tacoma, Washington

Lisa Ebert, RN, BSN, CEN
Emergency Department Charge Nurse &
Stroke Coordinator for the Aspirus System
Aspirus Wausau Hospital
Wausau, Wisconsin

Cathy C. Fox, RN, CEN, CPEN, FAEN
Nurse Consultant
Department of Quality Management
ED, Cath Lab, and Cardiovascular Services
Naval Medical Center Portsmouth
Portsmouth, Virginia

Michael D. Gooch, DNP, RN, ACNP-BC, FNP-BC, ENP-BC, CFRN, CTRN, CEN, NREMT-P
Instructor of Nursing—Vanderbilt University School of Nursing
Flight Nurse—Vanderbilt University Medical Center
Emergency Nurse Practitioner—TeamHealth
Nashville, Tennessee

Renee Semonin Holleran, FNP-BC, PhD, CEN, CFRN (Ret), CTRN (Ret), FAEN
Nurse Practitioner Holistic Medicine
George E. Wahlen VA Medical Center
Salt Lake City, Utah

Valerie Mack, BSN, RN, CEN, CPEN
Care Team Leader
University of Wisconsin Hospital and Clinics, Emergency Department
Madison, Wisconsin

Tami Morin, MS, RN, NEA-BC
Director, Emergency Services
University of Wisconsin Hospital & Clinics
Madison, Wisconsin

Jean A. Proehl, RN, MN, CEN, CPEN, FAEN
Emergency Clinical Nurse Specialist, Proehl PRN, LLC
Editor, *Advanced Emergency Nursing Journal*
Emergency Nurse, Dartmouth-Hitchcock Medical Center, Lebanon, New Hampshire
Emergency Nurse, Gifford Medical Center, Randolph, VT
Cornish, New Hampshire

Laura Smolinski, PhD, RN
Clinical Assistant Professor
University of Wisconsin—Oshkosh
Oshkosh, Wisconsin
Staff Nurse, ThedaCare, Neenah, Wisconsin

Bradley Thompson, MSN, RN-BC, PMHCNS-BC
Clinical Nurse Specialist, Inpatient Mental Health Services
CHI Franciscan Health—St Joseph Medical Center
Tacoma, Washington

Ann White, MSN, APRN, CCNS, CEN, CPEN
Clinical Nurse Specialist Emergency Services
Department of Advanced Clinical Practice
Duke University Hospital
Clinical Associate Faculty, Duke University School of Nursing
Durham, North Carolina

Preface

When considering components of a useful certification book, a first thought may be questions with answers including rationale. We had this thought as well. But what if the reader would like to review the elements of a neuro exam or signs and symptoms of the various types of hepatitis? Wouldn't it be more interesting if one book contained a review of content from the CEN exam blueprint *and* Q&A with rationale, all inside the same cover?

The aim of this book is to provide an overview of content for the CEN exam, followed by critical-thinking questions to help prepare for the exam. Along with serving as a preparation guide for the CEN certification exam, this book also serves as a clinical reference. Achieving specialty certification is a journey requiring diligent study and persistence. We know this book will be a valuable resource for you.

The system-specific chapters are presented in a concise format designed for easy reading. The content is designed to reflect the 2016 CEN blueprint as well as including current guidelines and evidence-based practice.

We thank the contributors to this book. As they wrote (and rewrote), they never complained about our requests—not even the last-minute ones. Thank you for sharing your knowledge and experience.

We appreciate the reviewers who provided their expertise in ensuring that the content was current and relevant. Thank you for generously sharing your time and work.

Also, thank you to the editors and staff at McGraw-Hill, who have provided support and guidance throughout this project.

Finally, we want to additionally dedicate this book to our readers and to all nurses who are working toward or maintaining their emergency nursing certification. Your desire for personal growth and dedication to our profession creates safer emergency departments for all patients.

— Jayne and Andi

Getting Ready for the CEN

Andi Foley, DNP, RN, ACCNS-AG, CEN

Congratulations on taking the next steps toward earning or maintaining your credential as a Certified Emergency Nurse (CEN®).

From the first test date in July 1980 through 2016, more than 30,000 nurses have earned the CEN mark of distinction.[1] This book, *Emergency Nursing Certification*, provides emergency nursing content based on topics suggested in the CEN test blueprint and includes more than 300 unique CEN preparation questions written and reviewed by experts in emergency nursing and related fields.

Why Certify?

Reasons to strive for the CEN credential can be as individual as each nurse taking the test. Common reasons may include dedication to the profession of emergency nursing, validation of emergency nursing expertise, a commitment to continued learning, external motivators from your employer, such as recognitions, financial bonus, or an increased pay rate, or simply because you want to challenge yourself.

Certified nurses improve patient outcomes. Specifically, certification has been associated with decreased rates of infection and decreased patient fall rates.[2,3] Certification is also positively correlated with perception of empowerment in the workplace, meaning that nurses with their CEN credential feel more empowered in their departments.[4] Nurses holding a professional certification are also more likely to feel informal power to lead or make clinical decisions in the workplace.[5,6] Certified nurses report feelings of pride, accomplishment, achievement, confidence, and credibility specifically related to the earned certification.[6]

The CEN test is recognized as a high-level nursing certification credential by the Accreditation Board for Specialty Nursing Certification.[1] Some states recognize specialty nursing certification, such as the CEN, as proof of continued competency or required continuing education credits.[7] Check with your state board to see if this applies in your state.

About the Test

In 2016, the CEN is earned by passing a 175-question test, of which 150 are scored questions and 25 are unscored questions undergoing validation. Proctored at *Pearson VUE®* testing centers throughout the United States, applicants have 180 minutes to take the test with the time starting after a brief computer tutorial. The Board of Certification for Emergency Nursing (BCEN) recommends, but does not require, two years of experience as an emergency nurse before testing.[1]

The CEN test was developed to evaluate specialized content and is a challenging certification to earn. It was not designed to be easy. Treat your preparation seriously with the respect and commitment that emergency nursing as a professional specialty deserves.

Resources for the CEN Test

The current test blueprint and the candidate handbook, two essential resources for CEN test preparation, are found on the BCEN website. Containing content recommended by the 2016 blueprint, the book is structured into functional physiological chapters more closely resembling common Emergency Nurses Association (ENA) resources, such as the Core Curriculum, Trauma Nursing Core Course (TNCC), and Emergency Nurse Pediatric Course (ENPC).

This Book As a Resource

This book is written to be an overview of content included in the CEN exam and provides more than 300 questions with rationalized answers to practice test taking while continuing to learn from correct and incorrect responses. Whether used as a self-assessment or a standard review, *Emergency Nursing Certification* is a study guide. This book is not intended to be a stand-alone resource, but rather to build on your current knowledge, enhance your internal culture of professional curiosity, and assist you in preparing for success on the CEN examination.

Electronic Resources

Online sources with questions and rationalized answers, such as the fee-based pre-tests available from BCEN, may be of interest to some and can be used to identify specific areas of content in which you need additional study. Various social media sites, including YouTube© and Facebook©, offer content that is specific to CEN review. Mobile applications are also available to review emergency nursing content and to answer certification-level questions. Podcasts and blogs cover evidence-based practice and current research from perspectives of emergency nurses or emergency providers. As long as the nurse remains astute about the source, emerging online resources offer free open access nurse education (FOANed) and free open access medical education (FOAMed) sites, blogs, or podcasts specifically directed to nursing or medicine content adding to knowledge leading to CEN success. However, critically evaluate the date of the online resource and the references used by the blog or podcast. While many FOANed and FOAMed sources are well researched and strongly evidence-based, some are intended primarily to share opinions of the author. When using online sources to study for CEN, think critically about the source because not all online sources are peer-reviewed.

In-Person Class Resources

Classes for CEN preparation are offered through various venues. Some hospitals offer classes using local CEN educators or contract professional CEN speakers as a teaching tool to offer support within the workplace. ENA chapters or state councils may also sponsor CEN review classes. Courses developed and sponsored by ENA, such as TNCC, ENPC, and GENE, are also helpful for CEN preparation.

Printed Resources

While you have already made an excellent choice for CEN review preparation by purchasing this book, other printed resources used for CEN preparation are also broadly available and varied in content. Current editions of publications referenced within the chapters of this book are recommended supplements to any CEN preparation. Professional emergency nursing publications, such as the *Journal of Emergency Nursing*, may also contain articles of interest, current research, and certification review questions. Scholarly peer-reviewed journals, such as the *Journal of Emergency Nursing* and the *Advanced Emergency Nursing Journal*, contain a higher level of accuracy and currency compared to nonpeer-reviewed publications. Emergency nursing textbooks are available through a variety of sources, but do ensure that the book you choose is the most recent edition.

Preparing for the CEN Test

Once initial resources are chosen (thank you again for choosing this book as part of your study plan), studying continues, building on current knowledge and experience. While everyone prepares differently, preparation may make the difference between success and poor performance. This section contains tips on studying for the CEN as well as other test preparation tips.

Study Tips

When preparing for the CEN test, have a strategy and overstudy. For some, this means accomplishing a certain amount of content review by a certain date. For others, this may mean scheduling time to study each day or each week. See Appendix 1 for an example CEN preparation study schedule for a full-time night shift nurse. Regardless of how you choose to prepare, do so to create a personal process. Think about the day of the CEN test. What may make you feel most anxious? How can you best prepare to reduce testing anxiety? While specific strategies depend on your personal learning style, there are a few common test preparation methods to consider.

Possible Study Methods:

- Create a timeline
  - Study by chapter
  - Study by disease state
- Determine your personal study style
  - Many tools are available online or are paper-based from instructors
  - Compilation website from BCEN: http://www.learning-styles-online.com
  - From BCEN: http://vark-learn.com/the-vark-questionnaire/
  - Another option: http://www.personal.psu.edu/bxb11/LSI/LSI.htm
- Study with a group
  - Group study can provide perspective that individual study lacks
- Attend a CEN review class
- Answer many questions but focus on the areas where you feel less confident
  - Since the maximum testing time is 180 minutes, sitting for three hours to answer CEN test prep questions helps you prepare for that length of time
- Create notecards or flashcards
  - Handwriting memory aids may lead to retaining more information compared to purchasing or electronically creating them[8-9]
- Develop more training in a "weak" content area
  - For example, if you are not strong in disaster content, consider preparing a Disaster Review for your local ENA chapter or for your department staff meeting. You can develop your own knowledge by preparing to teach others
- Think positive thoughts about your success
- Visualize yourself with your new CEN name badge

In the Days Before the CEN Test

In the days before taking the CEN test, consider planning a drive to the testing site. This "test drive" may actually help reduce anxiety on the day of the test. Consider other "what if" scenarios and create contingency plans. What is the plan if the car does not start or if the babysitter is sick? If the drive to the testing center may be a problem, consider planning for a nearby hotel the night before. Just as with patients, critically think through possible scenarios and plan your interventions.

The day before the test follow your "normal" schedule as much as possible. Avoid alcohol or any food creating GI upset. Avoid anything known to disrupt your rest. Do not take a new medication, especially a medication to sleep if you are not positive about how your body may react to it. Get the sufficient amount of rest you need to help yourself perform at your best. Lack of sleep can cloud your memory and slow your decision-making skills. Set yourself up for success.

On the Day of the CEN Test

Continue your journey toward success by eating breakfast. Give your brain the nutrients needed to critically think and your body fuel to push through any stress or anxiety you may feel. Avoid excessive caffeine to prevent jitters during the test. Carefully monitor your fluid intake. Your goal is enough fluid for your body to function without needing frequent trips to the restroom during the test. However, if you need them, the 180-minute time limit does include breaks. Dress in layers if you need to as you best understand how your body reacts to stress. Many personal items, including cell phones and coats, are not allowed in the testing center. Food, drink, and chewing gum are also prohibited. Plan enough time for your drive to arrive slightly early, but no more than 15 minutes early, with all needed personal identification documents and your authorization to test that day.[10] Do not plan further review for testing day. You followed your strategy for preparing and you are ready. In three hours or less from your start time, you will know the results of your hard work and preparation. Relax and do your best.

Test-Taking Tips

Undoubtedly, you already have many tools in your toolbox for successful testtaking. This section reviews but also adds some elements for you to consider while you are testing.

- Read the whole question
  - What is actually being asked?
  - Do you know the answer before reading the answer options? If so, is that answer one of your options?
- Read only the question as written
  - If you are thinking "well, the patient could also be "_____" (diabetic, hypotensive…), you are adding information and are overthinking the question
- Are there clues?
  - Details are added because they are needed and important. If the question references a specific time, it is important. It is a clue
  - Are there key words such as "always" or "priority" to guide you?
    - Consider writing the key word on the provided scratch paper
    - In a question such as, *"Which response indicates the need for further teaching?,"* the correct response is the one that is wrong. In this case, *"further teaching"* are the key words. Pay close attention to what the question is asking
- An incorrect answer may be partially correct
  - Incorrect options may be technically correct but not answer the question posed. What is the question asking?
  - While the incorrect answer might be partially correct, only the correct answer is *fully correct*, given the question being asked
  - There is always a best answer
- There are no patterns in the correct answers
  - Questions are randomly generated. If you have five "*D*" answers in a row, this is simply a coincidence
- Trust your first instinct
  - If you are contemplating changing your answer, ask yourself why the right answer is right. Why are the wrong answers wrong?
  - Before you change an answer, ask yourself, "Would I bet $50 that my new answer is right?" If you cannot answer "yes," reconsider
- If you do not know the correct answer
  - Narrow your options. Use a process of elimination
    - Consider treating each option as a true or false statement
  - Still do not know? Guess. Althougha blank answer is 100% wrong, a blind guess still has a 25% chance of being right. If you have narrowed your answer options, your chances of being right improve

With thorough preparation and thoughtful testing strategies, you will join over 30,000 CEN who are making a difference for patients everyday. You have already taken the first steps. Now, it is time to continue on your journey of preparation and readinessso you are successful on the CEN exam.

Appendix 1

Example CEN study plan for a night shift emergency nurse.

CEN Study Plan: February

Sunday	Monday	Tuesday	Wednesday	Thursday	Friday	Saturday
Jan 29 Family Day!	Jan 30 1300–1500 **Finish** Neuro Ch	Jan 31 1100–1300 **Start** Env/Tox	February 1 Work 7p-7a	2 Work 7p-7a	3 1900–2100 Env/Tox…	4 Work 7p-7a
5 Work 7p-7a	6 Work 7p-7a	7 Work 7p-7a	8	9 1300–1500 Env/Tox	10 1300–1500 Finish Env/Tox	11
12 0930–1200 **Start** Medical Ch **(LAST Chapter!!)**	13 1300–1500 Medical	14 1300–1500 Medical	15 Work 7p-7a	16 Work 7p-7a	17 1900–2100 Medical	18 Work 7p-7a
19 Work 7p-7a	20 Work 7p-7a	21 Work 7p-7a	22 ?? CEN study??	23 1300–1500 Medical	24 1300–1500 **Finish** Medical	25 **1430** Retake CEN prep test & analyze score
26	27 1300–1500 Review based on test score	28 1300–1500 Review based on test score	Mar 1 Work 7p-7a	Mar 2 Work 7p-7a	Mar 3 1700–1830 Review based on test score	Mar 4 Work 7p-7a
Mar 5 Work 7p-7a	Mar 6 Work 7p-7a	Mar 7 Work 7p-7a	Mar 8 1500–1600 Final review Good night sleep!	Mar 9 **TEST DAY!** **1430**	Mar 10	Mar 11

Test Day: March 9 @ 1430

REFERENCES

1. Board of Certification for Emergency Nursing (BCEN) website. https://www.bcencertifications.org/Home.aspx. Published 2016. Accessed March 8, 2016.
2. Boyle DK, Gajewski BJ, Miller PA. A longitudinal analysis of nursing specialty certification by Magnet® status and patient unit type. *J of Nursing Administration*. 2012;42(12):567–573. doi: 10.1097/NNA.0b013e318274b581
3. Boyle DK, Cramer E, Potter C, et al. The relationship between direct-care RN specialty certification and surgical patient outcomes. *AORN journal*. 2014;100(5):511–528. doi: 10.1016/j.aorn.2014.04.018
4. Fitzpatrick JJ, Campo TM, Gacki-Smith J. Emergency care nurses: certification, empowerment, and work-related variables. *Journal of Emergency Nursing*. 2014;40(2):e37–e43. Accessed http://dx.doi.org/10.1016/j.jen.2013.01.021
5. Krapohl G, Manojlovich M, Redman R, et al. Nursing specialty certification and nursing-sensitive patient outcomes in the intensive care unit. *American Journal of Critical Care*. 2010;19(6):490–498. doi:10.4037/ajcc2010406
6. Schroeter K, Byrne MM, Klink KA, et al. The impact of certification on certified perioperative nurses: a qualitative descriptive survey. *ORNAC Journal-Operating Room Nurses Association of Canada*. 2012:30(3):34.
7. Wolters Kluwer: Lippincott Nursing Center. State requirements for CE. http://www.nursingcenter.com/ceconnection/ce-state-requirements. Published 2016. Accessed April 20, 2016.
8. Alton S. Learning how to learn: Meta-learning strategies for the challenges of learning pharmacology. *Nurse Education Today*. 2016;38;2–4. doi:10.1016/j.nedt.2016.01.003
9. Li JX, James KH. Handwriting generates variable visual output to facilitate symbol learning. *J of Experimental Psych*. 2016;154(3):298–313. http://dx.doi.org/10.1037/xge0000134
10. Board of Certification for Emergency Nursing (BCEN). Candidate Handbook. https://www.bcencertifications.org/BCENMain/media/BCEN/BCEN-Candidate-Handbook-160210.pdf. Published on 2016. Accessed March 31, 2016.

Cardiovascular Emergencies

Tammy Kasprovich, PhD, RN, CEN

Acute Coronary Syndrome

Acute coronary syndrome (ACS) is described as a condition reducing coronary blood flow causing myocardial ischemia or infarction. The common cause of ACS is an unstable thin, fibrous plaque that ruptures causing a thrombosis to form.[1,2] This thrombosis partially or completely obstructs the coronary artery, which decreases the blood flow to the myocardium. The lack of blood flow deprives the myocardium of oxygen leading to cell damage and death.

If the ischemic episode is short, the myocardium may survive without injury.[1] However, if the ischemic episode is prolonged, the myocardium will infarct.[1] Necrosis from the infarction can be detected through specific cardiac biomarkers, troponins or creatine kinase–MB. Risk factors include men older than 45 years, postmenopausal women older than 55 years, individuals with diabetes, elevated cholesterol levels, cigarette smoking, obesity, sedentary lifestyle, hypertension, and stress.[2]

ACS Involves[3]

- Non-ST-segment elevation ACS (formally referred to as unstable angina and non-ST segment elevation myocardial infarction)[3]
  - A continuum occurs between unstable angina (UA) and non-ST segment elevation myocardial infarction (NSTEMI) and cannot be distinguished on initial presentation[3]
  - If an elevation in the biomarkers (cardiac troponins or creatine kinase–MB) does not occur, there is a confirmation of unstable angina[3]
  - A similar clinical guideline for non-ST-segment elevation ACS management has been crafted[3]
- ST-segment elevation myocardial infarction[3] (STEMI)

A commonly used medication for ACS is nitroglycerin. Nitroglycerin is a venous and arterial vasodilator that reduces myocardial oxygen demand by decreasing the preload and improving coronary blood flow. Preload is the degree of myocardial stretch prior to contraction.

Non-ST-Segment Elevation ACS

Prinzmetal (variant) angina was first identified in the late 1950s as a variant form of angina. Prinzmetal angina is associated with coronary arteries spasm and tobacco cessation can reduce the spasm.[4] Other modifiable risk factors for Prinzmetal angina are stress, cold weather exposure, and cocaine use. Calcium channel blockers alone or in conjunction with long acting nitrates are recommended treatment for this vasospastic type of angina.[3]

Unstable angina (UA) is chest pain that may increase in intensity and duration and is not relieved with rest. The pain may subside or become refractory. The main cause of angina is a thrombosis partially or intermittently occluding the coronary artery.[2] Other causes of unstable angina include vasospasm or spontaneous coronary artery dissection. UA can lead to NSTEMI or STEMI. Clinical guidelines for the care of patients with unstable angina and other causes of chest pain continue to be reviewed and updated in the literature.[5] Urgent invasive diagnostic angiography (with possible revascularization if needed) is strongly recommended for refractory angina, hemodynamic, or electrical instability absent of serious comorbidities.[3]

Assessment/Analysis

- History of chest pain occurring
  - At rest
  - During sleep
  - With exercise
  - After cold exposure
- Syncope
- Dyspnea
- Palpitations
- Diaphoresis
- Nausea or vomiting
- Dizziness/lightheadedness
- Tachycardia
- Tachypnea
- Hypotension or hypertension
- 12 lead ECG should be implemented for chest pain or other symptoms of ACS[3]
  - Within 10 minutes of arrival to the emergency department (and/or symptom onset), the patient should be evaluated for ischemic changes
  - Consider serial ECGs (such as 15 to 30 minute intervals for the first hour) if the first ECG is not diagnostic and the patient continues to have symptoms suggestive of ACS

- 18-lead may also be acquired for additional views of myocardial conduction
- Laboratory studies
  - CBC with differential
  - Serum chemistries
  - No elevation in cardiac enzymes, i.e., creatine kinase (CK), creatine kinase MB (CK-MB), and Troponin I or T[1,2]
  - Consider serial assessments for cardiac troponin every 3 to 6 hours after initial onset[3]
  - Coagulation profile
- Portable Chest X-ray

Interventions
- Cardiac and pulse oximetry (SpO_2) monitoring
- Oxygen
  - Routine administration of oxygen for a patient with normal oxygenation levels may not provide a benefit. Consider not administering supplemental oxygen for the non-hypoxic patient[6]
  - If less than 94%, start oxygen via nasal cannula and titrate, as needed
- Establish IV access for crystalloids/blood products/medications as needed
- Nitrates
  - Nitroglycerin can be administered in various forms including sublingual (SL), IV, topical ointment, transdermal, or translingual metered spray
  - Non-ST-segment elevation ACS with ongoing ischemic pain
    - Nitroglycerin (0.3 to 0.4 mg) every 5 minutes, sublingual or aerosol, up to 3 doses for unrelieved ischemic pain[6]
    - If pain persists after 3 doses, reassess need for IV nitroglycerin, if no contraindications
  - Contraindicated in[6]
    - Hypotension (SBP < 90)
    - Heart rate < 50 or > 100
    - Inferior wall MI with right ventricular infarction (V4R)
  - Do not administer to patients who have taken a Phosphodiesterase Inhibitor within the preceding 24 hours (such as sildenafil) or within 48 hours for tadalafil[3]
- Morphine IV: for chest pain unrelieved by nitrates
  - Preferred analgesic with a STEMI[6]
- Aspirin 160 mg to 325, if not given by EMS[6]
- Beta-blockers should be initiated within the first 24 after the onset of ACS providing there are no contraindications such as cardiogenic shock or presence of cocaine and/or methamphetamine[3]
  - Beta-blockers inhibit the $\beta 1$ adrenergic receptors in the heart therefore decreasing myocardial contractility and heart rate ultimately reducing myocardial oxygen demand
- Angiotensin-converting enzyme (ACE) inhibitor added for patients with reduced left ventricular ejection fraction (LVEF less than 0.40), hypertension, diabetes, or stable chronic kidney disease[3]
  - Angiotensin-converting enzyme (ACE) inhibitor decreases water reabsorption therefore decreasing the preload and afterload
  - The afterload is the force the contracting heart muscle must generate to eject blood from a filled heart
- Prepare for possible hospital admission

Evaluation
- Relief of chest pain
- No dysrhythmias or changes in cardiac rhythm
- Hemodynamic stability
- Reduction in controllable risk factors
  - Smoking cessation education
  - Follow up with primary care physician for management

Non-ST Elevation Myocardial Infarction (NSTEMI)

NSTEMI has signs and symptoms similar to angina, but patients may have increased chest pain intensity and/or duration, and elevated cardiac enzymes. NSTEMI is caused from a partially or intermittently occluded coronary artery.[2] Patients may need a diagnostic cardiac catheterization with possible percutaneous coronary intervention to increase perfusion to the myocardium.

Assessment/Analysis[1,2]
- Chest pain/pressure
- Radiation of pain to the left arm or jaw
- Dyspnea
- Diaphoresis
- Nausea
- Tachycardia
- Tachypnea
- Hypotension or hypertension
- Dizziness/lightheadedness
- Syncope
- ECG changes
  - ST depression
  - T wave inversion (may not always be present)
- Laboratory studies
  - CBC with differential
  - Serum chemistries
  - Elevation in cardiac enzymes, i.e., creatine kinase (CK), creatine kinase MB (CK-MB), and Troponin I or T
  - Coagulation studies
- Portable Chest x-ray

Interventions
- Similar to Non-ST-segment elevation ACS
- Cardiac and pulse oximetry (SpO$_2$) monitoring
- Oxygen
  - Routine administration of oxygen for a patient with normal oxygenation levels may not provide a benefit. Consider not administering supplemental oxygen for the non-hypoxic patient[6]
  - If less than 94%, start oxygen at 2 to 4 liters via nasal cannula and titrate, as needed
- Establish IV access for crystalloids/blood products/medications as needed
- Nitrates
  - Nitroglycerin can be administered in various forms including sublingual (SL), IV, topical ointment, transdermal, or translingual metered spray
  - Non-ST-segment elevation ACS with ongoing ischemic pain
    - Nitroglycerin (0.3 to 0.4 mg) every 5 minutes, sublingual or aerosol, up to 3 doses for unrelieved ischemic pain[6]
    - If pain persists after 3 doses, reassess the need for IV nitroglycerin, if no contraindications
  - Contraindicated in[6]
    - Hypotension (SBP < 90)
    - Heart rate < 50 or > 100
    - Inferior wall MI with right ventricular infarction (V4R)
  - Do not administer to patients who have taken a Phosphodiesterase Inhibitor within the preceding 24 hours (such as sildenafil) or within 48 hours for tadalafil[3]
- Morphine IV: for chest pain unrelieved by nitrates
- Aspirin 160 to 325 mg, if not given by EMS[6]
- Heparin IV or low molecular heparin subcutaneous (Enoxaparin™)
- Glycoprotein IIb/IIIa or P2Y$_{12}$ Inhibitor may be administered[3]
  - Clopidogrel (Plavix™)
  - Prasugrel (Efficent™)
  - Ticagrelor (Brilinta™)
- Prepare for inpatient admission

Evaluation
- Relief of chest pain
- Hemodynamically stable
- Repeat cardiac enzymes
- No cardiac dysrhythmias

ST Elevation Myocardial Infarction (STEMI)

A STEMI is caused from a thrombosis that completely occludes a coronary artery. Other less common causes of a STEMI include vasospasm, cocaine use, chemotherapeutic agents, serotonin receptor agonists, spontaneous coronary dissection, or aortic dissection.[7] A patient is diagnosed with a STEMI if there is ST segment elevation in two or more leads (see Table 2-1).[8] Pathophysiologically, it is important for a positive patient outcome that blood flow is restored to myocardium within 20 minutes to prevent irreversible damage.[9] However, CMS guidelines recommend reperfusion in no longer than 60 minutes from symptom onset.

Since all patients who have had a STEMI are considered to be at high risk, the plan of care will include secondary prevention strategies. Some of these recommended strategies tailored for individual patient needs, include cardiac rehabilitation, aspirin, and other medications such as lipid-lowering agents, beta-blockers, and ACE inhibitors.[5]

Assessment/Analysis[2,6,7]
- Chest pain/pressure
- Dyspnea

TABLE 2-1 STEMI Location, ECG Leads Elevated, and Likely Affected Cardiac Artery

Location	EKG Leads	Likely Artery Affected
Inferior wall	II, III, & AVF	Right coronary
Lateral wall	I, AVL, V$_5$, V$_6$	Left circumflex
Anterior wall	V$_3$ and V$_4$	Left anterior descending
Septal wall	V$_1$ and V$_2$	Left anterior descending
Anterior septal wall	V$_1$, V$_2$, V$_3$, V$_4$	Left anterior descending
Right ventricular wall	V4R Right-sided ECG recommended	Right coronary
Left Posterior Wall	V7, V8, V9 Posterior ECG recommended	Left posterior descending

Data from Wagner GS, Macfarlane P, Wellens H, et al: AHA/ACCF/HRS recommendations for the standardization and interpretation of the electrocardiogram: part VI: acute ischemia/infarction: a scientific statement from the American Heart Association Electrocardiography and Arrhythmias Committee, Council on Clinical Cardiology; the American College of Cardiology Foundation; and the Heart Rhythm Society: endorsed by the International Society for Computerized Electrocardiology, *Circulation*. 2009;119(10):e262–e270.

- Diaphoresis
- Radiation of pain
- Nausea
- Vomiting
- Tachycardia
- Tachypnea
- Hypotension
- Dizziness/lightheadedness
- Syncope
- ECG changes in 2 contiguous leads
  - ST elevation
  - New left bundle branch block
- Laboratory studies
  - CBC with differential
  - Serum chemistries
  - Elevation in cardiac enzymes
    - creatine kinase (CK)
    - creatine kinase MB (CK-MB)
    - Troponin I or T
  - Coagulation studies
- Portable Chest x-ray

Interventions
- Cardiac and pulse oximetry (SpO$_2$) monitoring
- Oxygen
  - Routine administration of oxygen for a patient with normal oxygenation levels may not provide a benefit. Consider not administering supplemental oxygen for the non-hypoxic patient[6]
  - If is less than 94%, start oxygen at 2 to 4 L/min via nasal cannula and titrate, as needed
- Establish IV access for crystalloids/blood products/medications as needed
- Nitrates
  - Nitroglycerin can be administered in various forms including sublingual (SL), IV, topical ointment, transdermal, or translingual metered spray
  - Non-ST-segment elevation ACS with ongoing ischemic pain
    - Nitroglycerin (0.3 to 0.4 mg) every 5 minutes, sublingual or aerosol, up to 3 doses for unrelieved ischemic pain[6]
    - If pain persists after 3 doses, reassess need for IV nitroglycerin, if no contraindications
  - Contraindicated in[6]
    - Hypotension (SBP < 90)
    - Heart rate < 50 or > 100
    - Inferior wall MI with right ventricular infarction (V4R)
  - Do not administer to patients who have taken a Phosphodiesterase Inhibitor within the preceding 24 hours (such as sildenafil) or within 48 hours for tadalafil[3]
- Morphine IV: for chest pain unrelieved by nitrates
- Aspirin 160 to 325 mg, if not given by EMS[6]
- Antiplatelet medications: reduces coronary reocclusion
  - Aspirin chewed, 160 to 325 mg PO (if not already administered by EMS)
    - Aspirin 300 mg rectal if unable to take orally
  - Glycoprotein IIb/IIIa Inhibitor medications—Administer as early as possible or at time of percutaneous coronary intervention (PCI)[5]
    - Clopidogrel (Plavix™)
    - Prasugrel (Efficent™)
    - Ticagrelor (Brilinta™)
    - Potent inhibitors of platelet aggregation
- Anticoagulant therapy such as Heparin IV or Low Molecular Weight Heparin subcutaneous (Enoxaparin™)[6]
- Percutaneous coronary intervention (PCI) within 90 minutes of medical evaluation[7]
- Prepare for inpatient admission

Evaluation
- Improvement in myocardial perfusion
- Relief of chest pain
- Hemodynamic stability
- No cardiac dysrhythmias

Aortic Aneurysm

An aortic aneurysm is a weakening of the inner lining of the aortic wall that leads to outpouching and stretching of the vessel. The primary cause of aortic aneurysm is hypertension resulting from the continual pressure on the aortic wall causing the wall to weaken and develop a bulge. Other causes include atherosclerosis, chronic cocaine use, and cardiac surgery.[9,10]

Assessment/Analysis[9,10]
- Pain
  - Chest pain
  - Thoracic pain
- Laboratory studies
  - CBC with differential
  - Coagulation studies
  - Type and Screen/cross
- Bedside ultrasound
- CT scan of the chest

Interventions[9,10]
- Establish IV access for crystalloids/blood products/medications as needed
- Monitor blood pressure and symptoms
- Medically manage the blood pressure, i.e., antihypertensives
- Surgical consultation

Evaluation
- Monitor for aneurysm rupture (see the next section Aortic Dissection)
  - Pain may be abrupt and feel like a ripping or tearing
  - Syncope
- Hemodynamically stability

Aortic Dissection

When the aortic wall weakens or bulges, this can lead to dissection, which is a leaking or tearing of the vessel wall. An ascending aortic dissection is more common than a descending aortic dissertation. Ascending aortic dissection most commonly occurs in patients who are in their fifth and sixth decade of life whereas descending aortic dissection affects patients in their sixth and seventh decade of life.[11,12] The most common risk factors include hypertension, atherosclerosis, hyperlipidemia, and tobacco use because it leads to a break down in the medial vessel wall. An aortic dissection is a life-threatening condition that causes internal bleeding which can quickly lead to death. Complications arising from aortic dissection include aortic rupture, ischemic stroke, visceral ischemia, cardiac tamponade, and circulatory failure.[11]

Assessment/Analysis[11,12]
- Sudden severe chest/back pain
- Aortic murmurs
- Dyspnea
- Signs and symptoms related to heart failure
- Pulse deficits
- Hemiplegia
- Dysphasia
- Syncope
- Seizures
- ECG changes
  - ST elevation
  - Q-waves present
- Chest x-ray
- Contrast enhanced CT of the chest
- Magnetic resonance imaging (MRI)
- Transesophageal echocardiography (TEE) or transthoracic echocardiography (TTE)

Interventions[11,12]
Ascending aortic dissection: surgery is the preferred method because it decreases patient mortality.
- Cardiac and pulse oximetry monitoring
- Establish IV access for crystalloids/blood products/medications as needed
- Analgesics for pain
- Blood pressure control, i.e., antihypertensives (systolic pressure between 100 to 120 mm Hg)
- Beta-blockers (to reduce myocardial contractility)
- Prepare for surgery

Descending aortic dissection: medical management is preferred due to an increase in patient mortality with surgery.
- Cardiac and pulse oximetry monitoring
- Establish IV access for crystalloids/blood products/medications as needed
- Analgesics for pain
- Blood pressure control, i.e., antihypertensives (systolic pressure between 100 to 120 mm Hg)
- Beta-blockers (to reduce myocardial contractility)
- Percutaneous treatment for descending aortic dissection
  - Endovascular graft

Evaluation
- Hemodynamically stability
- Decrease in blood pressure
- Relief of pain

Cardiopulmonary Arrest

Cardiopulmonary arrest occurs when the cardiac and respiratory centers are no longer functioning. The patient is without a pulse and respirations. Cardiopulmonary arrest is a medical emergency and immediate interventions are necessary to increase the chance of survival for the patient.[13] The most common cause of adult cardiopulmonary arrest is ventricular fibrillation.

Assessment/Analysis
- Unresponsive
- No pulse
- No respirations
- No blood pressure
- Skin is pale or cyanotic
- Laboratory studies
  - CBC with differential
  - Serum chemistries
  - Cardiac enzymes
- Arterial blood gas
- Chest x-ray

Interventions[14]
- Cardiopulmonary resuscitation (CPR)
  - Family presence recommended with support of faculty policy and available dedicated staff
- Attach cardiac monitor/defibrillator
- Monitor capnography: if $EtCO_2$ < 10 mm Hg, improves quality of compressions
- Defibrillation
  - Monophasic 360 J
  - Biphasic at 120 to 200 J
- Oxygen, i.e., bag-mask device, advanced airway/capnography

- Establish IV/IO access for crystalloids/blood products/medications as needed
  - Intravenous fluids
  - Medications: depends on the cardiac rhythm
    - Epinephrine 1 mg IV for ventricular tachycardia, ventricular fibrillation, pulseless electrical activity, and Asystole
    - Amiodarone 300 mg IV for pulseless ventricular tachycardia and ventricular fibrillation

Evaluation[14]
- Returns of spontaneous circulation (ROSC)
  - Maintain oxygen saturation ≥ 94%
  - Consider an advanced airway with capnography
  - Intravenous fluid bolus: normal saline or lactated ringers
  - Vasopressors (for systolic blood pressures < 90 mm Hg)
    - Epinephrine 0.1 to 0.5 mcg/kg/min
    - Dopamine 5 to 10 mcg/kg/min
    - Norepinephrine 0.1 to 0.5 mcg/kg/min
  - Targeted temperature management
    - Temperature should be between 32° to 36°C for at least 24 hours
    - Ice bags in cervical region, axilla, and groin
    - Surface or intravascular cooling devices
- Hemodynamically stability
- No ROSC: resuscitation efforts terminated and patient expired

Dysrhythmias

Dysrhythmias are classified as a change in the normal electrical conduction pathway. The electrical impulses may be too slow, too fast, irregular, erratic, or nonexistent.[15] Dysrhythmias can have no effect or be life-threatening depending on if the dysrhythmias affect the atria or ventricles of heart.[15] Commonly, dysrhythmias can cause a decrease in cardiac output. Signs and symptoms of decreased cardiac output include palpitations, chest pain, dyspnea, dizziness/lightheadedness, decrease in level of consciousness (LOC), syncope, and hypotension. Dysrhythmias are discussed in greater detail later in this chapter.

Sinus Bradycardia

Sinus bradycardia is commonly noted in patients who are sleeping or in trained athletes. However, sinus bradycardia can be indicative of a serious medical problem such as an acute inferior wall myocardial infarction, reperfusion rhythm after cardiac catheterization, hyperkalemia, hypothermia, hypothyroidism, and increased intracranial pressure due to increase pressure on the cardiac center in the brain stem.[16] Common cardiac medications, such as digoxin, beta blockers, and calcium channel blockers can cause sinus bradycardia.[16] Treatment should be initiated for patients who have symptomatic bradycardia (Figure 2-1).

Assessment/Analysis
- Syncope
- Dizziness/lightheadedness
- Weakness
- Fatigue
- Altered mental status
- Hypotensive
- Diaphoretic
- ECG: regular rhythm and heart rate 40 to 60 beats per minute
- 12 lead ECG
- Laboratory studies
  - Serum chemistries
  - Thyroid stimulating hormone (TSH)

Interventions[14]
- Cardiac and pulse oximetry monitoring
- Correct the underlying cause
- Establish IV access for crystalloids/medications as needed
  - Atropine 0.5 mg IV
  - Dopamine or Epinephrine IV (if waiting for a pacemaker)[12]
    - Dopamine infusion 2 to 20 mcg/kg/min. Titrate for patient response
    - Epinephrine infusion 2 to 10 mcg/min. Titrate for patient response
- Consider transcutaneous or transvenous pacing

Evaluation
- Hemodynamically stability
- Increased heart rate
- Relief of symptoms

Sinus Tachycardia

Common causes of sinus tachycardia include fever, pain, stress, anxiety, and dehydration. The treatment for sinus tachycardia is to correct what caused the rhythm (Figure 2-2).

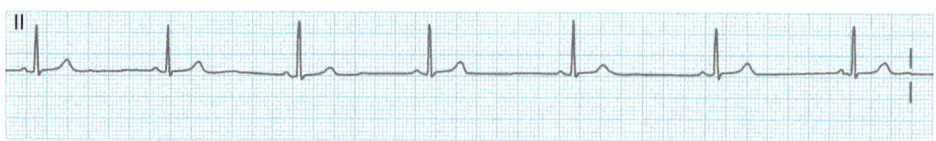

FIGURE 2-1 Sinus Bradycardia Rhythm

Reproduced with permission from Tintinalli J, Stapcyzynski J, Ma OJ, et al: Tintinalli's Emergency Medicine: A Comprehensive Study Guide, 8th ed. New York: McGraw-Hill Education; 2015.

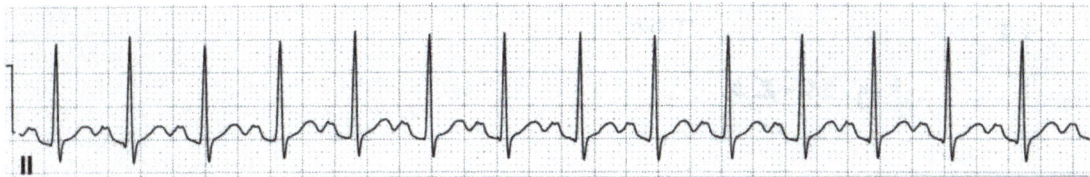

FIGURE 2-2 Sinus Tachycardia Rhythm
Reproduced with permission from Stone CK, Humphries R: CURRENT Diagnosis & Treatment Emergency Medicine, 7th ed. New York: McGraw-Hill Education; 2011.

Assessment/Analysis[16]
- Palpitations
- Dyspnea
- Weakness
- Fatigue
- ECG: regular heart rate over 100 beats per minute

Interventions[9,16]
- Cardiac and pulse oximetry monitoring
- Establish IV access for crystalloids/medications as needed
- Oxygen: if SpO_2 is less than 94%, start oxygen at 4 liters per nasal cannula and titrate, as needed
- Identify and treat causes
   - Fever, i.e., acetaminophen or ibuprofen
   - Dehydration, i.e., IV fluids
   - Pain, i.e., pain medication
   - Anxiety, i.e., benzodiazepines

Evaluation
- Hemodynamically stable
- Heart rate less than 100
- Relief of symptoms

Sinus Arrhythmia

A common cause of sinus arrhythmia is the respiratory pattern. The sinus node releases impulses faster during inspiration and slower during expiration.[16] Other causes include caffeine, cold medications, and stress (Figure 2-3).

Assessment/Analysis[16]
- Patients are typically asymptomatic
- ECG: irregular rhythm and heart rate 50 to 100
- 12 lead ECG

Interventions[16]
- Cardiac and pulse oximetry monitoring
- Monitor the patient
- Identify and treat the underlying causes

Supraventricular Tachycardia (SVT)

Common types of tachycardia are atrioventricular nodal reentry circuit and atrioventricular reentry mediated by an accessory pathway.[17] SVT has an abrupt onset and termination. Common causes of SVT include hypoxia, ischemia, heart failure, myocardial infarction, mitral valve prolapse, caffeine, alcohol, recreational drugs, and hyperthyroidism (Figure 2-4).[17,18]

Assessment/Analysis[14,16]
- Palpitations
- Chest pain
- Dyspnea
- Dizziness/lightheadedness
- Anxiety
- ECG: narrow complex regular rhythm

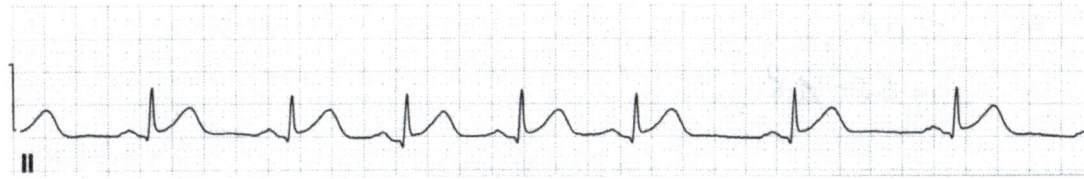

FIGURE 2-3 Sinus Arrhythmia Rhythm
Reproduced with permission from Stone CK, Humphries R: CURRENT Diagnosis & Treatment Emergency Medicine, 7th ed. New York: McGraw-Hill Education; 2011.

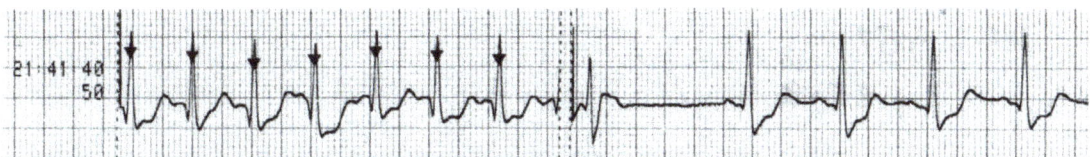

FIGURE 2-4 Supraventricular Tachycardia (SVT) Rhythm
Reproduced with permission from Stone CK, Humphries R: CURRENT Diagnosis & Treatment Emergency Medicine, 7th ed. New York: McGraw-Hill Education; 2011.

- Heart rates
  - Adults heart rate greater than 150 beats per minute
  - Children heart rate greater than 180 beats per minute
  - Infants heart rate greater than 220 beats per minute
- 12 lead ECG
- Laboratory studies
  - Thyroid stimulating hormone (TSH)
  - Serum chemistries
  - Possible toxicology screen, based on history

Interventions[14]
- Pulse oximetry and cardiac monitoring
- Attempt vagal maneuvers to stimulate the parasympathetic system
  - Bear down
  - Blow into an occluded straw
- Establish IV access, as proximal to the heart as possible. For crystalloids, use medications as needed
  - 1st dose: 6 mg rapid IV push with 20 mL normal saline flush
  - 2nd dose (after 1 to 2 min): 12 mg rapid IV push followed by 20 mL normal saline flush
- Synchronized cardioversion (if unstable)
- Beta blockers
- Calcium channel blockers

Evaluation
- Hemodynamically stability
- Return to normal sinus rhythm
- Resolution of symptoms

Premature Atrial Contractions (PACs) (Figure 2-5)

Assessment/Analysis[16]
- Palpitations
- ECG: irregular rhythm due to the premature atrial contractions. The underlying rhythm is regular
- 12 lead ECG
- Laboratory studies
  - Serum chemistries

Interventions
- Pulse oximetry and cardiac monitoring
- Identify and treat the underlying cause
  - Stress
  - Caffeine intake
  - Tobacco use
  - Alcohol intake
- Potassium replacement for hypokalemia[17]
- No interventions for infrequent PACs

Evaluation
- Hemodynamically stability
- No premature atrial contractions

Sinus Pause/Arrest

Sinus pause/arrest is used interchangeably to describe what is happening with the sinus node (SA). The sinus node fails to fire and conduct an impulse beat.[16] The failure of the impulse beat disrupts the timing of the normal conduction and the next impulse will have a delay in response. The SA node will send another impulse after the missed beat. Patients may or may not be symptomatic; it is dependent on how frequent the pauses are. Common causes include increase in vagal tone on the SA node, myocardial ischemia or infarction, and medications, i.e., digoxin, beta-blockers, or calcium channel blockers (Figure 2-6).[16]

Assessment/Analysis
- Dizziness/lightheadedness
- Altered level of consciousness

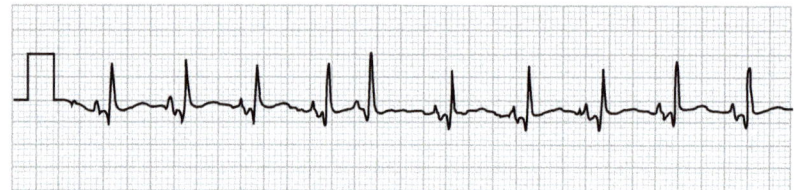

FIGURE 2-5 Premature Atrial Contractions (PACs) Rhythm (5th beat is PAC)
Reproduced with permission from Gomella L, Haist S: Clinician's Pocket Reference, 11th ed. New York: McGraw-Hill Education; 2006.

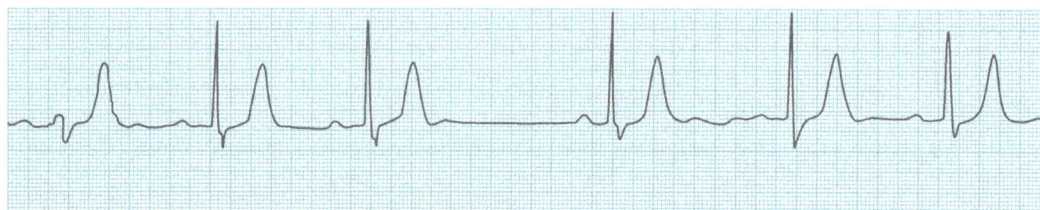

FIGURE 2-6 Sinus Pause/Arrest Rhythm
Reproduced with permission from Tintinalli J, Stapczynski J, Ma OJ, et al: Tintinalli's Emergency Medicine: A Comprehensive Study Guide, 8th ed. New York: McGraw-Hill Education; 2015.

- Bradycardia
- Hypotension
- Syncope
- ECG: missed beats and irregular rhythm, even though the underlying rhythm is sinus
- 12 lead ECG

Interventions[14,16]
- Cardiac and pulse oximetry monitoring
- Establish IV access for crystalloids/medications as needed
- Oxygen: if SpO_2 is less than 94%, start oxygen at 4 liters per nasal cannula and titrate, as needed
- Pacing (external, transvenous) may ultimately require permanent pacemaker

Evaluation
- Hemodynamically stability
- Increase in blood pressure
- Increase in heart rate
- No further syncopal episodes

Atrial Flutter

Atrial flutter is rarely seen in patients who have healthy hearts.[16] The most common causes include mitral and tricuspid valve disease, ischemic heart disease, pulmonary embolism, and alcohol intoxication (Figure 2-7).

Assessment/Analysis
- Palpitations
- Chest pain
- Dizziness/lightheadedness
- Syncope
- Hypotension
- 12 lead ECG

Interventions[16]
- Cardiac and pulse oximetry monitoring
- Establish IV access for crystalloids/medications as needed
  - Consider procedural sedation for cardioversion
- Oxygen: if SpO_2 is less than 94%, start oxygen at 4 L via NC/min and titrate, as needed
- Calcium channel blockers
- Beta blockers
- Antiarrhythmics, i.e., Amiodarone
- Synchronized cardioversion for patients who experience rate related complications such as[13]
  - Altered mental status
  - Ischemic chest discomfort
  - Acute heart failure
  - Hypotension

Evaluation
- Hemodynamically stability
- Return to normal sinus rhythm
- Controlled heart rate

Atrial Fibrillation

Atrial fibrillation is the most common benign rhythm and predisposes patients to thrombus formation in the atria, potentially leading to a cerebral vascular accident (CVA). Common risk factors for atrial fibrillation include cardiomyopathy, coronary artery disease, myocardial infarction, abnormal heart valves, hypertension, overactive thyroid, stress, fatigue, caffeine, alcohol, and tobacco use (Figure 2-8).[16]

Assessment/Analysis[16]
- Palpitations
- New onset may have uncontrolled rapid ventricular rate
- Chest pain

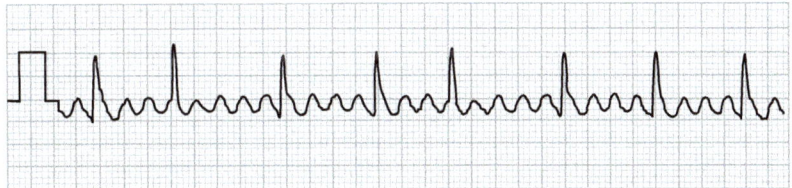

FIGURE 2-7 Atrial Flutter Rhythm
Reproduced with permission from Gomella L, Haist S: Clinician's Pocket Reference, 11th ed. New York: McGraw-Hill Education; 2006.

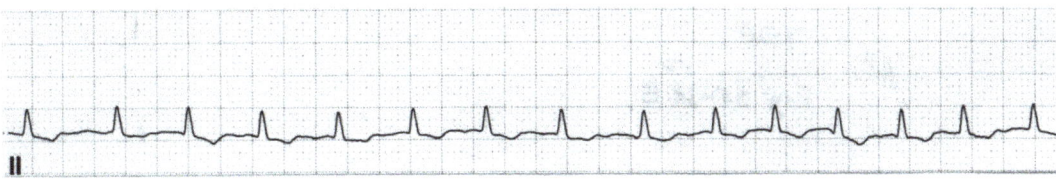

FIGURE 2-8 Atrial Fibrillation Rhythm (showing rapid rate ~130 bpm)
Reproduced with permission from Stone CK, Humphries R: CURRENT Diagnosis & Treatment Emergency Medicine, 7th ed. New York: McGraw-Hill Education; 2011.

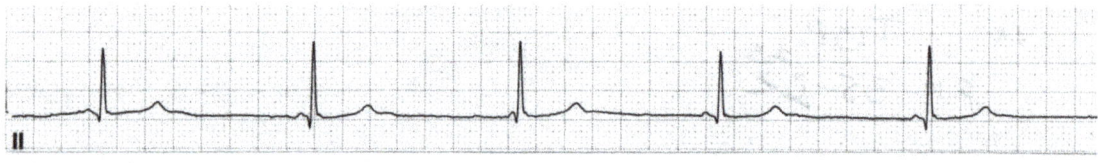

FIGURE 2-9 Junctional Rhythm
Reproduced with permission from Stone CK, Humphries R: CURRENT Diagnosis & Treatment Emergency Medicine, 7th ed. New York: McGraw-Hill Education; 2011.

- Dizziness/lightheadedness
- Dyspnea
- Altered level of consciousness
- ECG: irregular rhythm and no discernable P wave
- 12 lead ECG
- Laboratory studies
  - Serum chemistries

Interventions
- Cardiac and pulse oximetry monitoring
- Establish IV access for crystalloids/medications as needed
- Oxygen: if SpO$_2$ is less than 94%, start oxygen per nasal cannula and titrate, as needed
- Anticoagulants, i.e, warfarin, rivaroxaban (Xarelto™), and dabigatran (Pradaxa™)
- Calcium channel blockers, i.e., diltiazem
- Digoxin
- Patient/family education about anticoagulant therapy and risk of bleeding

Evaluation
- Return to normal sinus rhythm
- Controlled heart rate
- Hemodynamically stability

Premature Junctional Contractions (PJCs)

Common causes of PJCs include caffeine, alcohol, tobacco use, electrolyte imbalances, hypoxia, congestive heart failure, coronary artery disease, and digoxin.[16]

Assessment/Analysis[16]
- Palpitations
- ECG: premature junctional contractions and P waves absent, inverted, or within or after the QRS segment
- 12 lead ECG
- Laboratory studies
  - Serum chemistries

Interventions
- Cardiac and pulse oximetry monitoring
- Correct and treat the underlying causes

Evaluation
- Hemodynamically stability
- Return to normal sinus rhythm
- No premature beats

Junctional Rhythm

Junctional rhythm is an electrical impulse that originates below the atrioventricular (AV) node. Common causes of junctional rhythm include acute inferior myocardial infarction, third degree heart block, beta blockers, calcium channel blockers, digoxin, hypokalemia, and hypoxia (Figure 2-9).[16]

Assessment/Analysis[16]
- Palpitations
- Dizziness/lightheadedness: symptoms may be rate dependent
- Fatigue
- Syncope
- ECG: regular rhythm, P wave absent, inverted, or post QRS segment, and heart rate between 40 to 60 beats per minute
- 12 lead ECG
- Laboratory studies
  - Serum chemistries

Interventions[16]
- Cardiac and pulse oximetry monitoring
- Correct or treat the underlying cause(s)
- Atropine if patient symptomatic
- Replace potassium (if hypokalemia is present)
- Transcutaneous or transvenous pacing

Evaluation
- Hemodynamically stability
- Return to normal sinus rhythm

First Degree Atrioventricular Block (1st AV block)

First degree atrioventricular block (1st AV block) often occurs in conjunction with normal sinus rhythm and is seen when the impulse is slowed through the AV node.[16] The underlying rhythm is normal sinus and not clinically significant. Common causes include digoxin, beta blockers, and calcium channel blockers. Patients are typically asymptomatic and require no treatment (Figure 2-10).[16]

Assessment/Analysis[16]
- Asymptomatic
- Underlying rhythm is sinus rhythm
- ECG: PR interval > 0.20 and QRS < 0.12
- 12 lead ECG

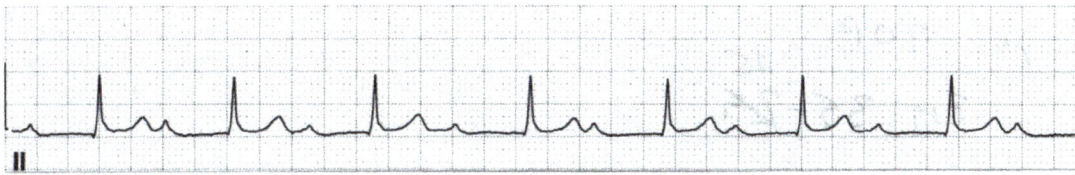

FIGURE 2-10 Normal Sinus Rhythm with First Degree Heart Block
Reproduced with permission from Stone CK, Humphries R: CURRENT Diagnosis & Treatment Emergency Medicine, 7th ed. New York: McGraw-Hill Education; 2011.

Interventions
- Cardiac and pulse oximetry monitoring
- Continue to monitor the patient

Second Degree Atrioventricular (AV) Block Type I (Mobitz I, Wenckebach)

Second degree AV block type I is not a clinically significant rhythm and most patients are asymptomatic. Common causes include athletic training, inferior myocardial infarction, beta blockers, calcium channel blockers, digoxin, and hyperkalemia (Figure 2-11).[16]

Assessment/Analysis[16]
- May be asymptomatic
- Palpitations
- Chest pain
- Dyspnea
- Dizziness/lightheadedness
- Syncope
- ECG: regular atrial rate, irregular ventricular rate, and varying PR interval
- 12 lead ECG
- Laboratory Studies
  - Serum chemistries

Interventions
- Cardiac and pulse oximetry monitoring
- Continued monitoring may be indicated if presence of the patient

Second Degree Atrioventricular (AV) Block Type II (Mobitz II)

Second degree AV block type II is less common than type I, but more clinically significant. This rhythm commonly leads to third degree heart block. Common causes include anterior wall myocardial infarction, myocarditis, hyperkalemia, beta blockers, calcium channel blockers, and digoxin (Figure 2-12).[16]

Assessment/Analysis[16]
- Palpitations
- Chest pain
- Dyspnea
- Dizziness/lightheadedness
- Decreased level of consciousness
- Hypotension
- Syncope
- ECG: regular atrial and irregular ventricular rate and PR interval varies
- 12 lead ECG
- Laboratory Studies
  - Serum chemistries

Interventions[16]
- Establish IV access for crystalloids/medications as needed
  - Atropine 0.5 to 1 mg IV, if symptomatic
  - Consider sedation for pacing, if patient condition allows
- Cardiac and pulse oximetry monitoring
- Transcutaneous or transvenous pacing
- Discontinue medications causing the AV block

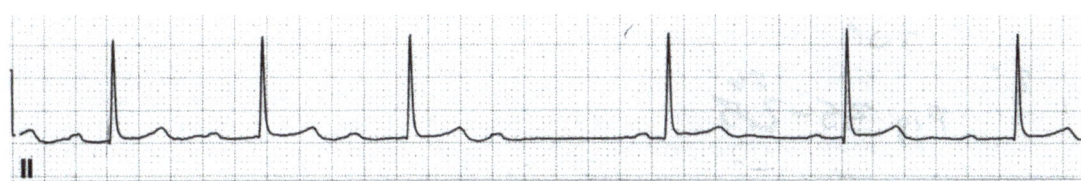

FIGURE 2-11 Second Degree Atrioventricular Block Type I
Reproduced with permission from Stone CK, Humphries R: CURRENT Diagnosis & Treatment Emergency Medicine, 7th ed. New York: McGraw-Hill Education; 2011.

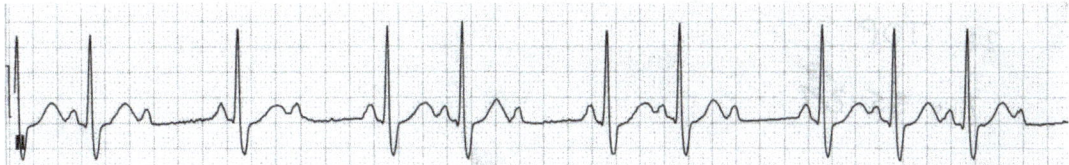

FIGURE 2-12 Second Degree Atrioventricular Block Type II
Reproduced with permission from Stone CK, Humphries R: CURRENT Diagnosis & Treatment Emergency Medicine, 7th ed. New York: McGraw-Hill Education; 2011.

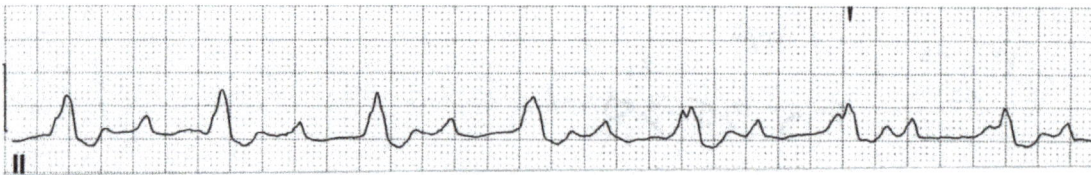

FIGURE 2-13   Third Degree Heart Block Rhythm
Reproduced with permission from Stone CK, Humphries R: CURRENT Diagnosis & Treatment Emergency Medicine, 7th ed. New York: McGraw-Hill Education; 2011.

Evaluation
- Hemodynamically stability
- No longer symptomatic

Third Degree Heart Block (Complete heart block)

Third degree heart block happens when the atria and ventricles are no longer functioning together. The atria receives the electrical impulse from the sinoatrial node. The impulse is blocked at the atrioventricular node (AV). Therefore, the ventricles receive the electrical impulse from below the AV node or the ventricles. Third degree heart block is clinically significant and needs immediate intervention if the patient is symptomatic. Common causes include inferior and anterior wall MI, beta blockers, calcium channel blockers, digoxin, and amiodarone (Figure 2-13).[16]

Assessment/Analysis[16]
- Airway patency
- Hemodynamic stability: pulse present and BP
- Chest pain
- Bradycardia
- Dyspnea
- Level of consciousness
- Dizziness/lightheadedness
- Syncope
- Hypotension
- ECG: P waves with a regular P to P interval, QRS segments with a regular R to R interval; no consistent P-R interval
- 12 lead ECG

Interventions[14,16]
- Establish IV access for crystalloids/medications as needed
  - Vasopressors (for systolic blood pressures < 90 mm Hg)
    - Epinephrine infusion 2 to 10 mcg/min. Titrate for patient response or alternative dose Epinephrine 0.1 to 0.5 mcg/kg/min and titrate for patient response
    - Dopamine infusion 2 to 20 mcg/kg/min. Titrate for patient response
- Cardiac and pulse oximetry monitoring
- Oxygen: if SpO_2 is less than 94%, start oxygen per nasal cannula and titrate for patient response
- Transcutaneous or Transvenous Pacing

Evaluation
- Hemodynamically stability
- Increase in blood pressure
- Increase in heart rate
- Increase in neurological functioning

Idioventricular Rhythm

Idioventricular rhythm is a wide and bizarre rhythm in which the impulses originate from the ventricles. A sustained idioventricular rhythm is typically seen with advanced heart disease.[16] This rhythm is called the dying heart because asystole follows shortly after this rhythm. Common causes of idioventricular include sinus arrest, sinus exit block, third degree heart block, and advanced heart disease (Figure 2-14).[16]

Assessment/Analysis[16]
- Airway patency
- Hemodynamic stability: pulse and BP present
- Level of consciousness (often patients are not hemodynamically stable in Idioventricular rhythm)
- Chest pain
- Bradycardia
- Dyspnea
- Diaphoresis
- Hypotension
- Dizziness/lightheadedness
- Syncope

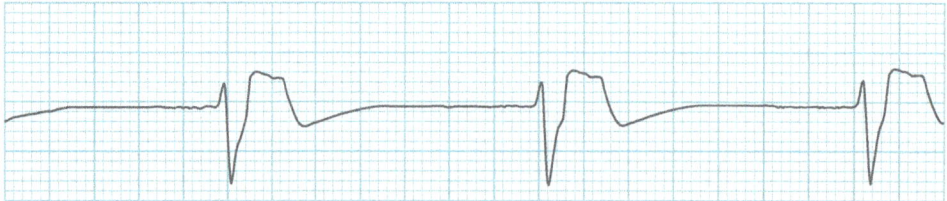

FIGURE 2-14   Idioventricular Rhythm
Reproduced with permission from Tintinalli J, Stapcyzynski J, Ma OJ, et al: Tintinalli's Emergency Medicine: A Comprehensive Study Guide, 8th ed. New York: McGraw-Hill Education; 2015.

- ECG: regular rate between 20 to 40 beats per minute
- 12 lead ECG

Interventions[16]
- Airway management
- Cardiac and pulse oximetry monitoring
- Establish IV access
- Atropine
- Vasopressors
  - Epinephrine infusion 2 to 10 mcg/min. Titrate for patient response or alternative dose: Epinephrine 0.1 to 0.5 mcg/kg/min
  - Dopamine infusion 2 to 20 mcg/kg/min. Titrate for patient response
- Transcutaneous or Transvenous Pacing

Evaluation
- Hemodynamically stability
- Increase in cardiac output

Premature Ventricular Contractions (PVCs)

Premature ventricular contractions (PVCs) are a common arrhythmia.[16] Common causes include emotional stress, alcohol, tobacco use, caffeine, myocardial infarction, cardiomyopathy, congestive heart failure, hypoxia, hypokalemia, digoxin toxicity, and after reperfusion therapy (Figure 2-15).[16]

Assessment/Analysis[16]
- Palpitations
- Chest pain
- Dyspnea
- Dizziness/lightheadedness
- Syncope
- ECG: underlying normally regular, but irregular with PVCs

- 12 lead ECG
- Laboratory Studies
  - Serum chemistries
  - Possible cardiac enzymes if positive cardiac history

Interventions[14,16]
- Cardiac and pulse oximetry monitoring
- Assess need for oxygen
- Establish IV access for crystalloids/medications as needed
  - Antiarrhythmics i.e. Amiodarone 150 mg IV over 10 minutes
- Identify and treat cause of PVCs

Evaluation
- Hemodynamically stability
- Resolution of symptoms
- No premature beats

Ventricular Tachycardia

Ventricular tachycardia (VT) is a wide complex regular rhythm in which the electrical impulse originates from the ventricles. VT commonly occurs in patients with underlying heart disease, coronary artery disease, acute myocardial infarction, cardiomyopathy, heart failure, electrolytes imbalances, especially potassium and magnesium, and cardiac trauma (Figure 2-16).[16]

Assessment/Analysis[14,16]
VT with a pulse
- Palpitations
- Chest pain
- Dyspnea
- Dizziness/lightheadedness
- Hypotension

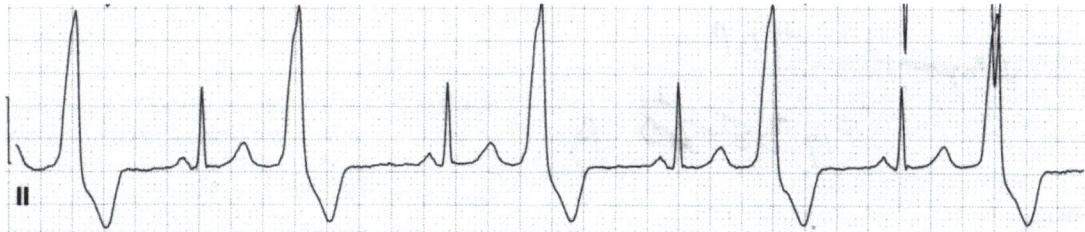

FIGURE 2-15   **Normal Sinus Rhythm with Premature Ventricular Contractions (Bigeminy)**
Reproduced with permission from Stone CK, Humphries R: CURRENT Diagnosis & Treatment Emergency Medicine, 7th ed. New York: McGraw-Hill Education; 2011.

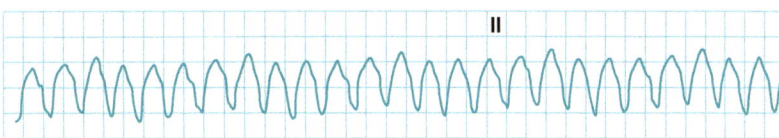

FIGURE 2-16   **Ventricular Tachycardia Rhythm**
Reproduced with permission from Tintinalli J, Stapczynski J, Ma OJ, et al: Tintinalli's Emergency Medicine: A Comprehensive Study Guide, 8th ed. New York: McGraw-Hill Education; 2015.

VT without a pulse
- Unresponsiveness
- Absent blood pressure, heart rate, and respiratory rate
- ECG: wide complex regular rhythm
- 12 lead ECG
- Laboratory studies
  - CBC with differential
  - Serum chemistries
  - Cardiac enzymes

Interventions[14,16]
VT with a pulse
- Cardiac and pulse oximetry monitoring
- Establish IV/IO access for crystalloids/medications as needed
  - Antiarrhythmics, i.e., Amiodarone 150 mg IV over 10 minutes
- Oxygen: if SpO_2 is less than 94%, start oxygen at 4 liters per nasal cannula and titrate, as needed

VT without a pulse[14]
- Begin CPR
- Cardiac monitor/defibrillator-immediately defibrillate
- As soon as the defibrillator is available: monophasic defibrillation 360 joules and biphasic defibrillation 120 to 200 joules
- Cardiac monitor and pulse oximetry
- Establish IV/IO access for crystalloids/medications as needed
  - Epinephrine 1 mg every 3 to 5 minutes IV push
  - Antiarrhythmics
    - Amiodarone 300 mg IV push
    - Lidocaine 1 to 1.5 mg/kg
  - Magnesium sulfate
    - Torsades de pointes
    - 1 to 2 grams IV over 15 minutes
- Identify and treat potential reversible causes
- Advanced airway/capnography

Evaluation
- Return of spontaneous circulation (ROSC)
- Hemodynamically stability
- Increase in blood pressure
- Decrease in heart rate

Ventricular Fibrillation

Ventricular fibrillation (VF) is described as a chaotic, disorganized, and irregular rhythm that is receiving impulses from various foci within the ventricles. In VF, the ventricles are no longer contracting, but fibrillating. The lack of contraction of the ventricles leads to no cardiac output and death is imminent. The common causes of VF include acute myocardial infarction, cardiomyopathy, heart failure, electrolyte imbalances, especially potassium and magnesium, and cardiac trauma (Figure 2-17).[16]

Assessment/Analysis[14,16]
- Absent blood pressure, heart rate, and respiratory rate.
- Unresponsiveness
- ECG: chaotic fibrillatory waves
- Laboratory studies
  - CBC
  - Serum chemistries
  - Cardiac enzymes
- Arterial blood gases

Interventions[14,16]
- Begin CPR
- Cardiac monitor/defibrillator: immediately defibrillate
- As soon as the defibrillator is available: monophasic defibrillation 360 joules and biphasic defibrillation 120 to 200 joules
- Administer oxygen per bag-mask device
- Establish IV/IO access for crystalloids/medications as needed
  - Epinephrine 1mg every 3 to 5 minutes IV push
  - Antiarrhythmics, i.e., amiodarone 300 mg IV push then 150 mg IV
  - Intravenous fluid bolus: normal saline or lactated ringers

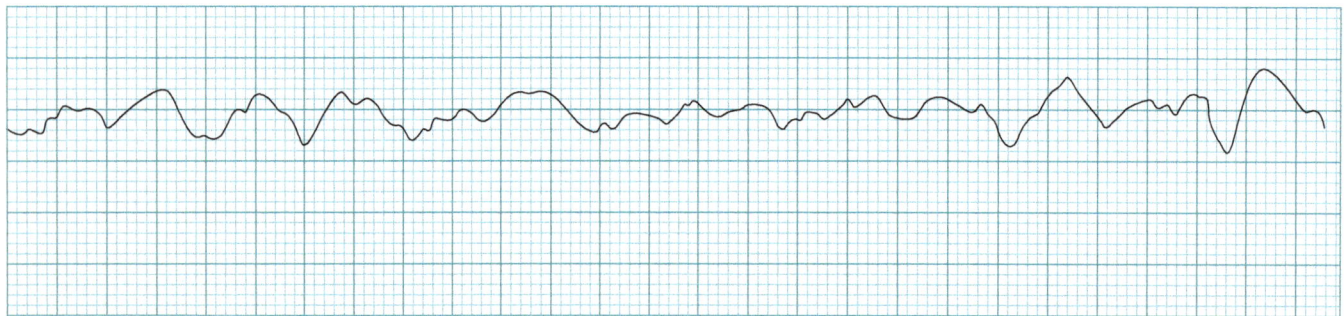

FIGURE 2-17 Ventricular Fibrillation Rhythm
Reproduced with permission from McKean SC, Ross JJ, Dressler DD, et al: Principles and Practice of Hospital Medicine. New York: McGraw-Hill Education; 2012.

- Vasopressors (for systolic blood pressures < 90 mm Hg)
  - Epinephrine 0.1 to 0.5 mcg/kg/min
  - Dopamine 5 to 10 mcg/kg/min
  - Norepinephrine 0.1 to 0.5 mcg/kg/min

Evaluation[14]
- Return of spontaneous circulation (ROSC)
  - Maintain oxygen saturation ≥ 94%
  - Consider an advanced airway with capnography
  - Consider for additional fluid resuscitation: 1 to 2 liters of normal saline or lactated ringers
  - Vasopressors (for systolic blood pressures < 90 mm Hg)
    - Epinephrine 0.1 to 0.5 mcg/kg/min
    - Dopamine 5 to 10 mcg/kg/min
    - Norepinephrine 0.1 to 0.5 mcg/kg/min
  - Targeted temperature management
    - Temperature should be between 32° to 36° for at least 24 hours
    - Ice bags to posterior or lateral neck, axilla, and groin
- Surface or intravascular cooling devices
- Hemodynamically stability
- Cessation of efforts
  - If ventricular fibrillation persists
  - If asystole develops without ROSC

Asystole

Asystole is the absence of electrical activity. Therefore, there is no mechanical activity or contraction, which leads to no cardiac output and imminent death. Conditions that can lead to asystole include ventricular tachycardia, ventricular fibrillation, idioventricular rhythm, pulseless electrical activity, defibrillation, and cardioversion (Figure 2-18).[16]

Assessment/Analysis
- Absent blood pressure, heart rate, and respiratory rate
- Unresponsiveness
- ECG: flat line
- 12 lead ECG
- Laboratory studies
  - CBC
  - Serum chemistries
  - Cardiac enzymes
- Arterial blood gases

Interventions
- Begin CPR
- Administer oxygen via bag-mask device
- Cardiac monitor/defibrillator
- Establish IV/IO access for crystalloids/medications as needed
  - Epinephrine 1mg every 3 to 5 minutes IV push
- Continue high-quality CPR
- Consider definitive airway
- Identify and treat potential reversible causes

Evaluation[14]
- Returns of spontaneous circulation (ROSC)
  - Maintain oxygen saturation ≥ 94%
  - Consider an advanced airway with capnography
  - Targeted temperature management
    - Temperature should be between 32° to 36° for at least 24 hours
    - Ice bags in cervical region, axilla, and groin
    - Surface or intravascular cooling devices
  - Fluid resuscitation: normal saline or lactated ringers
  - Vasopressors (for systolic blood pressures < 90 mm Hg)
    - Epinephrine 0.1 to 0.5 mcg/kg/min
    - Dopamine 5 to 10 mcg/kg/min
    - Norepinephrine 0.1 to 0.5 mcg/kg/min
- Hemodynamically stability
- Cessation of efforts
  - Asystole without ROSC

Infective (bacterial) Endocarditis (IE)

Infective endocarditis (IE) is an infection damaging the endocardial surface of the heart. IE are commonly caused from *viradans group streptococci* or staphylococci.[19,20] These microbial agents affect the heart valves, especially the aortic and mitral valves. After affecting the endocardium, systemic manifestations may occur. IE is uncommon, but carries high morbidity and mortality rates.[20]

Assessment/Analysis[19,20]
- Fever (90% of the patients)
- Chills
- Heart murmur (85% of the patients)
- Cough

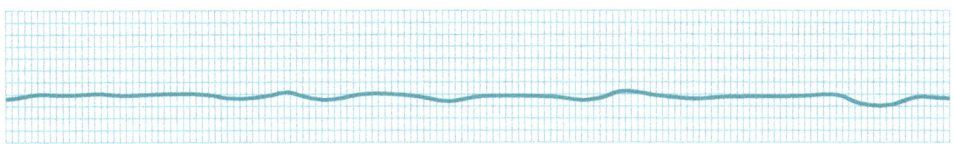

FIGURE 2-18 Asystole Rhythm
Reproduced with permission from Tintinalli J, Stapcyzynski J, Ma OJ, et al: Tintinalli's Emergency Medicine: A Comprehensive Study Guide, 8th ed. New York: McGraw-Hill Education; 2015.

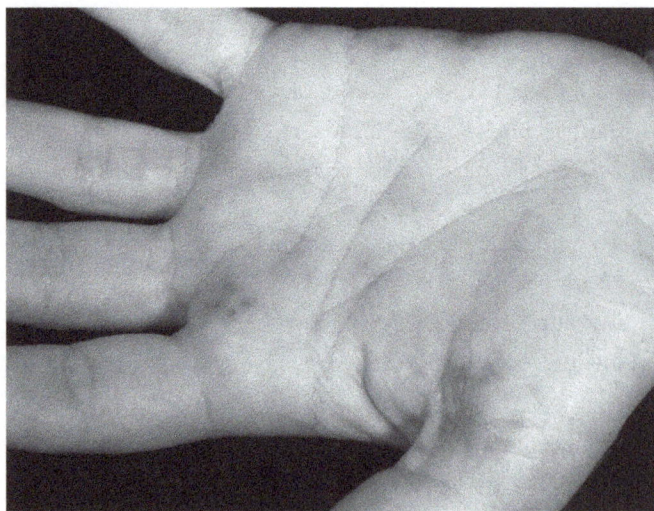

FIGURE 2-19 Olser nodes on the left hand
Used with permission from VisualDx.

- Dyspnea
- Arthralgia
- Anorexia
- Malaise
- Lethargy
- Osler nodes: painful hand or fingertip lesions. See Figure 2-19
- Small petechial hemorrhage
- Splinter hemorrhage in the nail beds
- 12 lead ECG
- Laboratory studies
  - CBC with differential—Elevated WBC
  - Serum chemistries
  - Cardiac enzymes
  - Increased erythrocyte sedimentation rate (ESR)
  - Increased c-reactive protein
  - Blood cultures
- Transthoracic echocardiography (TTE) and Transesophageal echocardiography (TEE)
  - Both of these diagnostic tests play an important role in managing and monitoring patients with IE
- Prevention[21]
  - At-risk patients who should receive antibiotics
    - Patients with prosthetic values
    - Previous episodes of IE
  - Antibiotics should be administered prior to
    - Surgery
    - Gastrointestinal procedures
    - Genitourinary procedures
    - Invasive dental procedures

Interventions[19-21]
- Cardiac and pulse oximetry monitoring
- Establish IV access for crystalloids/medications as needed
- Identify causative microorganisms
- Antibiotics
- Surgery for valve repair or replacement

Evaluation
- Hemodynamically stability
- Relief of signs and symptoms
- Monitor for the development of an embolic stroke
- Fever control[19]

Heart Failure

Heart failure is a result of structural or functional impairment of the myocardium. The sympathetic nervous system causes vascular vasoconstriction allowing the cells, tissues, and organs to receive an adequate amount of oxygen. However, over time the myocardium is weakened resulting in a decrease in cardiac output.[9]

Left-sided heart failure is more common than right-sided heart failure. Left-sided heart failure occurs when the left ventricle fails causing pressure to rise in the left atrium and pulmonary veins causing pulmonary congestion. This pressure rises as blood backs up behind the failing left ventricle. Common causes of left sided heart failure include myocardial infarction, cardiomyopathy, mitral stenosis or regurgitation, and aortic stenosis or regurgitation.[9]

Assessment/Analysis[9]
- Dyspnea with tachypnea
- Cough—productive or nonproductive
- Crackles with auscultation
- Tachypnea
- Blood tinged sputum
- Cyanosis
- Restlessness
- Tachycardia

Right-sided heart failure occurs when the blood from the right ventricle backs up into the right atrium then into the vena cava causing peripheral and organ edema. Common causes of right-sided heart failure include right ventricular infarction, persistent left-sided heart failure, pulmonary hypertension, tricuspid stenosis or regurgitation, and pulmonic stenosis or regurgitation.[9]

Assessment/Analysis[22]
- Fatigue
- Distended jugular veins[23]
- Ascites
- Anorexia and gastrointestinal distress
- Hepatomegaly and splenomegaly
- 12 lead ECG

- Laboratory studies
  - CBC with differential
  - Serum chemistries
  - Increased beta natriuretic peptide (BNP) or N-terminal pro-BNP (NT-proBNP)[23]
  - Cardiac enzymes
- Chest x-ray
- Echocardiogram

Interventions
- Pulse oximetry and cardiac monitoring
- Establish IV/IO access for crystalloids/medications as needed
- Oxygen, i.e., nasal cannula, mask, bilevel positive airway pressure (BiPAP), or continuous positive airway pressure (CPAP)
  - BiPaP and CPAP increase thoracic pressure therefore decreasing the preload and afterload within the heart[22]
  - Both BiPaP and CPAP are recommended for heart failure patients[22]
- Sodium and fluid restrictions
- Diuretics[23]
- ACE inhibitors[23]
- Digoxin

Evaluation
- Hemodynamically stability
- Improved breathing pattern and rate
- Clear breath sounds
- Improvement in intake and output

Hypertension

Hypertension is known as the silent killer because many people do not know they have the disease. When hypertension is undiagnosed or untreated, complications include cardiac hypertrophy, myocardial infarction, angina, cerebral vascular accident, seizures, kidney failure, and permanent blindness.[9]

Hypertension is elevated pressure within the arterial system. There are four classifications for hypertension.

- ❖ Essential hypertension: commonly known as primary hypertension, which occurs without evidence of other diseases
- ❖ Secondary hypertension: results from disease processes such as coarctation of the aorta, renal failure, renal artery stenosis, pheochromocytoma, Cushing syndrome, sleep apnea, obesity, oral contraceptives, and alcohol consumption
- ❖ Systolic hypertension: when the systolic pressure is continually above 140 mm Hg. The diastolic reading is less than 90 mm Hg[9]
- ❖ Hypertensive (crisis) emergency: an accelerated form of hypertension with sudden onset. Characterized by a systolic blood pressure of greater than 180 mm Hg and diastolic pressures greater than 120 mm Hg[24]

Assessment/Analysis[9]
- Headache (most common)
- Blurred vision
- Altered level of consciousness
- Numbness and tingling in the face and extremities
- Nausea
- Vomiting
- Chest pain
- 12 lead ECG
- Dyspnea
- CT scan of the head
- MRI of the brain

Interventions
- Treat underlying causes
- Monitor blood pressure
- Cardiac monitor
- Establish IV access for crystalloids/medications as needed
- Antihypertensives

Evaluation
- Decrease blood pressure slowly (no more than 25% within the first hour)[24]
- Relief of signs and symptoms
- Hemodynamically stability

Cardiac Tamponade

Cardiac tamponade is a condition in which blood or fluid accumulates in the pericardial sac. This accumulation places pressure on the heart and restricts the heart from pumping properly. The accumulation of the blood increases intracardiac pressure, causing a decrease in diastolic filling, and then a decrease in cardiac output. Pulsus paradoxus happens when there is a significant decrease in the systolic blood pressure during inspiration and is a key diagnostic finding with cardiac tamponade.[10] The decrease in blood volume leads to a decrease in cardiac output. The common causes of cardiac tamponade include trauma to chest, myocardial infarction, aortic dissection, cardiac surgery, and neoplasms.[24]

Assessment/Analysis[9,25]
- Chest pain
- Dyspnea
- Tachycardia
- Pulsus paradoxus
- Beck's Triad
  - Hypotension
  - Muffled heart sounds
  - Jugular vein distention

- Narrowed pulse pressure
  - A decrease in systolic blood pressure with a rise in diastolic blood pressure 12 lead ECG
- Laboratory studies
  - CBC with differential
  - Serum chemistries
  - Cardiac enzymes
- Chest x-ray
- Echocardiogram

Interventions
- Cardiac and pulse oximetry monitoring
- Establish IV access
- Oxygen: if SpO_2 is less than 94%, start oxygen per nasal cannula and titrate, as needed
- Focused Assessment with Sonography for Trauma (FAST) exam[26]
- Pericardiocentesis
- Prepare for surgery (pericardial window/pericardiotomy)

Evaluation
- Hemodynamically stable
- Increase in blood pressure
- Relief of signs and symptoms

Pericarditis

Pericarditis is an inflammation of the pericardium. The exact cause may be difficult to determine but several conditions can lead to pericarditis. These conditions include bacterial, viral, and fungal infections, along with systematic inflammatory disorders, neoplasms, myocardial infarction, cardiac trauma, and drug related. Mild pericarditis typically resolves spontaneously without intervention.[9]

Assessment/Analysis[27]
- Chest pain: relieved by leaning forward
- Fever
- Pericardial friction rub with auscultation
- 12 lead ECG
  - ECG changes: diffuse ST segment elevations, PR segment depression, and widespread T-wave inversion
- Laboratory studies
  - CBC with differential—leukocytosis
  - Serum chemistries
  - Elevated cardiac enzymes
  - Elevated erythrocyte sedimentation rate (ESR)
- Echocardiogram
- Chest x-ray
- CT scan of the chest (allows detection and confirmation of pericardial inflammation)
- Cardiac magnetic resonance imaging (allows detection and confirmation of pericardial inflammation)

Interventions[9,27]
- Cardiac and pulse oximetry monitoring
- Establish IV access for crystalloids/medications as needed
- Non-steroidal anti-inflammatory medications
  - Ibuprofen
  - Indomethacin
- Antipyretics
- Antibiotics
- Aspirin
- Weight adjusted colchicine as adjunct to NSAIDs improves remission rates and reduces recurrence rates
- Prednisone in low dosage for patients not responding to aspirin or NSAIDs

Evaluation
- Decreased inflammation of the pericardium
  - Decreased pain
  - Afebrile
  - Pericardial friction rub resolved
  - ECG changes returned to baseline
- Relief of signs and symptoms
- Hemodynamically stability

Peripheral Vascular Disease

Peripheral vascular disease commonly refers to disorders affecting the arterial or venous circulation of the extremities.[9] Disorders of the arterial system commonly affect the coronary and cerebral arteries, and may also affect the peripheral arteries. Disorders of the venous system are due to venous congestion of the affected tissues which predisposes the individual to deep vein thrombosis.[9] Peripheral vascular disease includes acute arterial occlusion, peripheral artery disease, Raynaud's disease, chronic venous insufficiency, and varicose veins.

Acute Arterial Occlusion

An acute arterial occlusion is a sudden event disrupting the blood flow to organs and/or tissues. Emboli and thrombosis are common causes of acute arterial occlusion. Emboli are free floating blood clots originating from a thrombosis. A thrombosis is a blood clot formed on the blood vessel wall causing an obstruction of blood return to the heart. Acute arterial occlusions to the organs or tissues can cause tissue death if blood flow is not restored in a timely manner.[8]

Assessment/Analysis[9]
- Five Ps
  - Pallor
  - Pulselessness
  - Pain
  - Paresthesia
  - Paralysis
- Skin is cold to touch

- Doppler to check pulses
- Ankle-Brachial Index (ABI)[28]
  - Compares the blood pressure in the ankle with the blood pressure in the arm
  - Low ABI indicates narrowed or blocked vessels
- Ultrasound of the extremities

Interventions
- Prepare for embolectomy
- Thrombolytic therapy

Evaluation
- Restoration of blood flow to the organs or tissues
- Relief of signs and symptoms
- Hemodynamically stability

Peripheral Artery Disease (PAD)

Peripheral artery disease (PAD) is caused by the development of atherosclerosis leading to the narrowing of an arterial lumen. The femoral or popliteal arteries are most commonly affected by PAD. The risks factors for developing PAD include increasing age, obesity, sedentary lifestyle, stress, cigarette smoking, hypertension, hyperlipidemia, and diabetes mellitus.[9]

Assessment/Analysis
- Intermittent claudication: ischemic muscle pain is precipitated by exercise such as walking
- Paresthesia
- Arteriography
- Doppler ultrasound of the extremities

Interventions[9]
- Identify and treat the causes
- Lifestyle changes
  - Smoking cessation
  - Daily exercise
  - Healthy diet
  - Control blood pressure

Evaluation
- Relief of signs and symptoms
- Decrease of cardiovascular risks

Raynaud's Disease

Raynaud's disease is an intense vasospasm of the arteries especially the arterioles in the fingers and less commonly in the toes.[9] Typically, younger women are more prone to Raynaud's disease. Strong emotions or being exposed to cold temperatures may precipitate the development of symptoms.[9]

Assessment/Analysis[9]
- Skin pallor or cyanosis
- A sensation of coldness
- Decreased palpable pulses in the affected extremity (possible)
- Period of hyperemia (return of blood flow): intense pain, redness, and paresthesia

Interventions[9]
- Cover fingers
- Abstinence from smoking
- Avoid cold medications because they can cause vasoconstriction, thereby worsening the symptoms
- Calcium channel blockers

Evaluation
- Decrease episodes of vasospasms

Chronic Venous Insufficiency (CVI)

Chronic venous insufficiency (CVI) affects the venous system, especially in the lower extremities.[29] The venous system returns blood back to the heart through the contraction of skeletal muscles and valves. When the return of blood becomes impaired, the veins quickly refill causing an increase in pressure in a low-pressure system.[29]

Assessment/Analysis[29]
- Dilated veins
- Edema
- Leg pain
- Skin discoloration
- Ulcerations as pictured in Figure 2-20
- Venous duplex imaging
- CT scan of the extremities
- MRI

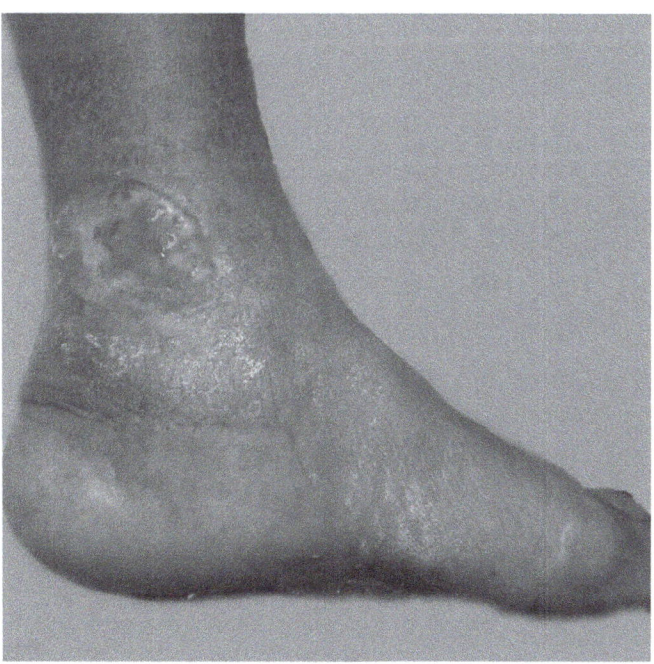

FIGURE 2-20 Ulceration from venous insufficiency
Used with permission from Dr. Steven Dean.

Interventions[29]
- Compression leg garments
  - Graded elastic compressive stockings
  - Paste gauze boots
  - Layered bandaging
  - Adjustable layered compression garments
- Exercise therapy
- Sclerotherapy for venous segments with reflux

Evaluation
- Improve venous blood flow
- Prevent tissue injury

Venous Thromboembolism (VTE)

Venous thromboembolism (VTE) is the formation of blood clots in the venous system. There are several causes of thromboembolic disease, such as prolonged bed rest, immobilization, long airplane rides, hypercoagulability of the blood, and vascular trauma.[9] An embolus can dislodge and travel through the heart into the lungs causing a pulmonary embolism.

Assessment/Analysis[9]
- Unilateral swelling of a lower extremity
- Skin warm to touch
- Pain of a lower extremity
- Deep muscle tenderness
- Laboratory studies-D-dimer[30,31]
  - Description: D-dimer is a crosslink between the fibrin being produced and the dissolution of the clot
  - Negative D-dimer can rule out VTE or Pulmonary Embolism (PE)
  - Elevated D-dimer levels can indicate thrombus or inflammatory issues
    - VTE
    - PE
    - Arterial or venous thrombosis
    - Neoplastic disease
    - Pre-eclampsia
    - Pregnancy (late and postpartum)
    - Thrombolytic or fibrinolytic therapy
- Ultrasound of the lower extremities

Prevention
- Ambulation
- Anti-embolism stockings

Interventions
- Anticoagulants
- Rest

Evaluation
- Decrease swelling and pain
- No signs and symptoms of pulmonary embolism

Trauma

Cardiac trauma is caused from a sudden, unexpected event disrupting the cardiac function or structure. The common causes of cardiac trauma include motor vehicle collision (MVC), falls, and blast injuries.[32] There is high mortality related to cardiac trauma. Most patients die on-scene and never make it to the emergency department.

Blunt Cardiac Trauma

Blunt cardiac trauma is typically caused from direct impact or compression.[32] This type of trauma has a high rate of mortality ranging from 50% to 86%.[33] The most common causes of blunt cardiac trauma are motor vehicle crashes, pedestrian struck by auto, motorcycle collision,[33] and work related injuries.[34] The right side of the heart is most commonly injured due to the close proximity to the chest wall.[35] Blunt cardiac trauma is often difficult to diagnose because multiple organs in the chest and abdomen are also injured. Suspect a cardiac injury when other organs are injured.[35]

Assessment/Analysis[32,35]
- Chest pain
- Dyspnea
- Ecchymosis to the chest wall
- Flail chest
- ECG abnormalities[36]
  - Sinus tachycardia (most common)
  - Premature ventricular contractions (PVCs)
  - Atrial fibrillation
  - ST segment changes
  - AV blocks
- 12 lead ECG[36]
  - ECG changes
    - ST segment elevation or depression
    - T wave inversion
    - Ventricular arrhythmias
- Laboratory studies
  - CBC with differential
  - Serum chemistries
  - Cardiac enzymes—Increased Troponin I or T levels
- Chest x-ray
  - Rib fractures
- Echocardiogram

Interventions
- Cardiac and pulse oximetry monitoring
- Establish IV access for crystalloids/medications as needed
  - IV fluids crystalloids to correct hypotension
- Correct any dysrhythmias

Evaluation
- Relief of signs and symptoms
- No abnormal ECG findings
- No increase in Troponin I or T
- Hemodynamically stability

See Shock chapter 5 for more information on Cardiogenic and Obstructive Shock.

REFERENCES

1. Trost JC, Lange RA. Treatment of acute coronary syndrome: Part 1: Non-ST-segment acute coronary syndrome. *Crit Care Med.* 2011;39(10): 2346-2353.
2. Overbaugh KJ. Acute coronary syndrome. *AJN.* 2009;109(5):42-52.
3. Amsterdam EA, Wenger NK, Brindis RG, et al. 2014 AHA/ACC Guideline for the Management of Patients With Non-ST-Elevation Acute Coronary Syndromes: a report of the American College of Cardiology/American Heart Association task force on practice guidelines [published online September 23, 2014]. *Circulation.* doi:10.1016/j.jacc.2014.09.017
4. Kinlay, S. Coronary artery spasms as a cause of angina. *Circulation.* 2014;129:1717-1719.
5. O'Gara PT, Kushner FG, Ascheim DD, et al. 2013 ACCF/AHA guideline for the management of ST-elevation myocardial infarction: a report of the American College of Cardiology Foundation/American Heart Association task force on practice guidelines. *Circulation.* 2013;127:e362-e425. doi: 10.1161/CIR.0b013e3182742cf6
6. O'Conner RE, Al Ali AS, Brady WJ, et al. American Heart Association guidelines for cardiopulmonary association and emergency cardiovascular care. Part 9: Acute Coronary Syndromes. *Circulation.* 2015;132:s483-s500.
7. Trost JC, Lange RA. Treatment of acute coronary syndrome: Part 2: ST-segment elevation myocardial infarction. *Crit Care Med.* 2012;40(9): 1939-1945.
8. Wagner G, Macfarlane P, Hein W, et al. AHA/ACCF/HRS recommendation for standardization and interpretation of the electrocardiogram. Part VI: acute ischemia/infarction. *Circulation.* 2009;119:e262-e270.
9. Grossman S, Mattson Porth C. *Porth's pathophysiology: Concepts of Altered Health States.* Philadelphia, PA: Lippincott Williams & Wilkins; 2014.
10. Simon A. Chest Pain. In: Tintinalli JE, Stapczynski J, Ma O, Yealy DM, Meckler GD, Cline DM, eds. *Tintinalli's Emergency Medicine: A Comprehensive Study Guide.* 8th ed. New York, NY: McGraw-Hill; 2016.
11. Tsai TT, Nienaber CA, Eagle KA. Acute aortic syndromes. *Circulation.* 2005;112:3802-3813.
12. Al'Aref SJ, Girard LN, Devenux R, et al. A contemporary review of acute aortic dissection. *Emerg Med (Los Angel).* 2015;5(274):2.
13. Link MS, Atkins DL, Passman RS, et al. Part 6: Electrical therapies: automated external defibrillators, defibrillation, cardioversion, and pacing 2010 American Heart Association guidelines for cardiopulmonary resuscitation and emergency cardiovascular care. *Circulation.* 2010;122: S706-S719.
14. Link MS, Berkow LC, Kudenchuk PJ, et al. American Heart Association guidelines for cardiopulmonary association and emergency cardiovascular care. Part 7: adult advanced cardiovascular life support. *Circulation.* 2015; 132:s444-s464.
15. "About Arrhythmia." *American Heart Association* 6 Nov. 2015. American Heart Association.org. Web. Accessed October 23, 2014.
16. Huff J (eds) *ECG Workout: Exercises in Arrhythmia Interpretation.* Philadelphia, PA: Lippincott Williams & Wilkins; 2012.
17. Delacretaz E. Supraventricular tachycardia. *N Engl Med.* 2006;354(9):1039-1051.
18. Criddle LM. Cardiovascular emergencies. In Hoyt KS, Selfridge-Thomas J, eds. *Emergency Nursing Core Curriculum.* 6th ed., pp. 187-247. St. Louis, MO: Elsevier/Saunders; 2007.
19. Hoen B, Duval X. Infective endocarditis. *N Engl J Med.* 2013;368:1425-1433.
20. Wilson W, Taubert K, Gewitz M, et al. Prevention of infective endocarditis. *Circulation.* 2007:1736-1754.
21. Habib G, Lancellotti P, Antunes MJ, et al. 2015 ESC guidelines for the management of infective endocarditis. *Eur Heart J.* 2015;36:3075-3123.
22. Scott MC, Winters ME. Congestive heart failure. *Emerg Med Clin N Am.* 2015;33:553-562.
23. Argulian E, McPherson C, Kukin M. Organ-specific responses to circulatory disturbances in heart failure: new insights. *Congest Heart Fail.* 2012;18(2):127-131.
24. Varon J. Treatment of acute severe hypertension. *Drugs.* 2008;68(3): 283-297.
25. Roy CL, Minor MA, Brookhart MA, et al. Does this patient with a pericardial effusion have cardiac tamponade? *JAMA.* 2007;297(16):1810-1818.
26. Yumoto T, Umei N, Kinami Y, et al. Cardiac tamponade associated with blunt cardiac injury: its definitive management in the emergency department. *Open Journal of Emergency Medicine.* 2015;3:9-12.
27. Imazio M, Gaita F, Lewinter M. Evaluation and treatment of pericarditis. A systematic review. *JAMA.* 2015;314(4):1498-1506.
28. Hong JB, Leonards CO, Endres M, et al. Ankle-brachial index and recurrent stroke risk. *Stroke.* 2016;47. http://stroke.ahajournals.org/lookup/supple/doi:10.1161/STROKEAHA
29. Eberhardt RT, Raffetto JD. Chronic venous insufficiency. *Circulation.* 2014:130:333-346.
30. D-dimer. Davis's drug guide. Nursing Central Web site. http://nursing.unboundmedicine.com/nursingcentral/index/Davis-Drug-Guide/All_Entries/A. Accessed March 21, 2015.
31. Kyrle PA, Eichinger S. Deep vein thrombosis. *Lancet.* 2005;365:1163-1174.
32. ENA. Emergency Nurses Association. *Trauma nurse core course.* Des Plaines, IL: Emergency Nurses Association; 2014.
33. Teixeira PGR, Georgiou C, Inaba K, et al. Blunt cardiac trauma: lessons learned from the medical examiner. *J Trauma.* 2009;67:1259-1264.
34. Genrich I, O'Mara S, Sulo S. Using a new evidence-based trauma protocol to improve detection and reduce costs in patients with blunt cardiac injury. *J Trauma Nurs.* 2015;22(1):28-34.
35. Marcolini EG, Keegan J. Blunt cardiac injury. *Emerg Med Clin N Am.* 2105;33:519-527.
36. Skinner DL, Hollander DD, Laing GL, et al. Severe blunt thoracic trauma: Differences between adults and children in a level I trauma centre. *S Afr Med J.* 2015;105:47-51.

Practice Questions

Question	Rationale
1. A patient enters the emergency department complaining of a racing heart, palpitations, and shortness of breath with an onset 30 minutes prior to arrival. The nurse places the patient on the cardiac monitor and notes that the heart rate is 190 bpm. What cardiac rhythm would the nurse expect to see? a. Normal sinus rhythm b. Sinus tachycardia c. Supraventricular tachycardia d. Ventricular fibrillation	*Answer: c* Supraventricular tachycardia is defined as a heart rate greater than 150, narrow complex, and regular rhythm. The signs and symptoms correlate with supraventricular tachycardia. Sinus tachycardia is a heart rate between 100 to 150. Normal sinus rhythm is a heart rate between 60 to 100. Ventricular fibrillation has no heart rate and the patient would be unresponsive.
2. A patient complains of chest pain unrelieved with rest. The ECG shows T wave inversion, but no elevation in his Troponin level. Based on the signs and symptoms, the patient is most likely experiencing? a. Stable angina b. Unstable angina c. Non-STEMI d. STEMI	*Answer: b* Unstable angina is defined as continued chest pain remaining after cessation of activity or chest pain relieved by nitroglycerin and without elevation in cardiac enzymes. Stable angina is characterized by chest pain relieved with cessation of the activity. Non-STEMI is defined as chest pain often with T wave inversion and/or ST segment depression and elevation in the cardiac enzymes. STEMI is characterized by chest pain with ST elevation and elevation in the cardiac enzymes.
3. A patient arrives to the emergency department with complaints of chest pain. On assessment, a pericardial friction rub and diffuse ST elevations are noted. The patient is most likely experiencing what condition? a. Pericarditis b. Non-STEMI c. STEMI d. Pericardial tamponade	*Answer: a* Pericarditis is an inflammation of the pericardial lining. Classic signs and symptoms include pain relieved when leaning forward, pericardial friction rub, and diffuse ST elevations. Non-STEMI signs and symptoms include ST depression or T wave inversions with elevation in cardiac enzymes. STEMI signs and symptoms include ST elevation in two or more leads, without the presence of a pericardial friction rub. Pericardial tamponade is an accumulation of fluid, pus, or blood in the pericardial sac compressing the heart preventing full myocardial expansion. The patient will have muffled heart sounds instead of a pericardial friction rub.
4. A 45-year-old female patient enters into the emergency department with complaints of intermittent chest pain that has happened at rest, during sleep, and with exercise. The patient was diagnosed with Prinzmetal's angina. What question should the nurse ask the patient? a. Do you smoke cigarettes? b. How long have you been exercising? c. Do you have any respiratory conditions? d. Does cold exposure relieve the chest pain?	*Answer: a* Cigarette smoking causes vasoconstriction which can cause vasospasm of the coronary arteries. The length of time exercising and any respiratory conditions does not directly address the causes of Prinzmetal's angina. Cold exposure causes vasoconstriction and would worsen rather than relieve the chest pain.

Question	Rationale
5. Ventricular tachycardia commonly leads to what rhythm? a. Third degree heart block b. Pulseless electrical activity (PEA) c. Supraventricular tachycardia d. Ventricular fibrillation	*Answer: d* Ventricular tachycardia commonly leads to ventricular fibrillation. Ventricular tachycardia does not commonly lead to third degree heart block, pulseless electrical activity (PEA), and supraventricular tachycardia.
6. A patient complains of chest pain, dyspnea, and dizziness for two hours prior to arrival. The patient is placed on the cardiac monitor. The patient's heart rate is 30 and the ECG shows asynchronous but regular P-to-P and R-to-R intervals. The patient is experiencing which of the following dysrhythmias? a. Normal sinus rhythm with first degree AV block b. Second degree AV block type 1 c. Second degree AV block type 2 d. Third degree heart block	*Answer: d* The patient symptoms of chest pain, dyspnea, and dizziness combined with the ECG findings indicate a third degree heart block. Normal sinus rhythm with first degree AV block is a prolonged PR interval and the heart rate is 60 to 100. The second degree AV block type 1 has a PR interval that varies with a QRS segment being dropped. The second degree AV block type 2 PR interval is not prolonged, but the QRS segment is dropped.
7. A patient arrives in the emergency department after being involved in a motor vehicle crash (MVC). The patient struck the steering wheel with her chest. The patient is diagnosed with blunt chest trauma and pericardial effusion and then becomes unresponsive and hypotensive. What is the priority intervention? a. Continue to monitor the patient b. Pericardiocentesis c. Administer Dopamine intravenously d. Needle-chest decompression	*Answer: b* The patient is unstable and needs immediate intervention such as a pericardiocentesis. If the RN simply continues to monitor the patient, the patient will become worse. Administering Dopamine intravenously may be needed, but it is not the priority intervention. The patient is not displaying signs or symptoms related to tension pneumothorax in which needle-chest decompression would be the recommended intervention.
8. A patient has a history of hypertension and hyperlipidemia and states that he developed sudden onset of upper back pain with dyspnea. The patient's blood pressure was 160/80 upon arrival with a heart rate of 104. A contrast CT scan was completed and an ascending aortic aneurysm was noted. What is the first priority to be completed for this patient? a. Administer intravenous fluids b. Administer an antihypertensive c. Administer a beta-blocker d. Administer analgesics	*Answer: b* To prevent aortic dissection, it is important to decrease the blood pressure keeping the systolic between 100 to 120 mm Hg. Adding intravenous fluids would further increase the vascular volume and increase the blood pressure. Administering a beta-blocker to reduce myocardial contractility and analgesics for the pain are necessary, but they are not the first priority.
9. A patient recently underwent a pericardiocentesis. What sign or symptom would indicate the procedure was unsuccessful? a. Narrowing pulse pressure b. Increased blood pressure c. Heart rate of 75 d. Increase in urine output	*Answer: a* A narrowed pulse pressure indicates poor heart function such as an unsuccessful pericardiocentesis. Signs and symptoms of cardiac tamponade include hypotension, muffled heart tones, and jugular vein distention. An increase in blood pressure and urine output indicates a successful procedure because there is an increase in blood flow to the heart, kidneys, and the rest of the body. Typically, patients with cardiac tamponade will have a rapid heartbeat greater than 100 bpm to compensate for the hypotension.

Question	Rationale
10. Four patients arrive at the front desk of the emergency department. Which patient should the RN assess first? a. 68-year-old male with chest pain, diaphoresis, pale skin, and vomiting b. 18-year-old male with chest pain worse upon movement and deep breathing c. 45-year-old female with abdominal pain, vomiting, and diarrhea d. 53-year-old female with pleuritic chest pain, productive cough, and dyspnea	*Answer: a* The symptoms of the 68-year-old male with chest pain, diaphoresis, and vomiting could indicate he is having an acute myocardial infarction and would be the first patient for the RN assesses. The 53-year-old female with pleuritic chest pain, productive cough, and dyspnea would be important to see, however not as important as the 68-year-old male patient. The 45-year-old with abdominal pain, vomiting, and diarrhea is not as critical as the 68-year-old male patient. The 18-year-old female patient with chest pain worsening with deep breathing and movement can wait to be seen.
11. A patient diagnosed with a deep vein thrombosis (DVT) suddenly becomes short of breath, tachycardic, tachypneic, and restless. What complication does the nurse suspect? a. Acute myocardial infarction b. Pulmonary embolism c. Pericardial tamponade d. Congestive heart failure	*Answer: b* Patients with DVTs are at high risk for pulmonary embolism. Sudden onset of shortness of breath, tachycardia, tachypnea, and restlessness are manifestations of pulmonary embolism. Acute myocardial infarction, pericardial tamponade, and congestive heart failure are not a complication of DVT.
12. A patient arrives in the emergency department complaining of chest pain, palpitations, and shortness of breath. The cardiac monitor displays supraventricular tachycardia (SVT). What common signs and symptoms would the nurse anticipate the patient to have? a. Dizziness and dyspnea b. Hypertension and nausea c. Clear mentation and respiratory rate of 16 d. Heart rate of 130 and respiratory rate of 28	*Answer: a* Dizziness and dyspnea are classic signs and symptoms of SVT. Patients may be hypertensive and nauseous when they are in SVT, but these are common signs and symptoms. Clear mentation and a respiratory rate of 16 are normal findings. Heart rate of 130 and a respiratory rate of 28 indicate tachycardia and tachypnea. However, the heart rate needs to be above 150 to be classified as SVT.
13. A patient complains of having two syncopal episodes at home. The patient is placed on the cardiac monitor and becomes unresponsive. The RN notices a third different episode of 10 to 20 second pauses on the cardiac monitor. What intervention will the RN expect the patient to receive? a. Intravenous fluids b. Beta-blocker medication c. Pacemaker d. CT of the head	*Answer: c* The patient is experiencing a sinus pause/arrest and requires a pacemaker as the SA node is not consistently generating an impulse. Intravenous fluids will not improve the sinus pause/arrest rhythm that caused the patient's syncope. Beta-blockers commonly cause sinus pause/arrest and therefore should not administer to the patient. The patient has an electrical conduction disorder and a CT of head is not recommended intervention for sinus pause/arrest.

Question	Rationale
14. A patient arrives to the emergency department after a minor MVC reporting chest pain. The nurse would suspect treatment interventions for blunt cardiac trauma, as opposed to STEMI care, due to which initial findings? a. ST segment changes, peaked T-waves, and increased Troponin I b. ST segment changes, T-wave inversion, and increased Troponin I c. ST segment changes, T-wave inversion, and normal Troponin I d. ST segment changes, T-wave flattening, and normal Troponin I	*Answer: c* Blunt trauma causes ST segment changes, T-wave inversion and normal Troponin levels. Peaked T-waves are common in hyperkalemia while flattened T-waves may be due to hypokalemia or coronary ischemia. Increased Troponin levels are more likely to be seen in STEMI than blunt cardiac trauma.
15. What common signs and symptoms would an RN expect to see in a patient with left-sided congestive heart failure? a. Syncope, palpitations, and dyspnea b. Tachypnea, dyspnea, and crackles in the lungs c. Anorexia, jugular vein distention, and fatigue d. Bradycardia, tachypnea, and headache	*Answer: b* Left-sided heart failure signs and symptoms include tachypnea, dyspnea, and crackles in the lungs due to the blood backing up into the lungs causing pulmonary congestion. Anorexia, jugular vein distention, and fatigue are signs and symptoms of right-sided heart failure. Syncope, palpitations, bradycardia and headache are not common in left-sided heart failure.
16. A patient complains of severe thoracic back pain radiating to the chest starting 2 hours prior to arrival. The patient has a history of hypertension and the initial blood pressure is 220/128. What condition does the nurse suspect? a. Hypertensive crisis b. Congestive heart failure c. Acute arterial occlusion d. Dissecting aortic aneurysm	*Answer: d* The patient is displaying signs and symptoms of a dissecting aortic aneurysm. When a patient is diagnosed with an aortic aneurysm, it is imperative to lower blood pressure to prevent dissection. The patient is hypertensive due to the body compensating for decreased cardiac output. The patient is not suffering from a hypertensive crisis. Congestive heart failure patients may be hypertensive due to fluid overload, but patients do not typically have severe thoracic back pain. Acute arterial occlusion signs and symptoms are pulseless, pallor, pain, paresthesia, and paralysis in the extremities, not in the thoracic region.
17. A patient is diagnosed with an aortic aneurysm. The patient displays the following vital signs: Blood pressure 200/98, heart rate 100 bpm, respirations at 24 per minute, temperature of 99.0°F, and pulse ox of 95% on room air. Which vital sign needs immediate attention? a. Blood pressure b. Heart rate c. Respiratory rate d. Temperature	*Answer: a* When a patient is diagnosed with an aortic aneurysm, it is imperative to lower blood pressure to prevent dissection. Even though the heart rate and respiratory rate are elevated, this compensatory mechanism is caused by the aortic aneurysm. The temperature is slightly elevated, but has no effect on an aortic aneurysm.

Question	Rationale
18. A patient enters the emergency department in cardiopulmonary arrest. The patient was intubated prior to arrival. The nurse auscultates the chest and hears breath sounds on the right side only. What intervention would the nurse expect the physician to order first? a. Arterial blood gases b. Chest x-ray c. CT scan d. Electrocardiogram	*Answer: b* The patient is intubated prior to arrival and one of the causes of absent breath sounds is displacement. The ET tube could be placed in the right mainstem bronchus. The physician would order a chest x-ray to verify placement of the endotracheal tube. If the endotracheal tube is in the correct place, an arterial blood gas may be ordered, but this is not the priority. A patient in cardiopulmonary arrest is unstable to go to CT scan. An electrocardiogram may be obtained if the patient has any electrical activity on the cardiac monitor, but this is not the priority.
19. A patient complains of dizziness/lightheadedness, palpitations, and dyspnea for the last two weeks. An electrocardiogram is performed with the following findings: irregular rate, unmeasurable PR interval, QRS < 0.12, QT interval 0.36. The nurse would interpret this cardiac rhythm to be? a. Sinus pause/arrest b. Normal sinus rhythm with premature ventricular contractions c. Atrial fibrillation d. Ventricular fibrillation	*Answer: c* An irregular rhythm with no measurable PR interval is characteristic of atrial fibrillation. Sinus pause/arrest is an irregular rhythm, but the PR interval is measurable. The patient is missing one or several beats. Normal sinus rhythm with premature ventricular contractions is an irregular rhythm, but the PR interval is measurable in the normal beats and usually within normal limits (0.12 to 0.20). Ventricular fibrillation is a chaotic rhythm that is irregular, but there is no heartbeat, no PR interval, no QRS segment, and no QT interval.
20. A patient is newly diagnosed with controlled atrial fibrillation. What intervention would the nurse expect the physician to order? a. Anticoagulants b. Aspirin c. Antithrombotics d. Atropine	*Answer: a* The patient is newly diagnosed with controlled atrial fibrillation and should be started on anticoagulants to prevent the development of a thrombosis. Aspirin is not as effective as anticoagulants in preventing a thrombosis. Antithrombotics are recommended for a thrombosis in the coronary arteries or brain it is not recommended for controlled atrial fibrillation. Atropine is recommended for sinus bradycardia and is not recommended for controlled atrial fibrillation.
21. A patient was found pulseless and apneic. Cardiopulmonary resuscitation was begun and a cardiac/defibrillator was applied. The patient's rhythm is asystole. What treatment would the nurse expect the physician to order? a. Atropine b. Epinephrine c. Amiodarone d. Defibrillation	*Answer: b* The American Heart Association recommends epinephrine as the medication to treat asystole. Atropine does not show any benefit to patients in asystole. Amiodarone is recommended for ventricular tachycardia and fibrillation and is not recommended for asystole. Adenosine is recommended for supraventricular tachycardia and not recommended for asystole.

Question	Rationale
22. A patient is diagnosed with infective endocarditis in the emergency department. What signs and symptoms will the patient display? a. Chest pain, dyspnea, and cough b. Syncope, bradycardia, and fever c. Fever, dyspnea, and anorexia d. Back pain, lethargy, and bradycardia	*Answer: c* Patients with infective endocarditis have fever, dyspnea, and anorexia due to the infectious process in the body. The patient with infective endocarditis does have dyspnea, but not a cough. The patient may have chest pain, but is not as common as fever and dyspnea. Patients with infective endocarditis have fevers and tachycardia, not bradycardia or syncope. While patients with infective endocarditis may be lethargic, back pain, and bradycardia are uncommon.
23. A patient with a history of Raynaud's disease presents to the emergency department with bilateral hand pain. The patient's hands are cold to the touch and pale, almost cyanotic. Following treatment, what patient education should the nurse provide? a. Make sure your hands remain covered during cold weather b. Apply ice to your hands when they began to hurt c. You can take cold medications as needed d. You need to take your antibiotics until they are gone	*Answer: a* It is important to help prevent exacerbations of Raynaud's by covering the hands when the weather is cold. If the patient applies ice to the hands, this will cause further vasoconstriction and make the condition worse. Cold medications cause vasoconstriction therefore exacerbating the patient's Raynaud's and should be taken with caution. Raynaud's disease does not require antibiotics.
24. A patient enters the emergency department with midsternal chest pain, nausea, and diaphoresis. The patient states the pain has increased in intensity over the last hour. An ECG was obtained and ST depression is noted. The patient has an elevation in cardiac enzymes. The patient is most likely experiencing? a. Stable angina b. Unstable angina c. NSTEMI d. STEMI	*Answer: c* In NSTEMI, the patient has elevation in cardiac enzymes with ST depression on the ECG. Stable angina does not have ST depression or elevation in cardiac enzymes. Unstable angina may have similar signs and symptoms, but patients do not have any elevation in cardiac enzymes. STEMI is classified as an elevation in cardiac enzymes along with ST elevation on the ECG.
25. A patient has been experiencing dizziness, fatigue, and a decreased level of consciousness. The patient's cardiac rhythm displays a P wave of 0.12, QRS <0.12, QT 0.48, and a heart rate of 38. What intervention would the nurse expect the physician to order? a. Atropine b. Amiodarone c. Cardioversion d. Defibrillation	*Answer: a* Atropine is the recommended treatment for symptomatic sinus bradycardia. Amiodarone, cardioversion, and defibrillation are not recommended for treatment of sinus bradycardia.

Question	Rationale
26. A patient has the following cardiac rhythm: inverted or missing P waves, narrow QRS segments, QT interval of 0.44, and a heart rate of 44 bpm. What is the rhythm? a. Atrial fibrillation b. Sinus bradycardia c. Idioventricular rhythm d. Junctional rhythm	*Answer: d* Classic junctional rhythms have no P wave or an inverted P wave, narrowed QRS segment, and a heart rate between 40 to 60. Atrial fibrillation has no discernable P waves, a narrowed QRS segment, and heart rate between 60 to 100 or greater than 100. Idioventricular rhythm has no P wave, wide and bizarre QRS segment, and heart rate between 30 to 40.
27. A patient developed chest pain, palpitations, dyspnea, and lightheadedness 2 days ago. The patient is currently on a beta-blocker for hypertension with a blood pressure of 140/74 mm Hg. The patient is placed on the cardiac monitor, which displays a second-degree heart block type II. What intervention would the physician order for treatment? a. Give epinephrine IV b. Discontinue the beta-blocker c. Continue to monitor the patient d. Give a calcium channel blocker	*Answer: b* One of the causes of a second degree heart block type II is beta-blockade. Removing the beta-blocker from the patient's medication regimen may help reestablish the previous cardiac rhythm. Epinephrine is recommended for patients who are hypotensive. This patient has normal blood pressure. Continuing to monitor the patient does not address the patient's change in cardiac rhythm, signs, or symptoms. It would not be recommended to give a calcium channel blocker, which may further worsen the second degree heart block type II.
28. A patient was found at home in cardiac arrest. The patient regained a pulse during EMS treatment. CPR is in progress as the patient enters the emergency department. After two minutes of CPR, a rhythm check reveals Asystole. What are the recommended interventions for Asystole? a. Defibrillation and Epinephrine b. CPR and Atropine c. Defibrillation and Atropine d. CPR and Epinephrine	*Answer: d* CPR and Epinephrine are the recommended interventions for Asystole. Atropine is not recommended to treat Asystole as there is no evidence of benefit for the patient. Defibrillation is not recommended because there is no electrical current with Asystole.
29. A patient presents to the emergency department with acute respiratory distress due to heart failure. The patient has audible crackles, tachypnea, tachycardia, and diaphoresis. The patient's vital signs consist of blood pressure 165/95 mm Hg, heart rate of 124 bpm, respirations at 32 per minute, and a pulse ox of 85% on room air. The patient was placed on oxygen for 5 minutes without improvement. What is the next priority for this patient? a. Bilevel Positive Airway Pressure (BiPAP) b. Electrocardiogram (ECG) c. Intravenous access with normal saline bolus d. Lasix intravenously	*Answer: a* The patient appears to be in acute respiratory distress and immediate action needs to be taken to address the patient's breathing such as Bilevel Positive Airway Pressure (BiPAP). An electrocardiogram (ECG) will be completed once the patient's breathing has been addressed. An IV will be inserted, but the patient should not receive a normal saline bolus as they appear to be in congestive heart failure. Lasix will be given after addressing the patient's breathing.

Question	Rationale
30. A patient has been having a headache and elevated blood pressure for the past three days. The patient's blood pressure upon arrival is 170/100 mm Hg. The patient has no allergies, takes no medications, and has no medical history. What is the patient's most likely condition? a. Essential hypertension b. Systolic hypertension c. Secondary hypertension d. Hypertensive emergency	*Answer: a* Essential hypertension occurs without evidence of other diseases and with a chronic elevation in blood pressure. Systolic hypertension occurs when the systolic pressure is continually elevated above 140 mm Hg, however the diastolic pressure is less than 90 mm Hg. Secondary hypertension results from diseases or processes occurring within the body. Hypertensive emergency is an accelerated form of hypertension suddenly displaying a systolic pressure greater than 180 mm Hg and a diastolic pressure greater than 120 mm Hg.
31. A patient enters the emergency department with pain, edema, and ulcer formation on the left lower leg. The patient states the edema has become worse over the past couple of days and the patient noticed skin discoloration on the left lower leg. What condition is most likely? a. Varicose veins b. Chronic venous insufficiency c. Deep vein thrombosis d. Raynaud's disease	*Answer: b* The patient is displaying signs and symptoms of chronic venous insufficiency. Varicose veins signs and symptoms consist of pain, edema, and dilated veins, not ulcer formation. Deep vein thrombosis signs and symptoms consist of unilateral swelling, skin is warm to touch, and pain in the lower extremity. However, ulcer formation is not a typical sign or symptom. Raynaud's disease is an intense vasospasm of the arteries in the fingers and toes, not in the lower extremities.
32. A patient presents to the emergency department with back pain and right lower leg pain. The nurse performs an assessment and discovers the right leg is pale and pulseless. The patient reports intense pain, paresthesia, and paralysis in the right leg. The patient is diagnosed with acute arterial occlusion. What would be the patient's priority intervention? a. Give the patient morphine for the pain b. Apply ice to the right leg c. Elevate the right leg d. Administration of tissue plasminogen activator (tPA)	*Answer: d* Blood flow needs to be immediately restored to the right leg and tissue plasminogen activator (tPA) or an embolectomy will restore the blood flow. Morphine is important, but will not restore the blood flow to the right leg. Applying ice to the right leg will cause vasoconstriction worsening the patient's condition. Elevating the right leg will not repair the obstruction of blood flow and could potentially worsen the condition.
33. An unrestrained driver was involved in a motor vehicle crash (MVC). The driver is responsive upon arrival to the emergency department and complaining of chest pain with a large area of ecchymosis on her anterior chest. The patient is placed on the cardiac monitor. What rhythm is most commonly associated with blunt cardiac trauma? a. Sinus tachycardia b. Third degree heart block c. Sinus bradycardia d. Premature ventricular contractions	*Answer: a* The most common arrhythmia seen in blunt cardiac trauma is sinus tachycardia. Third degree heart block is not a common arrhythmia related to blunt cardiac trauma. Sinus bradycardia may be seen if the patient is decompensating. However, this is not the most common arrhythmia. Patients could display premature ventricular contractions, but they are not the most common.

Question	Rationale
34. A 62-year-old patient is brought to the emergency department by his son. The patient has been complaining of severe headache for the past day, dizziness, shortness of breath, blurred vision and "…not feeling right." He denies chest pain or extremity weakness. His daily medications consist of Wellbutrin for depression and Captopril. The patient admitted he stopped taking Captopril about one week ago when the prescription "ran out," and he was "… coughing more." A 12 lead ECG shows sinus rhythm without ST segment or T wave abnormalities. Vital signs: Temp-98.6°F (37°C), Pulse- 88, Respirations- 22, BP-240/126, pulse oximetry-92% on room air. The nurse anticipates that any one of the following medications would be ordered right away *except* a. Nicardipine b. Benazepril (Lotensin™) c. Labetalol d. Nitroprusside	*Answer: b* Hypertensive emergencies can cause or worsen organ damage and immediate controlled treatment is imperative. Benazepril is an Angiotensin-converting enzyme (ACE) inhibitor class of antihypertensive medications and is only available in oral doses. The other three antihypertensive medications can be administered intravenously (IV). IV antihypertensive medications are indicated for hypertension emergencies as they can be titrated safely and reduce blood pressure more effectively. Patients are typically instructed to report a persistent cough while taking an ace-inhibitor, such as Captopril, as this can be one of the side effects. Nicardipine is a calcium channel blocker. Labetalol is an alpha/beta-adrenergic blocker and nitroprusside is a potent peripheral vasodilator.
35. A 55-year-old male presents to the emergency department with chest pain. He has a history of Type 2 diabetes and hypertension that has been well controlled with medication. He has no other past medical problems or history of chest pain. The medications he takes are hydrochlorothiazide and sildenafil (Viagra™). Pulse is 98, Respirations are 20, BP is 174/92 and pulse oximetry is 95% on room air. The following medication should not be administered while taking sildenafil a. Morphine b. Isosorbide c. Esmolol d. Fentanyl	*Answer: b* Isosorbide is an antianginal nitrate. Nitrates are contraindicated with phosphodiesterase 5 (PDE5) inhibitor class of drugs, such as sildenafil. The PDE5 class of pharmacological agents are prescribed for erectile dysfunction and if nitrates are administered while on this, cardiovascular collapse can occur. Esmolol is a beta-adrenergic blocker and often administered for hypertension. Morphine and Fentanyl are both opioids and given to patients with chest pain.
36. An 82-year-old female patient arrives via EMS following a low-speed collision. She was driving and the sole occupant in the car. She reports that suddenly she lost control and the car slid off the road hitting a parked car. Airway and breathing are intact and vital signs are stable. She is alert and oriented to person, place and time. She has a left-ankle deformity; otherwise, no obvious signs of injury. She complains of chest pain but denies any shortness of breath. The cardiac monitor shows ST-elevation in lead II, and a stat 12 lead ECG shows ST-elevation in leads II, III and AVF. What other information is needed to help determine the origin of her chest pain? a. Do you have any medication allergies? b. What medications do you take? c. Does the chest pain hurt worse with movement? d. Did the pain begin before you lost control of driving?	*Answer: d* All the above questions are needed information; however, her present signs of ST-segment elevation are suggesting that she is having an inferior-wall MI. The onset of her chest pain may help indicate if the crash is causing her chest pain (and possible MI) or if the chest pain precipitated her losing control of her car leading to the crash.

Question	Rationale

37. In pulsus paradoxus, the pulse during inspiration can be
   a. Palpated but not auscultated
   b. Auscultated but not palpated
   c. Auscultated and visualized on telemetry
   d. Auscultated but not visualized on telemetry
	Answer: b
	Pulsus paradoxus occurs during conditions such as cardiac tamponade and pericarditis in which the myocardium is able to conduct electricity and contract, but may not have enough force to create cardiac output strong enough for a palpable pulse, especially at the radial artery.

38. A patient who has been diagnosed with a NSTEMI is going for a diagnostic cardiac catherization and possible revascularization. He is receiving a heparin infusion. The emergency nurse would anticipate the following action
   a. Administer an oral dose of Dabigatran (Pradaxa™)
   b. Stop the heparin infusion until the procedure is completed
   c. Administer an oral dose of Clopidogrel (Plavix™)
   d. Administer IV Hydromorphone for his increased pain
	Answer: c
	Clopidogrel inhibits platelet aggregation by binding to the adenosine diphosphate P2Y12 receptor on platelets. This binding action inhibits the ADP-mediated formation of the glycoprotein GPIIb/IIIa complex activation that is necessary for platelet aggregation. Impeding platelet aggregation augments reperfusion. Heparin is not usually stopped for reperfusion therapy. Morphine decreases myocardial oxygen demand and is the first opioid analgesic of choice unless contraindicated for the patient.

39. A patient with ST-segment elevation in all ECG leads begins to rapidly decompensate with worsening vital signs. The emergency nurse knows to prepare for
   a. IV diuretics
   b. Repeat ECG
   c. IV Beta-Blocker
   d. Pericardiocentesis
	Answer: d
	Diffuse ST-segment elevation is indicative of Pericarditis. Significant vital sign decompensation may be an indication of cardiac compression requiring removal of fluid from around the heart. While diuretics may also be ordered, a pericardiocentesis would provide the most rapid relief of symptoms. A repeat ECG would not help with diagnosis or treatment and IV beta-blocker medications would not relieve the cause of the symptoms.

40. The nurse caring for a patient with chest pain notices Osler Nodes on the patient's fingertips and knows to expect an order for
   a. Aspirin
   b. Antibiotics
   c. Calcium
   d. Diuretics
	Answer: b
	Osler nodes are a sign of bacterial endocarditis, which requires treatment with antibiotic medications. Aspirin, calcium, and diuretics would not be a recommended treatment for bacterial endocarditis.

Respiratory Emergencies

Jamie Vranak, MSN, RN, CEN

Respiratory emergencies encompass all insults to the lungs including infections and injuries. Airway and breathing are the first two assessments made in any critical situation, and for good reason. Failure to secure the airway and ensure effective breathing can lead to rapid decline and death.

Considerations for Special Populations

Pediatrics

Children are at greater risk for airway compromise due to the smaller diameter of their neck and airway. Other physiologic differences, such as more mobile and delicate tissues in the tracheobronchial tissues, mediastinum, and chest wall also make them more susceptible to injury. Furthermore, children can rapidly decompensate and lose their respiratory drive due to tiring from respiratory efforts.[1]

Pregnancy

Pregnant women have increased oxygen needs to accommodate the growing fetus and increased cardiac output. As a result, $PaCO_2$ levels will drop to 27 to 34 mm Hg throughout pregnancy. The kidneys attempt to compensate for this acidotic state by excreting bicarbonate, so lower levels from 18 to 21 mEq/L can be anticipated.[2]

Geriatrics

Physiologic changes occur as a result of the aging process and are compounded by comorbidities more common in the elderly. These changes include decreased pliability and contractility of tissues, decreased muscle mass, and weakened bone structures. As a result, older patients are more susceptible to injury and less able to compensate for insults to the respiratory system.[3]

Aspiration

Aspiration is caused by inhalation of gastric or oropharyngeal matter into the lungs. There are several causes of aspiration. Aspiration of gastric contents can cause a chemical pneumonitis. When bacteria that is normally in the oral and nasal pharynx is inhaled, aspiration pneumonia may occur. Aspiration of toxic substances to the lower airway such as dust particles or gases can cause a chemical pneumonitis. If a patient inhales a foreign body such as a tooth or peanut, an airway obstruction may occur and pneumonia may result. Aspiration occurs in patients with a significant decrease in level of consciousness, which may be related to trauma, seizure, overdose, or other neurological deficit.[4] Patients who are emergently intubated are especially at risk.[4] Aspiration pneumonia predominately affects patients with dysphagia who are at increased risk for inhaling secretions, fluids, and food. The dysphagia decreases the patient's ability to cough and clear the aspirate, further complicating the problem. Dysphagia is extremely common in elderly patients and is a significant cause of morbidity and mortality.[4] Other patients who may be at risk for aspiration are those using a gastric feeding tube, have protracted vomiting, or a tracheostomy tube.

Assessment/Analysis

- Airway patency, effective breathing
- Clinical features are similar to pneumonia (fever, dyspnea, productive cough with purulent sputum)
- Lung sounds with auscultation
- Level of consciousness; ability to swallow
- Cyanosis
- Difficulty swallowing
- Chest pain
- Vocal changes, hoarseness
- Chest x-ray
- Swallow screening at bedside
- Evaluate for risk factors of aspiration
  - Age greater than 65, as the efficiency of the swallowing mechanism decreases[4]
  - Any neurological insult
    - Stroke
    - Intracranial bleed
    - Tumor of head or neck
  - Alzheimer's and/or dementia
  - Neurological diseases
    - Amyotrophic lateral sclerosis (ALS also known as Lou Gehrig's disease)
    - Parkinson's
    - Multiple sclerosis

- ○ Other diseases and disorders that increase esophageal acid
- ○ Impaired sensorium from intoxicants, and/or other drugs
- ○ Decreased level of consciousness

Intervention
- Tracheal suctioning to clear fluids of particulate matter
- Removal of the aspirated foreign body
- Supplemental Oxygen to maintain O_2 saturation to either 95% or patient's known baseline
  - ○ Noninvasive positive pressure ventilation (NPPV), such as biphasic positive airway pressure (BiPAP), or mechanical ventilation for severe cases
- Continuous pulse oximetry, cardiac monitor
- Medications
  - ○ Broad-spectrum antibiotics
- NG tube placement
  - ○ Should be done expediently in intubated patients to prevent aspiration

Evaluation
- Airway patency
- Effective breathing
- Patient/family education for chronic risk for aspiration
  - ○ Eat sitting upright
  - ○ Add a thickening agent to food and drinks to assist with swallowing

Asthma

Asthma is a common chronic condition for patients of all ages and is the most common childhood disease.[5] Asthma is characterized by inflammation and bronchoconstriction that results in wheezing and difficulty breathing, but is reversible with treatment.[5] It is important to collect the patient history including:

- ❖ Onset and duration of distress
- ❖ History of asthma
- ❖ Risk factors
  - ♦ Family history of asthma
  - ♦ Allergen exposure-cats, dogs, dust mites, or cockroaches
- ❖ Review medication history and compliance
- ❖ Possible triggers: exercise, cold air, exposure to allergens, cigarette smoking (or second-hand smoke), or work environment triggers
- ❖ Use of peak flow meter at home with personal best and current measures (if known)

Assessment/Analysis
- Dyspnea, tachypnea, cough, chest tightness, prolonged expiration, and wheezing
- Signs of infection, such as fever and productive cough
- Diminished breath sounds and wheezing
  - ○ Patients may begin with mild symptoms including dyspnea and end-expiratory wheezing
  - ○ As the exacerbation progresses, the distress is more evident with wheezing noted on inspiration and expiration, tachypnea, and tachycardia, and accessory muscle use
  - ○ Lack of wheezing with diminished breath sounds indicate severe obstruction of airflow and requires immediate intervention
- Hyperresonance to percussion
- Pulsus paradoxus of greater than 20 mm Hg may also be noted in severe exacerbations[5]
  - ○ See chapter 2 for further discussion on Pulsus Paradoxus

Intervention
- Supplemental oxygen to maintain O_2 saturation to either 95% or patient's known baseline
- Continuous pulse oximetry monitoring, consider cardiac monitor and capnography (see Appendix 3B) for high-risk patients
- Measure peak flow levels and compare to expected
- Medications
  - ○ β_2 adrenergic agonists (albuterol)
    - A sympathomimetic promoting relaxation of bronchial smooth muscle (bronchodilation), vasodilation, and ciliary clearance[5]
    - Side effects: skeletal muscle tremor, nervousness, anxiety, insomnia, headache, hyperglycemia, palpitations, tachycardia, and hypertension[5]
    - Metered-dose inhaler (MDI) inhaler or nebulized treatment (preferred), which may be given every 15 to 20 minutes as needed or continuously[5]
    - A spacer with MDI improves the amount of medication reaching the lungs
  - ○ Anticholinergics (atropine sulfate or ipratropium bromide)
    - Parasympatholytics promoting smooth muscle relaxation (bronchodilation) and reducing secretions
    - Side effects: dry mouth, thirst, pupil dilation, increased heart rate, and difficulty swallowing. Ipratropium bromide offers fewer side effects than atropine, and is therefore the preferred option[5]
    - Administered via MDI inhaler or nebulizer (preferred) which can be given simultaneously with albuterol[5]
  - ○ Corticosteroids (prednisone, methylprednisolone, or prednisolone)
    - Reduce inflammation and assist β_2 adrenergic agonists responsiveness
    - Side Effect: hyperglycemia
    - Oral and IV routes have similar onset of action
  - ○ Magnesium Sulfate
    - Promotes bronchodilation
    - May be indicated for severe exacerbations
    - 1–2 g IV given over 30 minutes[5]

- Systemic β₂ agonists (epinephrine or terbutaline)
  - Not frequently used[5]
  - No benefit over inhaled β₂ agonists (albuterol)
  - Side effects are the same as inhaled β₂ agonists
  - Arterial blood gas with severe exacerbations[5]
  - Chest x-ray-Identify possible triggering underlying infection
  - Pediatric considerations
- Use blow-by oxygen to reduce anxiety which may increase work of breathing
- Paradoxical respirations (abdominal breathing) are normal
- Non-standard methods for management[5]
  - Ketamine
  - Helium/oxygen mix
- Pregnancy considerations
  - Pregnant asthmatics are at increased risk for exacerbations[5]
  - Pregnancy causes an increased PaO₂ and decreased PaCO₂, a normal alkalosis, so asthma exacerbations are less tolerated and need rapid treatment to ensure oxygenation to the fetus[5]
  - β₂ Agonists and inhaled corticosteroids are recommended treatments for pregnant asthmatics

Evaluation
- Patent airway and effective breathing
- Decrease or resolution of wheezing
- Improved SpO₂ on room air and improved peak flows (greater than 70% of that predicted)[5]
- Consideration should be given to the patient's ability to manage themselves at home (medication availability and compliance) and other factors, such as comorbidities putting the patient at risk. Admission may be necessary for patients that have a poor response to treatment (peak flow levels less than 40% predicted) and persisting or progressing symptoms[5]
- Patient/family education
  - Arrange for and emphasize the importance of follow up with primary physician
  - Instruct on the proper use of inhaler with spacer and have the patient demonstrate understanding prior to discharge
  - Review use of peak flow meter and provide a diary to track measurements twice daily[5]
  - Smoking cessation and avoiding smoke in the home

Chronic Obstructive Pulmonary Disease

Chronic obstructive pulmonary disease (COPD) is a frequent cause for older patients' admission to emergency departments and carries a high morbidity and mortality rate. It is the third most common cause for hospital admission and the fourth most common cause of death in the United States, the only cause of death that is increasing.[6] COPD results in the progressive limitation of airflow and is not reversible. Those with COPD are often afflicted with chronic bronchitis (chronic inflammation and productive cough), while fewer are strictly afflicted with emphysema (degradation of bronchioles and alveoli).[6] COPD exacerbations are the result of inflammatory processes causing bronchoconstriction, pulmonary vasoconstriction, and mucus hyper secretion.[6] It is important to collect the patient history including:

- ❖ Onset and duration of distress
- ❖ History of asthma, including previous hospitalizations
- ❖ Review medication history, home oxygen, and compliance with use
- ❖ Immunizations, particularly influenza, and pneumococcal
- ❖ Triggers such as cold weather, beta blockers, narcotics, or sedative-hypnotics
- ❖ Smoking history or exposure to secondhand smoke
- ❖ Use of peak flow meter at home with personal best and current measures (if known)

Assessment/Analysis
- Hypoxemia/Altered mental status
- Dyspnea that worsens with exertion
- Difficulty speaking because of increased respiratory effort
- Cyanosis
- Tachypnea and tachycardia
- Chest tightness and cough
- Paradoxical chest wall movement
- Tripod position and/or pursed lip expiration
  - Patient creating positive end expiratory pressure or self-PEEP
- Prolonged expiration and accessory muscle use
- Assess sputum for color and consistency
- Signs of infection such as fever or productive cough
- Diminished breath sounds, crackles, expiratory wheezes, or rhonchi
- Hyper-resonance to percussion
- Signs of right-sided heart failure (cor pulmonale): jugular venous distension (JVD) and peripheral edema
- Pulsus paradoxus of greater than 20 mg Hg may also be noted
- Arterial blood gas: determines the severity of exacerbation and if hypercapnia is present
- Chest x-ray
  - More than 75% of COPD exacerbations are due to infection
    - Up to half are bacterial[6]
  - Rule out other complications such as pneumothorax, pleural effusion, or pulmonary thromboembolism[6]

- Laboratory studies
  - CBC with differential
  - Serum chemistries
  - Brain natriuretic peptide BNP to rule out CHF as a differential diagnosis
  - D-dimer: a negative result would rule out pulmonary embolus
  - Theophylline levels (as appropriate)
  - Troponin
- EKG

Intervention
- Supplemental O_2 to maintain SpO_2 >90% Caution for hypercapnia (CO_2 retention)
- Continuous SpO_2 measurement and cardiac monitor, consider capnography (see Appendix 3B)
- Measure peak flow and compare to predicted or personal best (if able)
- Medications change to
  - β_2 adrenergic agonists albuterol
  - Anticholinergics-ipratropium
  - Systemic glucocorticoids-prednisone
- Antibiotics if needed for underlying infection
- Anticipate set up of continuous positive airway pressure (CPAP) or bi-level positive airway pressure (BiPAP), which assists by maintaining open alveoli. See Figure 3-1 for an example of a patient wearing a BiPAP mask
  - Should only be used on alert and cooperative patients
  - Can improve outcomes: reduce need for intubation and decrease duration of hospitalization[6]
- Anticipate the need and set up for intubation if the patient fails NPPV
- Always review, when possible, the patient's Advanced Directives if intubation and mechanical ventilation is indicated

Evaluation
- Patent airway and effective breathing
- Decrease or resolution of wheezing and/or rhonchi
- Improved SpO_2 on room air
- Indications for hospital admission
  - Poor response to treatment in the ED
  - Development of new symptoms such as increased shortness of breath, cyanosis, or peripheral edema
  - Age of the patient
  - Co-morbidities such as congestive heart failure, diabetes, renal, or liver failure
- Consideration should be given to the patient's ability to manage at home. Evaluate medication availability and compliance, home O_2 assessment, and other comorbidities potentially placing the patient at risk
- Patient/family education
  - Encourage fluid intake to thin secretions
  - Instruct to limit the use of antihistamines, antitussives, and decongestants as they have a dehydrating effect
  - Encourage small, frequent meals as an overly distended abdomen decreases lung capacity
  - Encourage exercise as it helps to increase energy and endurance
  - Encourage the importance of influenza and pneumonia vaccine
  - Smoking cessation including nicotine replacement education

Infections

The respiratory system is often affected by infections; pneumonia is most common. Many infections are viral and require supportive treatment. Bacterial infections, such as streptococcus pneumonia, require antibiotic treatment.

Croup (Laryngotracheobronchitis)

Croup is an acute viral syndrome most commonly caused by the parainfluenza virus.[7] Croup is an inflammatory process of the upper airway typically affecting children up to three years. The illness is usually self-limiting and requires supportive treatment.[7]

Assessment/Analysis
- Barking cough that worsens at night
- Hoarseness
- Dyspnea and inspiratory stridor
- Drooling
- Hypoxemia
- Fever

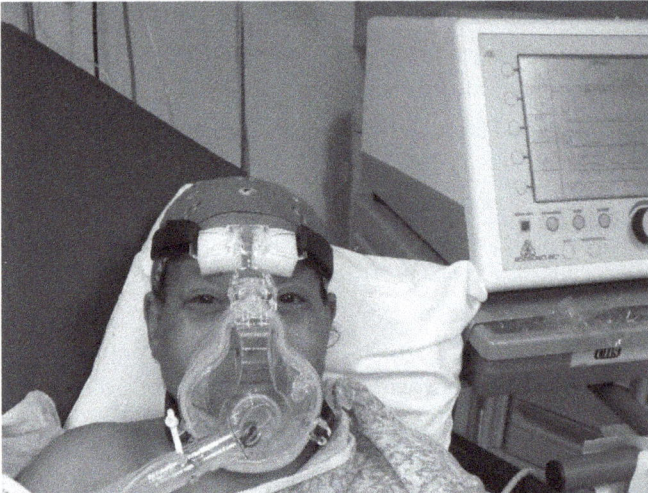

FIGURE 3-1 A patient is placed on BiPAP to assist breathing
Reproduced with permission from Knoop KJ, Stack LB, Storrow AB, et al: The Atlas of Emergency Medicine, 4th ed. New York: McGraw-Hill Education; 2016: Photo contributor: Steven J. White, MD.

- Croup Score
  - Mild croup
    - No stridor at rest
    - Baking cough at rest
  - Moderate croup
    - Stridor at rest
    - Little or no agitation
  - Severe croup
    - Stridor at rest
    - Severe retractions
    - Anxiousness and agitation
    - Pale
    - Fatigue
  - Impending Respiratory Failure
    - Fatigue and listlessness
    - Decreased or absent breath sounds
    - Altered mental status
    - Cyanosis
    - Increased heart rate

Intervention
- Humidified oxygen
- Minimize anxiety—allow the parent or caregiver hold the child
- Monitor pulse oximetry
- Observe for 3 to 4 hours
- Oral fluids as tolerated
- Intravenous fluids as needed
- Soft tissue radiograph of the neck to rule out epiglottitis
- Indications for admission
  - Poor air intake
  - Altered mental status
  - Need for supplemental oxygen
  - Poor response to treatment in the ED
  - Less than 6 months of age
  - Repeat ED visits
  - Inability for the family to care for the child
  - Medications
    - Antipyretic
    - Racemic epinephrine
    - Corticosteroids (dexamethasone)[7]

Evaluation
- Patent airway and effective breathing
- Fever reduction
- Patient/family education
  - Have the child breathe moist air either from a closed bathroom with a hot shower running or from going outside in the cool air
  - Cool mist humidifier in room at night
  - Encourage fluids
  - No smoking around the child
  - Fever management
  - Follow-up with primary care provider 24 hours post ED treatment

Bronchitis

Bronchitis is the inflammation of bronchi and/or trachea due to irritants or viral infection. Acute bronchitis is a cough greater than 5 days and chronic bronchitis is described as a cough longer than 3 months over 2 successive years.

Assessment/Analysis
- Harsh cough, may be productive
- Pleuritic chest pain
- Tachypnea and accessory muscle use
- Possible low grade fever
- History of causes of cough
  - Post nasal drip
  - Gastroesophageal reflux disease
  - Asthma
- Chest x-ray to rule out pneumonia

Intervention
- Medications
  - Expectorants (guaifensin)
  - Antitussives (dextromethorphan)
  - Inhaled β_2 Adrenergic agonists (albuterol)
  - Inhaled anticholinergics (ipratropium bromide)
  - Antipyretics
  - Corticosteroids
  - Antibiotics if bacterial cause is suspected

Evaluation
- Decrease pain and fever
- Patient/family education
  - Smoking cessation
  - Encourage fluids
  - Humidifier use
  - Hand hygiene
  - Explain why or why not antibiotics will be prescribed
  - Influenza vaccination

Epiglottitis

Epiglottitis is the swelling of the tissues just above the vocal cords, which is caused by either viral or bacterial infections. Since the swelling can completely occlude the airway, this illness can be immediately life threatening, particularly in small children.[8] See Figure 3-2.

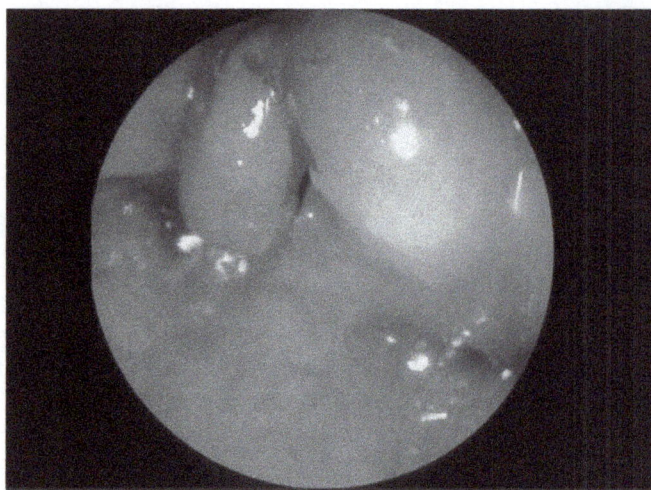

FIGURE 3-2 Swelling of the epiglottis and surrounding tissue that is almost completely obstructing the trachea, as viewed by laryngoscopy

Reproduced with permission from Knoop KJ, Stack LB, Storrow AB, et al: The Atlas of Emergency Medicine, 4th ed. New York: McGraw-Hill Education; 2016: Photo contributor: Department of Otolaryngology, Children's Hopsital Center, Cincinnati, OH.

Assessment/Analysis
- Fever, irritability, and sore throat
- Dyspnea with stridor
- Drooling
- Sitting upright and forward with open mouth breathing
- Muffled voice
- Sore throat
- Vaccination status
- X-ray soft tissue neck

Intervention
- Keep the child calm; allow him or her to be held by the parent or caregiver
- Avoid inserting any objects into the mouth as that may worsen swelling
- Assist with airway securement
  - Anticipate endotracheal intubation
  - Prepare for cricothyrotomy/surgical airway
- Medications
  - Antibiotics

Evaluation
- Patent airway and effective breathing
- Transfer or admission to the critical care unit

Influenza

Influenza is a viral infection affecting the respiratory system, typically in the winter months. High morbidity and mortality rates are experienced, particularly in the very young, elderly, or immunocompromised populations. Treatment is generally supportive for the young, healthy patient.

Assessment/Analysis
- Sudden onset of high fever, chills, myalgias, cough, rhinorrhea, sore throat, and headache
- Influenza vaccination status
- Respiratory distress concurrent or following severe illness
- Chest x-ray to rule out concurrent pneumonia
- Pregnancy test for women of child bearing age

Intervention
- Supplemental oxygen to maintain O_2 saturation to either 95% or patient's known baseline
- Influenza A and B testing
- Antipyretics
- Antivirals (if symptom onset <48 hours)
  - If the patient is pregnant, follow the CDC Guidelines
  - Reduce the duration and severity of symptoms
  - Oseltamivir PO (Tamiflu™)
  - Zanamivir inhaled—Not recommended for patients with asthma or COPD[9]
  - Rehydration with oral or intravenous fluids if there are signs and symptoms of dehydration

Evaluation
- Decrease pain and fever
- Patient/family education
  - Importance of immunization
  - Encourage fluids and rest
  - Fever management
  - Hand hygiene

Pertussis

Highly contagious upper respiratory infection also known as "whooping cough" because of the cough's sound of those who are infected. It is caused by the pathogen *Bordella pertussis*.

Assessment/Analysis
- Sore throat, rhinorrhea, and sneezing
- More common in adolescents and adults as previous immunizations diminish[9]
- 3 stages of Pertussis
  - Catarrhal (1 to 2 weeks): mild cough and upper respiratory infection (URI) symptoms
  - Paroxysmal (week 2): severe, forceful non-productive cough that may induce vomiting
    - "Whooping" sound in children—deep inspiration following coughing[9]
  - Convalescent (2 to 3 months): ongoing cough, which gradually reduces
- Persistent and forceful coughing can cause hernia, pneumothorax, rib fractures, and weight loss[9]
- Laboratory studies
  - Culture of the posterior nasopharynx, polymerase chain reaction (PCR), and serology[9]
- Other possible causes for chronic cough to explore if suspected
  - ACE inhibitor use

- Gastroesophageal reflux disease (GERD)
- Allergies and/or asthma

Intervention
- Fluids to prevent dehydration from coughing
- Good hand washing
- Cough hygiene
- Medications
  - Antibiotics—Do not affect the illness course, but reduces the risk that pertussis will infect others
  - Should provide antibiotics to others with close contact[9]

Evaluation
- Patient/family education
  - Encourage vaccination with Tdap every 10 years

Pneumonia

Pneumonia is an infection in the alveoli and bronchioles of the lung accounting for millions of hospitalizations each year.[17] Community-acquired pneumonia (CAP) is usually caused by Streptococcus *pneumoniae, Haemophilus influenza,* and *Moraxella catarrhalis.* Health care associated pneumonia (HCAP) can effect patients who have had intravenous therapy for other infections or wound care within the past 30 days; patients in nursing or extended care centers; have been hospitalized within the past 90 days or have been receiving renal dialysis. Mortality rates are greater for people over age 65, immunocompromised, or those with comorbidities. It is the sixth leading cause of death for older adults.[10]

Assessment/Analysis
- Cough, dyspnea, fever, and chills
- Chest pain (pleuretic—worse with inspiration)
- Tachypnea and tachycardia
- Thick, purulent, yellow or green sputum
- Auscultation of the lungs reveals coarse crackles or rhonchi
- Hypoxemia
- Weakness or altered mental status, especially in older adults[10]
- Laboratory studies
  - CBC with differential
  - Blood cultures
  - Arterial Blood Gases (ABGs)—See Appendix 3A for interpreting ABGs
  - B-type natriuretic peptide (BNP) to rule out CHF as a differential diagnosis
  - Sputum culture with gram stain
- Chest x-ray—Infiltrate

Intervention
- Supplemental oxygen to maintain O_2 saturation to either 95% or patient's known baseline
- Continuous pulse oximetry
- ECG if accompanying chest pain, cardiac history, older age, or other comorbidities
- Cardiac monitoring
- Fluids oral or intravenous
  - Medications
    - Antibiotics within 4 hours of arrival to the emergency department (ED)
    - Antipyretics
    - Inhaled β_2 adrenergic agonists (albuterol)
    - Glucocorticoids

Evaluation
- Effective breathing
- Reduction in pain and fever
- Older patients often require hospital admission
- Patient/family education
  - Encourage pneumococcal and influenza vaccine
  - Take all antibiotics as prescribed and until gone
  - Encourage fluids and rest
  - Use a cool mist humidifier
  - Antipyretics
  - Encourage expectorants and avoid antitussives unless needed to sleep
  - Hand hygiene

Respiratory Syncytial Virus

Respiratory Syncytial Virus (RSV) is a common cause for respiratory infection in young children, with 90% of children infected by age two. It is the most common cause for bronchiolitis, an inflammatory obstruction of the lower respiratory tract. RSV typically peaks in the winter months (November to April in the northern hemisphere) and can cause severe illness in premature infants less than 6 months, and those with congenital heart defects or lung diseases.[11]

Assessment/Analysis
- Tachypnea and tachycardia
- Low grade fever
- Cough
- Difficulty feeding and irritability (infants)
- Crackles and diffuse wheezing with auscultation
- Retractions and accessory muscle use
- Grunting and nasal flaring in infants
- Signs of dehydration
- Laboratory studies
  - Nasopharyngeal wash for RSV antigen
  - CBC with differential, chemistry, and blood cultures for severe illness
- Chest x-ray
- Concomitant otitis media

Intervention
- Blow by humidified O_2
- IV fluid if signs of dehydration are present

- Differential diagnosis: parainfluenza, rhinovirus, pertussis, and other viral and bacterial infections[11]
- Medications
  - β agonists and anticholinergics
  - Racemic epinephrine
  - Corticosteroids

Evaluation
- Admission should be considered if there is minimal clinical improvement with interventions, risk factors for complications (prematurity, infant less than 6 months, congenital defects), or a concomitant bacterial infection
- Discharge is common for otherwise healthy children who respond to treatment
- Patient/family education
  - Instruct on inhaler or nebulizer use (if indicated)
  - Fever management
  - Hand hygiene
  - Cough hygiene
  - Avoidance of exposure to tobacco or other smoke

Inhalation Injuries

Inhalation of smoke and chemicals causes damage to the cells of the lungs, pulmonary edema, bronchospasm, and atelectasis.[12] More than half of burn patients develop acute respiratory distress syndrome (ARDS). Edema of the upper airway can occur rapidly. Exposure to fire also exposes the patient to noxious chemicals (such as carbon monoxide (CO) and cyanide), which are particularly damaging to the lungs.[12] Inhalation injury is the primary cause of death in burn patients.[13]

Assessment/Analysis
- History of exposure to
  - Heat
  - Smoke
  - Chemicals
- Dyspnea
- Wheezes, rales, and rhonchi
- Indication of airway injury include
  - Facial burns, singed nasal hair, and soot around mouth or nose
  - Hoarseness
  - Extreme anxiety
  - Carbonaceous sputum
  - Stridor
- Headache (most common symptom with CO poisoning)
- Anxiety and agitation
- Altered mental status
- Nausea and vomiting
- Dizziness
- Malaise
- Skin color
  - Pale
  - Cherry red (rare)
- Laboratory studies
  - Carboxyhemoglobin levels
    - Non-smokers <1, smokers 4 to 6%, and significant exposure >10%
  - Arterial blood gas
  - CBC with differential
  - Serum chemistries
  - Urinalysis for myoglobinuria
  - Chest x-ray

Intervention
- Oxygen—Humidified 100% non-rebreather
- SpO_2 monitoring
  - Note: pulse oximeters cannot distinguish between oxyhemoglobin and carboxyhemoglobin, so readings are not reliable indicators of tissue oxygenation[12]
  - If carbon monoxide exposure is suspected, obtain a serum carboxyhemoglobin level
- Establish IV
- Endotracheal intubation immediately if
  - Facial, neck, or perioral burns
  - Respiratory distress
  - Altered mental status
  - Upper airway edema
  - Concerns about ability to maintain airway patency
- Cardiac monitor; 12-lead ECG
- Careful fluid resuscitation to avoid pulmonary edema
- Removal of any contaminated clothing
- Bronchoscopy
- Medications
  - Bronchodilators
- Cyanide poisoning antidote when cyanide poisoning suspected
  - Sodium thiosulfate
  - Hydroxocobalamin
- Hyperbaric oxygen treatment

Evaluation
- Airway patency and effective breathing
- Improvement of vital signs
- Patients at risk for developing respiratory failure should be admitted to the hospital for at least 24 hours for observation of respiratory status
- Reversal of toxicity from exposure

Obstruction

Airway obstruction is a medical emergency with the potential to cause immediate death if not treated. Obstruction can occur in the upper airway (mouth, nasopharynx, or larynx), central airway (trachea or mainstem bronchi), or lower airway (from diseases such as asthma and COPD).[14] See Figure 3-3 for the anatomical reference.

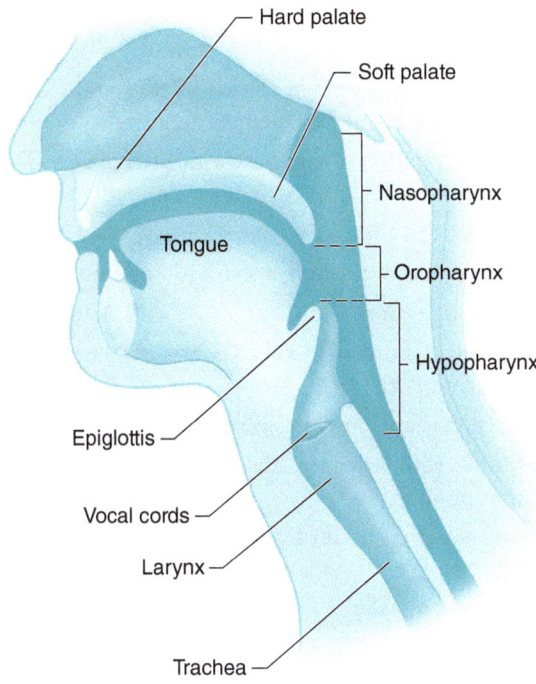

FIGURE 3-3　Diagram of the upper airway
Reproduced with permission from Butterworth J, Mackey DC, Wasnick J: Morgan and Mikhail's Clinical Anesthesiology, 5th ed. New York: McGraw-Hill Education; 2013.

- Anatomical causes
  - Macroglossia (enlarged tongue)
  - Micrognathia (abnormally small jaw)
  - Neck masses
    - Malignancies
    - Enlarged thyroid
    - Large tonsils
    - Large adenoids
- Infectious causes
  - Tonsillitis
  - Peritonsillar abscess
  - Retropharyngeal abscess
  - Pretracheal abscess
  - Epiglottitis
  - Laryngitis/respiratory syncytial virus
  - Ludwig's angina
- Medical causes
  - Cystic fibrosis
  - Angioedema
  - Laryngospasm
    - Airway muscle relaxation
    - Inflammatory
    - Asthma
    - Esophageal foreign bodies
  - Trauma/Tumor
    - Laryngeal trauma
    - Hematoma/masses
    - Smoke inhalation
    - Thermal injuries
    - Foreign body/hemorrhage[15]

Assessment/Analysis
- Extreme anxiety, audible wheezing or stridor, and cough (upper airway)[15]
- Dyspnea, cough, hemoptysis, and wheezing (central airway)[14]
- Tachypnea and tachycardia
- Complete obstruction results in no breathing sounds
- Position patient and open airway; jaw thrust, "sniffing position" by placing a folded towel under the head
- Chest x-ray and/or chest CT

Intervention
- Assist with opening and securing the airway
- Anticipate endotracheal intubation
- Prepare for cricothyrotomy
- Bronchoscopy
- Administration of antibiotics if an infectious agent is suspected

Evaluation
- Patent airway and effective breathing
- Hemodynamic stability

Pleural Effusion

A pleural effusion is the collection of increased fluids in the pleural space (see Figure 3-4). It can be caused by transudates (commonly heart failure), exudates (commonly pneumonia or cancer), empyema, and hemothorax.[16]

Assessment/Analysis
- May be asymptomatic
- Pleuretic pain
- Dyspnea and cough
- Diminished breath sounds
- Dullness to percussion over effusion
- Egophony—Hearing an "ah" sound when the patient makes a long "e" sound, with auscultation. The "ah" sound is heard over areas that have fluid[17]
- Chest x-ray or CT scan of chest
- Lab
  - Examination of pleural fluid

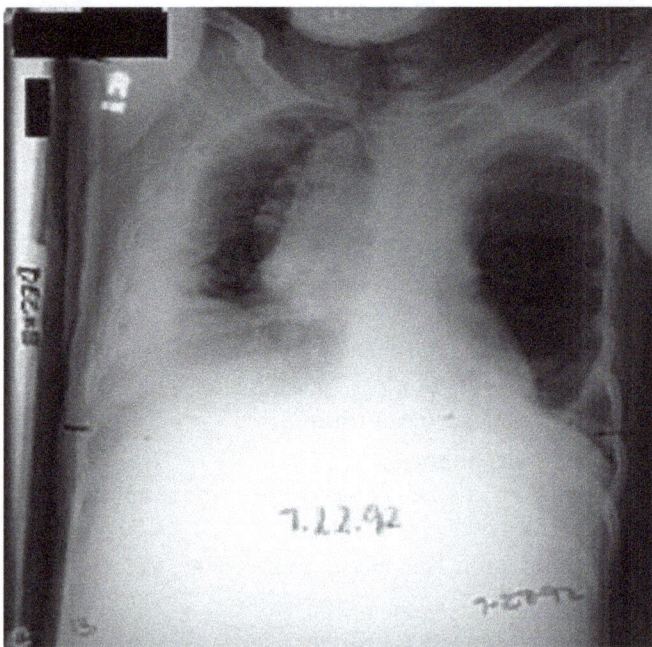

FIGURE 3-4 This chest x-ray illustrates the diminished capacity of the right lung due to pleural effusion
Reproduced with permission from Papadakis MA, McPhee S, Rabow MW: Current Medical Diagnosis & Treatment 2016. New York: McGraw-Hill Education; 2016.

Intervention
- For transudative pleural effusions, treatment should focus on the underlying cause
- Thoracentesis—Either diagnostic or therapeutic if indicated, often with ultrasound assistance

Evaluation
- Effective breathing
- Pain relief
- Chest x-ray post thoracentesis

Pneumothorax

A pneumothorax develops when air enters the pleural space. This can occur as a result of trauma or spontaneously. An iatrogenic pneumothorax occurs as a result of a procedure, such as a subclavian central line insertion. Primary spontaneous pneumothorax occurs in otherwise healthy individuals and typically affects young adult males of tall and thin stature, with an increased risk for smokers. Secondary spontaneous pneumothorax is a result of an underlying lung disease, such as COPD.[18] Recurrence is common.

Assessment/Analysis
- Presenting symptoms relate to the size of the pneumothorax and any underlying disease processes
- Weakness
- Dyspnea, especially on exertion
- Pleuritic chest pain on side of pneumothorax
- Cyanosis
- Past medical history of lung disease or smoking
- History of recent chest trauma
- History of primary spontaneous pneumothorax
- Tachypnea, tachycardia, hypotension, and hypoxemia
- Lung sounds: normal for small pneumothorax but unilaterally diminished or absent when larger
- Chest x-ray/Chest CT
- Laboratory studies
  - ABGs if severe distress
- EKG—Can cause ST changes and T-wave inversion[18]

Intervention
- Significantly diminished or absent breath sounds are an emergency that require immediate attention
  - Needle aspiration of the chest with 14-gauge needle or larger
  - Insertion of a chest tube
- Small pneumothorax may resolve without intervention
  - Needle aspiration
  - Insertion of a catheter using a commercial needle thoracentesis kit
- O_2, IV, cardiac and continuous pulse oximetry
- Chest tube, with water seal, insertion for larger pneumothoraces
  - Water seal prevents air from re-entering thoracic cavity
  - Repeat chest x-ray

Evaluation
- Effective breathing
- Pain relief
- Improvement of vital signs
- Patient with a small pneumothorax may be discharged with close follow up
- Patients with a chest tube will need to be admitted for observation
  - Utilize the mnemonic DOPE to troubleshoot
    - D—Dislodgement: ensure the tube is still in place
    - O—Obstruction: ensure there is no obstruction or kinking of the tube
    - P—Pneumothorax: monitor for signs of tension pneumothorax development or re-expansion pulmonary edema, a rare complication[18]
    - E—Equipment failure: ensure all equipment is properly attached and functioning[19]
  - Monitor chest tube for signs of air leak. Should be expected initially as a result of the pneumothorax. However, a persisting air leak needs to be investigated
  - Patient/family education
    - Referral and close follow up
    - Smoking cessation to decrease risk of recurrence
    - Instruct patient not to fly until pneumothorax is resolved and scuba diving must be avoided

Pulmonary Edema, Noncardiogenic

Noncardiogenic pulmonary edema is the accumulation of fluid in the alveolar space without cardiac etiology. This accumulation leads to decreased lung capacity, dyspnea, and hypoxemia. The major cause of noncardiogenic pulmonary edema is acute respiratory distress syndrome (ARDS). Other causes of pulmonary edema are high altitude pulmonary edema (HAPE), neurogenic, and re-expansion, salicylate toxicity, opioid overdose, pulmonary embolism and viral infections.[12]

High altitude pulmonary edema (HAPE) is the result of rapid accent to high elevations.[19] It develops a few days after arrival due to susceptibility to pressure changes with altitude. Neurological pulmonary edema occurs within a few hours of a neurological insult. Re-expansion pulmonary edema occurs after re-expansion of a collapsed lung. The risk increases with the size of the pneumothorax, but presenting symptoms can be delayed up to a day. In all of these cases, the response is typically self-limiting and responds well to treatment.

Assessment

- History is essential to distinguish cardiogenic from non-cardiogenic source of edema
- Overall assessment is typically normal, especially in the early stages
  - Headaches may be early symptom
- Dyspnea, especially when lying flat or with exertion
- Tachypnea and tachycardia
- Hypoxemia
- Auscultation may be normal, but will progress to diffuse crackles
- Pink frothy sputum
- Hypoxemia that persists despite supplemental oxygen
- Labs to determine severity of illness and identify cause change to
  - ABGs
  - CBC with differential
  - Serum chemistries
  - BNP (to rule out CHF as a differential diagnosis)
  - Lactic Acid
  - Blood cultures X 2 (if infection is suspected)
  - Urinalysis
- Chest x-ray—Observe for diffuse bilateral infiltrates and normal heart size[21]
- Chest CT

Intervention

- Supplemental oxygen to maintain O_2 saturation to either 95% or patient's known baseline
- Intubation and mechanical ventilation
- Establish IV access for crystalloids/medications, as needed
  - Fluid management
- Medications as indicated by the cause of the edema
  - Sedation
  - Antibiotics
  - Dexamethasone
  - DVT prophylaxis
- HAPE Management[19]
  - Oxygen
  - Rest
  - Slow decent from altitude
  - Hyperbaric therapy
  - Medications such as sildenafil

Evaluation

- Airway patency
- Effective breathing
- Hemodynamic stability
- Return to baseline neurological status

Pulmonary Embolus

Pulmonary emboli (PE) are the result of thrombus, air, fat, or amniotic fluid migrating to the pulmonary artery. They are most frequently formed from deep venous thrombosis (DVT), typically from the lower extremities. It can be a life-threatening complication for patients as 10% of patients with an acute PE die within 60 minutes.[22] Patients that experience venous stasis, venous endothelial injury, and hypercoagulability states are at increased risk.

Risk factors include

- ❖ Immobility, long plane or car rides
- ❖ Pressure on the popliteal artery from the edge of a seat during prolonged sitting
- ❖ Pregnancy, contraceptive use, and estrogen therapy
- ❖ Cigarette smoking
- ❖ Genetic predisposition or previous DVT or PE
- ❖ Recent surgery, particularly orthopedic surgery of the lower extremities[21]
- ❖ Trauma, lower extremity fracture, and spinal cord injury
- ❖ Advanced age >60 years

PE leads to vasoconstriction and bronchoconstriction, impaired gas exchange, and an increased vascular resistance. These physiological changes eventually result in a decrease in cardiac output and the development of pulmonary hypertension and right-sided heart failure.

Assessment/Analysis

- Pleuritic chest pain, especially with respiration
- Unexplained sudden onset of dyspnea and tachypnea at rest or exertion
- Tachycardia
- Hypotension possible
- Hypoxemia without CO_2 retention and cyanosis
- Hemoptysis and/or petechia on the chest are possible, but uncommon
- Lung sounds vary: normal, crackles, or pleural rub
- Cough possible

- Past medical history prior PE or DVT, evaluate for risk factors
  - Calf or thigh swelling, redness, edema, and tenderness
  - Laboratory studies
    - CBC with differential
    - Erythrocyte sedimentation rate
  - ABGs—May reveal respiratory alkalosis[22]
    - D-dimer testing
    - Troponins
    - BNP
  - See Appendix 3A for ABG interpretation
- Radiology
  - CXR—Difficult to detect PE
  - CT scan—Preferred
  - Ventilation/perfusion scan (VQ scan)—Highly specific, but takes several hours. Preferred alternative for patients that have contrast allergy or renal insufficiency
- EKG—May show ST or T-wave abnormalities

Intervention
- Supplemental O_2, cardiac and continuous pulse oximetry
- Establish IV access for crystalloids/medications as needed
- Differential diagnosis: pleural effusion, pneumonia, pneumothorax, or pulmonary edema, COPD or asthma exacerbation, CHF, and MI[22]
- Medications
  - Anticoagulants (Depending on bleeding risk)
    - Heparin
    - Low molecular weight heparin (Lovenox™)
    - Direct factor Xa and thrombin inhibitors, for example rivroxaban which is an oral medication
  - Vitamin K antagonist (warfarin)
  - Thrombolytic therapy (unstable patients)
  - Vasopressors to increase blood pressure in unstable patients requiring resuscitation
- Inferior vena cava (IVC) filters for recurrent clotting despite treatment[22]
- Stable patients who may be able to be discharged from the ED
  - No requirement for oxygen
  - No signs of respiratory distress
  - No serious co-morbidities
  - Able to care for themselves
  - No active DVT

Evaluation
- Effective breathing
- Pain relief
- Improvement of vital signs
- Consider admission, particularly those that are hemodynamically unstable, have a large PE, or other comorbidities[23]
- Patient/family education
  - Instruct on use of anticoagulants and risks—Signs of hemorrhagic stroke to observe for
  - Compression stockings
  - Smoking cessation
  - Risk factors to avoid clot formation
    - Stand up and walk around every 2 hours
    - Shift position frequently when seated
    - Drink fluids to keep hydrated
    - Wear loose-fitting clothes
    - Avoid alcohol or medications that can depress one's activity level

Respiratory Distress Syndrome

Acute respiratory distress syndrome (ARDS) encompasses many clinical conditions causing lung injury leading to the rapid onset of non-cardiogenic pulmonary edema and respiratory failure. ARDS can be caused by anything disrupting lung function, such as severe pneumonia, aspiration, drowning, pulmonary emboli, trauma, or inhalation injury. In addition, inflammatory processes from conditions such as sepsis, peritonitis, pancreatitis, burns, and trauma can instigate lung injury leading to ARDS.[21] The lung injury causes inflammation and fluid leakage from the alveoli which leads to flash pulmonary edema. Presenting symptoms are severe and progressive respiratory distress with hypoxemia unresolved with oxygen supplementation. The mortality rate for ARDS can exceed 50%.[21]

Assessment/Analysis
- Sudden onset of severe respiratory distress
  - Dyspnea, tachypnea, and hypoxemia
  - Diaphoresis
  - Cough may or may not be present
  - Cyanosis
- Tachycardia
- Accessory muscle use
- Fine to coarse crackles
- Sputum
- JVD
- Increase in weight gain
- Lower extremity edema
- Laboratory studies for initial management
  - ABGs
  - CBC with differential
  - Serum chemistries
  - BNP (to rule out CHF as a differential diagnosis)
  - Lactic Acid

- Blood culture samples
- Urinalysis
- Chest x-ray—Observe for diffuse bilateral infiltrates and normal heart size[21]

Intervention
- Supplemental oxygen to maintain O_2 saturation to either 95% or patient's known baseline
  - NPPV (BiPAP)
  - Endotracheal and mechanical ventilation
- Continuous SpO_2 measurement and cardiac monitor, consider capnography (see Appendix 3B)
- Hemodynamic monitoring
- Medications
  - Steroids to reduce inflammation
  - Sedation and paralysis to decrease oxygen consumption in the ventilated patient

Evaluation
- Effective breathing
- Improvement of vital signs
- Plan for ICU admission with mechanical ventilation. Survival is improved with mechanical ventilation using tidal volume carefully titrated to protect the lungs from further injury and progression of the syndrome[21]

Tension Pneumothorax

A tension pneumothorax is the result of chest trauma and is life threatening. Blunt trauma can cause rib fractures that penetrate the pleural space, allowing air in on inspiration that cannot escape.[23] The increasing air causes a mediastinal shift away from the affected side, compressing the heart and great vessels. This rapidly leads to obstructive shock and requires immediate intervention.

Assessment/Analysis
- Evidence of chest trauma
- Dyspnea and tachypnea
- Tachycardia, hypotension, and hypoxemia
- Cyanosis
- Diminished or absent lung sounds with hyper-resonance to percussion on affected side
- Crepitus or subcutaneous emphysema on affected side
- Distended neck veins
- Tracheal deviation away from affected side is the hallmark sign
- Chest x-ray/Chest CT
- Laboratory studies
  - ABGs if severe distress
  - CBC
  - Chemistry

Intervention
- Immediate needle decompression
  - Insert 14-gauge needle into the second intercostal space, just above the rib, at the mid-clavicular line. See Figure 3-5
- Airway support with oxygen to maintain O_2 saturation
- Establish IV access for crystalloids/ blood products/ medications as needed

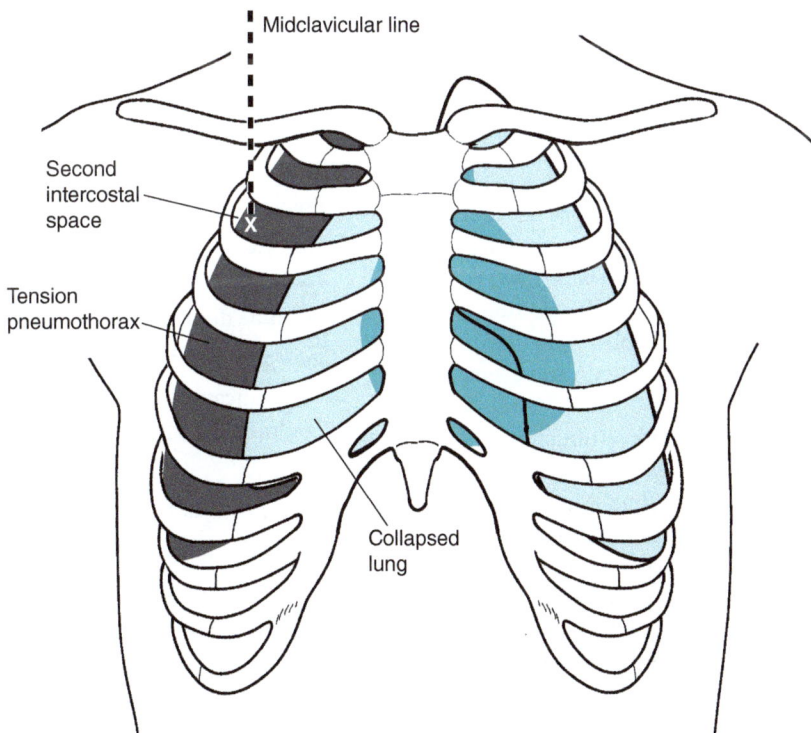

FIGURE 3-5 **Anatomical reference for needle decompression of tension pneumothorax**
Reproduced with permission from Reichman EF: Emergency Medicine Procedures, 2nd ed. New York: McGraw-Hill Education; 2013.

- Cardiac monitoring
- Continuous SpO₂ monitoring
- Chest tube insertion for larger pneumothoraces and after needle decompression has been performed
- Repeat chest x-ray

Evaluation
- Effective breathing
- Improvement of vital signs

Trauma

Thoracic trauma encompasses a wide range of injuries from minor to immediately life threatening and include blunt and penetrating trauma. Blunt trauma damages internal tissues through direct force, compression, or acceleration/deceleration forces.[23] Initial efforts should be performed according to current evidence-based guidelines, with airway and breathing part of the primary survey.[19] Prompt securement of the airway is of primary concern as hypoxemia and hypoventilation are preventable causes of mortality.[23] Life threatening injuries include tension pneumothorax, hemothorax, and flail chest. Any thoracic trauma has the potential to lead to acute respiratory distress syndrome, with the likelihood increasing in correlation to the severity of the injury.

Hemothorax is the collection of blood within the pleural space. It can be caused by penetrating trauma, or blunt trauma that ruptures blood vessels. Significant blood loss in the chest leads to hypovolemia, creates pressure on the great vessels, and diminishes lung capacity.

An open pneumothorax occurs when there is penetration of the chest wall which allows air to enter the pleural space surrounding the lung. Known as a "sucking chest wound," it is critical to immediately cover the wound with a dressing secured on three sides to prevent air from entering, but allowing air to escape. Complete occlusion of the wound can lead to a tension pneumothorax.[23]

A flail chest is the result of two or more fractures per rib in three or more adjacent ribs (see Figure 3-6) that break continuity of the rib section to completely. This "floating rib section" creates a paradoxical movement of the chest wall—inward with inspiration and outward with exhalation. See Figure 3-6.

This increased work of breathing coupled with the injury to the lung itself can lead to respiratory fatigue and eventually failure.[23]

Pulmonary contusion most often results from blunt force to the chest. It causes inflammation and edema to the lung tissue. Reperfusion efforts, such as blood and fluid administration to maintain hemodynamic stability, and can complicate pulmonary contusion as fluid seeps out of the damaged cells.[23]

Tracheobronchial injuries are often the result of rapid deceleration. This injury should be suspected if chest tube insertion fails to evacuate the trapped air. It most often requires surgical repair.

Injuries to the diaphragm are most frequently the result of penetrating trauma, but a rupture of the diaphragm can occur from significant blunt trauma. Smaller diaphragmatic injuries can be hard to detect. In larger injuries, abdominal organs can herniate into the lung space.

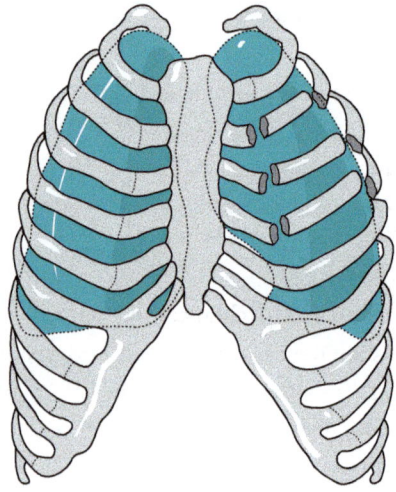

FIGURE 3-6 **Example of flail chest**
Reproduced with permission from Doherty G: CURRENT Diagnosis & Treatment: Surgery, 14th ed. New York: McGraw-Hill Education; 2015.

Rib and clavicle fractures are often uncomplicated injuries. However, displaced fractures can injure the lungs or vessels. Furthermore, fractures may indicate a more significant injury. Fractures to the first three ribs are a sign of high-energy trauma.[23] Because rib fractures are not always apparent on initial imaging; determination for treatment should be made based on clinical impression.

Assessment/Analysis
- Primary survey to include airway assessment
  - Dyspnea and tachypnea
- Vital signs including pulse oximetry
  - Hypotension, tachycardia, and hypoxemia
- Establish IV access for crystalloids/blood products/medications as needed
- Radiology
  - FAST exam (Focused Assessment with Sonography in Trauma)
    - Can be done rapidly at bedside by trained providers
  - Chest x-ray—Mark any penetrating wounds
    - Opacification, especially in later x-rays indicates pulmonary contusion[23]
  - CT Chest
- Laboratory studies
  - CBC with differential
  - Blood type and cross/screen
  - Serum chemistries
  - Coagulation studies
  - Consider toxicology screening including blood alcohol
  - ABGs
- Evaluate mechanism of injury

- Location of pain—Often at site of injury, but can be referred to back or shoulders
- Inspect the chest wall and neck for signs of trauma
  - Abrasions, contusions, and open wounds
  - Paradoxical breathing indicates flail chest
  - Ipsilateral decrease chest wall movement can be the result of a hemothorax or pneumothorax
- Assess for jugular vein distension (JVD)—May not be evident if the patient is hypovolemic
- Auscultate the lungs for diminished or absent breath sounds
  - Bowel sounds in the chest indicate a ruptured diaphragm
- Palpate for tenderness, crepitus, or subcutaneous emphysema
  - Subcutaneous emphysema in the neck or upper chest indicates a tracheobronchial injury and/or pneumothorax
- Percuss the chest—Dullness indicates fluid (such as hemothorax) and hyper-resonance indicates air trapping (pneumothorax)

Intervention
- Open and secure the airway
  - If the patient is in severe distress, assist with endotracheal (ET) intubation
    - Immediately following intubation, auscultate the epigastric area and observe the chest wall for the rise and fall with ventilation. Then auscultate the lungs for bilateral breath sounds
      - Unilateral absence of breath sounds indicate the endotracheal tube could be in the right bronchus[23]
    - Attach an exhaled CO_2 detector and observe for color change. It should change from purple to yellow with exhaled CO_2. Consider capnography (see Appendix 3B)
    - Obtain chest x-ray to verify ET tube placement[19]
  - Other considerations for intubation
    - Multiple injuries
    - Altered mental status
    - Hypovolemic shock
- Elderly patient or chronic lung disease
- Respiratory rate greater than 35 breaths per minute[23]
- Continuous pulse oximetry
- Establish IV access for crystalloid fluids/blood products/medications as needed
- Pain management
- Assist with chest tube insertion for large hemothorax
  - If greater than 1500 mL of blood return initially or greater than 200 mL per hour for 4 hours, patient requires emergency thoracotomy[23]
  - Autotransfusion may be considered

Evaluation
- Patent airway
- Effective breathing
- Improvement of vital signs
- Normothermic temperature
- Stabilization of bleeding
- Patients who suffer from major trauma will require stabilization and transfer to a trauma center
- Patients with significant injury are at risk to develop complications, such as pneumonia, infection, and acute respiratory distress syndrome
- Patients who appear stable may need to be admitted for observation
  - Pulmonary contusions can worsen over the first 24 hours and should be observed
    - Patients with multiple rib fractures have difficulty breathing and coughing due to pain and are at risk for developing pneumonia, particularly the elderly or those with a pre-existing disease[23]
- Patient/family education
  - Encourage deep breathing and cough exercises
  - Signs and symptoms related to need for immediate follow-up care
    - Shortness of breath
    - Altered mental status
    - Increasing pain

Appendix 3A

ABG Interpretation

Normal Range	pH (7.35–7.45)	PaCO$_2$ (35–45 mm Hg)	HCO$_3$ (22–26 mEq/L)	Causes
Respiratory Acidosis	<7.35	>45 mm Hg	Normal or increased with compensation	Ineffective respiration (CO$_2$ retention), airway obstruction
Respiratory Alkalosis	>7.45	<35 mm Hg	Normal or decreased with compensation	Hyperventilation, anxiety, fever
Metabolic Acidosis	<7.35	Normal or decreased with compensation	<22 mEq/L	Salicylate toxicity, kidney failure, sepsis, diabetic ketoacidosis
Metabolic Alkalosis	>7.45	Normal or increased with compensation	>26 mEq/L	Vomiting, ingestion of alkaline medications

Appendix 3B

Capnography

In the acute setting, capnography, or end tidal carbon dioxide (ETCO$_2$) monitoring, is useful to monitor for critical patients or those at risk of airway compromise. It can help to determine:

- Ventilation—How effectively CO$_2$ is being eliminated by the pulmonary system
- Perfusion—How effectively CO$_2$ is being transported through the vascular system
- Metabolism—How effectively CO$_2$ is being produced by cellular metabolism

Capnography allows real time feedback about the patient's ventilatory status. Comparatively, continuous pulse oximetry (SpO$_2$) has a delay in reporting lower levels and the feedback only provides information about the oxygenation level and not the ventilation or perfusion at the cellular level.
CO$_2$ wave form consists of four phases.

- See Figure 3B-1
- Phase 1 represents the beginning of exhalation where the dead space is cleared from the upper airway
- Phase 2 represents the rapid rise in CO$_2$ as air reaches the upper airway
- Phase 3 represents the CO$_2$ concentration reaching a uniform level as exhalation continues. The end tidal CO$_2$ occurs at the end point, when inhalation begins, and is the number that will be displayed on the monitor. Normal values range from 35 to 45 +/− 6%
- Phase 4 Inhalation

> Note: the taller the waveform, the more CO$_2$ is being exhaled. The longer the waveform, the more time it takes to exhale.

- Patients with COPD and asthma exacerbations will have a wave form that appear like a "shark fin" as the CO$_2$ is slow to escape during exhalation due to alveolar trapping

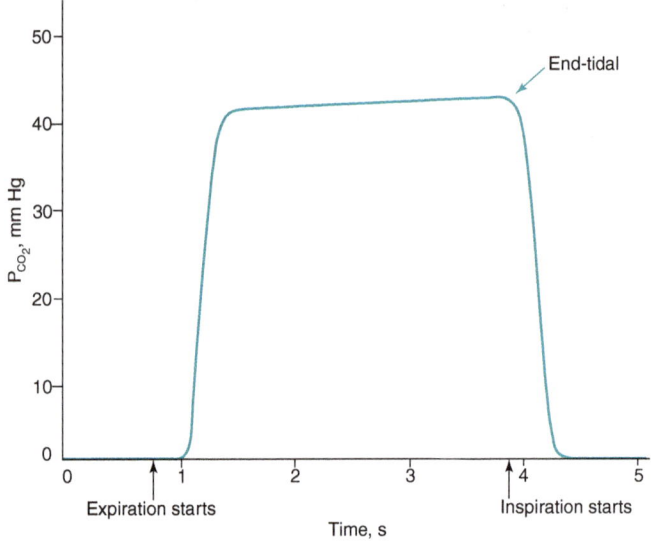

FIGURE 3B-1 **Illustration of a normal capnography wave form**
Reproduced with permission from Levitsky MG: Pulmonary Physiology, 8th ed. New York: McGraw-Hill Education; 2013.

REFERENCES

1. Gutiérrez CE. Pediatric trauma. In: Tintinalli JE, Stapczynski J, Ma O, et al, eds. *Tintinalli's Emergency Medicine: A Comprehensive Study Guide.* 8th ed. New York, NY: McGraw-Hill; 2016.
2. Patterson KC, O'Connor MF, Hall JB, et al. Critical illness in pregnancy. In: Hall JB, Schmidt GA, Kress JP, eds. *Principles of Critical Care.* 4th ed. New York, NY: McGraw-Hill; 2015.
3. Fleischman RJ, Ma O. Trauma in the elderly. In: Tintinalli JE, Stapczynski J, Ma O, et al, eds. *Tintinalli's Emergency Medicine: A Comprehensive Study Guide.* 8th ed. New York, NY: McGraw-Hill; 2016.
4. Marik PE. Aspiration-related pulmonary disorders. In: Grippi MA, Elias JA, Fishman JA, et al, eds. *Fishman's Pulmonary Diseases and Disorders.* 5th ed. New York, NY: McGraw-Hill; 2015.
5. Cydulka RK. Chapter 72. Acute asthma in adults. In: Tintinalli JE, Stapczynski J, Ma O, et al, eds. *Tintinalli's Emergency Medicine: A Comprehensive Study Guide.* 7th ed. New York, NY: McGraw-Hill; 2011.
6. Bates CG, Cydulka RK. Chapter 73. Chronic obstructive pulmonary disease. In: Tintinalli JE, Stapczynski J, Ma O, et al, eds. *Tintinalli's Emergency Medicine: A Comprehensive Study Guide.* 7th ed. New York, NY: McGraw-Hill; 2011.
7. Dolin R. Common viral respiratory infections. In: Kasper D, Fauci A, Hauser S, et al, eds. *Harrison's Principles of Internal Medicine,* 19th ed. New York, NY: McGraw-Hill; 2015.
8. Mittiga MR, Gonzalez del Rey JA, Ruddy RM. Chapter 14. Pediatric conditions. In: Knoop KJ, Stack LB, Storrow AB, et al, eds. *The Atlas of Emergency Medicine.* 3rd ed. New York, NY: McGraw-Hill; 2010.
9. Stern SC, Cifu AS, Altkorn D. Cough, fever, and respiratory infections. In: Stern SC, Cifu AS, Altkorn D, eds. *Symptom to Diagnosis: An Evidence-Based Guide.* 3rd ed. New York, NY: McGraw-Hill; 2014.
10. Emerman CL, Anderson E, Cline DM. Chapter 68. Community-acquired pneumonia, aspiration pneumonia, and noninfectious pulmonary infiltrates. In: Tintinalli JE, Stapczynski J, Ma O, et al, eds. *Tintinalli's Emergency Medicine: A Comprehensive Study Guide.* 7th ed. New York, NY: McGraw-Hill; 2011.
11. Levin MJ, Weinberg A. Infections: viral & rickettsial. In: Hay WW, Jr., Levin MJ, Deterding RR, et al, eds. *CURRENT Diagnosis & Treatment: Pediatrics.* 22th ed. New York, NY: McGraw-Hill; 2013.
12. Schwartzstein RM. Dyspnea. In: Kasper D, Fauci A, Hauser S, et al, eds. *Harrison's Principles of Internal Medicine.* 19th ed. New York, NY: McGraw-Hill; 2015.
13. Drigalla D, Gemmill J. Chapter 45. Burns & smoke inhalation. In: Stone C, Humphries RL, eds. *CURRENT Diagnosis & Treatment Emergency Medicine.* 7th ed. New York, NY: McGraw-Hill; 2011.
14. Won C, Michaud G, Kryger MH. Upper airway obstruction in adults. In: Grippi MA, Elias JA, Fishman JA, et al, eds. *Fishman's Pulmonary Diseases and Disorders.* 5th ed. New York, NY: McGraw-Hill; 2015.
15. Roman A. Chapter 28. Noninvasive airway management. In: Tintinalli JE, Stapczynski J, Ma O, et al, eds. *Tintinalli's Emergency Medicine: A Comprehensive Study Guide.* 7th ed. New York, NY: McGraw-Hill; 2011.
16. Chesnutt MS, Prendergast TJ. Pulmonary disorders. In: Papadakis MA, McPhee SJ, Rabow MW, eds. *Current Medical Diagnosis & Treatment 2016.* New York, NY: McGraw-Hill; 2016. http://accessmedicine.mhmedical.com/content.aspx?bookid=1585&Sectionid=96303413. Accessed November 22, 2015.
17. Kritek P, Choi A. Approach to the patient with disease of the respiratory system. In: Kasper D, Fauci A, Hauser S, et al, eds. *Harrison's Principles of Internal Medicine.* 19th ed. New York, NY: McGraw-Hill; 2015.
18. Humphries RL, Young W, Jr. Chapter 71. Spontaneous and iatrogenic pneumothorax. In: Tintinalli JE, Stapczynski J, Ma O, et al, eds. *Tintinalli's Emergency Medicine: A Comprehensive Study Guide.* 7th ed. New York, NY: McGraw-Hill; 2011.
19. Emergency Nurses Association. Chapter 11. Thoracic and neck trauma. In: *Trauma Nursing Core Course (TNCC): Provider Manual.* 7th ed. Des Plaines, IL: Emergency Nurses Association; 2007:137–150.
20. Jerrard, D. Noncardiogenic pulmonary edema. In: Schaider JJ, Barkin RM, Wolfe RE, et al, eds. *Rosen & Barkin's 5–Minute Emergency Medicine Consult.* 4th ed. Philadelphia, PA: Lippincott Williams & Wilkins; 2011.
21. Matuschak GM, Lechner AJ. Acute lung injury and the acute respiratory distress syndrome: pathophysiology and treatment. In: Lechner AJ, Matuschak GM, Brink DS, eds. *Respiratory: An Integrated Approach to Disease.* New York, NY: McGraw-Hill; 2015.
22. Sachdeva A, Matuschak GM. Pulmonary embolism. In: Lechner AJ, Matuschak GM, Brink DS, eds. *Respiratory: An Integrated Approach to Disease.* New York, NY: McGraw-Hill; 2015.
23. Brunett PH, Yarris LM, Cevik A. Chapter 258. Pulmonary trauma. In: Tintinalli JE, Stapczynski J, Ma O, et al, eds. *Tintinalli's Emergency Medicine: A Comprehensive Study Guide.* 7th ed. New York, NY: McGraw-Hill; 2011.

Practice Questions

Question	Rationale
1. A 2-year-old patient presents to the emergency department (ED) with a fever, barky cough, stridor, and retractions. Initially, the most beneficial treatment is a. A nebulizer with β_2 adrenergic agonists and anticholinergic b. Cool, humidified oxygen c. An antipyretic d. High flow oxygen	*Answer: b* This child is showing symptoms of croup causing respiratory distress. Oxygen is needed to manage the hypoxemia. Cool, humidified oxygen keeps the airway moist and prevents drying, which can help symptoms. In this case, a nebulizer with racemic epinephrine would be the first line drug along with corticosteroids. An antipyretic will help lower the fever, but it is not the initial intervention.
2. A 62-year-old female is in the ED for shortness of breath and has vital signs of P-114; R-28; BP-96/54; SpO_2-89% on room air, which increases to 93% on 2 liters oxygen by nasal cannula. ABG results are returned with a pH of 7.47, $PaCO_2$ of 32 mm Hg, HCO_3 of 24 mEq/liter. What do these results indicate? a. Metabolic alkalosis b. Respiratory acidosis c. Respiratory alkalosis d. Her ABGs are within normal limits	*Answer: c* The patient's pH is elevated, the $PaCO_2$ is low, and the HCO_3 is normal. The elevated pH indicates alkalosis. The decreased $PaCO_2$ and normal HCO_3 level indicates a respiratory component that is not being compensated for. These results, combined with the assessment, indicate the patient is in non-compensated respiratory alkalosis. Respiratory alkalosis can result from any condition causing hyperventilation, including fever and sepsis.
3. A 22-year-old male arrives to the ED following an all terrain vehicle (ATV) accident. What initial assessment finding requires the most immediate intervention? a. Abrasions across the chest b. Respiratory rate of 26 c. Complaints of pain to palpation across lower rib border d. Trachea deviated to the left	*Answer: d* A deviated trachea indicates a tension pneumothorax. This requires immediate intervention with needle decompression to prevent further respiratory compromise. Abrasions to the chest indicate trauma, as would pain to the lower rib border, but those findings alone do not require the most immediate intervention. Tachypnea can indicate chest injury, but can also be elevated due to pain or anxiety.
4. Your patient has been diagnosed with pulmonary edema. He is alert and talking, but has difficulty maintaining a SpO_2 greater than 90% with oxygen by nasal cannula. The most effective airway management for this patient is a. Non-rebreather mask at 10 LPM b. NPPV (BiPAP) c. Bag mask device with 100% oxygen d. Endotracheal intubation and mechanical ventilation	*Answer: b* Although oxygen support is necessary, a non-rebreather mask will not maintain positive pressure, which is necessary to prevent respiratory fatigue and possible failure. Non-invasive pressure support ventilation, such as BiPAP maintains positive pressure in the airway, which prevents the alveoli from collapsing, increases patient comfort, and may prevent acute respiratory failure. A bag-valve mask device, followed by endotracheal intubation and mechanical ventilation would be indicated if the patient demonstrated signs of progressive hypoxemia, such as altered mental status.

Question	Rationale

5. The emergency nurse knows that discharge instructions for a patient with asthma is effective when he states
  a. "I should return to the ED if I need a refill of my inhaler"
  b. "I will get better results from the medicine if I use a spacer with my inhaler"
  c. "I should avoid exercise to prevent asthma attacks"
  d. "It would help if I switched to light cigarettes"
	Answer: b
	The use of a spacer improves the amount of medication that reaches the lungs. Patients should follow up with their primary physician to improve continuity of care, and coordinate any necessary referrals. Exercise is important to strengthen the lungs and can actually reduce the frequency of attacks. Smoking of any kind is not recommended as it can instigate asthma attacks and leads to irreversible lung damage.

6. When using egophony as part of your assessment, an "ah" sound is heard through auscultation, at the left lower lung field, this is indicative of
  a. Inhalation injury
  b. Pulmonary emboli
  c. Pleural effusion
  d. Tension pneumothorax
	Answer: c
	Egophony is noted over areas where fluids are present, as with a pleural effusion. It is not noted over areas of air, such as with tension pneumothorax. Egophony would not be noted with inhalation injuries or pulmonary emboli as independent clinical findings.

7. A 30-year-old female patient presents to the emergency department with complaints of increasing shortness of breath over the last few days and pain over the right side of her chest. In assessing for potential risk factors for pulmonary embolus, all would be of concern *except*
  a. She takes birth control pills
  b. She is a marathon runner
  c. She smokes one pack of cigarettes per day
  d. She reports recent travel to Fiji
	Answer: b
	Frequent and regular exercise is not a risk factor for pulmonary emboli. Immobility from sedentary behaviors, long travel, or illness does increase the risk due to venous stasis which allows for clot formation. Cigarette smoking damages the vascular lining, which can promote clot formation. Birth control pills elevate hormone levels, which can increase coagulability.

8. Which of the following patients is NOT at risk for aspiration?
  a. A 72-year-old male with increasing weakness and confusion
  b. A 24-year-old trauma victim that is intubated
  c. A 42-year-old female with a history of Multiple Sclerosis
  d. A 58-year-old male with history of Bell's Palsy
	Answer: d
	Although symptoms mimic those of a TIA or stroke, Bell's Palsy affects the seventh cranial nerve and is limited to the face, therefore does not impair the swallowing mechanism. Advanced age, neurological disorders, such as Multiple Sclerosis, and endotracheal intubation are risk factors for aspiration.

9. A 63-year-old patient has evidence of pulmonary edema. Which of the following findings would indicate this pulmonary edema is *noncardiogenic* in nature?
  a. Chest x-ray shows normal heart size
  b. BNP level is 650 pg/mL
  c. Bilateral basilar crackles are heard on auscultation
  d. Shortness of breath increases when laying down
	Answer: a
	Cardiogenic pulmonary edema is the result of heart failure; therefore, the finding on x-ray that the heart size is normal would indicate heart failure is not likely the cause. A BNP level of 650 pg/mL is elevated and would indicate heart failure. Assessment findings on patient presentation and auscultation are similar for cardiogenic and noncardiogenic causes of pulmonary edema. For that reason, it is important to do lab and imaging tests to differentiate.

Question	Rationale
10. An emergency nurse knows it is important to never fully occlude an open pneumothorax or clamp a chest tube because occlusion would a. Put the patient at increased risk for infection b. Cause a pleural effusion c. Cause a tension pneumothorax d. Irritate the diaphragm	*Answer: c* Occlusion of a chest wound or clamping the chest tube prevents air and/or fluid from escaping the chest, which can lead to a tension pneumothorax. Although a chest tube can predispose the patient to an infection, such as an empyema, clamping it or occluding a wound would not increase that risk, nor irritate the diaphragm. A pleural effusion would not result from these actions either.
11. Pertussis is most commonly found in the following age group a. Less than 2 years b. 2 years to 5 years c. 5 years to 15 years d. Over 15 years	*Answer: d* Pertussis is most likely to affect adolescents and adults as the vaccination immunity diminishes. The Tdap vaccine protects against tetanus and pertussis and should be given to adults at least every 10 years to protect against illness.
12. A 72-year-old female presents to the ED with increasing weakness and confusion. She has a low grade fever, appears in mild respiratory distress with a room air SPO_2 of 94%. She is coughing up sputum that is thick and yellow in color. What is the most likely diagnosis? a. Pneumonia b. COPD c. Pulmonary edema d. Bronchitis	*Answer: a* The patient most likely has pneumonia based on the presenting symptoms. Pneumonia causes fever, chills, and productive cough with yellow, green, or purulent sputum. Elderly patients can present with weakness or confusion as a result of the underlying infection. COPD and pulmonary edema do not present with fever unless there is an underlying infection, which may be pneumonia. Bronchitis is possible, but the patient is showing signs of an infectious process more consistent with pneumonia.
13. Pulsus paradoxus may be noted on a patient with a. Pulmonary contusion b. Flail chest c. Severe asthma exacerbation d. Pneumothorax	*Answer: c* Pulsus paradoxus is a condition in which the systolic blood pressure changes significantly on inspiration. There are several cardiac etiologies of this phenomenon. Respiratory etiologies include severe asthma and COPD exacerbation. This phenomenon is observed when the systolic BP decreases greater than 20 mg Hg during expiration.
14. All of the following physical assessment findings are common with COPD *except* a. Leaning forward on outstretched arms b. Decreased resonance to percussion over the chest c. Accessory muscle use of neck and shoulders d. Barrel shaped chest	*Answer: b* Physical assessment finding for patients with COPD commonly include sitting in positions to decrease dyspnea, accessory muscle use, pursed lip breathing, barrel-shaped chest, and prolonged expiration. Hypoxemia and dyspnea worsening with exertion is expected with COPD. Decreased resonance to percussion over the chest would be a finding consistent with fluid in the lungs, not specific to COPD.

Question	Rationale

15. When considering airway options for patients with COPD, Noninvasive positive pressure ventilation (NPPV) such as BiPAP is beneficial because it
    a. Can be used on patients that are unconscious
    b. Creates negative pressure within the lungs
    c. Is easily tolerated by most patients
    d. Can reduce the need for intubation and improve outcomes
	Answer: d
	NPPV, such as BiPAP maintains continuous positive pressure in to maintain open alveoli. It should only be used on alert and cooperative patients. The tight mask seal can be uncomfortable and is not always tolerated by patients. However, it can improve outcomes by reducing the need for intubation and decrease duration of hospitalization.[3]

16. Treatments for RSV include all of the following *except*
    a. Racemic epinephrine
    b. Antibiotic administration
    c. Corticosteroids
    d. β_2 agonists and anticholinergics
	Answer: b
	RSV is a virus; therefore antibiotics would not be indicated. Treatment for RSV includes racemic epinephrine, β agonists, and anticholinergics to open the bronchioles. Corticosteroids are used to reduce pulmonary inflammation in children over 24 months of age.

17. A 46-year-old patient is diagnosed with pertussis and is being discharged. Further teaching is needed when the patient states
    a. "I will need to make sure my family also takes the prescribed antibiotics"
    b. "I should get the Tdap vaccination every 10 years"
    c. "The antibiotics will help me to feel better in a few days"
    d. "I can expect to have this cough for 2 to 3 months"
	Answer: c
	Pertussis is an infection that more often affects adolescents and adults as immunization duration decreases. Antibiotic use does not shorten the course of the illness, which typically lasts 2 to 3 months, but will reduce the spread to others. Those in close contact should also complete a course of antibiotics to reduce the spread of the illness. It is important to teach patients the importance of vaccination every 10 years to ensure immunity.

18. A 72-year-old patient presents with complaints of a mild fever and productive cough. A chest x-ray reveals a lower left infiltrate. After addressing the ABCs, a priority intervention with this patient is
    a. Prepare for administration of antibiotics
    b. Obtain an ECG
    c. Obtain ABGs
    d. Prepare the patient for admission
	Answer: a
	This patient has a lower left pneumonia based on the chest x-ray interpretation. A priority intervention is to prepare for administration of antibiotics, which must be done within 4 hours of arrival to the ED. An ECG and ABGs may be warranted based on patient presentation and comorbidities, but are not a generally a priority for patients with pneumonia. Elderly patients often do require admission, but it is important to ensure antibiotics are started first.

19. A 22-year-old patient was rescued from a house fire. Upon arrival to the ED, the patient is alert and talking. Which assessment findings may indicate the need for immediate endotracheal intubation?
    a. SpO_2 of 88% on room air
    b. Carboxyhemoglobin level of 6%
    c. Second degree burns noted to the anterior neck
    d. Wheezing and crackles noted in all lung fields
	Answer: c
	Endotracheal intubation should be immediately considered if the patient has facial, neck, or perioral burns. A decreased SpO_2 of 88% should be closely monitored, but without other signs of respiratory distress, this finding alone would not indicate the need for immediate endotracheal intubation. Carboxyhemoglobin levels of 6% may be normal in a patient that is a smoker. A patient with significant carbon monoxide exposure would have levels greater than 10%. Wheezing and crackles may be present in a patient with exposure to smoke and should be monitored for other signs of respiratory distress.

Question	Rationale
20. A 64-year-old female patient presents with a significantly swollen tongue and lips. She is extremely anxious and is drooling. The emergency nurse positions the patient and opens the airway with a jaw thrust. The priority intervention for this patient is a. Insert an oral airway b. Prepare for cricothyrotomy c. Apply oxygen via non-rebreather mask d. Obtain SpO$_2$ measurement	*Answer: b* The patient is showing symptoms of airway obstruction associated with angioedema. Insertion of an oral airway is dangerous as it could cause further swelling and completely obstruct the airway. It is important to anticipate immediate intubation and prepare for cricothyrotomy as insertion of an endotracheal tube may not be possible. Patients with an airway obstruction often have extreme anxiety and placement of a non-rebreather mask may worsen it. Although SpO$_2$ measurement is helpful and may be done simultaneously with other interventions, the priority is airway securement.
21. Which of the following tests is NOT helpful in distinguishing non-cardiogenic pulmonary edema from congestive heart failure (CHF)? a. ABGs b. Chest x-ray c. CT chest d. BNP	*Answer: a* Presentation of patients with pulmonary edema is similar whether it is cardiogenic or non-cardiogenic in nature. Radiological and laboratory tests help to distinguish the two. Patients with cardiogenic pulmonary edema, such as CHF will show a widened mediastinum on a chest x-ray and a CT chest. In addition, they will show an elevated BNP level. ABGs are not reliable to distinguish as they may be abnormal due to either cause.
22. A 35-year-old female presents with dyspnea and tachycardia. Her history includes use of birth control pills, cigarette smoking, and a severe iodine allergy. In addition to a D-dimer test, the nurse would anticipate an order for a. A chest x-ray b. An ECG c. A CT scan d. A ventilation/perfusion scan	*Answer: d* This patient has risk factors for a pulmonary embolus (PE), which are difficult to diagnose with a chest x-ray. An ECG may be ordered to rule out other causes for her symptoms, but would not definitively diagnose a PE. A CT scan is the most reliable test, but is contraindicated because of her iodine allergy. In this case, a ventilation/perfusion scan would be the preferred alternative.
23. A 32-year-old male patient involved in a motorcycle crash presents with multiple injuries. He was wearing a helmet and does not appear to have any head or facial trauma. He is dyspneic, tachycardic, and tachypneic with road rash and redness to his anterior chest. Close inspection reveals tracheal deviation to the left with diminished lung sounds on the right. The priority intervention is to a. Perform immediate needle decompression to the right 2nd intercostal space b. Prepare for immediate endotracheal intubation c. Perform immediate needle decompression to the left 2nd intercostal space d. Anticipate chest tube insertion	*Answer: a* Tracheal deviation is the hallmark sign of a tension pneumothorax. It is identified by absent or diminished lung sounds on the affected side and tracheal deviation away from the affected side. Immediate needle decompression is the primary intervention. In this case, the assessment indicates the tension pneumothorax is on the right side. Once needle decompression is successful, additional interventions would include preparing for endotracheal intubation and chest tube insertion.

Question	Rationale
24. A focused assessment with sonography in trauma (FAST) exam is the preferred radiological exam in trauma because it a. Requires minimal training to perform b. Can be done quickly at bedside to identify internal trauma c. Is more definitive than other radiological exams d. Is less expensive than other tests	*Answer: b* A FAST exam can be performed at the bedside and requires a skilled provider to perform the test. This ultrasound screening test is helpful in identifying blood (internal bleeding), such as a hemothorax. Although there are other radiological exams that provide clearer pictures, such as CT. The FAST exam is beneficial as it can be done rapidly and does not require moving the patient to another location.
25. A 25-year-old female patient was involved in a head on collision with significant chest wall trauma. A tracheobronchial injury is suspected when a. There is a contusion noted to the upper chest b. The patient is unable to speak c. The chest tube insertion fails to evacuate subcutaneous emphysema d. The patient has increasing dyspnea	*Answer: c* Tracheobronchial injuries are often the result of rapid deceleration. They should be suspected when chest tube insertion fails to evacuate subcutaneous emphysema. Contusions to the chest wall and increasing dyspnea can be indicative of many injuries and is therefore not specific to tracheobronchial injuries. The inability to speak would be indicative of a laryngeal injury.
26. A chest tube is placed in a patient to evaluate blood from a hemothorax following a significant chest trauma. An emergency thoracotomy is indicated when a. There is greater than 750 mL of initial blood return b. There is no blood return, but increasing dyspnea c. Blood return is greater than 200 mL per hour for 4 hours d. A second chest tube needs to be placed	*Answer: c* Emergency thoracotomy would not be required for an initial blood return of 750 mL. It is required if chest tube insertion results in greater than 1500 mL of blood return initially, or greater than 200 mL per hour for 4 consecutive hours. Autotransfusion-returning the shed blood, may be another intervention to consider. If there is no blood return, placement of the chest tube should be questioned, especially with increasing dyspnea, but an emergency thoracotomy would not be warranted. The need for a second chest tube, particularly if it is on the opposite side, does not require immediate thoracotomy unless there is significant blood loss.
27. Which of the following findings would be of concern immediately following endotracheal intubation? a. The color on the exhaled CO_2 indicator is yellow b. Upon auscultation, sounds are heard over the epigastrium c. Bilateral chest rise and fall is noted with ventilation d. Chest x-ray shows the tip of the endotracheal tube just above the right main bronchus	*Answer: b* Auscultation of the epigastrium should be performed immediately following endotracheal intubation. Sounds heard over the epigastrium with the absence of chest rise and fall indicates intubation of the esophagus. The next step should be auscultation of the lungs, with bilateral breath sounds indicating proper placement. Evaluation of the color on the CO_2 indicator should reveal a change from purple to yellow. Finally, a chest x-ray should be performed to confirm placement of the endotracheal tube. Because the right main bronchus is superior to the left, it is more common to enter. This would be indicated by diminished lung sounds on the left. To resolve, gently pull pack on the endotracheal tube so it rests just above the right main bronchus.

Question	Rationale
28. A patient suffered severe abdominal and chest wall trauma. During the initial assessment, abdominal sounds are auscultated in the lower left chest. The nurse suspects the patient has a. A ruptured diaphragm b. A tension pneumothorax c. A flail chest d. Hyper-resonant abdominal sounds	*Answer: a* A ruptured diaphragm is more likely to occur on the left side of the chest as there are not solid organs (such as the liver) to protect it from blunt or penetrating force. When this occurs, the intestines herniate into the chest cavity, displacing the lungs. Therefore, abdominal sounds may be heard. This phenomenon will not occur with a tension pneumothorax or flail chest.
29. What should be done expediently in intubated patients to prevent aspiration? a. Obtaining a chest x-ray b. Elevating the head of the bed c. Gastric tube placement d. Providing IV sedation	*Answer: c* Gastric tube placement should be performed immediately following endotracheal intubation to decompress the stomach and reduce the risk of aspiration. A chest X-ray is helpful in confirming tube placement, but will not reduce the risk of aspiration. Elevating the head of the bed is helpful to reduce aspiration and ventilator-associated pneumonia (VAP), but can be performed prior to intubation. Sedating intubated patients helps to reduce the risk of dislodgement and discomfort to the patient.
30. Which of the following findings indicate a patient with an asthma exacerbation is not improving? a. Peak flow levels are 75% of predicted b. Lung sounds are diminished throughout and without wheezing c. There is audible end expiratory wheezing noted d. SpO_2 measurements have improved	*Answer: b* Lack of wheezing with diminished breath sounds indicates severe obstruction of air flow and requires immediate intervention. Evaluations that show improvement of symptoms include an improved peak flow greater than 70% of predicted, improvement of SpO_2 measurements, and a transition from wheezing on inspiration and expiration to end expiration only.
31. A patient with angioedema related to smoke inhalation has the following ABG values pH 7.35, CO_2 53, HCO_3 28. These values show a. Compensated respiratory acidosis b. Uncompensated respiratory acidosis c. Compensated respiratory alkalosis d. Uncompensated respiratory alkalosis	*Answer: a* The patient has a pH on the low end of normal with an elevated CO_2, indicating respiratory acidosis. The elevated HCO_3 indicates the body is compensating, otherwise the pH would be even lower. It is helpful to remember that CO_2 is an acid and HCO_3 is an alkaline. The body uses these to balance the pH. If the CO_2 gets to high or the HCO_3 is too low, the pH drops. If the CO_2 gets too low or the HCO_3 gets too high, the pH increases.
32. A patient with extreme anxiety and hyperventilation has the following ABG values pH 7.48, CO_2 27, HCO_3 25. These values show a. Compensated respiratory acidosis b. Uncompensated respiratory acidosis c. Compensated respiratory alkalosis d. Uncompensated respiratory alkalosis	*Answer: d* The patient has an elevated pH and a decreased CO_2, which indicates respiratory alkalosis. The HCO_3 is within normal range, so the body is not compensating.

Question	Rationale
33. Patient teaching for patients with COPD should include all of the following *except* a. Encourage adequate fluid intake b. Limit the use of antihistamines, antitussives, and decongestants c. Avoid exercise as it may exacerbate symptoms d. Encourage small, frequent meals	*Answer: c* It is important to encourage exercise as it helps to increase energy and decrease shortness of breath. COPD patients should drink plenty of fluids to help thin secretions; limit the use of medications that have a dehydrating effect; and eat small meals frequently to minimize abdominal distension that can reduce lung capacity.
34. Which of the following types of shock can occur from a tension pneumothorax? a. Hypovolemic b. Cardiogenic c. Distributive d. Obstructive	*Answer: d* Tension pneumothorax causes a mediastinal shift away from the affected side. This compresses the heart and great vessels decreasing cardiac output. Despite the cardiac implications, it is considered obstructive shock as the cause of origin is non-cardiac. Hypovolemic shock is caused by excessive blood or fluid loss; cardiogenic shock is caused by decreased cardiac function/failure related to cardiac injury/illness; distributive shock is caused by ineffective vascular tone such as with anaphylaxis or sepsis.
35. A patient with respiratory distress is placed on capnography. The following wave forms would be anticipated with COPD? a. Flat and extended b. Tall and narrow c. "Shark fin" shaped d. Curved	*Answer: c* Patients with COPD and asthma exacerbations will have a wave form that appear like a "shark fin" as the CO_2 is slow to escape during exhalation due to alveolar trapping. This waveform usually correlates with a higher CO_2 level. ABG assessment is a good correlation tool with capnography. A flat and wider waveform may indicate little ventilation and perfusion occurring (lower CO_2 level). Other abnormal waveforms require assessing the patient's breathing pattern, rate, and depth of respirations. If the patient is mechanically ventilated or receiving supplemental oxygen, assuring that the tubing and circuitry are connected and working properly.
36. The emergency nurse knows the patient understands discharge homecare instructions for treatment and monitoring of a small (<10%) pneumothorax when the patient states a. "I'm glad I can go home; I am flying to Hawaii in two days" b. "I'm glad I can keep practicing my snorkeling in the local pool" c. "I need to come back in two days to have a tube placed in the side of my chest" d. "If I cut back on my smoking, this will never happen again"	*Answer: b* Patients discharged with a small pneumothorax should be counseled not to fly or dive but surface snorkeling will be safe as long as the patient is warned not to free dive while snorkeling. The patient would only require chest tube if the pneumothorax increases in size and the patient starts having symptoms of shortness of breath. Smoking will increase risk but reduction will not eliminate risk of recurrence.

Question	Rationale
37. A 34-year-old male being treated for an acute asthma exacerbation is showing improvement after treatment. However, he is tachycardic and complaining of dry mouth. His pupils appear dilated. This is likely a side effect of a. Albuterol b. Prednisone c. Magnesium sulfate d. Atropine sulfate	*Answer: d* Atropine sulfate is an anticholinergic, a parasympatholytic causing dilated pupils, decreased salivation, and tachycardia. Anticholinergics also dilate the bronchi and stimulate the release of epinephrine and norepinpherine, which is why medications such as atropine may beneficial in reactive airway diseases. Albuterol is a β_2 adrenergic agonist, a sympathomimetic that causes skeletal muscle tremors, anxiety, tachycardia, headache, palpitations, and hypertension. Prednisone can cause hyperglycemia, and magnesium sulfate can cause irregular heartbeat, hypotension, or muscle weakness.

Neurologic Emergencies

Edward Hunt, BS, RN, CEN

There is no system in the human body that can function without neurological stimulation and feedback. Neurological emergencies can present in many different ways. Insult to neurological function can be subtle or profound, chronic or acute. For the purposes of review, it is important to understand the general neurological concepts, as well as effects of chronic disease, acute infection and injury—including trauma—on the peripheral and central nervous system.

General Neurological Concepts

The primary neurological assessment begins with the level of consciousness using the AVPU scale.

Alert: are their eyes open?
Verbal: do they respond only to verbal stimuli?
Painful: do they respond only to painful stimuli?
Unresponsive: are they unresponsive?

If the patient is alert, are they oriented? Do they know the date; where they are; what day or month it is; the events that led to their ED visit? Alert and Oriented to (1) Person, (2) Place, (3) Time, and (4) Events would be considered A&Ox4. Orientation deteriorates in an orderly fashion with events being the first to be lost.

The **Glasgow Coma Scale** (GCS) is a tool for objectively assessing and measuring neurological responses and can have predictive value in the presence of an actual or suspected neurological insult. The three best eye opening, verbal, and motor responses are scored according to the level of response. Originally developed to assess head trauma, the GCS is now frequently applied as an effective neurological assessment tool. See Table 4-1.

A GCS of less than 8 is considered "**severe**"; between 9 to 12 is considered "**moderate**" and greater than 13 "**minor**."

Remember:

A patient who is alert with no deficits scores 15

A patient scoring 8 or less is considered comatose (less than 8: intubate)

A totally unresponsive patient scores a 3 (the lowest possible score)

Change in the **level of consciousness** is the first sign in neurological deterioration.

Assess the patient for motor and sensory function and any weakness or altered sensation. If the patient's consciousness does not allow cooperation with the exam, use painful stimuli to assess the patient's reaction.

- **Localizing pain:** reaching toward the painful stimulus
- **Withdrawal:** moving away from the painful stimulus
- **Decorticate posturing:** abnormal posture with the arms wrists and fingers flexed, legs fully extended and internally rotated, and plantar flexion of the feet
- **Decerebrate posturing:** abnormal extension with the arms extended and hands pronated outward
- **Flaccid:** no motor response

Deep tendon reflexes may also be used to examine neurological status. They should be assessed and compared bilaterally. Grade 0 is no response, 2+ is considered normal, and 4+ is hyperactive.

TABLE 4-1 **Glasgow Coma Score**

Eye Opening	Verbal Response	Best Motor Response
Spontaneous = 4	Alert and Oriented = 5	Obeys Commands = 6
To Speech = 3	Confused/Disoriented = 4	Moves to Localize Pain = 5
To Pain = 2	Inappropriate Words = 3	Withdraws from Pain = 4
No Response = 1	Incomprehensible sounds = 2	Abnormal Flexion = 3
	No Response = 1	Abnormal Extension = 2
		No Response = 1

Terms to know:

- **Paresis**—A weakness to an area of the body (i.e., hemiparesis)
- **Plegia**—Indicates paralysis to an area of the body (i.e. paraplegic)
- **Ipsilateral**—Same side
- **Contralateral**—Opposite side
- **Decorticate posturing**—Hands turned in toward the "core" of the body
- **Decerebrate**—Hands extended away from body
- **Grasp reflex**—Patient grasps when the palm is stimulated
- **Babinski reflex**—Great toe extends when the lateral aspect of the foot is stroked

Cranial Nerves

Twelve pairs of nerves emerge from the bottom (ventral) portion of the brain above the spinal cord. See Figure 4-1 and Table 4-2. These cranial nerves are important for sensory and motor functions particularly in the head and neck area.[1]

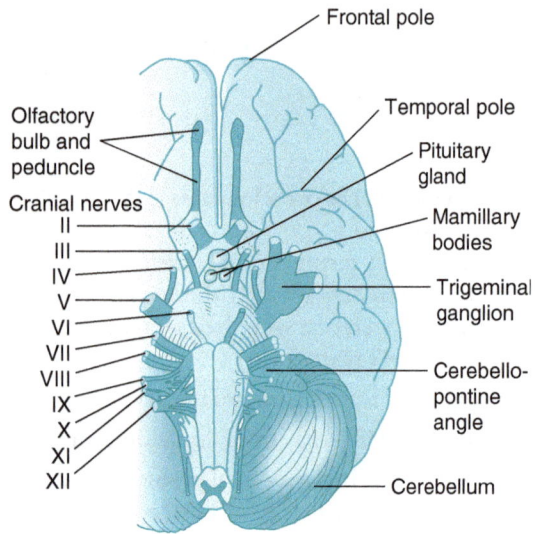

FIGURE 4-1 **Brain stem view of brain with cranial nerves**
Reproduced with permission from Waxman S: Clinical Neuroanatomy, 27th ed. New York: McGraw-Hill Education; 2013.

Alzheimer's Disease/Dementia

Loss of memory and cognitive abilities were once seen as a natural part of the aging process. As people age, it was expected there would be an accompanying erosion of mental acuity.

Research on aging populations has supported more distinct causes for mental decline in the elderly population. Distinguishing pathology from mental processing changes associated with aging occurs frequently in the emergency department. Differentiating between acute and chronic mental status deterioration is therefore an important skillset for the ED nurse.

Alzheimer's Disease

Alzheimer's disease is a type of dementia causing problems with memory, thinking, and behavior. It progresses slowly and is incurable. Alzheimer's is the sixth leading cause of death in the United States, accounting for 60 to 80% of dementia cases[2]. Definitive diagnosis of the disease requires an autopsy. However, clinical criteria allow a diagnosis of probable Alzheimer's with approximately 90% accuracy. Early progression may go unnoticed, but in late stages one can see the loss of the patient's ability to interact with the outside world or participate in basic activities of daily living. Change can be stressful for the Alzheimer patient, particularly changes in environment and caregivers.

Assessment/Analysis
- Early Behavioral Changes
  - Irritability
  - Anxiety
  - Depression
- Late Stages or Progressive Behavioral Changes
  - Anger
  - Agitation
  - Aggression
  - General emotional stress
  - Physical or verbal outbursts

TABLE 4-2 **Cranial Nerve Functions**

CN	Name	Significance	General Function
I	Olfactory	Smell	Sensory
II	Optic	Sight	Sensory
III	Oculomotor	Eye movement, eye lids, pupil constriction	Motor
IV	Trochlear	Downward and inward eye movement	Motor
V	Trigeminal	Mastication, pain touch and temperature	Both (Sensory and Motor)
VI	Abducens	Inward eye movement	Motor
VII	Facial	Facial expression, saliva, tears, lips	Both
VIII	Vestibulocochlear	Hearing, balance	Sensory
IX	Glossopharyngeal	Gag reflex, tongue movement, taste, swallowing	Both
X	Vagus	Heart, lungs, intestines	Both
XI	Spinal Accessory	Trapezius and sternocleomastoid movement	Motor
XII	Hypoglossal	Speech movements of the tongue, swallowing	Motor

- Hallucinations
- Delusions
- Sleep disturbances

Interventions
- Identify and address needs of the patient
- Provide a safe environment such as high fall risk precautions
- As the disease progresses, the patient will have difficulty expressing their needs
- Common medications for slowing progression of the disease
  - Cholinesterase inhibitors (Aricept™, and Exelon™)
  - N-Methyl-D-Aspartate (NMDA) receptor antagonist (Memantine, which is Namenda™)
- Medications to manage behavior
  - Antidepressants
  - Anxiolytics
  - Antipsychotic medications

Vascular Dementia

Vascular dementia is the second most common type of dementia after Alzheimer's, accounting for 20 to 30% of all cases.[3] Vascular dementia occurs when thinking skills decline caused by interruption of oxygenated blood flow to the brain. Vascular dementia may occur concurrently with Alzheimer's. Cognitive abilities may suddenly be impaired following strokes or other conditions that block major brain blood vessels. Mild changes may also worsen gradually as the result of multiple minor strokes or other conditions affecting smaller blood vessels result in cumulative damage. Vascular cognitive impairment (VCI) is a newer term emphasizing the dynamic nature of this condition.[3]

Both forms of dementia may go unnoticed in early stages when memory, attention, and concentration are affected in subtle ways erroneously attributed to stress or other causes. Because dementia is a chronic progressive disease, it is essential for the emergency nurse to determine whether the patient's presentation is a change from their baseline mental status.

Chronic Neurological Disorders

Multiple Sclerosis

Multiple sclerosis (MS) is a chronic autoimmune disease characterized by relapses brought on by stress, viruses, pregnancy, and warmer weather. Onset typically begins between ages 20 and 40 years. MS is characterized by periods of exacerbations followed by remissions. With each new relapse, symptoms tend to be worse. Currently, there is no cure.

Assessment/Analysis
- Vision changes
  - Blurred or double vision
  - Visual color distortion
  - Unilateral blindness
- Motor function
  - Weakness
  - Coordination problems
  - Loss of balance
- Numbness
- Pain
- Speech difficulties
- Tremors

Interventions
- Corticosteroids: because of the autoimmune nature of the disease, steroids are often a treatment choice for immunosuppressant effects
- Intereferon Beta (Rebif™) may also be prescribed
- Plasmapheresis may be initiated in the emergency department or during an inpatient stay
- Safety measures: provide assistance with ambulation and other protective measures
- Baclofen: for muscle spasms, rigidity, and pain
- Tricyclic antidepressants are often ordered for pain
- Anticonvulsants: phenytoin, gabapentin, and carbamazepine

Evaluation
- Pain management
- Safety: due to sensory and motor disturbance

Myasthenia Gravis

Myasthenia gravis presents as significant muscle weakness exacerbated with activity. This weakness can become so significant that the ability to speak and swallow is affected. In some cases, respiratory depression and arrest can occur.

Assessment/Analysis
- Drooping eyelids
- Double vision (diplopia) which improves when one eye is closed
- Altered speaking
- Difficulty swallowing
- Problems chewing
- Limited facial expressions

Interventions
- Support patent airway and effective breathing
- Corticosteroids
- Immunosuppressants: azathioprine, mycophenolate mofetil, and tacrolimus
- Cholinesterase inhibitors, such as pyridostigmine

Evaluation
- Adequate ventilation
- Hemodynamic stability
- Infection risk increases with use of immunosuppressants and steroids

Parkinson's Disease

Parkinson's disease is caused by the loss of dopamine-producing cells in the brain presenting as tremors, speech and movement difficulties, and eventual muscle rigidity. Patients with this chronic condition may present to the emergency department with associated depression, trouble speaking or swallowing, problems voiding, constipation, or falls. Parkinson's disease is usually not a medical emergency; emergency department care is supportive in nature.

TRAP (a common acronym used to describe common symptoms in Parkinson's disease) = **T**remors **R**igidity **A**kinesia and **P**ostural instability = Parkinson's

Guillian–Barré Syndrome

Guillian–Barré syndrome (GBS) is an acute inflammatory nerve syndrome affecting the motor functioning of the peripheral nerves. It is an autoimmune response provoked by a preceding infection with a key feature of an ascending (bottom up) weakness and paralysis, possibly requiring respiratory support—including ventilation—until resolved. One-third of patients with GBS require intubation, mechanical ventilation, and admission to ICU.[4]

Progression
- Mild febrile illness 2 to 3 weeks prior to onset of GBS symptoms
- Ascending neuropathy—weakness and paralysis—starting in the lower extremities that is symmetrical. Patients may present with absent or depressed deep tendon reflexes
- Ascending to the diaphragm and intercostal muscles leads to respiratory insufficiency
- Typically progresses over hours up to about a 2 week period[4]

Assessment/Analysis
- Stage in progression (see the preceding)
- Shortness of breath
- Possible altered gait
- Possible lower extremity weakness
- Labs often analyzed to rule out other causes
  - CBC with differential
  - Serum chemistries
  - Thyroid function testing
  - Erythrocyte sedimentation rate (ESR)
  - Serology studies for causative organism
- Lumbar puncture
  - Common: elevated CSF protein with normal WBC level[4]

Interventions
- Support airway and breathing
  - Avoid depolarizing neuromuscular blocking agent succinylcholine with GBS because of the risk of hyperkalemia
- Cardiac monitoring with continual pulse oximetry
- Establish IV access for crystalloids/medications as needed
- Hospital admission for respiratory support which may include intubation and respiratory support
- Plasmapheresis or IV Immunoglobulin therapy can shorten recovery time[5]

Evaluation
- Patent airway
- Stable hemodynamic status
- Recovery goal: patient is able to return to baseline neurological and motor function

Headaches

Migraine Headache

Migraine headaches affect approximately 6% of men and 15% of women over a 1-year time period.[6] Migraines often reoccur following a trigger, and this trigger seems to activate the onset of symptoms associated with the migraine. Migraines can last for days and can be incapacitating without treatment.

Photophobia distinguishes a migraine headache from cluster type headaches.

Assessment/Analysis
- History of similar symptoms
  - Presence of aura
  - Typical precipitating factors
- Headache description—Two or more of the following descriptors for pain[6]
  - Unilateral pain
  - Throbbing pain
  - Aggravated by movement
  - Moderate to severe intensity
- Nausea and vomiting
- Photophobia
- Sensitivity to sound or movement
- Reported triggers[6]
  - Glaring lights, sounds, or other received (afferent) stimuli
  - Hunger
  - Period immediately following high stress
  - Physical exertion or lack of sleep
  - Weather changes
  - Hormonal fluctuations during menstrual cycles

Interventions
- Place patient in a dark and quiet room
- Establish IV access for crystalloids/medications as needed
- Analgesic treatment: some of the classifications of medications used[6]
  - NSAIDs: most effective when taken early in onset
  - Serotonin Receptor Agonists: sumatriptan (Imitrex™)
  - Ergot Alkaloids: nonselective receptor agonists (Ergotamine, D.H.E. 45™)
  - Dopamine receptor antagonists: highly effective when administered parenterally or combined with other anti-migraine agents (Haloperidol)

- Anti-emetic medications
- Prevention medications
  - Cardiovascular medications
    - Beta blockers: propranolol
    - Calcium channel blockers: verapamil
    - Tricyclic antidepressants: amitriptyline
    - Anti-seizure medication: divalproex (Depakote™)

Evaluation
- Follow up with medical provider
- Patient teaching: "headache diary" identifying triggers, obtain adequate sleep and a healthy diet, stress reduction, and avoidance of other triggers

Cluster Headaches

Cluster headaches are a rare and disabling form of unilateral headache. They can occur in cycles of "clusters" with periods of remission. A series of one to two unilateral headaches may occur daily for 4 to 5 months, followed by a pain-free interval that may last about 1 year.[6]

Assessment/Analysis
- History of similar symptoms
- Headache history with ipsilateral symptoms: pain, lacrimation (tearing), nasal congestion, or even ptosis[6]
- Unilateral photophobia and phonophobia (sensitive to sounds) occurring on the same side of the pain
- Restlessness
  - May appear frantic or agitated; striking affected side of head
- CT scan of the head or MRI of the brain

Intervention
- Oxygen therapy
  - Low flow and high flow oxygen delivery effective for pain management in up to 78% of patients[7]
- Establish IV access for crystalloid fluids and medications as needed
- Place the patient in a dark and quiet room
- Medications[6]
- Course of prednisone may suspend the cycle of the headache pain
- Lithium
- Verapamil (also as preventative treatment)

Evaluation
- Pain relief
- Patient teaching about medications and management
- Follow up with medical provider

Temporal Arteritis

Temporal arteritis—also known as Giant cell arteritis—affects adults over the age of 50 years. It is a chronic vasculitis of the large and medium vessels. Temporal arteritis should be considered in patients over the age of 50 presenting with a complaint of new headaches. Temporal arteritis, if left undiagnosed, can lead to irreversible blindness.[8]

Assessment/Analysis
- Presenting symptoms include: double vision, loss of vision in one eye, temporal headache and tenderness
- No history of similar symptoms
- Laboratory studies
  - CBC with differential
  - Erythrocyte sedimentation rate: elevated
- CT scan or head/brain or MRI of the brain

Interventions
- Analgesia
- Immediate initiation of glucocorticoid therapy
- Evaluation
- Pain relief
- Patient teaching about medications and management
- Follow up with medical provider

Intracranial Pressure

The skull is a closed inflexible container. Inside this container is the cranium, which is composed of blood, the brain, and cerebrospinal fluid (CSF). An increase in one intracranial element increases pressure and requires a decrease in the other two elements, a concept called the Monro-Kellie doctrine.[9] When a change occurs within the volume of the intracranial elements, the intracranial pressure (ICP) is affected. ICP is impacted by three intracranial components.[10]

- Brain parenchyma (<1300 mL in the adult)
- CSF (100 to 150 mL)
- Intravascular blood (100 to 150 mL)

As one of these components increases, a homeostatic reduction occurs in the volume of another component. If this reduction does not occur, an elevation in the ICP ensues. Increased ICP is life threatening and can lead to Cushing reflex (triad).

Cerebral perfusion pressure (CPP) maintains brain perfusion and oxygen demands and is regulated by ICP and mean arterial pressure (MAP). CPP = MAP – ICP. A CPP of less than 60 mm Hg borders the lower limit of this regulation process that maintains adequate cerebral perfusion. Consequently, hypotension and/or increased ICP impedes the autoregulation process resulting in low perfusion and cerebral ischemia.[10]

Increasing the pressure in the intracranial space can lead to severe neurological consequences. Death can occur if the pressure becomes significant enough to displace the brain, a process called herniation.

ICP Measurements
- Normal pressure is <15 mm Hg inside the cranium
- Greater than 20 mm Hg is considered increased ICP
- Early increased ICP is elevated pressures without herniation
- Late increased ICP is elevated pressure with herniation

Cushing's triad is a set of three abnormal vital signs that emerge with advancement of increasing intracranial pressure. It is a compensatory response as the body tries to provide cerebral perfusion in the presence of increasing ICP.

- Hypertension with *widening pulse pressure* (increasing systolic and falling diastolic)
- Bradycardia
- Irregular breathing patterns

Assessment/Analysis
- Patient airway, breathing pattern
- History of present illness/injury
- Level of consciousness
- GCS
- Vital signs including temperature
- Motor responses and posturing to stimulus
- Signs of increased intracranial pressure (see Table 4-3)
- Signs of transtentorial herniation[10]
  - Ipsilateral or bilateral pupillary dilation
  - Hemiparesis
  - Motor posturing
  - Neurological deterioration
- Laboratory studies
  - CBC with differential
  - Serum chemistries
  - Arterial blood gas
  - Coagulation studies
  - Type/screen for crossmatching blood
  - Possible toxicology study
- CT of head and neck

Interventions
- Support the airway and maintain effective breathing-possible ventilator support
  - Cardiac monitor and continuous SpO_2
  - Consider capnography
    - Maintain PCO_2: 35 to 45 mm Hg
    - Avoid hyperventilation—Causes cerebral vasoconstriction leading to decreased perfusion[10]
  - Cervical spine precautions if suspected or actual spinal injury
  - Head of the bed should be elevated to 30 to 45 degrees in the absence of suspected spinal injury
  - Head midline to allow for jugular vein drainage
  - Prevent and/or treat seizures
  - Reduce noxious stimuli
  - Maintain temperature (normothermia)
  - Manage pain
  - Establish IV access for crystalloid fluids, blood products, and medications as needed
  - Medications for reducing ICP
    - Mannitol IV[11]
      - Osmotic diuretic that is excreted by the kidneys[11]
      - Requires in-line filter for precipitates
      - Dose-0.5 to 1 g/kg over 5 to 15 minutes; can be redosed every 4 to 6 hours
    - 3% NaCl (hypertonic saline)
      - 250 mL IV over 30 minutes[10]
      - Monitor serum sodium and serum chemistries
      - For continuous infusions, >2% NaCl, central IV access is highly recommended[11]
  - Insertion of a CSF drainage catheter may be necessary and/or surgical decompression

Evaluation
- ICP trending toward normal
- Neurologic symptoms resolving
- Patent airway and supported breathing
- Hemodynamic stability
- Intake and output

Shunt Dysfunctions

Hydrocephalus can be treated with a shunt system that drains CSF and relieves increased intracranial pressure. While effective, this treatment modality can present complications as an estimated 50% of all shunts in pediatric patients fail within 2 years of placement.[12]

Shunt malfunction is a partial or complete blockage of the shunt, which causes CSF to accumulate and result in symptoms associated with untreated hydrocephalus (increasing ICP). Another shunt malfunction, although more rare, is when the shunt drains too much CSF. Whether the shunt is draining too much CSF or is obstructed, either patient condition presents with symptoms of increased ICP.[13] Patients with ventriculoperitoneal (VP) shunts are also at risk for developing abdominal complications such as hernias and bowel perforations.[12]

TABLE 4-3 **Early and Late Signs of Increased Intracranial Pressure (ICP)**

Early Signs of ICP	Late Signs of ICP
Confusion, restlessness, lethargy. Progressive disorientation	Responds only to deep pain or unarousable. (Stupor, coma)
Pupils = sluggish response to light	Pupils = fixed or dilated
Motor = decreased strength noted	Motor = Posturing or no response
Vitals = Tachycardia, hypertensive	Vitals = Cushing's Triad

A shunt infection is most often caused by the patient's normal flora. The most common organisms are *Staphylococcus Epidermidis* and *Staphyloccus aureus*.[13] Shunt infections are rare with an incidence of 0.3%, and usually develop within the first few months after a placement or revision.[13]

Assessment/Analysis
- Shunt malfunction
  - Altered mental status
  - Lethargy and somnolence
  - Abnormal gait
  - Symptoms associated with increased ICP
    - Irritability
    - Headache
    - Neck pain
    - Bulging fontanels in infants
    - Seizure
    - Vomiting
    - Decreased pupillary response and/or dilated pupils
- Shunt infection
  - Fever
  - Signs of surgical site infection
  - Redness, edema, and tenderness along the skin over the shunt
  - Signs of peritonitis (VP shunts)
- Shunt overdrainage
  - Depressed fontanels
  - Overlapping skull bones
  - Headache increases when HOB elevated
  - Headache decreases when supine

Interventions
- Airway and breathing support
- Airway protection: suction, anticipate need for intubation
- Establish IV access for crystalloids/medications as needed
- Cardiac monitor and continuous SpO_2
- Shunt series: radiography of the shunt system[13]
- CT and/or MRI of head
- Laboratory studies
  - CBC with differential
  - Serum chemistries
  - Blood cultures (if suspected infection)
  - Coagulation studies, if anticipated surgical repair[13]
- Shunt malfunction
  - Treat increased ICP
  - Supportive therapy
  - Seizure management
  - Surgery to replace shunt if necessary
- Shunt infection
  - Antibiotics after blood cultures
  - Fever management
  - Analgesia
  - Consult patient's neurologist for recommendations on shunt management

Meningitis

Meningitis is an infection and inflammation in the meningeal layers surrounding the brain and spinal cord.

> The meninges **PAD** the brain and consist of three layers: **p**ia mater (innermost), **A**rachnoid space, **D**ura mater (outermost, nearest the skull).

Bacterial, fungal, or viral infectious agents may be the cause.
- ❖ **Bacterial meningitis** is life threatening and has acute onset
  - ♦ Subarachnoid space fills with infectious material which increases ICP through obstruction of CSF
  - ♦ Common organisms include *Strep Pneumoniae, H. flu,* and *N. meningitides*[14]
- ❖ **Viral meningitis** is mild and short lived, gradual in onset and non-contagious
- ❖ **Fungal meningitis** is rare and mainly associated with immunocompromised patients
  - ♦ Common organisms include *Aspergillus* and *Candida*[14]

Bacterial infection starts with bacterial organisms invading the host through the upper airway and may present as a sinus infection that appears to resolve some days prior to the development of meningitis symptoms. Sepsis, basilar skull fractures, infected facial structures, and brain abscesses can also lead to bacterial meningitis. The infecting organisms cause an inflammatory cascade and brain swelling in the fixed volume space of the skull. CSF fluid is inhibited and overall the pressure (ICP) in the skull increases.[14]

Assessment/Interventions
- Headache, especially occipital
- Fever at SIRS criteria levels
  - See the sepsis discussion in Medical (chapter 9) or Shock (chapter 5) chapters
- Neck stiffness (nuchal rigidity)
- Altered mental status
- Purpura or petechial rash on torso and legs (meningococcal)
- *Infant assessment*
  - Bradycardia in neonates
  - High pitched cry
  - Restlessness and inconsolability
  - Tense or bulging fontanel[15]
- Resistance (and pain) with *passive neck flexion*
- **Brudzinski sign**—Flexion of the hips and knees in response to neck flexion

- **Kernig sign**—Contract of the hamstrings in response to knee extension while the hip is flexed
- Head CT scan *before* lumbar puncture to rule out space occupying lesions that could cause brain herniation during spinal tap
- Lumbar Puncture results with CSF that appears cloudy and results with elevations in white blood cells and protein are consistent with bacterial meningitis
- Cerebral Spinal Fluid (CSF) from a lumbar puncture can yield an array of findings
  - Initial cloudy appearance of CSF may indicate the presence of white blood cells or bacteria
  - Healthy CSF should be clear and colorless with a glucose level two-thirds that of blood
  - CSF Analysis[14]
    - Gram stain, culture, and differential analysis of the WBCs helps determine infecting organism whether bacterial, fungal, or viral
    - Protein: 150 to 1000 mg/dL for bacterial. May be over 1000 mg/dL in fungal. Slightly increased in viral
    - White blood cells: varies from normal (under 5 WBCs/mm^3) to over 1000/mm^3 in all three types
    - Glucose: decreased in bacterial. Generally normal in viral. May be normal or decreased in fungal
- Other laboratory studies
  - CBC with differential
  - Serum chemistries with liver function tests
    - Monitor for hyponatremia[14]
  - Blood cultures
  - Elevated procalcitonin: may indicate bacterial versus viral meningitis

Interventions
- Isolate the patient in a negative pressure room and droplet precautions
  - The patient should wear a surgical mask when traveling outside of room
- Seizure precautions for patient safety
- Consider prophylactic antibiotics
  - Family and friends in prolonged close contact
  - Caregivers engaged in procedures such as intubation or breathing treatments
  - Choice of antibiotics depends on suspected organism[14]
- Reduce ICP
  - Elevate the head of the bed
  - Antiemetics to prevent vomiting
  - Barbiturates or diuretics
- Assist with lumbar puncture
- Antibiotics
  - Do not delay for confirmatory tests such as neuroimaging or lumbar puncture
- Dexamethasone may be indicated to reduce CNS inflammation in some cases[16]

Evaluation
- Mental status
- Hemodynamic status
- Resolving signs and symptoms

Seizure Disorders

Seizures are temporary neurologic dysfunctions resulting from abnormal electrical neuronal activity in the cerebral cortex of the brain. Seizures originate from either a primary CNS dysfunction or could be a manifestation as an unaddressed metabolic problem.[17]

Seizures have different presentations based on motor involvement and severity.

- ❖ **Focal** or **partial seizures** affect only one area of the brain. The patient may or may not be aware of the seizure activity
- ❖ **Generalized seizures** cause impairment of consciousness and involve disruption of the electrical activity of the whole brain
- ❖ **Unclassified seizures** are not able to be placed into a category due to a lack of information.[17] Neonatal seizures consisting of swimming motions, lip smacking, or eye rolling is one example
- ❖ **Postictal state** is a brief period of confusion, disorientation, or agitation following a generalized seizure and lasting several minutes. The postictal state may also indicate ongoing non-convulsive seizures

<u>Febrile seizures</u> occur in children between the age of 6 months and 5 years, usually on the first day of a febrile illness such as a simple cold virus or an ear infection (>100.4°F/38°C). The convulsions last for less than 10 minutes and occur in the first hour of illness; often the seizure is the first noticed indication that the child is sick.[18] Febrile seizures can be very frightening to parents who need to be reassured that febrile seizures do not cause any long-term harm to the child and often run in families. Treatment is usually antipyretics.

Approximately two-thirds of patients will only experience a single febrile seizure in their lifetime.[18] These convulsions are usually self-limiting and treatment is often unnecessary. If the seizure lasts more than 15 minutes, anti-seizure medications may be used as treatment. Providers may also wish to evaluate patients for CNS infections as a differential diagnosis.

Assessment/Analysis
- **Partial seizures**
  - May be unilateral
  - Involve focal motor activity
  - Somatic sensory experiences
  - Vision, smell, taste, or hearing disturbances
  - May evolve to generalized seizures[17]
- **Generalized seizures**
  - May be preceded by an *aura*: an awareness of the impending seizure in the form of strange odor, taste, or vision[17]

- Loss of consciousness followed by tonic stiffening and clonic jerking motor action of the extremities
- Biting of the tongue
- Loss of bladder control
- Loss of bowel control—rarely seen
- Sudden loss of muscle tone
  - May be called atonic seizures
- Postictal state following seizure
  - Absence seizures often do not have a postictal state afterward and occur most often in patients between the ages of 1 to 8 years old[19]
- Prolonged or so close together that there is no time for recovery[20]
  - Status epilepticus (SE)
  - Life-threatening condition
  - Seizures can continue for 30 minutes or longer[20]
  - Prolonged postictal states
- Missed or changed dose of antiseizure medications
- Change in pattern of seizure activity
- CT scan or MRI of the head if there is no seizure history
- Lumbar puncture to rule out meningitis
- Laboratory studies
  - CBC with differential
  - Serum chemistries
  - Toxicology studies for substance use/abuse or medication levels

Interventions
- Airway: to prevent aspiration
- Safety: pad bed rails and protect head from striking hard objects
- Supplemental oxygen, if indicated by SpO_2
- Undress for cooling if a febrile seizure
- Establish IV access for crystalloid fluids and medications as needed
  - Benzodiazepines to stop active seizure activity
    - Lorazepam and diazepam
  - Anticonvulsants to prevent recurrence
    - Phenytoin (Dilantin™): rate of 50 mg/minute or less
    - Fosphenytoin (Cerebyx™) in phenytoin equivalents
    - Dextrose 50% if hypoglycemic
    - Thiamine and other nutritional supplements if deficient
- Oral anticonvulsants depending on seizure type[17]
  - Partial: carbamazepine, lamotrigine, oxcarbazepine, and phenytoin
  - Generalized: valproate, phenytoin, carbamazepine, and lamotrigine

Evaluation
- Mental status
- Hemodynamic status
- Prolonged seizure or postictal state
- Glucose monitoring for hypoglycemia

Stroke

A stroke or cerebral vascular accident (CVA) is an interruption of blood flow to the brain possibly causing permanent deficits through infarction of brain tissue. A stroke may be alternatively referred to as "brain attack," a term that references the immediate care publicly associated with heart attacks. Like a heart attack, the majority of strokes are caused by ischemia of brain tissue secondary to a thrombus or emboli blocking a cerebral blood vessel. Treatment with thrombolytics is time limited starting at the onset of symptoms.

Strokes can also be hemorrhagic when bleeding from a ruptured vessel presents in either the subarachnoid or intracranial space. Location of the bleeding determines symptoms and deficit.

Transient Ischemic Attack (TIA) is a sudden onset of stroke-like symptoms, typically lasting less than 60 minutes and rarely more than 24 hours. It differs from a stroke only in that symptoms resolve without intervention. A TIA is a stroke until symptoms resolve and thus should activate hospital stroke protocols. Unilateral deficits, aphasia, and other symptoms usually resolve within the first 30 minutes after onset. Sometimes symptoms resolve in as little as 5 minutes. TIAs are warning signs of stroke. One-third of patients who experience a TIA go on to have a stroke within the next 12 months.[21]

Stroke presentation often exhibits unilateral symptoms but may vary based on the location of the occluded blood vessel within the brain.

- **Broca's aphasia** (expressive aphasia) is an inability to speak fluently when a stroke or injury occurs in the dominant frontal lobe. Language may be limited to short 4-word utterances or no ability to speak at all. Language comprehension, however, often remains intact. Damage causing Broca's aphasia is usually in the left frontal hemisphere[22]
- **Wernicke's aphasia** (receptive aphasia) is the inability to understand language in spoken or written form. Patients can speak fluently, but are unable to recognize when their speech lacks meaning. Inability to understand what is being said inhibits the patient's ability to follow commands in the acute setting and is secondary to damage in the dominant temporal lobe

The emergency nurse conducts rapid assessment and facilitates diagnostic studies to determine the cause of symptoms and initiate treatment aimed at restoring or reversing blood supply causing ischemia or hemorrhage.

Stroke Assessment Scales

Cincinnati Prehospital Stroke Scale (CPSS) is used to identify patients who may be suffering a stroke in the prehospital setting or quickly upon arrival to the emergency department.[23] It involves three brief tests: facial symmetry, arm strength, and speech ability.

The FAST evaluation is a simplified version of the CPSS developed to increase early identification of ischemic strokes outside the hospital setting.

- ❖ **Facial Droop:** have the patient smile or show his or her teeth and watch for droop or weakness on one side
- ❖ **Arm Drift:** have the patient hold up his or her arms and close the eyes. Watch for unilateral drift or weakness
- ❖ **Speech:** have the patient say, "you can't teach an old dog new tricks" or some other simple phrase. Note slurred words or difficulty speaking certain words
- ❖ **Time:** when was the patient last seen normal?[23]

National Institute of Health Stroke Scale (NIHSS) is a much more detailed neurologic exam used to evaluate the effect of acute CVA in the hospital setting. It has been evaluated as appearing to be a good predictor of patient outcomes.[24] The baseline exam is followed by repeated assessment at regular intervals during the hospital course. NIHSS evaluates the following elements.[23]

- Level of consciousness
- Gaze
- Visual fields
- Facial movement
- Motor function of extremities
- Limb ataxia
- Neglect
- Motor function
- Dysarthria/language
- Sensory loss

Assessment/Analysis
- Ischemic stroke
  - Sudden numbness or weakness of the face, arm, or leg, especially on one side of the body
  - Sudden confusion, trouble speaking, or understanding
  - Sudden trouble seeing in one or both eyes
  - Sudden trouble walking, dizziness, lack of balance, or coordination
  - Sudden severe headache with no known cause
  - Note "last seen normal" or "last known well" as time of onset and start of 3 hour window for tissue plasminogen activator (tPA) administration
- ECG
  - 60% of embolic strokes are associated with atrial fibrillation or acute MI[17]
  - Laboratory studies for initial management
    - CBC with differential
    - Serum chemistries with liver function tests
    - Coagulation studies
    - Troponin I to rule in/out Acute MI
  - Head CT to rule out bleed is prioritized
    - Within 25 minutes of arrival with official result within 45 minutes of arrival[17]
  - Bedside glucose testing
    - Hypoglycemia can mimic symptoms of a stroke
  - Stress and anxiety of the patient
    - Inability to speak or understand what is happening can greatly increase
- Hemorrhagic stroke
  - Described as "Thunderclap headache" or "Worst headache of my life"
    - Sudden and maximal at onset
  - Head CT/CTA is prioritized
  - Signs of increasing ICP
    - Nausea or vomiting
    - Level of consciousness changes
  - Photophobia
  - Sudden seizure
  - Unilateral deficits
  - Meningeal signs (fever and nuchal rigidity)

Interventions
- Maintain airway
- Supplemental oxygen, as indicated
- Establish IV access for crystalloid fluids and medications as needed
  - Labetalol IV to keep Systolic blood pressure <185 mm Hg[17]
    - Avoid hypotension which reduces cerebral perfusion
  - Consider tPA if symptom onset is <3 hours
    - Alteplase is FDA approved for <3 hours from onset but studies have shown it can be effective up to 4.5 hours and some facilities are extending this window
- Trauma, bleeding, or stroke within the last 3 months or neurological surgery are issues that may rule a patient out as a tPA candidate[23]
- Treatment includes reducing ICP
  - Elevate the head of the bed
  - Keep the head in neutral alignment with the spine to facilitate drainage
- If the patient is on anticoagulants, consider reversal agents as appropriate
  - Vitamin K
  - Fresh Frozen Plasma (FFP)
  - Prothrombin Complex Concentrates (PCC)[25]
- Surgical intervention to control hemorrhage
- Address causative factors such as hypertension and carotid atherosclerosis

Evaluation
- Level of consciousness
- Maintain airway
- Hemodynamic status
- Monitor for signs of increasing ICP

- Home medication therapy needed or continued per primary care
  - Antiplatelet (aspirin or clopidogrel)
  - Anticoagulation therapy (heparin or warfarin)

Trauma

All traumatic injuries begin with a primary survey: **A**irway, **B**reathing, **C**irculation (including massive bleeding control), **D**isability. Some will include **E**xposure (to allow inspection for other injuries), as part of the primary survey.[26] Neurological trauma can affect the central and peripheral nervous system in many ways. Primary injury may occur to the brain or spinal cord. Following a traumatic event, secondary injury, such as from hypotension, hypoxia, or cerebral edema may occur. General assessment and analysis concepts are common to most neurological trauma.

Assessment/Analysis: General Neurologic Trauma
- Spontaneous respiratory effort
- Patient movement
  - Paraplegia or quadriplegia indicates spinal cord injury
- Disability using GCS or FOUR Score[27]
  - FOUR score evaluates eye response, brainstem reflexes, motor response, and respiratory response on a scale of zero to four each, for a total score of 16
- Pupils
  - Size, symmetry, and reactivity
- CT scan of the head or of the cervical, thoracic, or lumbar spine as appropriate

Concussion

Concussion is a traumatic, reversible neurological deficit including a temporary loss of consciousness and retrograde amnesia.

Assessment
- Transitory loss of consciousness following blunt head trauma
- Temporary deficits in cognition that improve over time
- Retrograde amnesia
- Dizziness
- Nausea
- Uncoordinated movement, including gait

Interventions
- Decreasing brain stimulation (brain rest)
- Prohibiting contact sports or vigorous activities that risk re-injury until asymptomatic (at least 24 to 72 hours)[27]
- Acetaminophen for headache pain
  - Aspirin or ibuprofen may increase risk of bleeding
- Patient/family teaching regarding **post-concussive syndrome**
  - Symptoms lasting days or years
  - Personality changes
  - Prolonged fatigue
  - Inability to concentrate
  - Changes in sleep pattern
  - Changes in smell or taste[28]
  - Importance of primary care follow-up[27]

Evaluation
- Signs and symptoms of increasing ICP
- Altered level of consciousness
- Seizures
- Observation with frequent checks for decreasing level of consciousness (LOC)

Diffuse Axonal Injury

Diffuse axonal injury (DAI) is a serious traumatic brain injury involving disruption of the cerebral axons creating a disconnection between the brain stem and the cortex. DAI is caused by axonal stretching to the point of disconnection by acceleration/deceleration or rotational forces. Severe DAI often results in a persistent vegetative state or death.

Assessment/Analysis
- Maintain airway
- Monitor vital signs
  - Hypertension
  - Hyperthermia
- Immediate and prolonged (days to months) unconsciousness
- The patient often will not regain consciousness in the emergency setting and may remain in a coma
- Consider assault or abusive head trauma
- Loss of brainstem reflexes in severe cases
- Decorticate or decerebrate posturing
- Excessive sweating due to autonomic dysfunction
- CT Head or MRI: injury may be greater at the microscopic level than imaging can detect
- Electroencephalogram (EEG)
- Laboratory studies
  - CBC with differential
  - Serum chemistries
  - Coagulation studies
  - ABGs, if respiratory compromise

Interventions
- Intubation and airway management if necessary
- Maintain adequate oxygenation and ventilation[27]
- Capnography
- Establish IV access for crystalloid fluids, blood products, and medications as needed
- Maintain normothermia to decrease metabolic demands of the brain
- Prevent seizures to minimize additional brain insult
- Interventions to prevent secondary injury from elevated ICP
  - See "ICP Interventions" noted previously in this chapter

Evaluation
- Patent airway
- Monitor vital signs and temperature
- Monitor for hypoxemia, hypercarbia and hypocarbia, hypoglycemia and hyperglycemia

Hemorrhage

Intracerebral hemorrhage is bleeding in and around the brain manifests in different ways depending on the location and nature of the bleeding, whether *venous* or *arterial*.

Epidural hemorrhage occurs between the skull and the dura mater and is often involved in the middle meningeal artery secondary to temporal skull trauma.

Subdural hemorrhage occurs below the dura and above the arachnoid meningeal layers. Usually the bleeding is from small bridging veins. Since the bleeding is venous rather than arterial, the manifestation and progression is much slower.[19]

Assessment/Analysis
- Headache
- Hemiparesis (opposite side of injury)
- Pupil dilation (same side as injury)
- Signs of increasing ICP
- Epidural *pattern* of mental status
  - A period of unconsciousness
  - Lucid, often asymptomatic period for minutes to hours
  - Rapid deterioration into unconsciousness
- If bleeding is venous, there is brief or no loss of consciousness and the patient may initially appear "fine"
- Laboratory studies
  - CBC with differential
  - Serum chemistries
  - Coagulation studies
- CT of head

Interventions
- Monitor for changes in LOC
- Intubation and airway management if necessary
- Maintain adequate oxygenation and ventilation[27]
- Consider invasive ICP monitor
- Interventions to prevent secondary injury from elevated ICP
  - Elevate the head of the bed
  - Keep head in neutral alignment with spine to facilitate drainage
  - Avoid vomiting—Consider prophylactic antiemetics
  - Assist with insertion of ventricular drain as needed
  - Prevent seizures—Consider anticonvulsants[28]
- If patient is on anticoagulants, consider reversal agents as appropriate
  - Vitamin K
  - Fresh Frozen Plasma (FFP)
  - Prothrombin Complex Concentrates (PCC)[25]
- Surgical intervention to control hemorrhage

Evaluation
- Maintain airway
- Hemodynamic status
- Reassess neurologic symptoms frequently
- Monitor for deterioration of level of consciousness

Basilar Skull Fracture

Basilar skull fractures occur at the base of the skull and may present with CSF leakage. The brain tissue can be torn or punctured from the fractured skull creating an opening for the CSF leak. Other signs of a basilar skull fracture include:

- CSF Otorrhea: fluid from the ears that contains CSF. Indicates damage to the middle fossa
- CSF Rhinorrhea: fluid from the nose that contains CSF
- Battle Sign is ecchymosis behind the ear due to bruising of the mastoid sinus, as pictured in Figure 4-2. Indicates damage to the posterior fossa in a Basilar skull fracture
- Raccoon Eyes: periorbital ecchymosis secondary to intra-orbital bleeding, as pictured in Figure 4-3. Indicates damage to the anterior fossa

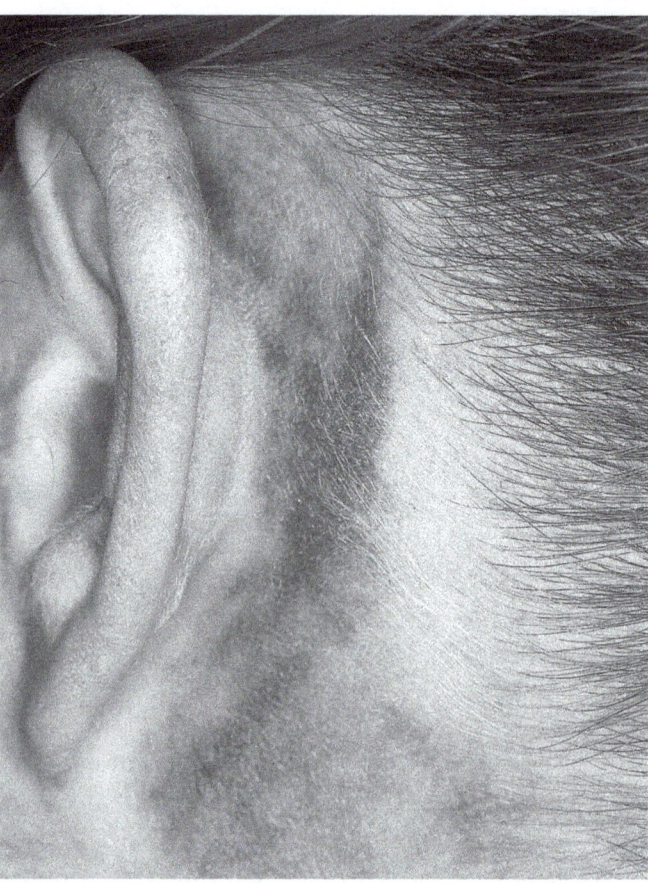

FIGURE 4-2 Mastoid ecchymosis, more commonly referred to as Battle Sign

Reproduced with permission from Knoop KJ, Stack LB, Storrow AB, et al: The Atlas of Emergency Medicine, 4th ed. New York: McGraw-Hill Education; 2016: Photo contributor: Frank Biriny, MD.

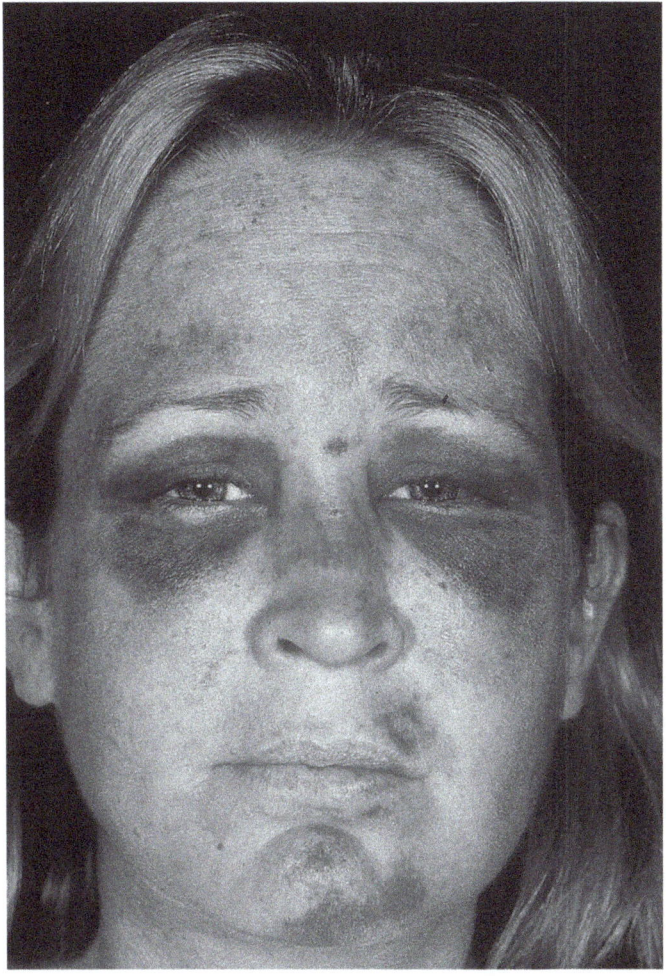

FIGURE 4-3 Periorbital ecchymosis, more commonly referred to as Raccoon eyes
Reproduced with permission from Knoop KJ, Stack LB, Storrow AB, et al: The Atlas of Emergency Medicine, 4th ed. New York: McGraw-Hill Education; 2016: Photo contributor: Frank Biriny, MD.

Assessment/Analysis
- Mental status
- Pain
- Presence of surface trauma: lacerations, avulsions
- If drainage is noted from the ears or nose, two tests are used at bedside to determine possible CSF leak
  - Halo Test (ring): allow blood from the ear to drop on a piece of gauze. If CSF is in the blood, a yellow "halo" will form outside the blood-stained portion of the gauze
  - Glucose Test: collect clear drainage from the nose on a glucose strip. CSF is high in glucose; generally nasal drainage is not[27]
  - Both tests can produce false positives and are not reliable[27]
  - β_2–Transferrin: involves a laboratory study on the fluid for detecting the presence of CSF. This test is the most reliable[27]
- Laboratory Studies
  - ABGs, if indicated
- CT scan of the head and possible MRI scan

Interventions
- Maintain airway
- Antibiotics if an open skull fracture
- Monitor ICP and treat increased ICP
- Instruct patient to avoid blowing nose or sneezing
- Avoid nasogastric tubes, nasal cannula, or nasal intubation
- Severe cases may require surgical intervention

Evaluation
- Patent airway
- Hemodynamic status
- Reassess for changes in the LOC
- Monitor and maintain normal ICP
- Assess for cranial nerve damage

Spinal Cord Injuries

Spinal cord injuries vary in presentation based on the level of injury on the spine and the portion of the spinal cord that is injured.

Complete Cord Injuries

In complete cord injuries, there is a transection of the cord. Patients have no sensory or motor function below the level of injury. See Figure 4-4 for the level of spinal cord and correlating function.

Partial/Incomplete Spinal Cord Injuries
- **Anterior cord:** complete motor loss below the lesion. Loss of pain and temperature perception with intact vibration, light touch, and positioning perception[29]
- **Posterior cord:** loss of light touch, proprioception, and vibration, but not pain or motor function
- **Central cord syndrome:** quadriparesis with greater loss of motor function in *upper extremities* rather than in lower extremities, variable sensory loss
- **Brown-Sequard syndrome:** loss of motor function on the *same side* as the injury. Sensory loss (pain and temperature) on the opposite side
- **Cauda equina syndrome:** damage to the lower spinal cord resulting in bowel, bladder, and sexual dysfunction

Assessment/Analysis
- Complete Cord
  - No motor or sensory function below the injury
  - No reflexes below the injury
  - Loss of autonomic nervous system functioning[29]
    - Hypotension due to venous pooling
    - Bradycardia with normal or strong pulse
    - Loss of bowel or bladder control
    - Poikilothermia: inability to regulate body temperature
  - Respiratory depression

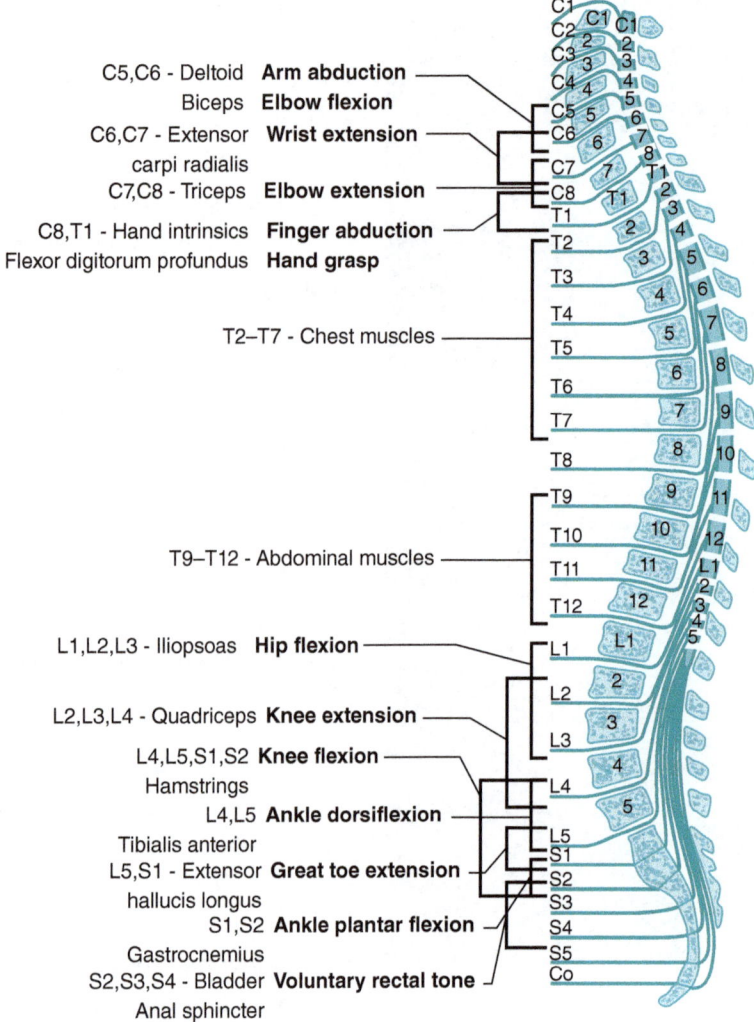

FIGURE 4-4 **Spinal Cord level with corresponding function. Each spinal nerve is named for its corresponding vertebrae**
Reproduced with permission from Tintinalli J, Stapcyzynski J, Ma OJ, et al: Tintinalli's Emergency Medicine: A Comprehensive Study Guide, 8th ed. New York: McGraw-Hill Education; 2015.

- Partial/incomplete cord
  - Assessment findings vary by the location of the injury, as previously described
  - Sacral sparing
    - Intact sensation in the perianal area
    - Voluntary control over the anal sphincter
    - Purposeful control over the great toe flexion
- Shallow or decreased work of breathing indicates high-level injury
- Laboratory studies
  - CBC with differential
  - Serum chemistries
  - Coagulation studies
  - Blood bank analysis (Type and Screen/Cross), if a transfusion is likely
- Lateral and oblique spinal X-rays
- CT scan or MRI of cervical, thoracic, and lumber spine

Interventions
- Maintain airway
- Monitor hemodynamic status
- Establish IV access for crystalloid fluids/blood products/ medications as needed
  - Caution with IV fluids: assess for pulmonary edema
  - If no improvement after fluid bolus, consider inotropic support
  - IV atropine for symptomatic bradycardia[28]
  - Consider IV steroids: steroid use is falling out of favor due to conflicting evidence, but may still be in local hospital protocols[30]
- Maintain temperature stability
- Prepare for admission or transfer

Evaluation
- Airway patency
- Hemodynamic status
- Changes in sensation or movement

Spinal Shock

Spinal Shock results from damage to the nerve fibers of the spinal cord resulting in a *temporary* loss of sensation and movement. Spinal shock does *not* result in circulatory collapse and should not be confused with neurogenic shock. The term refers to a "shock" to any level of the spinal cord through trauma. In injuries to the spinal cord above T6, neurogenic shock can occur.[31]

Assessment/Analysis
- Symptom onset shortly after injury
- Temporary loss of
  - Sensory function
  - Motor function
  - Reflexes
  - Bowel and bladder dysfunction
- May take hours for all symptoms to fully present
- Variable duration of symptoms; hours to years for complete resolution[29]
- Laboratory studies
  - CBC with differential
  - Serum chemistries
  - Coagulation studies
- CT scan or MRI of cervical, thoracic, and lumber spine

Intervention
- Maintain airway
- Hemodynamic monitoring
- Spinal precautions to prevent further injury
- Establish IV access for crystalloid fluids, blood products, and medications as needed
  - Steroids (methylprednisolone) to reduce inflammation in the first 8 hours (30 mg/kg bolus over 15 minutes followed 45 minutes after infusion by a 5.4 mg/kg/hr drip)
  - Steroid use is falling out of favor due to conflicting evidence, but may still be in local hospital protocols[30]
- Surgical spinal decompression may be indicated
- Spinal stabilization, often surgical fixation, until injury is healed
- Laboratory studies
  - CBC with differential
  - Serum chemistries
  - Coagulation studies
- CT scan and/or MRI of cervical, thoracic, and lumber spine

Evaluate
- Maintain airway
- Hemodynamic status
- Maintain spinal precautions as appropriate
- Reassess neurological status after any movement
- Monitor progression of symptoms

Neurogenic Shock

Neurogenic shock is the loss of sympathetic tone resulting from damage to sympathetic nerve fibers. It is most associated with spinal injuries above the level of T6. Neurogenic shock is a life-threatening event and is treated using shock protocols. See the Shock chapter (chapter 5) for additional information.

Assessment/Analysis
- Hypotension
- Bradycardia (not tachycardia as in other forms of shock)
- Shallow breathing
- Warm, normal skin color
- Priapism
- Inability to regulate core body temperature
- Laboratory studies
  - CBC with differential
  - Serum chemistries
  - Coagulation studies
- CT chest and abdomen
  - Look for a concurrent occult hemorrhage in chest and abdomen that may also be present

Interventions
- Maintain airway
- Monitor hemodynamics, pulse oximetry, and capnography
- Spinal protection precautions
- Establish IV access for crystalloid fluids, blood products, and medications as needed
- Interventions to treat shock: including isotonic IV fluids (see Shock chapter [chapter 5])
- Warming measures to prevent hypothermia

Evaluate
- Airway and hemodynamic status
- Spinal protection precautions
- Monitor for fluid overload with fluid volume replacement in the presence of bradycardia

Autonomic Dysreflexia

Autonomic dysreflexia, or hyperreflexia, is a life threatening complication of spinal cord injury (usually above T6) presenting when cord injured patients experience a vasoactive crisis secondary to noxious stimuli. Vasoconstriction results below the level of the injury increasing blood pressure in the upper part of the body. Baroreceptors sense the sudden increase in blood pressure and respond by inducing bradycardia and vasodilation above the level of the injury.[28] Autonomic dysreflexia should be suspected in patients with complete spinal cord injuries.

Assessment/Analysis
- Assess for noxious stimuli and resolve as soon as possible
  - Full bladder: possibly from an indwelling catheter
  - Full rectum
  - Acute abdomen

- Decubitus ulcer
- Renal calculi
- Cystitis
- Symptoms
  - Sudden severe headache
  - Anxiousness
  - Nasal congestion
  - Dizziness
  - Confusion
  - Dilated pupils
  - Hypertension
  - Dysrhythmias: primarily bradycardia
  - Flushing above the injury
  - Clamminess below the injury

Interventions
- Find and treat the cause of autonomic dysreflexia by removing noxious stimuli
  - Drain the distended bladder
  - Checking for kinked or clogged catheter tubing
  - Assist the patient into the sitting position to allow blood flow to the lower extremities
  - Resolving fecal impaction
- Establish IV access for crystalloid fluids, blood products, medications as needed
- Treat systolic blood pressure over 150 mm Hg[32]
  - Nifedipine (Procardia™)
    - Caution with adverse effect of extreme hypotension
  - Prazosin (Minipress™)
  - Captopril
  - Hydralazine
  - Nitrates
- Elevate head of bed
- Plan for hospital admission or transfer

Evaluation
- Resolution of symptoms
- Airway patency
- Hemodynamic status for hypertension and cardiac arrhythmias
- Skin for signs of ulcers or infection
- Circulation below the level of the injury

REFERENCES

1. Waxman SG. Chapter 8. Cranial nerves and pathways. In: Waxman SG, ed. *Clinical Neuroanatomy*. 27th ed. New York, NY: McGraw-Hill; 2013.
2. *What is Alzheimer's?*, Alzheimer's Association Web Site, http://www.alz.org/alzheimers_disease_what_is_alzheimers.asp. Accessed November 8, 2015.
3. Vascular Dementia, Alzheimer's Association Web Site, http://www.alz.org/dementia/vascular-dementia-symptoms.asp. Accessed November 8, 2015.
4. Vriesendorp F. *Treatment and prognosis of Guillain-Barre syndrome in adults*. Upto Date Website, http://www.uptodate.com/contents/treatment-and-prognosis-of-guillain-barre-syndrome-in-adults. Updated January 3, 2015. Accessed November 3, 2015.
5. Andrus P, Guthrie J. Acute peripheral neurologic disorders. In: Tintinalli JE, Stapczynski J, Ma O, et al, eds. *Tintinalli's Emergency Medicine: A Comprehensive Study Guide*. 8th ed. New York, NY: McGraw-Hill; 2016.
6. Goadsby PJ, Raskin NH. Migraine and other primary headache disorders. In: Kasper D, Fauci A, Hauser S, et al, eds. *Harrison's Principles of Internal Medicine*. 19th ed. New York, NY: McGraw-Hill; 2015.
7. Petersen A, Barloese M, Jensen R. Oxygen treatment of cluster headache: a review. *Cephalalgia*. 2014;34(13):1079–1087. http://www.ncbi.nlm.nih.gov/pubmed?term=24723673. Accessed December 3, 2015.
8. Hunder G. *Treatment of giant cell (temporal) arteritis*, UptoDate Website, http://www.uptodate.com/contents/treatment-of-giant-cell-temporal-arteritis?source=see_link. Updated November 2, 2015. Accessed November 20, 2015.
9. McLaughlin JC. Brain, cranial, and maxillofacial trauma. In: Emergency Nurses Association. *Trauma Nursing Core Course, Provider manual*. 7th ed. Des Plaines, IL: Author;2014:105–122.
10. Wright DW, Merck LH. Head trauma. In: Tintinalli JE, Stapczynski J, Ma O, et al, eds. *Tintinalli's Emergency Medicine: A Comprehensive Study Guide*. 8th ed. New York, NY: McGraw-Hill; 2016.
11. Brophy GM, Human T, Shutter L. Emergency neurological life support: pharmacotherapy. *Neurocrit Care*. 2015;23:S48–S68. doi: 10.1007/s12028-015-0158-1
12. Complications of Shunt Systems. Hydrocephalus Association Web Site, http://www.hydroassoc.org/complications-of-shunt-systems/. Accessed December 3, 2015.
13. Horton C, Byrd L, Lucht H, et al. Emergency care of children with high-technology neurologic disorders. *Clin Pediatr Emerg Med*. 2012;13(2):114–124. doi:10.1016/j.cpem.2012.04.004
14. Peard AS. Communicable and infectious disease emergencies. In: Hoyt KS, Selfridge-Thomas J, eds. *Emergency Nursing Core Curriculum*. 6th ed. St. Louis, MO: Saunders/Elsevier; 2007:438–482.
15. Muller M. *Pediatric Bacterial Meningitis Clinical Presentation* Medscape. http://emedicine.medscape.com/article/961497-clinical. Published August 19, 2015. Accessed December 1, 2015.
16. Van de Beek D, Farrar JJ, de Gans J, et al. Adjunctive dexamethasone in bacterial meningitis: a meta-analysis of individual patient data. *The Lancet Neurology*. 2010;9(3):254–263.
17. Baxter CS. Neurological emergencies. In: Hoyt KS, Selfridge-Thomas J. *Emergency Nursing Core Curriculum*. 6th ed. St. Louis, MO: Saunders/Elsevier; 2007:510–535.
18. Kaneshiro N. *Febrile Seizures*. US National Library of Medicine Medline Plus Website, https://www.nlm.nih.gov/medlineplus/ency/article/000980.htm. Updated February 26, 2014. Accessed December 3, 2015.
19. Golder D. Childhood illness. In: Emergency Nurses Association. *Emergency Nurse Pediatric Course. Provider Manual*. 4th ed. Des Plaines, IL: Author; 2012:147–170.
20. Segan S. Absence seizures: epidemiology. MedScape. http://reference.medscape.com/article/1183858-overview#a3. Updated November 23, 2015. Accessed April 17, 2016.
21. American Stroke Association. *Why Rush? TIA is an Emergency Stroke Connection Published January/February 2009*. http://www.strokeassociation.org/STROKEORG/AboutStroke/TypesofStroke/TIA/Why-Rush-TIA-is-an-Emergency_UCM_310729_Article.jsp#.VxOEK2PGLdk. Updated October 2012. Accessed April 17, 2016.
22. American Heart Association/American Stroke Association. *Types of aphasia*. http://www.strokeassociation.org/STROKEORG/LifeAfterStroke/RegainingIndependence/CommunicationChallenges/Types-of-Aphasia_UCM_310096_Article.jsp#.VxN_IGPGLdk. Updated March 6, 2015. Accessed April 17, 2016.
23. Jauch EC, Saver JL, Adams HP, et al. Guidelines for the early management of patients with acute ischemic stroke. *Stroke*. 2013;44:870–947. doi: 10.1161/STR.0b013e318284056a

24. Bruno A, Saha C, Williams LS. Percent change on the National Institutes of Health Stroke Scale: a useful acute stroke outcome measure. *Journal of Stroke and Cerebrovascular Disease*. http://www.strokejournal.org/article/S1052-3057(08)00182-1/abstract. Published January 18, 2009. Accessed April 12, 2016.
25. Mathew A, Kumar A. Focus On: Reversal of Anticoagulation. *ACEP News*. https://www.acep.org/Clinical—Practice-Management/Focus-On–Reversal-of-Anticoagulation/. Published June 2010. Accessed April 12, 2016.
26. Dries D, Chief Editor, Geibel J, et al. Initial Evaluation of the Trauma Patient. *Medcape*. http://emedicine.medscape.com/article/434707-overview#a3. Updated January 31, 2014, Accessed November 29, 2015.
27. McLaughlin JC. Brain, cranial, and maxillofacial trauma. In: Emergency Nurses Association. *Trauma Nursing Core Course, Provider manual*. 7th ed. Des Plaines, IL: Author; 2014:105–122.
28. Smith DA. Neurologic trauma. In: Hoyt KS, Selfridge-Thomas J, eds. *Emergency Nursing Core Curriculum*. 6th ed. St. Louis, MO: Saunders/Elsevier; 2007:820–847.
29. Crowley, M. Spinal cord and vertebral column trauma. In: Emergency Nurses Association. *Trauma Nursing Core Course, Provider manual*. 7th ed. Des Plaines, IL: Author; 2014:173–192.
30. Hulbert R, Hadley MN, Walters BC, et al. Pharmacological therapy for acute spinal cord injuries. *Neurosurgery*. Chapter 8. 2013:72;93–105. http://www.metrolinatrauma.org/Neurosurg_2013_-_Pharmacologic_Management.pdf. Accessed April 2016.
31. Popa C, Popa F, Grigorean VT, et al. Vascular Dysfunctions Following Spinal Cord Injury. *J Med Life*. 2010;3(3):275–285. http://www.ncbi.nlm.nih.gov/pmc/articles/PMC3019008/. Accessed April 12, 2016.
32. Krassioukov A, Warburton DE, Teasell R, Eng JJ; Spinal Cord Injury Rehabilitation Evidence Research Team. A systematic review of the management of autonomic dysreflexia after spinal cord injury. *Arch Phys Med Rehabil*. 2009;90(4):682–695.

Practice Questions

Question	Rationale
1. A patient presents to the emergency department with hypertension, left side weakness, and an inability to speak. The patient appears frustrated and anxious but is able to follow commands. The emergency nurse understands the patient has likely had a stroke in what area of the brain? a. Huntington's area: Located in the left Parietal lobe b. Cushing's area: Located in the right Limbic lobe c. Broca's area: Located in the dominant frontal lobe d. Wernicke's area: Located in the right temporal lobe	*Answer: c* Interruption of blood flow to Broca's area affects the motor component of speech. The patient is able to understand and follow commands so the patient can still processes speech. Inability to understand commands would indicate a receptive aphasia secondary to damage in Wernicke's area. Huntington and Cushing's area do not exist as anatomical features of the brain.
2. A patient is brought into the emergency department by EMS. EMS states the patient's car was hit on the driver's side by another vehicle. The patient's head shattered the side window and there is a laceration on the left side of the skull. EMS states the patient was unconscious at the scene but was alert and talking on the way in. He complained of a severe headache and had weakened grips on the right side. Upon arrival, however, the patient has again lost consciousness and has a left fixed and dilated pupil. The ED nurse suspects the patient has a. A subdural bleed b. An epidural bleed c. A diffuse axonal injury d. A concussion	*Answer: b* Epidural bleeds are associated with trauma and often have a lucid period prior to rapid deterioration. Because the bleeding is arterial, usually from the middle meningeal artery, with a hematoma developing between the skull and tough covering of the brain. Injury side pupil dilation and opposite side motor weakness is consistent with this type of injury.
3. A 38-year-old male presents to the emergency department complaining of weakness and numbness of the lower extremities. He had a fever with "the flu" a few weeks ago, but no other medical history. He states the numbness started in his feet but has now progressed to the level of his hips and he is so weak he can barely stand. Exam shows depressed deep tendon reflexes and symmetrical weakness of the lower extremities. The ED nurse anticipates this patient will need a. Admission to the ICU on an insulin infusion b. Ultrasound cardiovascular exam of bilateral lower extremities for arterial occlusion c. Lumbar puncture to rule out meningitis d. Admission to the ICU and mechanical ventilation	*Answer: d* Ascending symmetrical weakness and numbness with loss of deep tendon reflexes indicates Guillain-Barré Syndrome. One quarter of all patients with Guillain-Barre require mechanical ventilation due to respiratory failure as the syndrome progresses to breathing muscles. The patient's history does not suggest he has hyperglycemia and would need an insulin infusion. He is not exhibiting signs of arterial occlusion in the lower extremities or signs associated with meningitis.

Question	Rationale
4. Upon entering a room with a patient complaining of a headache, the patient is found to be pacing the room and refusing to lie on the bed. The patient complains of sharp pain behind the right eye. The right eye is swollen and drooping with tear production noted. What medication is considered to be most effective for this type of headache? a. Hydromorphone IV with a Normal Saline bolus b. Proparacaine drops to the affected eye c. High flow oxygen through a non-rebreather mask d. Compazine™/Benadryl™/Toradol™ combination	*Answer: c* The unilateral pain behind the right eye, inability to sit still, and agitation are indicative of a cluster headache. High flow oxygen is the preferred treatment for cluster headaches. Compazine™/Benadryl™/Toradol™ combination is the treatment for a migraine headache, which involve bilateral pain, nausea, and photophobia. Opioids are not usually the first line treatment for suspected cluster headaches, and proparacaine eye drops would not be indicated.
5. A seven-month old girl is brought into the emergency department by her mother. The mother states the little girl was fine at daycare today, but tonight she found the toddler "jerking her arms and legs with her eyes rolled back in her head." The child is warm to the touch with a rectal temp of 100.9°F (38.3°C), rhinorrhea, and tachycardia. Otherwise the child has clear lung sounds and appears well hydrated. The ED nurse reassures the patient's mother by telling her a. There was nothing the mother could do to prevent the illness b. Two-thirds of patients will never experience a second episode c. Anti-seizure medications are very effective these days d. A CT scan is non-invasive and will reveal any brain damage	*Answer: b* The patient is presenting with a febrile seizure. CT scans and anti-seizure medications are not appropriate for this patient since febrile seizures rarely cause permanent damage to the brain, and often do not recur.
6. A patient with a history of T6 cord injury presents with a headache, high blood pressure, nasal congestion, and appears flushed and diaphoretic. The first action would be to a. Start two large bore IVs and initiate a fluid bolus b. Give IV Mannitol 0.9 mg/kg with 10% of the total dose as a bolus followed by an infusion of the rest over the next 60 minutes c. Check the patient's indwelling urinary catheter for kinks d. Obtain a 12 lead ECG	*Answer: c* This patient appears to be suffering from autonomic dysreflexia, a dangerous complication of spinal cord injuries that can be triggered by something as simple as a distended bladder. Of the given answers, unkinking the catheter tubing is the only intervention that would remove a stimulus that could trigger autonomic dysreflexia.

Question	Rationale
7. A 53-year-old patient presents to the emergency department by ambulance with a chief complaint of nausea and dizziness with headache. EMS started an IV and gave a 500 mL normal saline bolus and 4 mg of Zofran™ prior to arrival. Vital signs are P-70; R-20; BP-169/59, SPO$_2$ 99% on room air. The patient states his main complaint is his headache, which has been going on for a few days but is now much worse. He also states he's been "bumping into things, lately and I might need my glasses checked." Eyes are reactive, but the left pupil is 2 mm larger than the right. On exam the ED nurse notes no unilateral deficits. The priority is to a. Obtain labs, ECG, and a full set of vitals b. Notify the emergency provider with anticipating an order for a stat non-contrast head CT c. Obtain a visual acuity exam and collect a detailed medical history d. Apply high flow oxygen via non-rebreather mask	*Answer: b* This patient has symptoms of a posterior stroke, which can often be missed because they do not present with unilateral weakness. Headache with nausea and visual disturbance coupled with the difference in pupil size (anisocoria) should raise the nurse's concern of a cerebrovascular accident. Other options such as obtaining labs and a visual acuity exam are not the priorities for this. High flow oxygen is treatment for cluster headaches.
8. A patient presents to the ER through triage with a headache. She was seen at urgent care 6 days ago for a sinus infection but now reports "I thought I was all better, but suddenly tonight it is much worse." The patient is febrile at 103.6°F (39.8°C) and complains of a stiff neck, which is a very painful to move. The triage nurse prioritizes which interventions for this patient? a. IV access, labs, and blood cultures followed by antibiotics b. Lumbar puncture and head CT scan, followed by antibiotics c. Head CT scan, followed by LP and antibiotics only after CT results d. Lumbar puncture, head CT scan with antibiotics after LP results	*Answer: a* The question asks the nurse to prioritize interventions for a patient with suspected bacterial meningitis. Initiation of antibiotics in these patients should not be delayed while waiting for neuroimaging or LP results. Head CT would be performed prior to lumbar puncture to rule out the risk of herniation secondary to a space-occupying lesion.

Question	Rationale
9. A patient returns from CT with a change in condition. Earlier the patient was confused and restless but now the patient only responds to a sternal rub. The patient's pulse has decreased from 120 bpm to 64 bpm. Blood pressure was 150/70 mm Hg and is now 180/40 mm Hg. Breathing has become increasingly irregular in both rate and depth. The nurse recognizes that a. This is Cushing's Triad: increasing pulse pressure with systolic hypertension, bradycardia, and irregular respirations, a sign of increasing pressure inside the skull b. This is Honing's Sign: hypertension, tachypnea with a normal pulse rate, and a sign of increasing intracranial pressure c. This is Kehr's Sign: indication that there is bleeding inside the peritoneal cavity, possibly a ruptured spleen d. This is Homer's Triad: deterioration in mentation with a decrease in heart rate indicates bleeding in the brain	*Answer: a* Increasing hypertension with a widening pulse pressure, bradycardia, and irregular respiratory patterns is Cushing's Triad. Don't be fooled by the "normal" pulse of 64 bpm. It clearly is trending down from previous tachycardia. Kehr's sign is pain in the left shoulder when the patient is prone. Honing's Sign and Homer's Triad are not actual clinical signs.
10. What medications are expected to be ordered for the patient with Cushing's Triad? a. Atropine b. Mannitol c. Octreotide d. Hypotonic solution IV, such as 0.45% NaCl	*Answer: b* Mannitol is an osmotic diuretic that decreases intracranial pressure. A Hypotonic IV solution such as 0.45% NaCl would not have an osmotic diuretic effect. Atropine and octreotide would not be appropriate.
11. A young patient presents to the emergency department with her mother. The patient has a history of hydrocephalus and had a shunt placement 4 months ago. The patient is now complaining of a severe headache whenever she is sitting up and her fontanels are depressed. The concern for this patient is a. Shunt malfunction, which is common in the first 2 years after placement b. Shunt infection, which is caused by the patient's normal flora and can lead to septic shock c. Overdrainage of the shunt, which requires supportive therapy, seizure protocols, and surgery to replace the shunt d. Shunt dislodgement: the distal end of the shunt has moved	*Answer: c* The depressed fontanels and headache when she is sitting up are signs that the shunt is draining too much. If the patient had signs of increasing intracranial pressure (ICP) such as increased irritability and changes in her level of consciousness, a malfunctioning shunt would be a more likely cause for symptoms.

Question	Rationale
12. A patient is brought in by ambulance with aphasia and right-sided weakness. The stroke protocol was activated in the field. EMS states the patient lives alone, and had been seen working in her garden 2 hours prior to the 911 call. The patient can follow commands but only repeat the words "no, not." Her right-sided hand grasps are significantly weaker than her left, and she has some moderate right-sided arm drift. She cannot hold her right leg up against gravity at all. The doctor is in the room on patient arrival and listens to the EMS report. The doctor asks the paramedic, "Did you check a blood sugar?" Why was this question asked? a. Hypertension and diabetes increase the risk for stroke b. High blood sugar can inhibit the effectiveness of alteplase (tPA) c. Hypoglycemia can mimic stroke symptoms, but is easily reversible d. Hyperglycemia can increase the chances of hemorrhagic stroke	*Answer: c* Low blood sugar should be checked on patients presenting with altered mental status including symptoms associated with stroke. While a history of hypertension and diabetes are risk factors for stroke, reducing potential stroke mimics, such as hypoglycemia is a more immediate priority.
13. A patient is brought in by ambulance after having a seizure in the local discount store. When EMS arrives, the patient is lethargic and confused but is able to speak in sentences and answer questions. The patient states that he has a history of seizures and doesn't like going to the hospital. The nurse should ask that patient a. Have there been any changes in your medications, or have you missed taking your medication recently? b. Has there been increased stress in your life? c. Have you recently suffered a head injury or viral illness? d. Do you regularly check your blood sugar?	*Answer: a* Changes is seizure medications or missed doses can lead to subtherapeutic levels. Subtherapeutic levels place the patient at an increased risk for more seizure activity or changes in the pattern of seizure activity. Stress is not a cause for actual seizures. Seizures may be a symptom of an illness, injury or severe hypoglycemia; however, knowing that this patient has a known seizure disorder, initial history should focus on the patient's medications and seizure history.
14. A patient presents to the emergency department through triage. The patient tells the ED nurse that he has "…the worst headache of my life, and I never even get headaches." He is nauseated and has photophobia. He has no history of recent trauma and no unilateral deficits are detected. Based on his presentation, the ED nurse anticipates a. High flow oxygen will be ordered prior to any pain medication b. The patient will be placed in a dark room and given IV fluids, narcotic pain medication and antiemetics c. A stat head CT scan will be ordered d. IV fluids, ketorolac, prochlorperazine, and diphenhydramine	*Answer: c* The description of "worst headache of my life" and no history of recurrent headaches increases the suspicion that this patient's presentation could be experiencing a hemorrhagic stroke. High-flow oxygen is a treatment for a cluster headache, which presents often with unilateral pain behind the eye. IV fluids and medications such as ketorolac and diphenhydramine are often used to treat migraine headaches.

Question	Rationale
15. A patient presents to the emergency department by ambulance for stroke-like symptoms including left-side weakness and facial droop lasting approximately 25 minutes. On arrival, her neuro exam is normal. Vitals are stable and blood sugar is 120 mg/dL. She states this is the third time she has experienced similar symptoms in the past week; the first two times, symptoms lasted only a few minutes and she did not call the ambulance. The nurse understands a. This patient is diabetic and suffering from low blood sugar b. This patient is exhibiting signs of recurrent partial seizure activity c. This patient is faking it to get attention and wasting EMS resources d. This patient is describing a TIA and is at high risk for ischemic stroke	*Answer: d* TIA is highly correlated with ischemic stroke within 12 months if left untreated. Hypoglycemia can mimic stroke like symptoms, but low blood sugar is incorrect because the blood sugar is normal without intervention.
16. A trauma patient is brought into the emergency department after being assaulted outside a casino. He smells of ETOH and is bleeding from the back of his skull. He does not open his eyes to pain but withdraws his arm when an IV start is attempted. He does not speak or answer questions but makes incomprehensible sounds. The ED nurse assesses this patient as having a Glasgow Coma Scale of a. 3 b. 5 c. 7 d. 15	*Answer: c* 7: Eye opening = 1, incomprehensible sounds = 2, withdraws from pain = 4. 15 is normal and 3 is the lowest possible score on GCS.
17. A patient was driving his car at high speeds and was involved in a head-on collision with a truck. The emergency nurse collects some of the drainage on a clean gauze and observes a ring around it. To confirm the drainage is cerebral spinal fluid (CSF), the B_2-Transferrin lab test is sent, and the results confirm the presence of CSF. The following injury is suspected a. Basilar skull fracture b. Increased ICP c. Subdural hemorrhage d. Diffuse axonal injury	*Answer: a* The halo sign has an appearance of a ring around drainage from the nose or ear when CSF is present. CSF also contains glucose and the drainage will reveal a positive glucose although glucose is also present in nasal drainage. Since both tests can produce a false positive, the most reliable test is the B_2-Transferrin that requires laboratory testing. A basilar skull fracture can result in a tear to the brain tissue causing a CSF leak. Other concomitant injuries such as a subdural hemorrhage or diffuse axonal injury could be present; however, these injuries alone do not cause CSF to leak. Increased ICP can result from cerebral ischemia.

Question	Rationale
18. A patient having problems with hearing and balance may have damage to which cranial nerve? a. V: Trigeminal b. X: Vagus c. VIII: Vestibulocochlear d. II: Optic	*Answer: c* The VIII cranial nerve is responsible for hearing and balance. The optic nerve is responsible for sight and the Vagus nerve is involved in control of the heart, lungs, and digestive functions. The trigeminal nerve is involved in mastication.
19. The emergency nurse suspects that a patient's neurological status is changing. The best indicator for assessing this change is a. Widening pulse pressure b. Level of consciousness c. Blood glucose d. Deep tendon reflexes	*Answer: b* A person's level of consciousness is the first indicator of a changing neurologic status. While the other parameters may all be assessed to evaluate neurological function, a change in level of consciousness is the first sign in neurological deterioration.
20. A 70-year-old man arrives in triage. He is a recovering alcoholic. He started complaining of a headache early this morning and has become increasingly disoriented over the past 10 hours. No known trauma has occurred, but his wife states that he has had increasing problems with balance and memory over the past 2 weeks. He has difficulty staying awake in triage. The ED nurse suspects a. Elevated blood alcohol level b. Hypoglycemia c. Subdural hemorrhage either subacute or chronic d. Elevated Ammonia levels	*Answer: c* All the listed answers may cause deteriorating mental status but the patient's history of alcohol abuse increases his risk for a chronic subdural bleed. Subdural bleeding usually is from small bridging veins. These bridging veins can weaken with chronic heavy alcohol use. Memory loss, headache, and somnolence are also consistent with a subdural bleed.
21. The ED nurse responds to a patient's room to find the patient actively seizing with full tonic-clonic activity. The first priority is a. Be sure the bed rails are up and padded, and if possible place patient on his or her left side to reduce risk of aspiration b. Reassuring family saying, "It will be over soon" c. Having the medical provider observe the seizure to identify the cause d. Inserting an oral airway into the patient's mouth so he does not swallow or bite his tongue	*Answer: a* Patient safety is the priority in most situations. Here the nurse should make sure that secondary trauma, injury or aspiration, does not occur during the seizure. False reassurance and oral airway insertion are not appropriate and seeking prompt provider evaluation could be delegated while the nurse assures patient safety.

Question	Rationale
22. The patient has a closed head injury. Pupils are noted to be fixed and dilated. This indicates damage to which cranial nerve (CN)? a. Optic: CN II b. Oculomotor: CN III c. Abducens: CN VI d. Trochlear: CN IV	*Answer: b* There are four cranial nerves innervating the eyes, but only one is associated with the pupils. The third cranial nerve (oculomotor) controls pupil constriction and dilation and eye movement. The optic nerve is a sensory nerve involved with sight. Abducens and Trochlear nerves control the movement of the eye itself.
23. A patient has a spinal injury. Upon assessment, greater loss of motor function in his upper extremities compared to his lower extremities is noted. This is consistent with a. Central cord syndrome b. Brown-Sequard syndrome c. Cauda equina syndrome d. Posterior cord syndrome	*Answer: a* Central Cord Syndrome manifests as quadriparesis with greater motor function lost in the upper limbs. Brown-Sequard Syndrome is loss of motor function on the same side as the injury with sensory loss on the opposite side. Cauda equina Syndrome is a lower cord injury that results in loss of bowel, bladder, and sexual function. Posterior Cord Syndrome is a loss of light touch and sensation but no loss of pain or motor function.
24. A patient is brought in by EMS after being thrown from a horse. The patient is in cervical-spine precautions. Vital signs are P-56; R-8; BP-88/45 mm Hg. Priapism is noted. The ED nurse suspects a. The patient has suffered massive internal bleeding and is in hypovolemic shock b. The patient has suffered a spinal injury and is in neurogenic shock c. The patient has suffered a massive head injury with increasing ICP d. The patient should have been intubated in the field	*Answer: b* This is neurogenic shock secondary to spinal trauma. Priapism would not manifest in hypovolemic shock alone but rather is a finding in neurogenic shock. Internal bleed is still a possibility on this patient. Increasing ICP would yield bradycardia with hypertension rather than hypotension.
25. Raccoon eyes and Battle sign are indications of what type of injury? a. Domestic violence b. Subdural hematoma c. Diffuse axonal injury d. Basilar skull fracture	*Answer: d* Battle sign (mastoid ecchymosis) and raccoon eyes (periorbital ecchymosis) are associated with basilar skull fractures. Other answer options are injuries that would not exhibit raccoon eyes or battle signs.
26. The ED nurse is asked to conduct a FAST assessment on a patient who presents in triage with stroke-like symptoms. What is assessed? a. Fasting glucose, articulate speech, smile, and touch sensitivity b. Facial droop, arm strength, speech difficulty, and time since onset c. Facial droop, arm drift, smile, and touching finger to nose d. Fine motor skills, accurate memory, sensitivity to touch, and time since onset	*Answer: b* FAST is an acronym for Facial droop, Arm strength, Speech difficulty, and Time since onset. FAST is a somewhat simplified version of the Cincinnati Prehospital Stroke Scale. Either is useful in detecting the symptoms of ischemic stroke. The other answers are not correct acronyms.

Question	Rationale
27. A patient arrives at the emergency room after being hit in the head with a falling pipe from scaffolding. Coworkers say he briefly lost consciousness at the scene but on arrival he states he is fine; he is only here because "work" made him come in and get checked out. After waiting in the waiting room for one hour, the patient comes up to the triage desk and states his vision is now blurry. The triage nurse a. Requests a urine sample for drug screening b. Should reassess the patient's neuro status c. Should reassess a visual acuity check d. Rechecks vital signs	*Answer: b* Given the mechanism of injury and the brief loss of consciousness, the patient is at risk for a close head injury. The blurred vision may be an early sign of increasing ICP and so reassessment of neurological status is warranted. An employer may require drug screening, if the injury is work-related however; this is not a priority until a changing neurological status has been assessed. Visual acuity is not a top priority either and vital signs may warrant reassessing after assessing the patient's neuro status.
28. The emergency nurse knows widening pulse pressures occur with increased intracranial pressure due to a. Increased cerebral autoregulation b. Decreased cardiac output c. Increased cerebral perfusion d. Decreased pulmonary return	*Answer: a* Patients experiencing increased intracranial pressure will exhibit Cushing's response, which is widening pulse pressure, bradycardia, and decreased respiratory effort. Widening pulse pressures occur when increased intracranial pressure (ICP) impedes blood flow to the brain. Cerebral autoregulation is the brain's mechanism to ensure sufficient nutrient delivery. Because of autoregulation, systolic blood pressure increases attempting to maintain adequate brain perfusion despite the increased ICP. Bradycardia can decrease cardiac output but generally does not affect widening pulse pressures. Cerebral perfusion would most likely decrease due to changes in MAP (mean arterial pressure) and ICP. Decreased pulmonary return is a distractor.
29. A patient with a history of Guillain-Barre arrives to the emergency department in severe respiratory distress requiring emergent intubation. In preparing for rapid sequence intubation, the emergency nurse knows which medication is contraindicated? a. Rocuronium b. Etomidate c. Succinylcholine d. Propofol	*Answer: c* For patients with Guillain-Barre, succinylcholine is contraindicated due to the risk of severe hyperkalemia. Hyperkalemia occurs due to the muscle atrophy from Guillain-Barre that can lead to increase of acetylcholine receptors and alterations in the sodium-potassium pump causing an increased sensitivity to succinylcholine. There is no known contraindication with the other medications listed for Guillain-Barre.
30. A mother arrives with her 3-month-old infant. The child is febrile with a new high-pitched cry; she is restless and inconsolable. When examining the child for signs of dehydration, a tense, bulging fontanel is noted. The ED nurse suspects a. Pulmonary atresia b. Meningitis c. Supraventricular tachycardia d. Dehydration	*Answer: b* Infants cannot verbalize when they have a headache or stiff neck. A high-pitched cry, inconsolability, and bulging fontanels indicate increased intracranial pressure. This child needs blood cultures and antibiotics as soon as possible. The other options may cause a child to be restless but would not generally cause a tense, bulging fontanel.

Question	Rationale
31. A 17-year-old boy who suffered a brief loss of consciousness while playing football is being discharged. The ED nurse knows that the patient and parents require additional discharge teaching when they state a. "I won't return to football until my doctor says it is OK" b. "I know I can't play football, and it's OK since I really wanted to join the wrestling team anyway" c. "I will avoid TV, video games, and all other technology for now" d. "We will bring him back to the emergency department for decreasing level of consciousness or projectile vomiting"	*Answer: b* Contact sports should be avoided and wrestling would be considered a contact sport. The other answers listed are part of current recommended treatment for concussion. Brain rest and avoiding repeated trauma to the brain are important to allow the brain to heal and reduce the risk of post-concussive syndrome. Decreasing mental status or vomiting are signs of increasing ICP and would warrant returning to the emergency department for emergent evaluation.

Shock

Jayne McGrath, MS, RN, CEN, CCRN, CNS-BC

Shock is a condition of inadequate tissue perfusion resulting from disequilibrium between the oxygenated blood supply and demand for metabolic processes. As decreased perfusion fails to meet metabolic requirements, cellular damage occurs and inflammatory mediators are produced. This inflammatory response causes changes to the vasculature, which further jeopardizes perfusion. A deteriorating cycle follows of maldistributed blood flow and hypoperfusion that eventually causes organ dysfunction and failure.

Intrinsic compensatory mechanisms, such as an increased heart rate, respond early in shock to maintain tissue perfusion. When these mechanisms fail to meet perfusion requirements, anaerobic metabolism occurs causing a lactic acidosis. Although nonspecific, symptoms such as resting tachycardia, anxiety, mental status changes, and tachypnea can be early signs of shock.

A variety of triggers can begin the deteriorating process of shock. Knowing the precipitating cause of shock can improve the effectiveness of treatment. These varied causes are grouped into four different types or classifications of shock: cardiogenic, obstructive, distributive, and hypovolemic.

Cardiogenic Shock

Cardiogenic shock occurs with ineffective cardiac pump function. Decreased cardiac output ensues resulting in decreased tissue perfusion. Cardiogenic shock occurs in about 5 to 7% of patients with an ST-segment elevated myocardial infarction (STEMI)[1] but can also occur with traumatic injuries such as transection of a coronary structure. Other causes associated with cardiogenic shock can include heart failure and cardiomyopathy.

Assessment/Analysis
- Confusion, altered level of consciousness
- Hypotension
- Tachycardia
- Cool extremities
- Pallor
- Weak peripheral pulses
- Decreased urine output (oliguria)
- Symptoms associated with heart failure
  - Dyspnea
  - Decreased cardiac index
  - S3 and S4 heart sounds[2]
  - Crackles auscultated in lung fields
  - Jugular venous distention
  - Edema
- ECG
  - Possible elevated ST-segment reflective of acute MI pattern
  - Left ventricular hypertrophy pattern suggestive of heart failure
- Chest X-ray may reveal pulmonary congestion
- Transthoracic echocardiogram: impaired contractility of the left ventricle
- Elevated cardiac biomarkers
- Elevated serum lactate
- Elevated B-type natriuretic peptide (BNP)[3]

Interventions
- Support airway, breathing, and circulation as needed
- Pulse oximetry and capnography
- Administer oxygen as needed for pulse oximetry <94%
- Cardiac monitoring
- Establish IV access for crystalloids/blood products/medications as needed
- Interventions tailored to patient response
  - Cautious approach with IV fluid administration especially in the presence of heart failure
  - Cautious use of vasopressors—Increases afterload, adding to increased end-diastolic pressure and workload of myocardium
  - Inotropic agents may improve cardiac output, particularly Dobutamine
  - Diuretics
- Immediate coronary intervention in cardiac catheterization lab or surgical/procedural area, may be indicated
- Intra-aortic balloon counterpulsation via Intra-aortic balloon pump (IABP) provides augmented hemodynamic support, then decreases afterload and improves cardiac output

Evaluation
- Effective breathing and perfusion
- Hemodynamic stability
- Cardiac monitoring, pulse oximetry, and capnography
- Urine output

Obstructive Shock

In obstructive shock, circulating blood volume is typically sufficient. However, the sufficient blood flow is "blocked" or "obstructed" by a mechanical cause. The obstruction leads to decreased cardiac output resulting in an ultimate lack of effective tissue perfusion. Similar to other types of shock, determining the cause is essential for appropriate interventions. The three causes of shock in this category are pericardial tamponade, tension pneumothorax, and pulmonary embolus.

Pericardial Tamponade

The pericardium, a fibrous covering encasing the heart, is comprised of two layers: the visceral and parietal layers. The visceral pericardium attaches to the epicardium and the outer layer is the fibrous parietal layer. Between the visceral and parietal layers is a serious fluid that helps protect the heart. Normally, there are about 50 milliliters of pericardial fluid.[4] The excess accumulation of fluid within the pericardial sac is known as a pericardial effusion. Often, the fluid collects slowly over time, and the patient may not experience significant symptoms.

If the pericardial effusion continues to increase, or occurs quickly such as with a traumatic injury, the accumulating pericardial fluid exerts increased pressure constricting the heart causing a pericardial tamponade. Ventricular filling and myocardial function are inhibited. Effective cardiac output is obstructed leading to inadequate tissue perfusion and shock. About 2% of penetrating trauma results in a pericardial tamponade. The most common cause of pericardial tamponade is a malignancy.[5]

Assessment/Analysis
- Chest pain, possibly pleuritic in nature
- Dyspnea; possible orthopnea
- Feeling of impending doom
- Tachycardia
- Pulsus paradoxus
- Skin cool and pale
- Cyanosis
- Hypotension
- Elevated central venous pressure (CVP)
- Beck's triad
  - Muffled or distant heart tones
  - Jugular venous distention (may be absent if hypovolemic)
  - Hypotension (narrowed pulse pressure)
- Laboratory studies
  - CBC with differential
  - Erythrocyte sedimentation rate (ESR) may be elevated
- FAST (Focused Assessment with Sonography for Trauma), if traumatic injury
- Chest X-ray
- Echocardiogram: showing pleural effusion
- CT Scan

Interventions
- Support airway, breathing, and circulation as needed
- Pulse oximetry; consider capnography
- Administer oxygen as needed
- Cardiac monitoring
- Establish IV access for crystalloid fluids, blood products, and medications as needed
- Anticipate and prepare for a pericardiocentesis-needle drainage of the pericardial fluid (see Figure 5-1)
  - Ultrasound often used to guide visualization
  - Small amount of aspirated fluid (30 to 50 mL) can improve hemodynamic stability[5]
  - May be temporary measure until surgical cardiac repair to cut a pericardial window

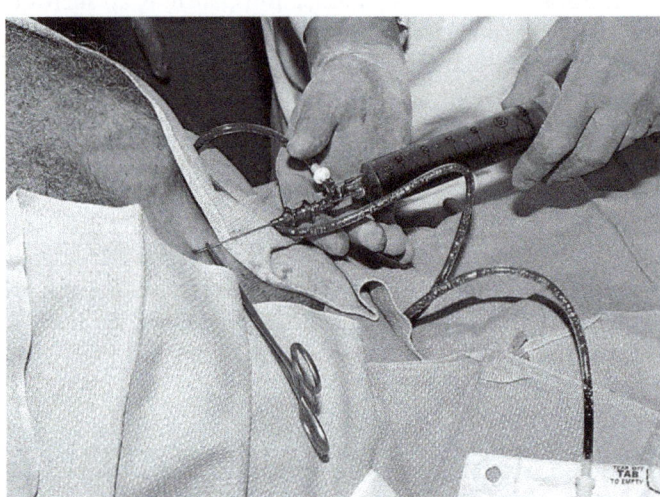

FIGURE 5-1 Emergency pericardiocentesis for a pericardial tamponade
Reproduced with permission from Knoop KJ, Stack LB, Storrow AB, et al: The Atlas of Emergency Medicine, 4th ed. New York: McGraw-Hill Education; 2016: Photo contributor: Lawrence B. Stack, MD.

Evaluation
- Patent airway and effective breathing and ventilation
- Hemodynamic stability
- Pain relief
- Blood loss

Tension Pneumothorax

Tension pneumothorax is a life-threatening emergency and requires immediate treatment. A tension pneumothorax occurs when air accumulates within the intrapleural space either through injury or a spontaneous pneumothorax and cannot escape. Pressure builds in the intrapleural space pushing on the mediastinum and compressing the vena cava, pulmonary vessels, heart, and eventually the unaffected lung. Cardiac output decreases from the obstruction of blood flow. Thus signs of hypoperfusion ensue for this type of obstructive shock.

Assessment/Analysis
- Restlessness, anxiety, feelings of impending doom
- Tachypnea
- Absent breath sounds on affected side with auscultation and hyperresonance with percussion
- Respiratory distress
- Tachycardia
- Subcutaneous emphysema
  - Detected on chest radiography; also maybe palpable
- Late signs
  - Tracheal deviation, toward the unaffected side
  - Distended neck veins on affected side (may not visualize if hypovolemic)

Interventions
- Supplemental oxygen
- Support airway if needed
- Cardiac monitoring, pulse oximetry
- Establish IV access for crystalloid fluids/blood products/medications as needed
- Emergent needle decompression to release air
  - Location #1: a 14-gauge needle (5 cm) is inserted, on the affected side, into the second intercostal space at the midclavicular line over the top of the third rib[6]
  - Location #2: a 14-gauge needle (8 cm) is inserted, on the affected side, into the fourth intercostal space at the anterior axillary line[7]
  - A hissing sound may be heard as air is released
- Insertion of chest drain with water-seal is the definitive treatment

Evaluation
- Patent airway and effective breathing and ventilation
- Auscultation of lung fields
- Hemodynamic stability
- Pain relief
- Fluid balance: intake and output

Pulmonary Embolus

About 60,000 to 100,000 Americans die of DVT/PE (venous thromboembolism) every year.[8] Venous thromboembolism begins with clot formation in distal peripheral veins. The clot travels through the venous circulation and lodges within an area of the pulmonary circulation, such as the main pulmonary artery or part of the lobar branches. The embolus impedes blood flow. The increased pulmonary pressure creates resistance to the right ventricle outflow of blood increasing the workload for the right side of the heart. As right-sided heart failure and decreased lung perfusion results, the patient experiences dyspnea and hypoxia. Cardiac output also decreases due to reduced left ventricular stroke volume causing diminished perfusion to vital organs and tissue.

Assessment/Analysis
- Risk Factors
  - Deep vein thrombosis (DVT)
  - Factor V Leiden defect: greater tendency for developing blood clots
  - Virchow's triad
    - Damaged vascular endothelium
    - Venous stasis
    - Hypercoagulability of blood[9]
  - History of smoking
  - Exogenous estrogen (oral contraceptives or hormone replacement therapy)
  - Obesity
  - Recent surgery
  - Pregnancy
- Dyspnea, at rest and/or with exertion
- Tachycardia
- Tachypnea
- Restlessness, anxiety, and feelings of impending doom
- Chest pain with possible radiation to shoulder
- Possible wheezing and possible diminished lung sounds with auscultation
- Elevated D-dimer (Quantitative: <250 ng/mL or <0.4 mcg/mL[10]; Qualitative-positive)
  - Fibrinolysis (breakdown of fibrin) and increased coagulability occur with acute clot formation. D-dimer is a fibrin degradation product that is made from fibrinolysis. Normally, plasma does not have detectable D-dimer fragments
  - Fibrin degradation products are also present with other conditions such as disseminated intravascular coagulation (DIC) and sickle cell anemia. Thus, a positive value identifies increased clotting formation but is non-specific[10]
  - A negative D-dimer indicates a strong predictability in ruling out acute clot formation (DVT/PE)
  - A positive D-dimer necessitates further testing for a DVT or PE
- Chest X-ray
- Venous doppler of the bilateral lower extremity
- Echocardiogram of the possible right ventricular (RV) dilation, reduced RV function
- Spiral CT scan of the chest with contrast
- Ventilation/perfusion (V/Q) lung scan (quantifies high or low probability for PE)[9]
- Pulmonary angiography

Interventions
- Support airway, breathing, and circulation
- Cardiac monitoring

- Pulse oximetry
- Establish IV access for crystalloid fluids, blood products, and medications as needed
  - Anti-coagulation (i.e., heparin) to prevent the existing thrombi (thrombus) from increasing in size[11]
  - Thrombolytic, such as Alteplase™ for massive pulmonary embolus
  - If hypotensive: IV fluids and vasopressor support

Evaluation
- Patent airway and effective breathing and ventilation
- Hemodynamic stability
- Patient teaching
  - Eliminating risk factors that can be controlled
  - Prevention and health promotion practices

Distributive Shock

Distributive shock occurs when there is a maldistribution of the circulating volume. Adequate circulating blood volume is dependent on effective systemic vascular resistance. When abnormal, maldistribution of blood flow can result. Despite an adequate circulatory volume, the decreased systemic vascular resistance results in reduced cardiac output and tissue perfusion.[12] Defects in the systemic vascular resistance can be caused by massive vasodilation, such as anaphylactic or septic shock, or a loss of autonomic sympathetic tone, as seen in neurogenic shock. Similar to other types of shock, decreased perfusion occurs leading to symptoms of decreased cardiac output such as hypotension and tachycardia.

Neurogenic Shock

Neurogenic shock occurs with a loss of sympathetic tone in cervical and upper thoracic complete spinal cord lesions. This loss of sympathetic tone leads to a decrease in peripheral vascular resistance and a loss of vascular tone.[13] A parasympathetic response dominates; hypotension and bradycardia develop.

Assessment/Analysis
- Spinal cord lesion above T6 level
  - Flaccidity and paralysis
  - Loss of sensation
  - Areflexia: absence of neurologic reflexes
- Skin temperature warm and dry due to peripheral vasodilation
- Bradycardia or lack of expected tachycardia response in trauma patients
- Hypotension: may not respond to fluid challenge due to decreased peripheral vascular resistance and loss of vascular tone
- Hypothermia due to peripheral vasodilation allowing for increased heat loss
- If other injuries present, may contribute to variable types of shock

Interventions
- Support airway, breathing, circulation, and spinal immobilization
- Cardiac monitoring
- Pulse oximetry
- Establish IV access for crystalloid fluids, blood products, medications as needed
  - Administer warm IV fluids
  - Vasopressors for refractory hypotension
  - Atropine for symptomatic refractory bradycardia
- Monitor vital signs with attention to patient temperature
- Prevent hypothermia

Evaluation
- Patent airway and effective breathing and ventilation
- Spinal protection
- Hemodynamic stability
- Pain management
- Intake and output

Anaphylactic Shock

Anaphylaxis is a medical emergency that is caused by an antigen-antibody reaction. A serious allergic reaction requiring immediate treatment may even lead to death despite appropriate emergency management.

The hypersensitive response to an antigen involves the release of immunoglobulin E (IgE). With initial exposure to the antigen, IgE antibodies form and join to mast cells in the connective tissue and basophils.[9] Antibodies are formed, and with subsequent antigen exposure, histamine is released, causing an immune response. This response can vary from mild to life-threatening anaphylactic shock.

Histamine is released during a systemic allergic reaction causing an increase in cellular permeability and vasodilation leading to the volume distribution problem in anaphylactic shock. Circulating volume moves from the vascular space into the interstitial spaces causing tissue edema. Cardiac output is reduced causing a decrease in tissue perfusion.

Assessment/Analysis
- Urticaria (hives)
- Conjunctivitis
- Rhinorrhea
- Tachycardia
- Wheezing with auscultated lung sounds (may be early sign)
- Decreased or silent auscultated lung sounds (usually a later sign)
- Angioedema: most common around eyes and lips as in Figure 5-2
  - Associated signs
    - Audible respiratory stridor
    - Stridor auscultated in pharynx area
    - Uvula edema
    - Respiratory distress

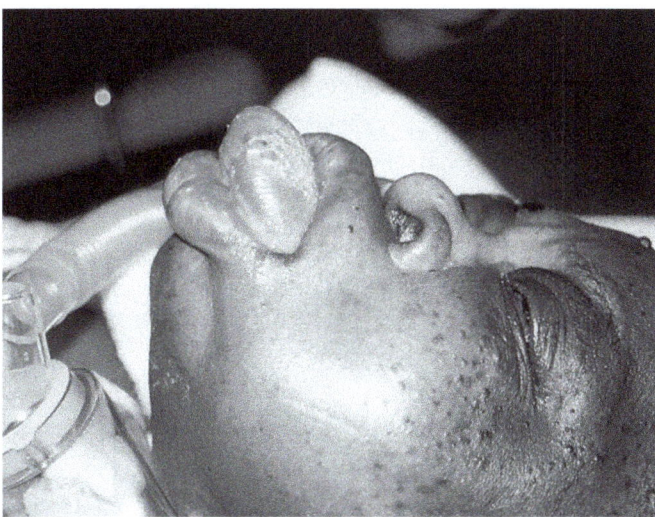

FIGURE 5-2 Angioedema leading to airway obstruction and requiring emergency cricothyrotomy
Reproduced with permission from Knoop KJ, Stack LB, Storrow AB, et al: The Atlas of Emergency Medicine, 4th ed. New York: McGraw-Hill Education; 2016: Photo contributor: W. Brian Gibler, MD.

- Cutaneous flushing
- Hypotension
- Bronchospasm
- Dyspnea
- Feeling of fullness in throat or throat swelling
- Cardiac dysrhythmias
- Anxiety
- Nausea, vomiting, and/or diarrhea
- Circumoral cyanosis

Interventions
- Airway stabilization
- Cardiac monitor and pulse oximetry
- Oxygen as needed
- Remove allergen, if known (i.e., bee stinger)
- Establish IV access for crystalloid fluids, blood products, and medications as needed
- Administering Epinephrine is *the most important treatment* for suspected anaphylaxis[14]
    - Epinephrine (1 mg/1 mL) recommended dose[15]
        - Adults and children weighing 30 kg or more: 0.3 milligram (mg) intramuscularly (IM)
        - Children 15 to 30 kg: 0.15 mg IM
    - A repeat dose may be beneficial if initial dose does not provide adequate relief, and advanced life support treatment is not available within 5 to 10 minutes
    - Epinephrine effects receptors that treat the symptoms of anaphylaxis and anaphylactic shock
        - Alpha 1 (α_1) adrenergic receptor: decreases mucosal edema and reverses vasodilation through vasoconstriction
        - Beta 2 (β_2) adrenergic receptor: relaxes bronchial airways
- Antihistamines
    - H1-histamine receptor antagonist
        - Diphenhydramine (Benadryl™)
        - Cetirizine (Zyrtec™)
    - H2-histamine receptor antagonist
        - Ranitidine (Zantac™)
    - Inhaled bronchodilators (nebulizer treatments)
        - Albuterol
        - Racemic epinephrine
    - Corticosteroids
    - Glucagon IV for patients on β-blocking medications with refractory hypotension

Evaluation
- Airway stabilization and effective breathing
- Lung sounds clear
- Hemodynamic stability
- Cardiac rhythm and vital signs
- Patient discharge education
    - Identification (avoidance) of allergen(s)
    - Proper use and carry of epinephrine auto-injector

Septic Shock

Sepsis is defined as a suspected or actual infection along with some of the diagnostic criteria of fever greater than 38.3°C. (100.9°F.), or hypothermia (core temperature less than 36.0°C or 96.8°F), heart rate greater than 90 per minute, tachypnea, altered mental status, significant edema, hyperglycemia (glucose >140 mg/dL in the absence of diabetes).[16] When sepsis leads to decreased tissue perfusion and organ dysfunction, severe sepsis is present. Septic shock results when hypotension, related to sepsis, is unresponsive to sufficient fluid challenges[16] and requires treatment with a vasopressor or inotropic agents. See Figure 5-3.

Sepsis is the ninth leading cause of disease-related deaths and kills more than 258,000 Americans each year.[17] About one in every

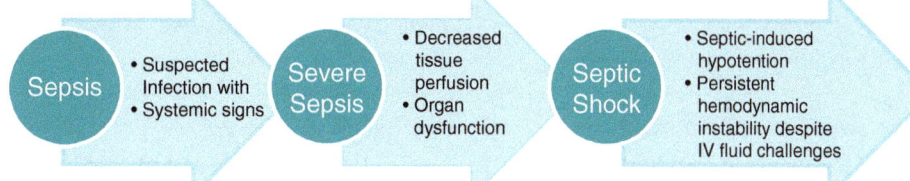

FIGURE 5-3 Progression of sepsis to septic shock

four patients presenting to the emergency department with sepsis will progress to septic shock within 72 hours.[18] Rapid recognition and appropriate treatment is essential for improving patient outcomes. Consistent screening for potentially infected patients allows septic patients to be identified and treated rapidly. In 2015, the Surviving Sepsis Campaign™ (SCC) published specific bundled interventions based on current evidence.[19] The interventions need to be implemented within a specific time frame beginning with initial patient presentation. For the emergency department, SCC defines the time of presentation at triage.[19]

SIRS criteria, refers to a systematic inflammatory response syndrome and may still be applied in some clinical settings for recognizing septic patients. Recent literature has suggested replacing SIRS with a clinical definition of organ dysfunction quantified by a sequential (sepsis-related) organ failure assessment (SOFA) score that increases by 2 or more points.[20] The quickSOFA (qSOFA) is a clinical score used for patients with a suspected infection to identify symptoms with an increased risk for a poor outcome. The symptoms with an increased risk for poor outcomes include a respiratory rate at or over 22 breaths per minute, an altered mental status, or a systolic blood pressure under 100 mm Hg.[20]

Assessment/Analysis
- SIRS criteria for potentially infected patients
  - SIRS has been defined as two or more of the following[20]
    - Temperature: >100.4°F (38.0°C) or <96.8°F (36.0°C)
    - Heart rate: >90 beats per minute
    - Respiratory Rate: >20 breaths per minute (or $PaCO_2$ <32 mm Hg)
    - WBC: >12,000 or <4,000/mm³, or >10% bands (immature WBC)
- General assessment findings
  - Mental status changes
  - Rigors
  - Elevated lactate level: sign of tissue hypoperfusion
  - Biomarkers procalcitonin and C-reactive protein (CRP)—Limited in value due to non-specificity[16]
  - Decreased urine output

Interventions
- Airway stabilization
- Cardiac monitor and pulse oximetry
- Oxygen, as needed (maintain pulse oximetry)

2015 SCC bundled interventions:[19]

To Be Completed Within 3 Hours of Time of Presentation

> 1. Measure lactate level
> 2. Obtain blood cultures prior to administration of antibiotics
> 3. Administer broad spectrum antibiotics
> 4. Administer 30 mL/kg crystalloid for hypotension or lactate ≥4 mmol/L

To Be Completed Within 6 Hours of Time of Presentation

> 5. Apply vasopressors (for hypotension that does not respond to initial fluid resuscitation) to maintain a mean arterial pressure (MAP) ≥65 mm Hg
> 6. In the event of persistent hypotension after initial fluid administration (MAP <65 mm Hg) or if initial lactate was ≥4 mmol/L, re-assess volume status and tissue perfusion and document findings (see the following documented reassessment)
> 7. Re-measure lactate if initial lactate elevated >2 mmol/L

- Vasopressor therapy for persistent hypotension refractory to fluid resuscitation
  - Norepinephrine infusion: preferred initial choice for vasopressor agents[21]
- Documented reassessment, following initial fluid resuscitation, with adherence to the SCC guidelines, requires[19]
  - A focused exam by a licensed independent practitioner
  - Exam includes: vital signs, cardiopulmonary, capillary refill, peripheral pulse evaluation, and skin findings
  - Or two of the following parameters should be included in the documented reassessment[19]
    - CVP measurement
    - Central venous oxygen saturation ($ScvO_2$) measurement
    - Bedside cardiovascular ultrasound
    - Assessment of fluid responsiveness with passive leg raises or fluid challenge

Evaluation
- Evaluation and continued monitoring
  - Airway stabilization, effective breathing and ventilation
  - Lung sounds, pulse oximetry
  - Hemodynamic stability and effective fluid resuscitation
  - Cardiac rhythm and vital signs
  - Lactate level, if initial level was elevated
  - Intake and output

Hypovolemic Shock

Massive bleeding, often induced by traumatic injury, is the leading contributor to hypovolemic shock. Other causes of massive blood loss can occur with epistaxis, gynecological/obstetric hemorrhage, and ruptured arterial bleeding such as aortic aneurysm.

Hemorrhagic shock is categorized according to the severity of symptoms related to blood loss in adult patients:[22]

❖ Class I: an adult can lose up to 15% of their circulating blood volume, be normotensive, and have a pulse less than 100 and other normal perfusion signs

- ❖ Class II: between 15 to 30% of circulating blood volume is lost. This stage is characterized by mild tachycardia, normal blood pressure (BP) with a decreased pulse pressure and a delayed capillary refill
- ❖ Class III: between 30 to 40% of circulating blood volume is lost. The pulse is greater than 120 with a decreased BP, pulse pressure and delayed capillary refill
- ❖ Class IV: more than 40% of the circulating blood volume is depleted. The pulse is greater than 140 with a decreased BP, pulse pressure, and delayed capillary refill[22]

Nonhemorrhagic causes such as hyperglycemia, severe burns, diabetes insipidus, and gastrointestinal (GI) losses by way of vomiting and diarrhea can also cause hypovolemic shock. Although some of these nonhemorrhagic causes may not be as common in the emergency department, replacing the fluid loss and treating the underlying cause are priorities.

Assessment/Analysis
- Mental status changes: decreased level of consciousness
- Tachycardia as a compensatory measure
  - Conditions that may prevent the development of tachycardia in hypovolemic shock include
    - Spinal injury and neurogenic shock
    - Patient medication history includes β-blockers
- Weak peripheral pulses
- Cool clammy skin
- Tachypnea
- Hypotension
- If traumatic injury: obtain history and mechanism of trauma
- External signs of bleeding
- Laboratory studies
  - CBC with differential
  - Coagulation studies
  - Thromboelastography (TEG)[23]
    - Point of care testing
    - An under-utilized coagulation study
    - Results in a visual graphic providing information about clotting process and coagulopathy
    - Information guides replacement of specific clotting factors
  - Serum chemistries
  - Liver function tests (if suspected abdominal source)
  - Consider blood bank analysis (Type and Screen/Cross), if a transfusion is likely
  - Possible arterial blood gas (ABG)
  - Serum lactate
  - Carboxyhemoglobin level (in burns)
  - Blood alcohol level
  - Toxicology screening: serum or urine

Interventions
- Support airway, breathing, and circulation as needed
- Hemorrhagic sources: control bleeding
  - Direct pressure
  - Splinting for long bone fractures
  - Pelvic binder if suspected unstable pelvic fracture
  - Apply tourniquet close to the injury to control extremity bleeding,[24] even without amputation
- Nonhemorrhagic sources: crystalloid fluids and treat underlying causes
- Pulse oximetry and capnography
- Administer oxygen as needed for pulse oximetry <94%
- Cardiac monitoring
- Establish IV access for crystalloids/blood products/medications as needed
- Identify source of bleeding as quickly as possible
  - FAST (Focused Assessment with Sonography for Trauma)
  - Radiography: chest, pelvis, other applicable areas based on pain, deformity, mechanism of injury, and history
  - CT scans: chest, pelvis, other applicable areas based on pain, deformity, mechanism of injury, and history
  - CT angiography: to detect the vascular source of bleeding[25]
- Damage Control Resuscitation: goal directed therapy focused on improving perfusion, minimizing bleeding, and preventing further complications of acidosis and coagulopathy[22]
  - Limiting crystalloids for fluid resuscitation. Administering aggressive blood products early such as 1:1:1 ratio of packed red blood cells (PRBCs) to fresh frozen plasma (FFP) to platelets[22]
  - Tranexamic Acid (TXA) IV: prevents clot breakdown and helps control hemorrhage[22]
  - Selective use of permissive hypotension
    - Infusing large quantities of IV fluid and expanding intravascular volume may impede clot formation or disrupt clots that have already formed[22]
    - Systolic BP <80 mm Hg during controlled amount of time, such as prehospital to surgery[26]
    - Not recommended for Class III or IV of hemorrhagic shock, traumatic brain injuries, and preexisting diseases such as angina or hypertension[26]
- Prevent hypothermia
  - Administer warm IV fluids
  - Keep the resuscitation room warm if independent temperature control is available
  - Keep the patient warm with blankets

Evaluation
- Airway stabilization, effective breathing, and ventilation
- Lung sounds, pulse oximetry

- Hemodynamic stability
- Cardiac rhythm and vital signs
- Intake and output
- Serial laboratory studies
  - CBC
  - Serum chemistries
  - Coagulation studies
- Need for preparation for emergency surgery

REFERENCES

1. Hochman JS, Ingbar DH. Cardiogenic shock and pulmonary edema. In: Kasper D, Fauci A, Hauser S, et al, eds. *Harrison's Principles of Internal Medicine*. 19th ed. New York, NY: McGraw-Hill; 2015.
2. Warise, L. Understanding cardiogenic shock. *Dimens Crit Care Nurs*. 2015; 34(2):67–78.
3. Weber JE, Peacock WF. Cardiogenic shock. In: Tintinalli J, ed. *Tintinalli's Emergency Medicine*. 7th ed. New York, NY: McGraw-Hill; 2011:385–389.
4. Hoit BD. Pericardial disease. In: Fuster V, Walsh RA, Harrington RA, eds. *Hurst's The Heart*. 13th ed. New York, NY: McGraw-Hill; 2011.
5. Schub T, Boling B. Cardiac tamponade. *Cinahl Information Systems*. 2015; March 27.
6. Emergency Nurses Association. Thoracic and neck trauma. *In Trauma Nursing Core Course*. 7th ed. Des Plains, IL: Emergency Nurses Association; 2014:137–150.
7. Change SJ, Ross SW, Kiefer DJ, et al. Evaluation of 8.0-cm needle at the fourth anterior axillary line for needle chest decompression of tension pneumothorax. *J Trauma Acute Care Surg*. 2014;76(4):1029–1034.
8. Center for disease control and prevention (CDC). *Venous Thromboembolism: Data and Statistics*. http://www.cdc.gov/ncbddd/dvt/data.html. Published June 22, 2015. Accessed November 7, 2015.
9. Ahrens TS, Prentice D, Kleinpell RM. *Critical Care Nursing Certification*. New York, NY: McGraw-Hill; 2010.
10. Pagana K, Pagana T, Pagana T. *Mosby's Diagnostic & Laboratory Test Reference*. 12th ed. St. Louis, MO: Elsevier; 2015.
11. Smithburger PL, Campbell S, Kane-Gill SL. Alteplase treatment of acute pulmonary embolism in the intensive care unit. *Crit Care Nurse*. 2013;33 (2):17–27. doi: http://dx.doi.org/10.4037/ccn2013626
12. Owens CD, Gasper WJ, Johnson MD. Blood vessel and lymphatic disorders. In: Papadakis MA, McPhee SJ, Rabow MW, eds. *Current Medical Diagnosis & Treatment 2016*. New York, NY: McGraw-Hill; 2016.
13. Summers RL, Baker SD, Sterling SA, et al. Characterization of the spectrum of hemodynamic profiles in trauma patients with acute neurogenic shock. *J Crit Care*. 2013;28:531.e1–531.e5. http://dx.doi.org/10.1016/j.jcrc.2013.02.002
14. Rowe BH, Gaeta TJ. Anaphylaxis, acute allergic reactions, and angioedema. In: Tintinalli JE, Stapczynski JS, Cline DM, et al, eds. *Tintinalli's Emergency Medicine*. 7th ed. New York, NY: McGraw-Hill; 2011.
15. Singletary EM, Charlton MP, Epstein JL, et al. First aid: 2015 American Heart Association and American Red Cross guidelines update for first aid. *Circulation*. 2015;132(suppl 2):S574–S589.
16. Dellinger RP, Levy MM, Rhodes A, et al. Surviving sepsis campaign: international guidelines for management of severe sepsis and septic shock: 2012. *Crit Care Med*. 2013;41(2):580–637.
17. Sepsis Fact Sheet. *Centers for Disease Control and Prevention*. http://www.cdc.gov/sepsis/basic/index.html. Published 2015. Accessed November 22, 2015.
18. Capp R, Horton CL, Takhar SS, et al. Predictors of patients who present to the emergency department with sepsis and progress to septic shock between 4 and 48 hours of emergency department arrival. *Crit Care Med*. 2015;43(5):983–988. doi: 10.1097/CCM.0000000000000861
19. Bundles: Surviving Sepsis Campaign. *Society of Critical Care Medicine*. http://www.survivingsepsis.org/bundles/Pages/default.aspx. Published April, 2015. Accessed May 31, 2016.
20. Singer M, Deutschman CS, Seymour C, et al. The third international consensus definitions for sepsis and septic shock (Sepsis-3). *JAMA*. 2016;315(8): 801–810. doi:10.1001/jama.2016.0287
21. Pollard S, Edwin SB, Alan C. Vasopressor and inotropic management of patients with septic shock. *P&T*. 2015;40(7):438–450.
22. Kobayashi L, Costantini TW, Coimbra R. Hypovolemic shock resuscitation. *Surg Clin N Am*. 2012;(92):1403–1423.
23. Emergency Nurses Association. ENA Topic Brief: Use of Thromboelastography (TEG) in The Emergency Department. https://www.ena.org/practice-research/Practice/Documents/Forms/DispForm.aspx?ID=34. Published October, 2015. Accessed April 30, 2016.
24. Pentecost DA, Smith S. Shock. In: *Trauma nursing core course (TNCC)*. 7th ed. Des Plaines, IL: Emergency Nurses Association; 2014:73–90.
25. Webster AM, Bratcher CM. Abdominal and pelvic trauma. In: *Trauma nursing core course (TNCC)*. 7th ed. Des Plaines, IL: Emergency Nurses Association; 2014:151–172.
26. Gourgiotis S, Gemenetzis G, Kocher HM, et al. Permissive hypotension in bleeding trauma patients: helpful or not and when? *Crit Care Nurse*. 2013;33(6):18–24.
27. Perrin A, Bergman C, Hart L. A 30-year-old industrial worker with upper back pain. *Adv Emerg Nurs J*. 2013;35(2):103–109.
28. Wadell JP, Drucker WR. Occult injuries in pedestrian accidents. *J Trauma*. 1971;(10):844–852.

Practice Questions

Question	Rationale
1. A patient arrives to the emergency department after sustaining second-degree burns over 30% of her body after falling into a campfire pit one hour prior to arrival. She is hypotensive, tachycardic, and restless. What type of shock is she experiencing? a. Neurogenic shock b. Anaphylactic shock c. Hypovolemic shock d. Septic shock	*Answer: c* Circulating plasma volume is diminished with severe burns. Protein and plasma leakage result from the cellular damage. Without adequate fluid resuscitation, the patient develops hypovolemic shock. Neurogenic shock occurs with spinal cord injuries. Anaphylactic shock results from severe anaphylaxis that follows an antigen-antibody reaction. A patient with severe burns would be at risk for developing an infection that may lead to septic shock. However, typically, this does not immediately follow the burn injury.
2. Identify one cautious use for vasopressor agents with cardiogenic shock a. Increases systemic vascular resistance b. Increases urine output c. Decreases afterload d. Decreases systemic vascular resistance	*Answer: a* Vasopressors cause vasoconstriction of the vasculature, which increases the SVR; hence, the heart has to increase the force of contraction when a higher SVR exists. A vasopressor agent, such as IV norepinephrine, will increase the workload on the reduced pump ability that accompanies cardiogenic shock. Urine output may decrease as blood flow is decreased to the kidneys through the vasoconstrictive effect of vasopressor agents. Afterload increases, as extra myocardial workload is required to overcome the resistance caused by a higher SVR.
3. A 56-year-old female patient who has history of lung cancer and metastasis to the bone arrives to the emergency department via EMS, with severe shortness of breath and chest pain. She is pale, and her vital signs are T-98.6°F (37.0°C) oral; P-110; R-34, BP-78/54; SpO$_2$-82% on room air. She is alert, and has an increased work of breathing. Physical assessment reveals bilateral clear lung sounds on auscultation and heart sounds are muffled. Based on her history and current symptoms, what condition and type of shock do her symptoms suggest? a. Severe sepsis and distributive shock b. Anaphylaxis and distributive shock c. Tension pneumothorax and obstructive shock d. Pericardial tamponade and obstructive shock	*Answer: d* Two common signs of pericardial tamponade are chest pain and dyspnea, and the most common cause is a malignancy. Auscultating heart sounds through the fluid surrounding the heart creates the muffled sounds that are heard. An abnormal temperature and infection usually accompany septic shock whereas muffled heart tones are not part of the clinical presentation for septic shock. Urticaria, angioedema, and respiratory stridor are classic symptoms in anaphylactic shock, and she is not presenting with these. She does not have unilateral decreased breath sounds with auscultation. This sign is classic for a tension pneumothorax.

Question	Rationale
4. A 75-year-old male has just arrived to the emergency department, following a MVC when his car, which he was driving, left the road and hit a telephone pole. He was restrained with no airbags to deploy. He is restless, complaining of chest pain and shortness of breath. His lung sounds are clear and equal and skin is cool and pale. His last set of vital signs are P-118; R-28; BP-88/40; SpO$_2$-86% on a non-rebreather mask with high-flow oxygen. While auscultating a manual BP, the nurse notes a significant drop (about 20 mm Hg) when he inhales. Identify the term describing this physical finding a. Muffled heart tones b. Pulsus paradoxus c. Pulsus alternans d. Diminished perfusion	*Answer: b* During normal inspiration, negative intrathoracic pressure increases resulting in increasing blood flow. However, in pericardial tamponade with the pericardial pressure already increased, adding more pressure during end-inspiration further weakens the stroke volume and decreases the blood pressure. Pulsus paradoxus occurs when the BP decreases (>10 mm Hg) during inspiration. Muffled heart tones can be a sign of pericardial tamponade and is one of the components of Beck's triad. However, the sound of muffled heart tones is heard through auscultating heart sounds and not the BP. Pulsus alternans describes a pulse pattern that alternates between strong and weak without a change in the pulse rate. Although this may be observed in a patient with an arterial line, pulsus alternans is not auscultated during a BP assessment. He is exhibiting signs of decreased perfusion such as hypotension, tachycardia, and restlessness. However, the variation is auscultating a BP related to the respiratory cycle does not indicate diminished perfusion.
5. A 41-year-old male presents with complaints of increasing dyspnea and chest pain. While collecting a history from a patient, the nurse notices documentation in the patient's health history that raises suspicion of a pulmonary embolism. What risk factor was noted? a. Factor V deficiency b. Von Willebrand's disease c. Factor V Leiden d. Fragile X Syndrome	*Answer: c* The natural clotting process contains intrinsic responses to slow or stop the clotting process to prevent abnormal blood clots. Factor V Leiden, also known as thrombophilia, is a mutated gene. People who have this gene have a greater tendency for developing blood clots. A hypercoagulable condition exists. The clotting system normally applies activated protein C (APC), an anticoagulant, to limit clot formation. With Factor V Leiden, a mutated gene causes resistance to APC.[27] Factor V plays a role in the normal clotting development by converting prothrombin to thrombin. People with a Factor V deficiency have a greater risk for bleeding, especially following surgery or childbirth. Von Willebrand's disease is an inherited condition and is caused by a lack of the Von Willebrand factor, one of the factors involved with clotting. Bleeding episodes can be severe for people who have Von Willebrand. Additional clotting factors may be required, such as fresh frozen plasma, for patients with Factor V deficiency or Von Willebrand's to decrease bleeding. Fragile X syndrome is an inherited condition from an altered gene. It affects both sexes and can cause severe cognitive and behavioral challenges.

Question	Rationale
6. A 22-year-old construction worker arrives via EMS after falling from a second story building. He was intubated prior to arrival. He is currently unresponsive to verbal stimuli and is not moving his extremities. FAST exam is negative. A total of 2 liters of crystalloid IV fluid has infused. His current vital signs are T-98.1°F (36.7°C); P-48; R-14 (assisted); BP-78/40. His skin is warm and dry. What type of shock is suggested by the symptoms? a. Neurogenic shock b. Hypovolemic shock c. Cardiogenic shock d. Obstructive shock	*Answer: a* This patient's mechanism of injury would raise the index of suspicion that he has sustained a spinal cord injury. Neurogenic shock occurs with a loss of sympathetic tone in cervical and upper thoracic complete spinal cord lesions, and the balance between the sympathetic nervous system (fight or flight) and the parasympathetic nervous system (slow and dilate) are not synergistic. Bradycardia and hypotension are the result of increased parasympathetic tone and are often present in neurogenic shock. Hypotension may not improve with fluid challenges, and a vasopressor infusion may be needed to improve perfusion. With hypovolemic shock, typically when the intravascular space is depleted, the heart responds with tachycardia. An exception to a tachycardic response would be if the patient were on a *B*-blocker or other heart slowing medication. Tachycardia and hypotension are two common symptoms for cardiogenic shock. The classification of obstructive shock includes pericardial tamponade, tension pneumothorax and pulmonary embolus. This patient's injury and presentation do not have the common presenting symptoms for obstructive shock.
7. Virchow's triad is a. Jugular venous dissention (JVD), muffled heart sounds, and hypotension b. Tachycardia, mental status changes, and decreased urine output c. Damaged vascular endothelium, venous stasis, and hypercoagulability of blood d. Lower extremity fracture, abdominal or thoracic, and head injuries	*Answer: c* Virchow's triad is a group of simultaneous factors that increases the risk for thrombosis development. A hypercoagulable state may follow recent surgery. Vascular endothelial injury may occur after catheter insertion or recent trauma, and venous stasis can result from pregnancy, immobility, or obesity. JVD, muffled heart sounds, and hypotension, referred to as Beck's triad, are a cluster of symptoms associated with pericardial tamponade. Tachycardia, mental status changes and decreased urine output can be early signs of shock. Waddel's triad describes an injury pattern that may occur when a pedestrian is struck by a car. A triad of injuries involving lower extremities, the abdomen or thorax, and head are potentially involved is this injury pattern.[28]
8. A mother drives her 6-year-old son, with a peanut allergy, to the emergency department after he developed urticaria. The child weighs 20 kg. The emergency nurse observes edema around his lips and hears inspiratory wheezes when auscultating lung sounds. The next action should be a. Establish an IV and administer a 400 mL 0.9 NS fluid bolus b. Apply a cardiac monitor and continuous pulse oximetry c. Administer 0.15 mL epinephrine IM (1 mg/mL concentration of epinephrine) d. Administer 0.015 mL epinephrine IM (0.1 mg/mL concentration of epinephrine)	*Answer: c* This child's allergic reaction is deteriorating to symptoms of anaphylaxis. He is developing angioedema, and his lung sounds have wheezing. Epinephrine is the most important treatment for suspected anaphylaxis. The correct concentration for epinephrine, when administered IM, is 1 mg/mL (or 1:1,000). The correct concentration is 0.1 mg/mL when epinephrine is administered IV (or 1:10,000). Cardiac monitoring and pulse oximetry are indicated but can immediately follow administration of epinephrine. IV establishment and a fluid bolus (20 mL/kg) may be indicated if the child's symptoms continue and anaphylactic shock is suspected.

Question	Rationale
9. A 31-year-old female arrives to the emergency department after being stung by a bee and she is "deathly" allergic to bee stings. She does not carry her epinephrine autoinjector with her. After stabilization, she responds to treatment. After a period of observation, she is ready for discharge. Part of discharge teaching should include a. The importance of calling 911 b. The instructions about where to obtain a first aid kit c. Education about administering a nebulizer treatment d. Instructions about availability and use of an epinephrine autoinjector	*Answer: d* Although calling 911 is an important teaching step, it does not stop the rapid immune response seen in anaphylactic shock. Epinephrine is the single most important administered medication to stop or slow the rapid evolving anaphylactic shock, and patient/family education about emergency treatment is essential.
10. A patient recently brought to the emergency department is demonstrating a clinical picture of cardiogenic shock following an acute MI. The ED nurse anticipates observing all of the following signs with this patient *except* a. Elevated brain natriuretic peptide (BNP) b. S3 heart sound c. Bradycardia d. Hepatomegaly	*Answer: c* With cardiogenic shock, tachycardia usually is part of the clinical picture as the heart attempts to increase cardiac output and tissue perfusion. One of the hallmarks of cardiogenic shock is heart failure and the signs and symptoms that accompany this. An elevated BNP, S3 heart sound and hepatomegaly are all indicative of heart failure.
11. A 45-year-old man arrives by EMS after being stabbed in the chest an hour earlier. Upon arrival, he is restless and complains of shortness of breath. He is on a non-rebreather mask with high flow oxygen. Vital signs are T-97.4°F (36.3°C); P-116; R-32; BP-82/56; SpO_2-81%. Diminished breath sounds are auscultated on his left side and tracheal deviation is noted toward his right side. What type of injury and shock are suspected? a. Pericardial tamponade (obstructive shock) b. Pericardial tamponade (distributive shock) c. Tension pneumothorax (obstructive shock) d. Tension pneumothorax (distributive shock)	*Answer: c* Obstructive shock is a classification of shock when blood flow is decreased. The hypoperfusion is caused by a pathological obstruction as seen with a tension pneumothorax, pericardial tamponade and pulmonary embolus.
12. A 41-year-old female patient presents to the emergency department with a suspected infection. The patient develops fever, tachycardia, rigors and hypotension. Her vital signs are T-102.6°F (39.2°C); P-118; R-20; BP-84/52; SpO_2-92% on room air. The following lab test is a sensitive marker for decreased tissue perfusion? a. Procalcitonin b. INR c. Lactate level d. ABG	*Answer: c* When a patient with a suspected or known infection develops sepsis with possible deterioration to septic shock, a serum lactate is a sensitive indicator for tissue hypoxia. The INR or international normalized ratio measures the clotting ability of varied clotting factors. Although procalcitonin is a marker of an inflammatory response, the lack of non-specificity minimizes the useful utility in identifying sepsis and septic shock. An ABG may not be immediately indicated as this patient is not in severe respiratory distress, and the patient has a pulse oximetry of 92% on room air.

Question	Rationale
13. A critically injured trauma patient arrives in the emergency department following ejection from the car that he was driving. He was unresponsive, hypotensive, and intubated at the scene. During transport via medical helicopter, he received 2 units of crystalloids, 2 units of packed red blood cells, 1 unit of fresh frozen plasma, and Tranexamic Acid (TXA) IV. Current vital signs are T-97.8°F (36.6°C); P-128; R-16 (assisted); BP-80/48. The emergency nurse anticipates the one of the following lab tests is needed for guiding blood product administration a. Hematocrit and hemoglobin b. INR c. Thromboelastography d. Platelet count	*Answer: c* Thromboelastography (TEG) provides a visual graphic about the clotting process. The graphic provides information about specific clotting factors that are deficient and can guide administration of blood components. The other lab tests do not provide complete information about any coagulopathy.
14. Damage control resuscitation for traumatic hypovolemic shock focuses on preventing all of the following complications *except* a. Infection b. Blood loss c. Coagulopathy d. Metabolic acidosis	*Answer: a* Damage control resuscitation does not prevent infection. Infection control measures include hand hygiene and aseptic technique. Administering combined blood products to replenish clotting factors and blood volume and maintaining adequate perfusion are part of damage control resuscitation interventions.
15. A 17-year-old male presents to the emergency department with complaints of weakness. He is tachypneic, tachycardia, and hypotensive. A glucometer check in the waiting room reveals a glucose reading of 406. The triage nurse anticipates which immediate action? a. Transport to ED treatment area b. Assess airway c. Establish IV d. Administer insulin	*Answer: b* This patient is presenting with symptoms of hypovolemic shock, possibly a nonhemorrhagic origin such as DKA. Although he would need all of the above interventions, a patent airway is the top priority.
16. A 68-year-old arrives via EMS with complaints of shortness of breath. Symptoms started about 3 hours prior to arrival. According to the patient's wife, he had flu-like symptoms for the past three days. He has no other significant past medical history. Upon arrival, he is on oxygen at 4 liters via nasal cannula. Vital signs are T-96.2°F (35.7°C); P-98; R-24; BP-110/62; SpO_2-93% on room air. According to his presentation, what condition would the nurse suspect? a. Pulmonary embolism (PE) b. Sepsis c. ARDS d. DIC	*Answer: b* This patient has a suspected infection, and sepsis is often diagnosed in the presence of a suspected or actual infection along with some of the following signs and symptoms: some of the diagnostic criteria of fever greater than 38.3°C. (100.9°F.), or hypothermia (core temperature less than 36.0°C or 96.8°F), heart rate greater than 90 per minute, tachypnea, altered mental status, significant edema, hyperglycemia (glucose >140 mg/dL in the absence of diabetes).[16] Although pulmonary embolism could be a possible diagnosis for this patient, none of the known risk factors are listed upon arrival such as recent surgery, history of blood clots, or DVT. Adult respiratory distress syndrome (ARDS) usually follows an acute illness or injury and results in extreme shortness of breath as the lungs become less compliant. Disseminated intravascular coagulation (DIC) is a coagulopathy involving systematic circulation and a rapid consumption of clotting factors.

Question	Rationale
17. A 45-year-old man arrives by EMS after being "accidently" stabbed in the chest by his girlfriend an hour earlier. Upon arrival, he is restless and complains of shortness of breath. He is on a non-rebreather mask with high flow oxygen. Vital signs are T-97.4°F (36.3°C); P-116; R-32; BP-82/56; SpO_2-81%. Decreased breath sounds are auscultated on the left side and a stat chest x-ray confirms a tension pneumothorax. What intervention should occur next? a. A needle thoracostomy b. Obtain a type and crossmatch lab c. A chest tube placement d. Prepare for surgery	*Answer: a* Immediate decompression of tension pneumothorax is a top priority with the goal of restoring adequate ventilation and perfusion to the lungs. Chest tube placement is the definitive treatment, after decompression to relieve the trapped air. Depending on the amount of internal blood loss and patient symptoms, blood products may be needed after his airway and breathing are stabilized. Surgical intervention may be required following his trauma resuscitation.
18. Afterload is increased by a. Increased preload b. Decreased preload c. Increased systemic vascular resistance d. Decreased systemic vascular resistance	*Answer: c* Afterload is the amount of "load" or resistance that the heart must beat against to generate a cardiac output, like trying to open a door against the wind. The resistance to the blood flow within the systemic circulation is referred to as systemic vascular resistance (SVR). SVR is increased in conditions such as vasoconstriction and aortic valve stenosis. SVR is decreased in vasodilation. Many antihypertensives decrease SVR. Preload is the filling pressures of the atria and ventricles at end diastole. Preload is influenced by many variables such as circulating blood volume and myocardial contractility.

Gastrointestinal Emergencies

6

Jayne McGrath, MS, RN, CEN, CCRN, CNS-BC

Chief complaints of abdominal problems are common in the emergency department (ED). In the United States, abdominal pain with various descriptions was the number one reason cited for all ED visits.[1] Symptoms and severity of gastrointestinal (GI) emergencies vary. A patient's history, symptoms, and physical findings guide interventions. Complaints may be localized in the abdomen or may be more diffuse. Dividing the abdomen into four quadrants with an understanding of anatomical structures can help identify potential diagnoses. See Figure 6-1.

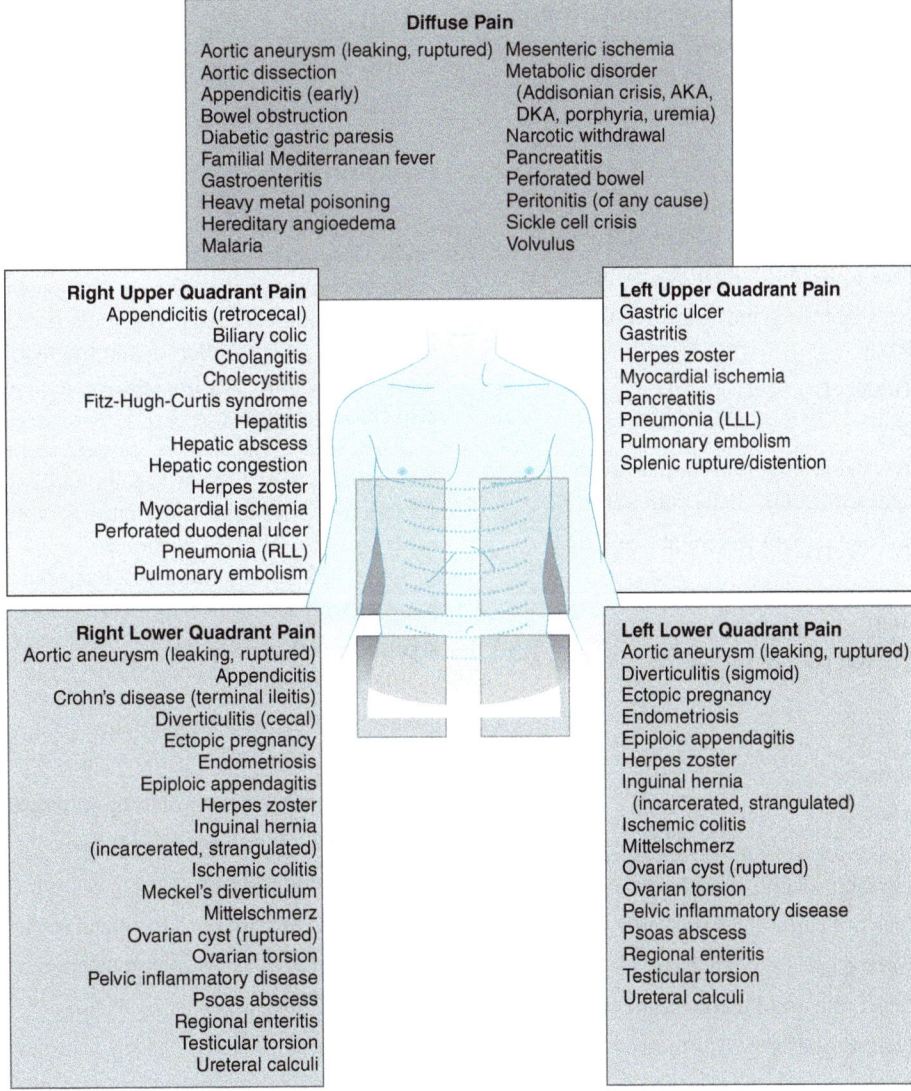

FIGURE 6-1 **Possible origins of abdominal pain**
Reproduced with permission from Tintinalli J, Stapcyzynski J, Ma OJ, et al: Tintinalli's Emergency Medicine: A Comprehensive Study Guide, 8th ed. New York: McGraw-Hill Education; 2015.

Acute Abdomen

An acute abdomen often begins with a sudden onset of pain. An infectious process may be involved and surgical treatment may be required. Some of the more common acute abdominal presentations are highlighted.

Appendicitis

Once thought to be more common among very young patients, increasing numbers of adults are presenting with appendicitis and the complication rate increases for the elderly (≥80 years).[2] Appendicitis continues to be a common presentation, especially for adolescence through young adulthood, and is truly a GI emergency. If symptoms have been present more than 48 hours, perforation is a likely risk.[3] If left untreated, peritonitis and severe sepsis will occur.

Appendicitis occurs when the vermiform appendix becomes obstructed and inflamed. Often the obstruction is caused by a fecalith (hard mass of fecal matter). However, other causes such as lymphatic tissue, tumor, or parasites can cause the obstruction.[4] As inflammation results from the obstruction, early onset of pain may be more diffuse or may localize to the periumbilical area. Increases in bacteria lead to more localized pain in the right lower quadrant (RLQ) of the abdomen.

Assessment/Analysis
- Pain
    - Early onset diffuse or localized to periumbilical area
    - Later pain localizes to RLQ (McBurney's point)[3]
    - Muscle rigidity and guarding: may be noted with palpation over RLQ
    - Rebound tenderness
- Positive Rovsing sign[6]
    - Applying pressure, like testing for rebound tenderness, in the left lower quadrant (LLQ), elicits pain in the RLQ
    - Common physical assessment test for appendicitis
- Anorexia
- Nausea and vomiting
- Possible change in bowel pattern such as constipation or diarrhea
- Possible fever
- Decreased bowel sounds
- CBC with differential
    - Elevated WBC in the presence of other suspecting symptoms has a greater diagnostic value for appendicitis
    - Normal WBC does not rule out appendicitis
- If female of childbearing age, pregnancy test
- Abdominal ultrasound may yield inconclusive results
- Abdominal computed tomography (CT) scan

Interventions
- Establish IV access for crystalloids/blood products/medications as needed
- Position of comfort
    - Movement may increase pain
    - Knee and hip flexion may decrease pain
- Analgesic administration
- Anticipate hospital admission
    - Maintain NPO status
    - IV fluids
    - Prepare for surgery
- If patient presents with an abscess, (>3 cm in diameter), drainage of the abscess may be initial treatment with appendectomy 6 to 12 weeks later after inflammation decreases[3]
- Patient/family education
    - Plan of care including anticipated surgery
    - Importance of remaining NPO

Evaluation
- Decreased pain
- Vital signs
- Afebrile
- Intake and output

Peritonitis

Peritonitis results from contamination within the peritoneal cavity. The causes are varied. Often the mechanism is contamination of bowel content through spillage from the hollow organ into the peritoneal cavity. The spillage can range from penetrating trauma to a misplaced percutaneous endoscopic gastrostomy (PEG) tube. An infected peritoneal dialysis catheter can also cause peritonitis.

Peritonitis may also be caused from a perforation of an abdominal organ such as the appendix, duodenum, or colonic diverticuli.[3] Intestinal obstructions, volvulus, and cancer are other causes leading to peritonitis.

Over 90% of spontaneous bacterial peritonitis is seen in patients with ascites or hypoproteinemia (<1 g/L).[3]

Assessment/Analysis
- Effective breathing
- Severe diffuse abdominal pain
- Fever
- Rebound tenderness noted upon palpation
- Abdominal guarding and rigidity
- Positive "cough test"[6]
    - Patient experiences a localized sharp pain with coughing
- Tachycardia, possible hypotension
- Elevated WBC
- Acidosis
- Abdominal X-ray: free air in a suspected perforation in about 80% of patients[5] and dilated bowel with associated edema of bowel wall[3]
- Hypoactive or absent bowel sounds

Interventions
- Establish IV access for crystalloids, blood products, or medications as needed
- Maintain NPO status
- Cardiac monitor and pulse oximetry
- Anticipate possible surgical emergency: prepare for surgery and hospital admission
- If patient is stable and has ascites, diagnostic paracentesis may be indicated[3]

Evaluation
- Effective breathing
- Hemodynamic stability
- Vital signs
- Decreased pain
- NPO status maintained
- Intake and output

GI Bleeding

The incidence of GI-related complications resulting in hospitalizations in the United States was studied and researchers found a slight decrease in the first decade of the 21st century compared to the 1990s. Hospitalizations related to GI bleeding arising from the upper GI tract accounted for 40%, 25% were from the lower GI tract, and 35% were from unidentified locations from 2001 to 2009.[7]

Bleeding can occur in variable locations within the GI tract with fluctuating symptoms and severity. Tachycardia, hypotension, and other shock-like symptoms, such as syncope, nausea, and thirst can signal a >20% reduction in circulating blood volume.[8] GI hemorrhage will precipitate hypovolemic shock.

Upper GI Bleeding

Upper GI bleed originates in the esophagus, stomach, and duodenum proximal to the ligament of Treitz. The ligament of Treitz is a smooth muscle attached to the junction of the duodenum and jejunum. More common causes of upper GI bleeds are peptic ulcers (about 50%).[8] Other common causes are erosive gastritis and esophagitis. Predisposing factors include salicylates, NSAIDs (nonsteroidal anti-inflammatory drugs), and alcohol.[9] Possible sources of infections can also lead to esophageal bleeding. These potential infectious sources include herpes simplex virus, human immunodeficiency virus, and cytomegalovirus.[9] Esophageal and gastric varices also cause upper GI bleeds.

Mallory–Weiss syndrome is a tear in the lower esophagus. Causes vary but may result from repeated vomiting, often from chronic alcohol use[10] and in patients with anorexia or bulimia eating disorders. A lower esophageal tear can also occur with a single episode of forceful vomiting.

Assessment/Analysis
- History of chief complaint
  - Pain, nausea, and vomiting
  - Bowel patterns and characteristics
  - Medication history (including history of NSAIDS, aspirin, and anticoagulants)
  - Pertinent past medical history including alcohol intake and tobacco use
- Laboratory studies
  - CBC with differential
  - Blood bank analysis (Type and Screen/Cross), if transfusion is likely
  - Serum chemistries with liver function tests
    - Increased blood urea nitrogen (BUN)[8]
  - Coagulation studies
  - Fecal occult blood test
- Abdominal ultrasound
- Hematemesis: vomiting blood or "coffee-ground" emesis
- Melena: black "tarry" stool from rectum
  - Can also occur with a lower GI-bleed (ascending colon)[8]
  - Ingestion of certain substances such as iron, beets, licorice, bismuth, and charcoal can cause pseudomelena[8]
- Signs of GI hemorrhage/shock: hypotension, tachycardia, decreased pulse pressure, and pale and cool skin color

Interventions
- Establish IV access for crystalloids/blood products/medications, as needed
- Maintain NPO status
- Cardiac monitor and pulse oximetry
- Patient education-avoidance of contributing factors
- Nasogastric insertion
  - Consider topical local anesthetic for insertion
  - If blood clots or bright red blood, gastric lavage may be indicated. Gently irrigate with room temperature water[9]
- Anticipate subsequent need for endoscopy or angiography[9]
- Other potential diagnostic studies
  - Upper GI barium radiography: about 80% accuracy with detecting pathology but does not identify source of bleeding[8]
  - Tagged red-cell scintigraphy[9] (Radioisotope scanning)
- Blood transfusion(s)
- If history of cirrhosis[8]
  - Albumin IV
  - If coagulopathy with cirrhosis
    - Fresh frozen plasma IV
    - Phytonadione (Vitamin K) (10 mg IV or subcutaneous)
- Patient/family education
  - Plan of care
  - Any needed dietary changes
  - Avoidance of alcohol and spicy foods
  - Medications, adding or avoiding
- Medication administration: see Table 6-1 for a summary of common treatments

TABLE 6-1 **Treatment of Upper GI Bleed**

Treatment	Dose	Comments
Blood transfusion		Transfuse if ≤7 grams/dL in most; ≤9 grams/dL in older patients or patients with comorbidities
Correct coagulopathy		Correct if INR is elevated or platelets <50,000; or if bleeding severe, correct coagulopathy unless contraindications to correction (e.g., stents)
Omeprazole	80-milligram IV bolus then infusion of 8 milligrams/h	Labeled use for ulcer bleeding
Octreotide	50-microgram bolus then infusion of 25–50 micrograms/h	Unlabeled use for varices; for elderly, begin at lower dose range of 25-microgram bolus and infusion of 25 micrograms/h
Antibiotics	Ciprofloxacin 400 milligrams IV or ceftriaxone 1 gram IV	Antibiotics for cirrhotics with UGI bleeding

Reproduced with permission from Tintinalli J, Stapcyzynski J, Ma OJ, et al: Tintinalli's Emergency Medicine: A Comprehensive Study Guide, 8th ed. New York: McGraw-Hill Education; 2015.

Evaluation
- Hemodynamic stability
- Pain management
- Laboratory values
- Intake and output
- Patient's understanding of possible needed diet and/or lifestyle changes

Lower GI Bleeding

The source of bleeding in a lower GI bleed is distal to the ligament of Treitz involving the jejunum, ileum, large intestine, and/or rectum. The risk for GI bleed increases with age and the most common cause is diverticulitis.[10] Other causes of lower GI bleeding can include colitis, carcinomas, and hemorrhoids. For the adolescent or young adult, the most probable causes are Meckel's diverticulum, inflammatory bowel disease, and polyps.[11] Locating the source of bleeding may be a challenge since 80 to 85% of lower GI bleeding resolve spontaneously.[11]

Assessment/Analysis
- History of chief complaint
  - Bowel patterns and characteristics including constipation and straining with bowel movements or any changes in bowel habits
  - Pain, nausea, and vomiting
  - Medication history (including history of NSAIDS, aspirin, or anticoagulants)
  - Recent colonoscopy
  - Insertion of foreign bodies
  - History of aortic graft (possible aortoenteric fistula)[12]
- Hematochezia
  - Bright red or maroon rectal bleeding
  - May occur with a rapid upper GI bleed of more than 1000 mL[8]
- Pain from diverticulitis
  - Possible cramping lower abdomen
  - Left lower quadrant (LLQ) pain indicates possible diverticulosis
  - LLQ tenderness upon palpation
  - Possibly no pain and may be asymptomatic
- Laboratory studies (see upper GI bleeding)

Interventions
- Administer IV crystalloid IV fluids, antibiotics, or analgesics
- Maintain NPO status
- Cardiac monitor and pulse oximetry
- Patient education-avoidance of contributing factors
- CT angiography
- If hemodynamic instability: anticipate hospital admission and a colonoscopy may be indicated
  - Can locate source of bleed
  - Allows for possible treatment of bleeding site, such as ablation[13]
- Possible emergency surgery for abdominal exploratory laparotomy
- Patient/family education
  - Plan of care
  - Any needed dietary changes
  - Medications, adding or avoiding

Evaluation
- Hemodynamic stability
- Pain management
- Laboratory values
- Intake and output
- Patient's understanding of possible needed diet and/or lifestyle changes

> **Some GI History to Digest**
>
> Dr. Barry Marshall, an Australian gastroenterologist, discovered that not only are peptic ulcers caused by a specific bacteria but that *Helicobacter pylori* is the most common cause of peptic ulcers.[14] Part of his research included infecting himself with the bacteria. Although he made this discovery in the early 1980s, it took about 10 years to convince the medical world a bacteria causes ulcers.[15] If left untreated, *H. pylori* can cause gastritis, peptic ulcers, and gastric cancer. Today, *H. pylori* infects about 30 to 40% of adults in the United States.[10]

Gastritis

Gastritis is an inflammation within the stomach lining that can be erosive leading to an upper GI bleed or other GI pathology. Causes include *H. pylori* infection, alcohol, tobacco use, stress, and certain medications, such as glucocorticoids, salicylates, or NSAIDs.

Acute gastritis can also stem from a severe illness such as shock, trauma, or organ failure.

Autoimmune factors destroying the gastric parietal cells could be a cause of chronic gastritis. This gastric parietal cell destruction could lead to a malabsorption of vitamin B_{12} consequently leading to pernicious anemia.[16]

Assessment/Analysis
- History of chief complaint
- Pain/Dyspepsia
  - Epigastric area
  - May be accompanied with nausea and bloating
  - Chronic or intermittently occurring
  - Gradual or sudden onset
  - As gastric contents empty, pain may return waking the patient at night[16]
- Diet and medication history
- Bowel sounds may be hyperactive
- Tenderness noted upon palpation

Interventions
- Establish IV access for crystalloids/medications as needed
- Administer medications, as ordered or indicated
  - Antiemetics
  - Analgesics
  - Antacids
  - Proton pump inhibitors (Omeprazole or Pantoprazole)
  - Histamine (H_2) receptor antagonist (Cimetidine or Famotidine)
- Patient education
  - Dietary changes: decrease or eliminate contributing factors such as alcohol or spicy foods
  - Avoid NSAIDs, explore other medication options
  - Managing stress
- Pain decreased
- Hemodynamic stability
- Patient understanding of illness

Ulcers

As acceptance and knowledge increased about the connection between *H. pylori* and peptic ulcers, hospitalization rates for peptic ulcer disease (PUD) decreased by 21%. In the United States, hospitals reported that 71.1/100,000 patients were admitted in 1998 with PUD, and in 2005, 56.5/100,000 patients were admitted with PUD.[17]

Other risk factors for ulcers include medications such as NSAIDs and aspirin. The risk increases when NSAIDs are used by patients with a history of alcohol consumption, *H. pylori* infection, older age, or with other medications such as aspirin, clopidogrel, selective serotonin reuptake inhibitors (SSRIs), and glucocorticoids.[18] Some conditions create a predisposition to PUD such as hereditary factors, smoking, renal disease or transplantation, chronic obstructive pulmonary disease (COPD), and cirrhosis.[16]

Complications of ulcers include bleeding, perforation, and gastric outlet obstruction. When an obstruction occurs at the gastric outlet, often from scarring and inflammation related to the ulcer, the patient often experiences severe symptoms. These symptoms include nausea, vomiting, abdominal distention, and fullness as well as dehydration and electrolyte imbalances.[16]

Assessment/Analysis
- History of chief complaint and present illness
- Diet, medication, and alcohol history
- History of chronic gastritis
- Lethargy or general malaise
- Epigastric pain
  - Episodic, burning (dyspepsia)
  - Occurs about 2 to 5 hours after meals, when the stomach is empty, or at night[18]
  - May be decreased with food or antacids
  - Increase in severity may be a sign of perforation
- Duodenal Ulcer (DU): characteristics may slightly differ from a gastric ulcer[18]
  - Pain may be more localized in the left upper quadrant (LUQ) or radiate into the back with large duodenal ulcers
  - Pain is more persistent for large DU and not relieved by food or antacids
  - First symptom may be a GI bleed; perforated DU is a surgical emergency (see Figure 6-2)
- Elderly patients
  - May not experience typical pain characteristics
  - Have greater chance of GI bleeding[18]
- Tenderness with palpation and muscle guarding
- Laboratory studies
  - CBC with differential
  - Serum chemistries

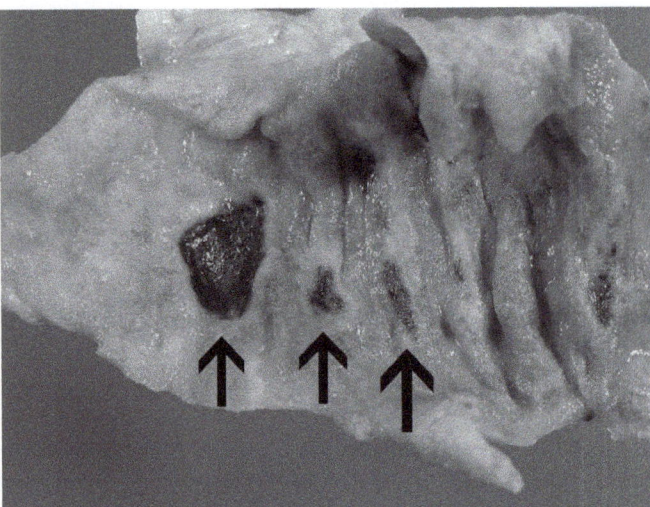

FIGURE 6-2 Duodenal ulcers. The arrows indicate superficial ulcers in the duodenum. Peptic ulcer disease is a chronic condition, often due to infection with Helicobacter pylori. Stress ulcers, as shown in the photograph, develop acutely, often due to burns, head injuries, or other forms of physical stress

Reproduced with permission from Kemp W, Burns D, Brown T: Pathology: The Big Picture. New York: McGraw-Hill Education; 2007.

- Liver enzymes tests
- Lipase and amylase
- Blood bank analysis (Type and Screen/Cross), if transfusion likely
- Coagulation studies, if on anticoagulants or bleeding is suspected
- Fecal occult blood test
- *H. pylori* test: different methods for testing
  - Urea breath test
  - Blood antibody test
  - Fecal antigen test
  - Biopsy sample
    - Tissue sample removed during endoscopy
    - Very accurate and most invasive
- Upper GI endoscopy for definitive diagnosis

Interventions

- Airway support and hemodynamic resuscitation for GI hemorrhage
- Establish IV access for crystalloids, blood products, and medications as needed
- Remove or discontinue offending agents (i.e., NSAIDs)
- Proton pump inhibitors
  - Most effective if taken 30 to 60 minutes before meal[16]
  - Heal ulcers faster than histamine (H_2) receptor antagonists[16]
  - Used in combination with antibiotics to treat *H. Pylori*
- Histamine (H_2) receptor antagonists
- Antiulcer, surface protectant (sucralfate)
- Antacids (short term)
- Nasogastric tube, if bleeding present or suspected. Gently irrigate with room temperature water or saline[9]
- Anticipate need for endoscopy and hospital admission for GI bleeding or other complications
- Interventional radiology or surgery for unstable bleeding
- Patient education: avoiding foods that may worsen pain, alcohol, and NSAIDs

Evaluation

- Hemodynamic stability
- Pain management
- Intake and output
- Discharge instructions: follow-up/referral
- Patient's perception and understanding of illness, warning symptoms for immediate medical care

Esophagitis

When an excessive reflux of acid and pepsin erode the esophageal mucosal lining, esophagitis occurs.[19] The reflux causes inflammation of the lining. The condition can be acute or chronic and may vary in severity. Severe esophagitis can lead to strictures and GI bleeding.[20] The severe strictures may require dilation.[19] Over time, the esophageal epithelium can change and is referred to as Barrett's esophagus. Barrett's esophagus is a pre-cancerous condition leading to esophageal adenocarcinoma which is rapidly increasing in the Western world.[19]

Gastroesophageal reflux disease (GERD) causes esophageal inflammation due to reflux of stomach acid. Certain medications such as NSAIDs and salicylates can also cause the inflammation associated with esophagitis. Esophageal injuries from swallowing pills have occurred causing esophagitis. Factors impacting type of injury include swallowing position, age, capsule size, and fluid intake.[21] Another type of esophagitis is eosinophilic esophagitis (EE). This condition can be seen in children as well as adults and occurs when eosinophils infiltrate the esophagus and provoke an inflammatory response. Infectious agents such as *Candidal* species, herpes simplex, or cytomegalovirus infection can cause esophagitis in the immunosuppressed patients.[21]

Assessment/Analysis

- History of present illness and chief complaint
- Epigastric pain
- Chest pain
- Dysphagia-difficulty swallowing
- Odynophagia-burning type of pain with swallowing
- Eructations (belching)
- Nausea
- Vomiting
- Abdominal pain
- Appearance of thrush or herpetic lesions in oral mucosa
- Regurgitation
- Definitive diagnosis: upper gastrointestinal endoscopy with possible biopsy

Interventions
- Establish IV access for crystalloids/medications as needed
- Antacids (aluminum hydroxide or calcium carbonate) may offer short-term relief if taken sparingly
- Proton-pump inhibitor (PPI) once to twice daily for 8 to 12 weeks[19]
- Patient education-life style changes including dietary changes, wearing loose-fitting clothing, and elevating head of bed

Evaluation
- Pain decreased
- Hemodynamic stability
- Patient understanding of illness

Cholecystitis

Acute cholecystitis results from a bacterial infection usually due to a gallbladder outlet obstruction.[22] The gall bladder becomes inflamed from the blockage of the cystic duct or common bile duct (cholangitis) (see Figure 6-3). Gallstones are the most common cause of the obstruction and if left untreated, gangrene and perforation may occur.[22] Cholelithiasis (presence of gallstones) is not typically painful. The pain and inflammation develops from obstruction.

Gallstones are more common in women than men, and the incidence increases with age.[23] Common risk factors for gallstones are obesity, diabetes, and a high-carbohydrate diet. Pregnancy, especially combined with obesity or insulin resistance, increases risk for gallstones.[23]

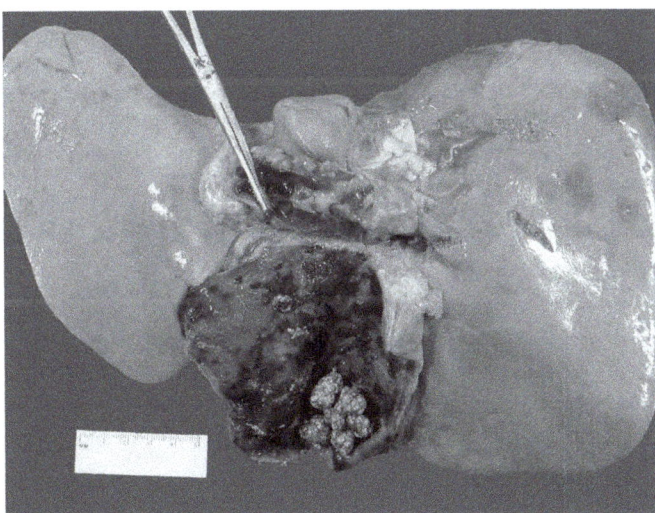

FIGURE 6-3 Acute cholecystitis and cholelithiasis. This gallbladder has been opened, revealing a thick edematous wall and an inflamed mucosa (acute cholecystitis). These inflammatory changes are due to the several calculi within the lumen of the gallbladder
Reproduced with permission from Kemp W, Burns D, Brown T: Pathology: The Big Picture. New York: McGraw-Hill Education; 2007.

Assessment/Analysis
- History of chief complaint and present illness
- Pain right upper quadrant (RUQ)[22]
  - May radiate to the flank and possibly right shoulder
  - Can present following consumption of high-fat meal
- Positive Murphy's sign[6]
  - Palpation along right costal margin
  - During palpation, patient experiences pain, and pause in inspiration
- Nausea and vomiting
- Possible fever
- Ultrasound-presence of gallstones
- Possible jaundice
- Laboratory studies
  - Elevated WBC
  - Pregnancy test
  - Liver function tests: often elevated[23]
- Gallbladder nuclear scanning (scintigraphy and HIDA scanning)[24]
- Possible abdominal CT scan
- Serum chemistries

Interventions
- Establish IV access for crystalloids/medications as needed
- IV antibiotics
- Analgesia (narcotic and non-narcotic)
- NPO
- Anticipate hospital admission with surgery if obstruction. If simple gallstones and adequate pain control, patient may be discharged and elective surgery planned
- Patient/family education: low-fat diet, plan of care

Evaluation
- Hemodynamic stability
- Pain management
- Intake and output
- Patient understanding of illness and plan

Cirrhosis

The pathology behind cirrhosis involves fibrosis (scar tissue) and regenerative nodules formed in response to liver injury. The hepatocellular mass decreases and alterations in blood flow occurs.[25] The distorted blood flow leads to an increased pressure within the portal vein. Fibrosis eventually leads to cirrhosis as the hepatocytes cycle through stages of healing and injury from chronic insults to the liver.[26]

Causes vary; however, more common causes are Hepatitis C, Hepatitis B, and alcoholism. Regardless of cause, patients with cirrhosis are at risk for developing complications. Portal hypertension is one of the earliest complications triggering further problems. Blood is shunted away from the liver cells to other abdominal venous circulation. Ascites and bleeding develop from esophagogastric varices. Continued loss of hepatocellular function leads to jaundice, coagulopathies, and hypoalbuminemia.[25]

Assessment/Analysis
- Fatigue and weight loss
- Abdominal pain

- Anorexia and nausea
- Hepatic encephalopathy: mental status changes and decreased cognitive function[25]
- Liver may be enlarged[25]
- Coagulopathies/Increased tendency for bleeding
  - Anemia
  - Decreased platelets
  - Prolonged prothrombin time
  - Decreased hemoglobin and hematocrit
- Laboratory studies
  - Increased liver function tests
  - Serum chemistries
  - Serum ammonia level: possibly increased
    - Result may be falsely elevated if tourniquet is placed too tight for a long duration[24]
    - Some facilities may require specimen to be sent to the laboratory on ice[24]
- Urine: dark tea color
- Jaundice
- Pruritus
- Palmar erythema: palms may have erythema on the periphery of the palms and pallor in the middle of the palm (see Figure 6-4)

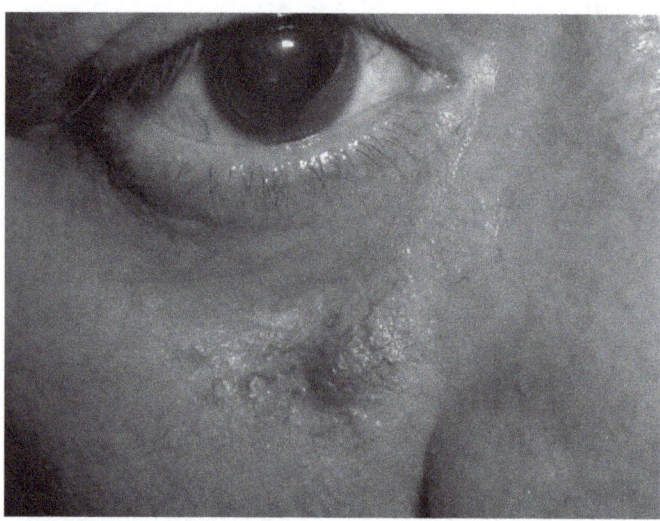

FIGURE 6-5 **Spider angioma on the face of a woman with cirrhosis secondary to chronic hepatitis C**
Reproduced with permission from Usatine RP, Smith MA, Chumley HS, et al: The Color Atlas of Family Medicine, 2nd ed. New York: McGraw-Hill Education; 2013. Photo contributor: Richard P. Usatine, MD.

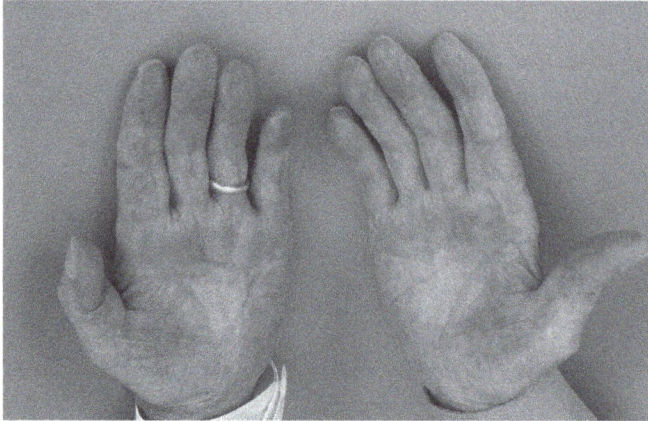

FIGURE 6-4 **Palmar erythema. This figure shows palmar erythema in a patient with alcoholic cirrhosis. The erythema is peripheral over the palm with central pallor**
Reproduced with permission from Kasper DL, Fauci AS, Hauser S, et al: Harrison's Principles of Internal Medicine, 19th ed. New York: McGraw-Hill Education; 2015.

- Ascites
- Dyspnea (with ascites)
- Spider Angiomas (see Figure 6-5)
- Hepatic encephalopathy
- Hypersplenism (from portal hypertension)[25]

Interventions
- Establish IV access for medication and crystalloids, blood products, medications as needed
- With end stage liver disease, medications are administered in reduced dosages
  - Reduced dosage of acetaminophen
    - Not more than 2 grams per day may be safer with short-term management of pain[27]
  - NSAIDS may increase toxicity and should be avoided[27]
  - If history of hepatic encephalopathy, cautious use of opioids[27]
- Patient education
  - Dietary sodium restriction with recommended intake <2 grams of sodium per day[25]
  - If cirrhosis is from alcoholism, explore options with patients for treatment and abstinence from alcohol abuse
- Diuretic therapy[26]
- Lactulose for hepatic encephalopathy (decreases ammonia level)
- Management of coagulopathies: vitamin K, fresh frozen plasma, and/or platelets[27]

Evaluation
- Hemodynamic status
- Signs of bleeding
- Mental status
- Reduced pain
- Intake and output

Hepatitis

Viral causes are the most common for hepatitis. Other causes include chronic alcohol ingestion and exposure to chemicals or industrial toxins.[28] Patients may be asymptomatic and have generalized complaints, such as malaise or fatigue. Viral hepatitis is classified based on the specific causative viral agent with varying routes of transmission and incubation periods as noted in Table 6-2. The symptoms and illness presentation are similar regardless of the cause.[29]

TABLE 6-2 Hepatitis Classifications

Classification	Mode of Transmission[28]	Incubation Period and Onset of Symptoms
Hepatitis A (HAV)	Oral-fecal route	Range of incubation time is 15–45 days.[29] Symptom onset may be immediate, but is typically self-limiting. Children less than 6 years of age often asymptomatic.[30]
Hepatitis B (HBV)	Blood and body fluids	Incubation from 6 weeks to 6 months.[30] About half of adults who contract HBV will be asymptomatic.[30] Symptom onset usually in about 2–6 weeks.[29] Different strains exist. If acute virus persists after 6 months, develops into chronic HBV.
Hepatitis C (HCV)	Blood and body fluids	Average incubation period is 7 weeks.[29] Initially, most adults will have mild symptoms or are asymptomatic[30]
Hepatitis D (HDV)	Blood and body fluids	Incubation period ranges from 1–6 months and only affects patients with history of HBV. Higher mortality rate of 20%.[30]
Hepatitis E (HEV)	Oral-fecal route	Incubation period ranges from 14–60 days.[29]

In the United States, hepatitis C is the most common blood borne disease and about 80% of individuals who contract the disease will eventually develop a chronic form of hepatitis. Hepatitis C can also lead to hepatocellular cancer.[30]

Assessment/Analysis
- History of chief complaint and present illness
- Anorexia, nausea, and vomiting
- Fatigue and weakness
- Abdominal pain
- Fever
- Hepatomegaly
- Possible splenomegaly
- Possible jaundice and pruritus
- Dark colored urine: from liver's inability to remove circulating bilirubin resulting in presence of bilirubin[28]
- Possible clay-colored stools
- Coagulopathy (may be later sign with hepatitis)
- Laboratory studies
  - Hepatitis serology tests: depending on the specific type of hepatitis can detect exposure and/or immunity
  - CBC with differential: may be within normal limits or show lymphocytosis
  - Elevated liver function tests
  - Coagulation studies

Interventions
- Establish IV access for crystalloids/blood products/medications as needed
- Post-exposure[30]
  - Immune globulin following exposure to HAV
  - HBV: if hepatitis B immunoglobulin (HBIg) is administered within two weeks of exposure, passive immunity may be effective for 75 to 95% non-vaccinated individuals
- Patient/family education
  - Strict proper hygiene including food handling and preparation
  - Not sharing any personal items, i.e., towels, razors, etc[28]
  - Risks of unprotected sexual contact and recommendations for safer contact[28]
  - Alcohol abstinence
  - Vaccinations for high-risk individuals
  - Indications for seeking immediate medical treatment or return to emergency department, i.e., increased pain, bleeding, and vomiting

Evaluation
- Pain management
- Intake and output
- Understanding of teaching

Esophageal Varices

The three major complications from portal hypertension are esophageal varices with hemorrhage, ascites, and hypersplenism.[25] As portal hypertension develops, an increased resistance to blood flow through the diseased liver occurs. Collateral channels of dilated veins, also called varices, extend into the stomach and esophagus. Varices result from the high resistance caused by the obstructed portal circulation. Esophageal varices occur in about half of all people with cirrhosis; hemorrhage occurs in about one-third of those with esophageal varices.[32] Patients with cirrhosis are often screened and monitored for esophageal varices using endoscopy.

Assessment/Analysis
- History of present illness and chief complaint
- Abdominal pain
- Other visible signs of liver disease
  - Jaundice
  - Ascites

- Hepatomegaly
- Splenomegaly
- Spider angiomas
- Palmar erythema
- Dark colored urine
- Coagulopathies/Increased tendency for bleeding
  - Anemia
  - Reduced platelets
  - Prolonged prothrombin time
  - Reduced hemoglobin and hematocrit
- Laboratory studies
  - CBC with differential
  - Serum chemistries
  - Liver function tests
  - Serum ammonia level
  - Coagulation studies
  - Fecal occult blood test
  - Blood bank analysis (Type and Screen/Cross), if transfusion is likely
- Abdominal imaging (CT or MRI)
- Hematemesis-color, frequency, or amount
  - Airway patency
  - Hemodynamic stability
  - Hypovolemic shock with hemorrhage
    - Tachycardia or hypotension
    - Decreased level of consciousness
    - Diaphoresis or pallor
    - Decreased urine output

Interventions
- Assist with airway management or oxygen delivery
- Suction for airway clearance
- Cardiac monitor, pulse oximetry, and frequent trending of vital signs
- Establish IV access for crystalloids, blood products, and medications as needed
- Maintain NPO status
- Blood transfusions and blood products (fresh frozen plasma and platelets)
- Anticipate and prepare for hospital admission
- Vitamin K
- Octreotide (vasoconstrictor properties) 25 to 50 mcg/hour continuous infusion[32]
- Emergent endoscopy (sclerotherapy and variceal band ligation)[25]
- Balloon tamponade (Sengstaken–Blakemore tube): when esophageal and gastric balloons are inflated, esophageal blood flow is decreased to tamponade the varices[32]

Evaluation
- Airway stability
- Hemodynamic status
- Level of consciousness
- Pain relief
- Intake and output
- Serial hematocrit and hemoglobin
- Nausea and vomiting

Diverticulitis

Diverticula are pockets within the colon wall. They typically range from 5 to 10 millimeter (mm) but can grow up to 20 mm in size.[33] The presence of these diverticula is referred to as diverticulosis and are typically benign and painless. The incidence of diverticulosis increases with aging. When the diverticula become inflamed, pain is commonly reported. The inflammation occurs when bacteria from fecal material become trapped. This can lead to abscess formation, obstruction, fistula formation, or perforation.[33]

Assessment/Analysis
- Chief complaint and history of current symptoms
- Pain localized in left lower quadrant (LLQ): pain in right lower quadrant (RLQ) is rare[33]
  - Intermittent or constant
  - Often associated with change in bowel habits such as diarrhea or constipation[33]
- Fever
- Nausea and vomiting
- Abdominal tenderness upon palpation in LLQ
- Laboratory studies
  - CBC with differential: increase in WBC and immature neutrophils (bands or stabs) indicating a bacterial infection
  - Fecal occult blood test
- Abdominal CT
- Possible ultrasound

Interventions
- Establish IV access for crystalloids, blood products, and medications as needed
- NPO status for bowel rest
- Antibiotic administration
- Pain management
- Anticipate hospital admission

Evaluation
- Hemodynamic stability
- Reduced pain and comfort
- Intake and output

Foreign Bodies

Esophageal Foreign Bodies

A foreign body in the esophagus occurs most often by children between ages 18 months to 4 years and in people with mental illness.[21] For some adults, loose partial dentures and food boluses can be more common foreign bodies. The risk of airway obstruction, perforation, or chemical corrosion (such as from button batteries) exists and may warrant immediate interventions. One hospital system reported treating various patients with foreign bodies from wire bristles from grill-cleaning brushes.[34] These wire bristles caused injuries to the GI tract. The authors recommended that people examine their grill surfaces for wire bristles before grilling.[34]

Assessment/Analysis
- Chief complaint and history of present illness
- Pain-may be localized
- Coughing, choking, and possible aspiration
- Dysphagia
- Vomiting
- Young children or children with developmental delay
  - History may be unclear[21]
  - Refusal to eat
  - Vomiting
  - Gagging, unable to eat, and choking
  - Pain in throat or neck
  - Stridor or drooling
- Inspect throat and nasopharynx region

Interventions
- Airway and breathing management
- Establish IV access for crystalloids/medication administration as needed
- NPO-anticipate potential procedural sedation and endoscopy for removal
- Radiography-plain films: effective if ingested object is radiopaque
- CT scanning provides superior diagnostic information to evaluate ingested object and possible injuries, such as perforation[21]
- Glucagon IV
  - Relaxes smooth muscle of GI tract
  - 1 to 2 mg IV (adult dose) relaxes lower sphincter allowing passage of foreign body[21]
- Endoscopy for airway compromise
  - See Table 6-3 regarding indications for emergent endoscopy

Evaluation
- Airway and breathing stabilization
- Lung sounds and work of breathing
- Pain management

TABLE 6-3 Indications for Emergent Endoscopy

Ingestion of sharp or elongated objects (including toothpicks, aluminum soda can tabs)
Ingestion of multiple foreign bodies
Ingestion of button batteries
Evidence of perforation
Coin at the level of the cricopharyngeus muscle in a child
Airway compromise
Presence of a foreign body for >24 h

Reproduced with permission from Tintinalli J, Stapczynski J, Ma OJ, et al: Tintinalli's Emergency Medicine: A Comprehensive Study Guide, 8th ed. New York: McGraw-Hill Education; 2015.

- Behavioral health consult, if applicable
- Patient/family education: safety and home environment
  - Follow-up for ill-fitting dentures
  - Child: eliminating small objects and choking hazards
  - If cleaning grill with bristle brush, inspect surfaces prior to grilling

Rectal Foreign Bodies

The most hazardous complication of a rectal foreign body is perforation of the rectum or colon.[35] Typically, the trapped foreign body was inserted, and the patient may offer a vague history or may be a victim of an assault. Signs of infection and pain can indicate peritonitis from a previous perforation.

Assessment/Analysis
- Pain in lower abdomen or perianal region
- Rectal bleeding
- Signs of local infection: purulent drainage, redness, and edema
- Fever
- CBC with differential: increase in WBC and immature neutrophils (bands or stabs) indicating a bacterial infection
- Abdominal X-ray: free air sign of possible perforation[35]
- Peritonitis: rigid abdomen, rebound tenderness with palpation

Interventions
- Chief complaint and history of present illness
- Reportable incident if vulnerable patient is believed to be a victim of an assault
- Monitor vital signs, especially pulse oximetry
- Establish IV access for crystalloids/blood products/medications as needed
- NPO-anticipate potential procedural sedation
- Lower GI endoscopy may follow removal to determine if perforation or laceration has occurred[35]
- If risk for perforation, prepare patient for surgery
- Sexual assault nurse examiner (SANE)/forensics nurse exam as applicable

Evaluation
- Hemodynamic stability
- Pain management
- Signs of bleeding and infection

Gastroenteritis

Acute gastroenteritis continues to be a common illness in the United States with an estimated 179 million occurrences each year. Norovirus was the known or suspected causative agent in 58% of reported cases.[36] Causes vary, including bacterial, protozoan, and viral or parasitic agents.

Assessment/Analysis
- History of current illness including any international travel
- Nausea and vomiting
- Diarrhea
- Fever
- Bloody stools
  - Fever and bloody stools are reported significantly more frequently when caused by *Salmonella* and *Shigella*[36]
- Abdominal cramping
- Headache
- Fatigue
- Bowel sounds hyperactive on auscultation

Interventions
- Establish IV access for crystalloids, blood products, and medications as needed
- Antiemetics
- Laboratory studies
  - CBC with differential
  - Serum chemistries
  - Stool for ova and parasites
- Antibiotics—if bacterial infection is suspected or confirmed
- Fluid replacement with oral rehydration–oral electrolyte solution
- Pediatric patients at greater risk for dehydration
- BRAT diet (bananas, rice, applesauce, and toast) after diarrhea has subsided[37]

Evaluation
- Intake and output
- Nausea and vomiting subsided: ability to drink oral fluids
- Pain and cramping decreased

Hernias

A hernia is a weakness or defect within the muscular tissues. This weakness enables an internal organ, such as a loop of the bowel, to bulge or protrude through the muscle wall.[38] Hernias are classified by location. Men have a 25% lifespan risk of developing a groin hernia (inguinal or femoral) compared to women who have a 5% lifespan risk.[38]

The following terms are used to describe hernias.[38]
- ❖ Reducible: the hernia can be easily returned into the body cavity
- ❖ Irreducible/incarcerated: a hernia that cannot be reduced
- ❖ Strangulated: the blood supply for the contents is impaired

The impaired blood supply results from the incarcerated hernia and a strangulated hernia is a surgical emergency.[39]

Assessment/Analysis
- Pain (a reducible hernia may be painless)
- Nausea and vomiting, especially with a strangulated hernia
- Laboratory studies
  - CBC with differential, possible leukocytosis
  - Serum chemistries
- Protrusion may be visible
- Hernias undetected while the patient is supine may be detected through inspection and palpation while the patient is standing[6]
- Ultrasound exam
- Abdominal CT provides a good diagnostic analysis[39]

Interventions
- Chief complaint and history of present illness
- Establish IV access for crystalloids/medications as needed
- Administered pain medication and assist to a position of comfort
- NPO with possible surgery
- Applying cold packs to hernia site reduces edema and may improve reduction if attempted by the medical provider[39]
- For strangulated hernia
  - Administer prescribed antibiotics
  - Anticipate a surgical consult
  - Prepare patient for a hospital surgical admission

Evaluation
- Hemodynamic stability
- Pain reduction
- Patient knowledge of potential hospital admission and plan

Inflammatory Bowel Disease

Inflammatory bowel disease (IBD) involves two types of chronic GI disorders: crohn's disease (CD) and ulcerative colitis (UC). A similarity of the two diseases is that both have periods of remissions and relapses and both affect more people from Westernized nations. IBD often has a peak onset between 15 to 30 years of age.[40] An increase in children aged 5 to 19 with IBD presenting to U.S. emergency departments has been observed.[41] The cause is unknown but believed to be part of an autoimmune response. Table 6-4 summarizes the more common symptoms of CD and UC.[42]

TABLE 6-4 **Common Symptoms of Crohn's Disease and Ulcerative Colitis**

Inflammatory Bowel Disease	Crohn's Disease (CD)	Ulcerative Colitis (UC)
Location of GI Tract Affected	• Can affect any part of the GI tract, but rarely involves the rectum. • Usually affects small bowel and colon; although, may involve the small bowel only. • Usually the ileum is affected when the small bowel is involved.	• Nearly all occurrences involve the rectum. • UC may extend beyond the sigmoid colon but does not affect the entire colon. • A smaller percentage of patients with UC will have a complete colitis.

Pathology of disease process	• The inflammation of Crohn's may expand through the entire colon wall layer leading to formation of fistulas, abscesses or strictures.
	• The inflamed areas are intermittent: Diseased tissue may exist between healthy non-affected tissue.
		• Mild inflammation, the mucosa appears erythematous.
		• Abdominal pain
		  ○ May be localized to lower abdomen and/or perirectal area
		  ○ Cramping

Assessment/Analysis Chief complaint and history of present illness	• Abdominal pain
	  ○ Colicky
	  ○ Defecation often relieves pain
	  ○ Often in right lower quadrant pain
	  ○ Pain may be more localized to area of inflammation in GI tract
	• Diarrhea
	• Anorexia and weight loss
	• Possible palpable mass
	• Fever
	• CBC with differential: Leukocytosis
	• Fecal lactoferrin[24]
	• Serum chemistries
	• C-reactive protein
	• Erythrocyte sedimentation rate (ESR)
	• As disease continues, bowel obstructions
	• Complications
	  ○ Obstructions
	  ○ Abscess formation
		• Rectal bleeding
		• Bloody diarrhea
		• Passage of mucus
		• Tenesmus—urgency with straining to defecate with little relief
		• CBC with differential: leukocytosis
		• Fecal lactoferrin[24]
		• Serum chemistries
		• Blood bank analysis (Type and Screen/Cross), if transfusion likely
		• C-reactive protein
		• Erythrocyte sedimentation rate (ESR),
		• Diagnosed through endoscopy and clinical symptoms
		• With severe disease, the bowel mucosa becomes very ulcerated and may lead to perforation.
		• Complications
		  ○ Toxic megacolon
		  ○ Peritonitis

Data from Kasper D, Fauci A, Hauser S: Harrison's Principles of Internal Medicine, 19th ed. New York, NY: McGraw-Hill; 2015.

Interventions
- Establish IV access for crystalloids, blood products, and medications as needed
- Administered prescribed analgesia
- Gastric tube for obstruction, peritonitis, or toxic megacolon[43]
- NPO-bowel rest
- Administer antibiotics, IV corticosteroids, as ordered
- Patient/family education
  - Plan of care
  - Dietary changes and medications
  - Support groups for patients with inflammatory bowel disease

Evaluation
- Hemodynamic stability
- Electrolyte balance
- Intake and output
- If discharged, follow-up with primary care provider

Intussusception

Intussusception occurs when a bowel segment folds over another loop of bowel creating a telescoping of the bowel. It is more predominate in children and usually stems from benign causes in pediatrics. Although rare, intussusception in adults may be idiopathic or due to a different etiology, such as a tumor.[44] With intussusception at any age, the bowel telescoping causes a mechanical obstruction and can lead to ischemia and infarction or perforation of the bowel.[44]

Assessment/Analysis
- Pediatric classic triad presentation[44]
  - Intermittent abdominal pain
  - "Red currant jelly" stool

- Palpable mass (may be sausage-shaped)
- Most common age group: 5 to 9 months
- Additional pediatric assessment findings[20]
  - Pain-spasmodic: will draw legs to the chest with sudden episodic pain that lasts a few minutes followed by a pain-free looking appearance
  - Vomiting bilious substance about 6 to 12 hours after onset
  - If a child is hemodynamically unstable, he or she may need immediate surgery
  - Ultrasound is preferred first to study in children with uncertain diagnosis
- Adults: abdominal pain often accompanied with nausea and vomiting[44]
- Abdominal guarding and rigidity
- Palpable mass
- Bowel sounds hyperactive, alternating with hypoactive sounds
- Laboratory studies
  - CBC with differential: possible leukocytosis with an increase in immature neutrophils
  - Serum chemistries
  - Positive fecal occult blood test
- Computed tomography (CT) scans: more common for adults with suspected intussusception[44]
- Pediatric Ultrasound-guided air enema: both diagnostic and therapeutic

Interventions
- Establish IV access for crystalloids/medications as needed
- Analgesics
- Pediatric patient
  - Ultrasound-guided air enema
  - Both diagnostic and often therapeutic with reduction of the intussusception[46]
- Anticipate surgery for child if the intussusception is not reduced with the air enema
- Anticipate surgery for adult
- Prepare for hospital admission: even if intussusception is reduced in pediatric patient, may be admitted to observe for any reoccurrence[46]

Evaluation
- Hemodynamic status
- Pain reduction
- Intake and output
- Auscultate bowel sounds

Bowel Obstructions

A bowel obstruction occurs with an interruption in the normal flow of food and bowel contents within the GI tract. Obstructions may be partial or complete and can occur in the small or large intestines. About 80% of mechanical obstructions occur within the small bowel and the most significant risk factor in the United States is previous abdominal surgery with subsequent postoperative adhesion formation.[46] Some other causes include tumors, intussusception, volvulus, fecal impactions, incarcerated inguinal hernia, and foreign bodies.

A nonmechanical type of obstruction is a paralytic ileus. Occasionally, this occurs postoperatively when propulsive movement decreases and may resolve with few interventions required. An ileus can occur in the non-postop setting as well. See Table 6-5 for a symptom comparison between ileus and bowel obstruction.

TABLE 6-5 Characteristics of Ileus and Bowel Obstructions

	Ileus	Bowel Obstruction
Pain	Mild to moderate	Moderate to severe
Location	Diffuse	May localize
Physical examination	Mild distention, ± tenderness, decreased bowel sounds	Mild distention, tenderness, high-pitched bowel sounds
Laboratory	Possible dehydration	Leukocytosis
Imaging	May be normal	Abnormal
Treatment	Observation, hydration	Nasogastric tube, surgery

Reproduced with permission from Wikiradiography.com

The more proximal the obstruction, the earlier the onset of symptoms. Anaerobic and aerobic bacteria accumulate proximal to the obstruction. Initially, peristalsis increases and more bowel secretions are released. Increased movement and secretions lead to worsening abdominal distension and bowel edema.[37] Malabsorption of nutrients, fluids, and electrolytes ensues. With a complete obstruction, subsequent ischemia and necrosis can lead to perforation causing peritonitis and sepsis.

Assessment/Analysis
- Nausea and vomiting: may worsen following oral intake
- Emesis: may have foul odor of feces
- Abdominal pain-intermittent and cramping, may be severe
- Abdominal tenderness and rigidity
- Abdominal distention
- Bowel sounds
  - High-pitched and hyperactive bowel sounds in early obstruction
  - Hypoactive or absent bowel sounds later in obstruction
- Diarrhea initially and after distal bowel is evacuated, constipation and inability to expel flatus develops[46]
- Possible fever and tachycardia

- Laboratory studies
  - CBC with differential: leukocytosis
  - Serum chemistries
- Upright abdominal X-ray with dilated fluid-filled loops of bowel[37]
- Ultrasound
- Abdominal CT scan helps determine severity, location, and cause of obstruction

Interventions
- Establish IV access for crystalloids and medications as needed
- NPO
- Analgesia, antiemetics, and antibiotics
- Gastric tube for decompression of stomach and help alleviate vomiting
- Surgical consult: prepare for hospital admission and possible urgent surgery

Evaluation
- Hemodynamic stability
- Decreased pain
- Intake and output

Pancreatitis

Pancreatitis involves an inflammation of the pancreas and may be confined to just the pancreas or may include surrounding tissue and other organs. The inflammation can be mild causing minimal symptoms or may be extensive. Two leading causes of pancreatitis are chronic alcohol intake and cholelithiasis.[47] Other causes are variable and occasionally the cause is unknown. Regardless of the cause, the progression of pancreatitis occurs when activated digestive enzymes are released into the pancreas and nearby tissue. The pancreatic autodigestion leads to injury of the pancreas. In response to the injury, inflammatory mediators are released leading to further inflammation. The inflammation may become systemic causing systemic inflammatory response syndrome (SIRS) and organ failure.[47]

Assessment/Analysis
- Chief complaint and history of present illness
- Persistent abdominal pain[47]
  - Often located in epigastric region
  - Radiates to the back, chest, and right shoulder or flanks
  - May increase with oral intake
  - Position of comfort may be sitting up with knees flexed
- Rebound tenderness and abdominal guarding
- Nausea and vomiting
- Abdominal distention
- Hypoactive bowel sounds
- Tachycardia; possible hypotension
- Tachypnea and shortness of breath
- Fever
- Laboratory studies
  - Elevated serum lipase and amylase
  - CBC with differential—leukocytosis
  - Serum chemistries
  - Liver function tests
- Abdominal ultrasound
- Abdominal CT scan
- MRI
  - Identifies any complications of pancreatitis
  - Detects choledocholithiasis (presence of gallstones in the common bile duct)

Interventions
- Establish IV access for crystalloids, blood products, and medications as needed
- Monitor hemodynamic status
- Administer analgesics and antiemetics
- NPO
- Antibiotics only if infectious process is suspected
- Surgical consult if pancreatitis cause is gallstones
- Prepare for hospital admission

Evaluation
- Hemodynamic stability
- Intake and output
- Patient/family education
  - Diet: when allowed to resume oral intake
  - Low-fat diet
  - Avoidance of alcohol

Abdominal Trauma

The most common mechanism for blunt abdominal trauma is motor vehicle crashes (MVC) and carries a higher mortality rate than penetrating abdominal trauma due to delayed injury detection. Additionally, blunt abdominal trauma is often associated with concurrent injuries of the head and/or chest.[48] Stabbings from a knife or any sharp object, gunshot wounds (GSW), or impaled objects from explosions are types of penetrating injuries. Severe internal bleeding from injuries within the abdominal cavity can be a large contributor to hemorrhage and death.[49]

Assessment/Analysis
- History of chief complaint and circumstances around trauma and patient information[49]
  - MVC: type of crash, patient restrained, airbag deployed, patient ejected, extent of vehicle damage, speed of car, and patient's location within the vehicle
  - Fall: how far patient fell, landing surface, and part of body impacted
    - Anticipate possibly severe injuries and transfer to trauma center
      - Children: falling over three times their height
      - Adult: over 11 feet

- Penetrating trauma: weapon or object used, if GSW- approximate distance from shooter and caliber and velocity, estimated blood loss
- Any penetrating injury to the lower chest, pelvis, flank, or back has the probability of entering the abdominal cavity until proven otherwise[50]
- Airway stability, effective breathing, and adequate circulation
- Vital signs and cardiac monitor
- Inspect abdomen: normal appearing abdomen does not exclude possibility of internal injuries
  - Seatbelt ecchymosis or abrasions as pictured in Figure 6-6
    - Appearance of a seatbelt sign in the emergency department indicates high level of force transferred during MVC

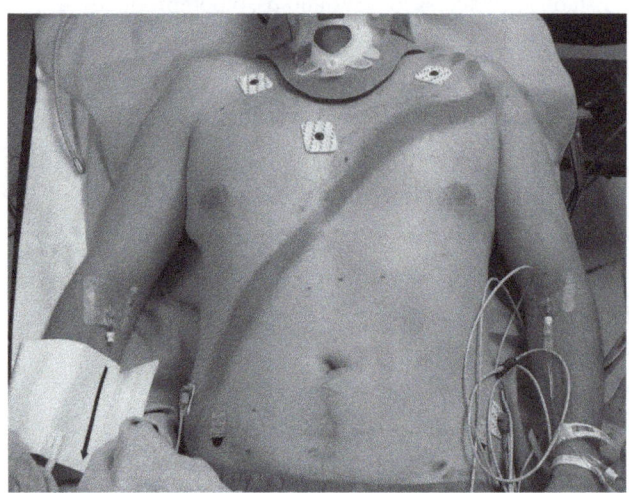

FIGURE 6-6 **Seatbelt sign**
Reproduced with permission from Knoop KJ, Stack LB, Storrow AB, et al: The Atlas of Emergency Medicine, 4th ed. New York: McGraw-Hill Education; 2016: Photo contributor: Brad Russell, MD.

  - Cullen's sign (periumbilical ecchymosis) and Grey Turner's sign (flank ecchymosis) delayed indicators for retroperitoneal bleeding[50]
  - See Figure 6-7 for Cullen's sign and Grey Turner's sign on the same patient

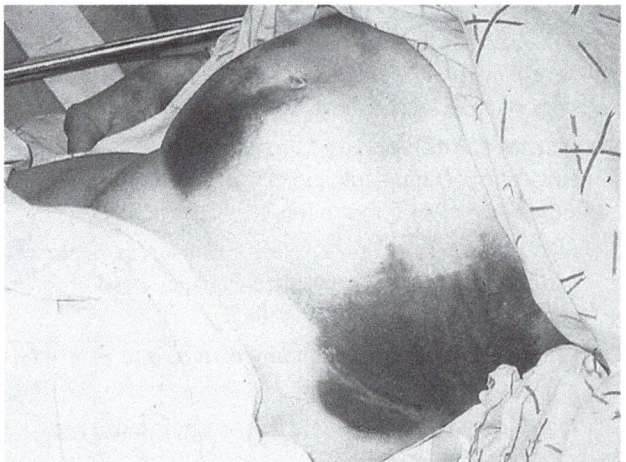

FIGURE 6-7 **Cullen's sign and Grey Turner's sign**
Reproduced with permission from Knoop KJ, Stack LB, Storrow AB, et al: The Atlas of Emergency Medicine, 4th ed. New York: McGraw-Hill Education; 2016: Photo contributor: Michael Ritter, MD.

- Auscultate for bowel sounds and characteristics
- Percuss abdomen
  - Tympany (air in hollow organ such as stomach or small bowel)
  - Dullness (fairly solid organ such as liver or spleen)[51]
- Palpate all four quadrants of abdomen noting tenderness, distention, or rigidity
  - Immediate pain and tenderness could indicate chemical irritation, from gastric acid contents, within peritoneum[50]
- Laboratory tests
  - CBC with differential
  - Serum chemistries and liver function tests
  - Coagulation profiles
  - Blood bank analysis (Type and Screen/Cross), if transfusion is likely
  - Amylase and lipase
  - Toxicology screen and blood alcohol
  - Urine for hematuria
- Other diagnostic studies
  - Abdominal/pelvic CT scan with IV contrast is gold standard for diagnosis of abdominal injuries[50]
  - Hepatic lacerations or hematomas are graded I–IV to illustrate the severity of injury with grade I as minor injury and grade VI as the most severe injury[49]
  - Splenic injuries are also graded for severity with grade I as the least severely injured and grade V is the most severely injured[49]
  - **F**ocused **A**ssessment with **S**onography for **T**rauma (FAST)
    - Can quickly evaluate for intra-abdominal blood or fluid (possible blood in abdomen)
    - Accuracy can be operator dependent
    - Ultrasound has replaced the diagnostic peritoneal lavage (DPL)/diagnostic peritoneal aspiration (DPA) in most American trauma centers[50]
  - DPA: after the indwelling urinary catheter is inserted, a small incision is made midline below the umbilicus. Aspiration is obtained with a catheter. If aspirate reveals gross blood, the DPA is considered positive. If no gross blood, a DPL may be performed[49]
  - DPL: one liter of fluid infused through catheter (insertion described in the previous DPA) and then drained out of peritoneal cavity into empty container using unvented tubing. Presence of blood indicates a positive DPL[49]

Interventions
- Support airway and effective breathing as needed
- Cardiac monitor, pulse oximetry, possible end-tidal CO_2 monitoring (if intubated or other compromised respiratory condition)
- Establish IV access for crystalloids, blood products, and medications as needed

- Prevent hypothermia: warm trauma bay, warm blankets, and warm fluids
- Analgesia
- NPO
- Possible gastric tube to prevent gastric distention (avoid nasogastric tube if facial fractures are suspected)
- Prepare for possible hospital admission and/or emergency surgery

Evaluation
- Airway stability; effective breathing
- Vital signs, signs of bleeding
- Pain management
- Laboratory values and focused assessments for trending

REFERENCES

1. National Hospital Ambulatory Medical Care Survey: 2011 Emergency Department Summary Tables. *CDC National Center for Health Statistics.* http://www.cdc.gov/nchs/fastats/digestive-diseases.htm. Published June 18, 2012. Accessed May 30, 2016.
2. Harbrecht BG, Franklin GA, Miller FB, et al. Acute appendicitis—not just for the young. *Am J Surg.* 2011;202:286–290. doi:10.1016/j.amjsurg.2010.08.017
3. Jacobs DO. Acute appendicitis and peritonitis. In: Kasper D, Fauci A, Hauser S, et al, eds. *Harrison's Principles of Internal Medicine.* 19th ed. New York, NY: McGraw-Hill; 2015.
4. DeKoning E. Acute appendicitis. In: Tintinalli JE, Stapczynski J, Ma O, et al, eds. *Tintinalli's Emergency Medicine: A Comprehensive Study Guide.* 8th ed. New York, NY: McGraw-Hill; 2016.
5. O'Brien MC. Gastrointestinal emergencies. In: Tintinalli JE, Stapczynski JS, Cline DM, et al, eds. *Tintinalli's Emergency Medicine.* 7th ed. New York, NY: McGraw-Hill; 2011:519–527.
6. Macaluso CR, McNamara RM. Evaluation and management of acute abdominal pain in the emergency department. *Int J Family Med.* 2012;5:789–797.
7. Laine L, Yang H, Chang S, et al. Trends for incidence of hospitalization and death due to GI complications in the United States from 2001 to 2009. *Am J Gastroenterol.* 2012;107:1190–1195.
8. Longo DL, Fauci AS, Kasper DL, et al. Gastrointestinal bleeding. In: Longo DL, Fauci AS, Kasper DL, et al, eds. *Harrison's Manual of Medicine.* 18th ed. New York, NY: McGraw-Hill; 2013.
9. Ziebell CM, Kitlowski A, Welch JM, et al. Upper gastrointestinal bleeding. In: Tintinalli JE, Stapczynski J, Ma O, et al, eds. *Tintinalli's Emergency Medicine: A Comprehensive Study Guide.* 8th ed. New York, NY: McGraw-Hill; 2016.
10. Curry K. The ins and outs of GI bleed. *Nurs Spectr.* January 2011:18–23.
11. Price TG, Armstrong ZE. Gastrointestinal bleeding. In: Stone C, Humphries RL, eds. *CURRENT Diagnosis & Treatment Emergency Medicine.* 7th ed. New York, NY: McGraw-Hill; 2011.
12. Byerly JC. A 68-year-old man with bright red emesis. *J Emerg Nurs.* 2012;38(4):357–259.
13. Lo BM. Lower gastrointestinal bleeding. In: Tintinalli JE, Stapczynski J, Ma O, et al, eds. *Tintinalli's Emergency Medicine: A Comprehensive Study Guide.* 8th ed. New York, NY: McGraw-Hill; 2016.
14. Cappell MS. Famous gastroenterology quotes. *Gastroenterol Nurs.* 2012;35(5):357–360.
15. Weintraub P. The Dr. who drank infectious broth, gave himself an ulcer, and solved a medical mystery. *Discover.* http://discovermagazine.com/2010/mar/07-dr-drank-broth-gave-ulcer-solved-medical-mystery. Published March 2010. Accessed May 30, 2016.
16. Gratton MC, Bogle A. Peptic ulcer disease and gastritis. In: Tintinalli JE, Stapczynski J, Ma O, et al, eds. *Tintinalli's Emergency Medicine: A Comprehensive Study Guide.* 8th ed. New York, NY: McGraw-Hill; 2016.
17. Feinstein LB, Holman RC, Yorita KL, et al. Trends in hospitalizations for peptic ulcer disease, United States, 1998–2005. *Centers for Disease Control and Prevention.* http://wwwnc.cdc.gov/eid/article/16/9/09-1126_article. Published September 2010. Accessed May 30, 2016.
18. Wadie NI. Peptic ulcer disease. *Prim Care.* 2011;38(3):983–994. doi:10.1016/j.pop.2011.05.001
19. Parasa S, Sharma P. Complications of gastro-oesophageal reflux. *Best Pract Res Clin Gastroenterol.* 2013;27:433–442. http://dx.doi.org/10.1016/j.bpg.2013.07.002
20. Rossoll L. Abdominal emergencies. In: Hoyt KS, Selfridge-Thomas J, eds. *Emergency nursing core curriculum,* 6e. St. Louis, MO: Elsevier; 2007:159–186.
21. Mendelson M. Esophageal Emergencies. In: Tintinalli JE, Stapczynski J, Ma O, et al, eds. *Tintinalli's Emergency Medicine: A Comprehensive Study Guide.* 8th ed. New York, NY: McGraw-Hill; 2016.
22. Saccomano SJ, Ferrara LR. Evaluation of acute abdominal pain. *Nurse Pract.* 2013;8(11):46–53.
23. Friedman LS. Liver, biliary tract, and pancreas disorders. In: Papadakis MA, McPhee SJ, Rabow MW, eds. *Current Medical Diagnosis & Treatment 2016.* New York, NY: McGraw-Hill; 2016.
24. Pagana KD, Pagana TJ, Pagana TN. *Mosby's diagnostic & laboratory test reference.* 12th ed. St. Louis, MO: Elsevier; 2015.
25. Bacon BR. Cirrhosis and its complications. In: Kasper D, Fauci A, Hauser S, et al, eds. *Harrison's principles of Internal Medicine.* 19th ed. New York, NY: McGraw-Hill; 2015.
26. Werner KT, Perez ST. Role of nurse practitioners in the management of cirrhotic patients. *J Nurse Pract.* 2012;8(10):816–821.
27. O'Mara SR, Gebreyes K. Hepatic disorders. In: Tintinalli JE, Stapczynski J, Ma O, et al, eds. *Tintinalli's Emergency Medicine: A Comprehensive Study Guide.* 8th ed. New York, NY: McGraw-Hill; 2016.
28. Harris H, Crawford A. Hepatitis goes viral. *Nursing 2013.* 2013; 43(11):38–43. doi: 10.1097/01.NURSE.0000435198.73152.01
29. Dienstag JL. Acute viral hepatitis. In: Kasper D, Fauci A, Hauser S, et al, eds. *Harrison's Principles of Internal Medicine.* 19th ed. New York, NY: McGraw-Hill; 2015.
30. Poole S. Update on the treatment and management of patients with hepatitis. *J Infus Nurs.* 2009;32(5):269–275.
31. Coomes J, Platt M. Abdominal pain. In: Stone C, Humphries RL, eds. *CURRENT Diagnosis & Treatment Emergency Medicine.* 7th ed. New York, NY: McGraw-Hill; 2011.
32. Smith MM. Variceal hemorrhage from esophageal varices associated with alcoholic liver disease. *Am J Nurs.* 2010;110(2):32–39.
33. Graham A. Diverticulitis. In: Tintinalli JE, Stapczynski J, Ma O, et al, eds. *Tintinalli's Emergency Medicine: A Comprehensive Study Guide.* 8th ed. New York, NY: McGraw-Hill; 2016.
34. Centers for disease control and prevention. Injuries from Ingestion of Wire Bristles from Grill-Cleaning Brushes—Providence, Rhode Island, March 2011–June 2012. *MMWR.* 2012;61(26):490–492.
35. Birnbaumer DM, Flowers LK. Sexually transmitted infections and anorectal conditions. In: Knoop KJ, Stack LB, Storrow AB, Thurman R, eds. *The Atlas of Emergency Medicine.* 3rd ed. New York, NY: McGraw-Hill; 2010.
36. Wikswo ME, Kambhampati A, Shioda K, et al. *Outbreaks of Acute Gastroenteritis Transmitted by Person-to-Person Contact, Environmental Contamination, and Unknown Modes of Transmission—United States, 2009–2013.* http://www.cdc.gov/mmwr/preview/mmwrhtml/ss6412a1.htm?s_cid=ss6412a1_w. Published December 11, 2015. Accessed May 30, 2016.
37. Herrington A. Gastrointestinal emergencies. In: Howard PK, Steinmann RA, eds. *Sheehy's Emergency Nursing: Principles and Practice.* 6th ed. St. Louis, MO: Elsevier; 2010:467–477.
38. Yeh DD, Hasan BA. Hernia emergencies. *Surg Clin N Am.* 2014;94:97–130. doi: http://dx.doi.org/10.1016/j.suc.2013.10.009
39. Byars D, Kayagil T. Hernias. In: Tintinalli JE, Stapczynski J, Ma O, et al, eds. *Tintinalli's Emergency Medicine: A Comprehensive Study Guide.* 8th ed. New York, NY: McGraw-Hill; 2016.

40. Horn AE, Ufberg JW. Appendicitis, diverticulitis, and colitis. *Emerg Med Clin N Am*. 2011;29:347–368. doi:10.1016/j.emc.2011.01.002
41. Chaitanya P, Deshpande A, Fraga-Lovejoy C, et al. Emergency department visits related to inflammatory bowel disease: Results from nationwide emergency department sample. *JPGN*. 2015:61(3):282–284.
42. Friedman S, Blumberg RS. Inflammatory bowel disease. In: Kasper D, Fauci A, Hauser S, et al, eds. *Harrison's Principles of Internal Medicine*. 19th ed. New York, NY: McGraw-Hill; 2015.
43. Kman NE, Werman HA. Disorders presenting primarily with diarrhea. In: Tintinalli JE, Stapczynski J, Ma O, et al, eds. *Tintinalli's Emergency Medicine: A Comprehensive Study Guide*. 8th ed. New York, NY: McGraw-Hill; 2016.
44. Lindor RA, Bellolio F, Sadosty AT, et al. Adult intussusception: Presentation, management and outcomes of 148 patients. *J Emerg Med*. 2012:43(1):1–6. doi:10.1016/j.jemermed.2011.05.098
45. Fleischman RJ. Acute abdominal pain in infants and children. In: Tintinalli JE, Stapczynski J, Ma O, et al, eds. *Tintinalli's Emergency Medicine: A Comprehensive Study Guide*. 8th ed. New York, NY: McGraw-Hill; 2016.
46. Bordeianou L, Yeh DD. Epidemiology, clinical features, and diagnosis of mechanical small bowel obstruction in adults. *UpToDate*. http://www.uptodate.com/home. Published June 2015. Accessed January 23, 2016.
47. Besinger B, Stehman CR. Pancreatitis and cholecystitis. In: Tintinalli JE, Stapczynski J, Ma O, et al, eds. *Tintinalli's Emergency Medicine: A Comprehensive Study Guide*. 8th ed. New York, NY: McGraw-Hill; 2016.
48. Bacidore V. Abdominal and genitourinary trauma. In: Howard PK, Steinmann RA, eds. *Sheehy's Emergency Nursing: Principles and Practice*. 6th ed. St. Louis, MO: Elsevier; 2010:301–312.
49. Webster AM, Bratcher CM. Abdominal and pelvic trauma. In: *Trauma nursing core course (TNCC)*. 7th ed. Des Plaines, IL: Emergency Nurses Association; 2014:151–172.
50. French L, Gordy S, Ma O. Abdominal trauma. In: Tintinalli JE, Stapczynski J, Ma O, et al, eds. *Tintinalli's Emergency Medicine: A Comprehensive Study Guide*. 8th ed. New York, NY: McGraw-Hill; 2016.
51. Jarvis C. *Physical Examination & Health Assessment*. 4th ed. St. Louis, MO: Saunders; 2004.

Practice Questions

Question	Rationale
1. A patient experiences point tenderness at McBurney's point during an abdominal assessment. What other findings may coincide with this symptom? a. History of chronic intermittent pain b. Hematochezia c. Elevated WBC d. Pain radiates to the right shoulder	*Answer: c* McBurney's point is located midway between the umbilicus and the anterior superior iliac crest in the RLQ. If point tenderness is localized at this point, it may be an indication of an acute appendicitis. An elevated WBC, in the presence of other suspecting symptoms, has a greater diagnostic value for appendicitis. Acute pain is associated with appendicitis. The risk of perforation increases if symptoms are present more than 48 hours. Hematochezia is bright red or maroon rectal bleeding and is suggestive of a lower GI bleeding or a massive upper GI bleed. Pain radiating to the right shoulder can be symptomatic for acute cholecystitis
2. The correct sequence of physical assessment for the abdomen is a. Palpation, inspection, percussion, auscultation b. Inspection, auscultation, percussion, palpation c. Auscultation, percussion, palpation, inspection d. Auscultation, inspection, percussion, palpation	*Answer: b* Inspecting the abdomen allows for assessing for distention, scars, and skin changes. Auscultation provides an assessment for the presence of bowel sounds and the characteristics of them. High-pitched bowel sounds may imply an intestinal obstruction. Dullness on percussion helps identify the liver and splenic borders, and tympany on percussion may suggest a dilated loop of bowel.[5] Reserving palpation for last allows a better opportunity to identify the area and degree of tenderness.
3. While palpating the abdomen of a patient, the emergency nurse observes rebound tenderness. Rebound tenderness raises the possibility for all of the conditions *except* a. Appendicitis b. A perforated colon c. Constipation d. Cholecystitis	*Answer: c* Although rebound tenderness does not have 100% sensitivity for appendicitis, peritonitis (a perforated colon) or cystitis, patients presenting with any of these conditions may have rebound tenderness noted during physical assessment. Some of the common symptoms associated with constipation are abdominal discomfort, bloating, and straining during bowel evacuation.

Question	Rationale
4. A 17-year-old male patient is being discharged from the emergency department. He had presented with abdominal pain in his right and left lower quadrants. Besides mild nausea and some tenderness with palpation in his lower abdomen, he has no other symptoms. His CBC, ultrasound, and CT scan results were negative for any findings. The ED nurse's discharge instructions should include a. Avoid greasy foods and consider an over-the-counter proton pump inhibitor, such as Omeprazole b. Increase your fiber intake and drink 6 to 8 glasses of water per day to relieve your constipation c. If symptoms continue or new ones develop, rest and follow-up with your primary care provider in 3 days d. If pain persists and/or worsens or a fever or vomiting appear, return to the emergency department	*Answer: d* This patient did not appear acutely ill; however, his symptoms could be in the early stage for appendicitis or small bowel obstruction. Given his age, there is a greater likelihood for an early appendicitis that could progress. Discharge instructions, both written and verbal, should emphasize returning for medical care should an acute infectious process, such as appendicitis, evolve. Avoiding greasy foods is encouraged if cholelithiasis is suspected. The patient does not report a history of colicky RUQ abdominal pain suggesting gallstones. Proton pump inhibitors are typically prescribed when a patient has a history of gastroesophageal reflux disease (GERD) or ulcer. Although increasing fiber and water intake is healthy, his symptoms and imaging results do not suggest constipation. The risk of a perforated appendix is likely with symptoms lasting more than 2 days. Waiting 3 days to follow-up with one's primary care provider, for new or continued symptoms, is too long of a wait with possible appendicitis.
5. An ill-appearing 50-year-old male arrives at the emergency department via EMS. His chief complaint is abdominal pain, vomiting, and fever of 101°F (38.3°C) for the past 12 hours. His abdominal pain is diffuse with muscle rigidity upon palpation of his abdomen. Past medical history is noncontributory except for a screening colonoscopy 24 hours earlier. This patient may be experiencing the following condition a. Appendicitis b. Diverticulitis c. Perforated ulcer d. Peritonitis	*Answer: d* A perforation may have occurred from the colonoscopy causing spillage of bowel contents into the peritoneal cavity. If left untreated, sepsis will ensue. His history of having a recent colonoscopy would raise the index of suspicion for a perforated colon. Typically pain from appendicitis becomes localized in the RLQ and pain from diverticulitis becomes localized in the LLQ. Although a ruptured appendix or perforated ulcer can cause diffuse abdominal pain with peritonitis, his history of a recent colonoscopy coincides with the potential cause of his peritonitis.
6. Hematochezia has the following characteristics a. Black or "tarry" blood from rectum often associated with upper GI bleeds b. Vomiting of blood or "coffee ground" emesis c. Bright red or maroon rectal bleeding and can be associated with upper or lower GI bleeding d. Bleeding from the ligament of Treitz	*Answer: c* Hematochezia is bright red or maroon rectal bleeding and is usually indicative of lower GI bleeding. However, hematochezia can also occur with a very rapid upper GI bleed (>1000 mL). Melena is black or "tarry" stool from rectum. Although melena is often associated with upper GI bleeding, it can also occur with intake of specific substances such as iron, licorice and beets (pseudomelena). Vomiting blood or "coffee ground" emesis is referred to as hematemesis. The ligament of Treitz is a smooth muscle that is connected to the junction of the duodenum and jejunum and is referred as a landmark separating an upper GI and lower GI bleed.

Question	Rationale
7. A 46-year-old patient comes to the emergency department with complaints of a "stomachache." She said the pain began about 12 hours prior to arrival and she suspects the cause as "some vegetables I ate." Vital signs are within normal limits and she ambulates without difficulty from triage to her room. Shortly after arrival, she has a black tarry stool in the bedside commode. What test does the nurse anticipate for a stool specimen? a. Hemoglobin and Hematocrit b. Orthostatic vital signs c. Fecal occult blood test d. Stool sample of ova and parasites	*Answer: c* A "pseudomelena" can occur as a result of ingesting certain substances such as iron, beets, licorice, bismuth, and charcoal. The stool may look "tarry" and black but testing for occult blood will be negative. Measuring the hemoglobin and hematocrit may be deferred until GI bleeding is confirmed. Orthostatic vital signs may be helpful if she were complaining of dizziness and weakness while ambulating. Stool for ova and parasites should be tested if an infectious process or ingestion of contaminated food or water is suspected.
8. A 62-year-old male complains of "… vomiting blood for days." He is pale and weak with cool and clammy skin. His past medical history (PMH) includes coronary artery disease (CAD), hypertension, benign prostatic hypertrophy (BPH), and alcohol abuse. Vital signs are: T-97.7°F (36.5°C), P-108, R-22, BP-168/96, SpO_2-94% on 2 liters per nasal cannula. Initial lab results: hemoglobin is 9.1 g/dL and hematocrit is 33.6 %. Considering his PMH, what test would the nurse anticipate is needed? a. 12-lead ECG b. Uric acid level c. Glycosylated hemoglobin (HbA_{1c}) d. Parathyroid hormone level	*Answer: a* Decreased oxygen delivery occurs with bleeding as evidenced by decreased hemoglobin and hematocrit. His history of CAD is a risk factor for ischemia to the coronary arteries. A 12-lead ECG would be warranted. Uric acid levels may be obtained if gout is suspected. Although increased uric acid levels can occur with alcoholism, his chief complaint and PMH do not reveal complaints of joint pain or swelling as seen with gout. Since there is no report of diabetes or hyperglycemia, glycosylated hemoglobin (HbA_{1c}) would not be indicated. A serum parathyroid hormone level is often measured with serum calcium and used for assessing the parathyroid function.
9. A driver of a car is transferred to a trauma center, after being involved in a head on collision with a truck. The emergency nurse suspects the patient has a retroperitoneal bleed when the following assessment finding is observed a. Grey Turner sign b. Virchow triad c. Beck's triad d. Rovsing sign	*Answer: a* Grey Turner sign is ecchymosis in the flank area and is often associated with a retroperitoneal bleed from abdominal and/or pelvic trauma. Virchow's triad relates to the three characteristics that can lead to an increase in thrombosis formation: Hypercoagulability of blood, damaged vascular endothelium, and venous stasis. Beck's triad may indicate pericardial tamponade. Beck's triad consists of muffled heart tones, jugular venous distention, and hypotension. Rovsing sign is tested by palpating for rebound tenderness in the LUQ, distant from the appendiceal area in the RLQ. Rovsing sign is positive if the patient experiences pain (rebound tenderness) in the RLQ, and this can be a possible sign for appendicitis.

Question	Rationale
10. The emergency nurse is preparing a 46-year-old male for discharge from the emergency department following his visit for complaints of "indigestion" and "stomach pain." He has a history of GERD and had stopped taking his proton pump inhibitor (Omeprazole) two weeks ago because he "…was feeling better." All of the following statements indicate the patient's understanding of his condition *except* a. I only take this pill when I am having pain b. I should consider putting my bed on blocks or sleeping on an elevated pillow to help decrease my reflux c. I should avoid drinking alcoholic beverages and spicy foods d. I need to lose about 20 pounds	*Answer: a* Acid reflux typically occurs with GERD, and proton pump inhibitors suppress gastric acid secretion. This action requires a consistent compliance with the medication schedule. Reflux may also be diminished with elevating the head of the bed, avoiding alcoholic beverages and spicy foods. Losing weight can help decrease reflux with patients who are overweight.
11. What is the bacteria responsible for causing a high incidence of peptic ulcers, gastritis, and stomach cancers? a. *Candida albicans* b. *Helicobacter pylori* c. *Listeria* d. *Clostridium perfringens*	*Answer: b* *Helicobacter pylori* can cause gastritis, peptic ulcers, and stomach cancers. *Candida albicans*, a fungus that is part of the normal flora within the colon, can cause opportunistic infections. *Listeria* and *Clostridium perfringens* are bacteria that can cause food poisoning.
12. A pale, anxious 32-year-old female presents to the emergency department complaining of chest pain and nausea that woke her. She describes the pain as sharp and denies vomiting or diarrhea. Vital signs: T-98.4° F (36.9°C), P-92, R-24, BP-116/68, SpO_2-97% on room air. Cardiac monitor shows sinus rhythm, ECG is within normal limits, and first set of cardiac enzymes is normal. Her medications consist of ibuprofen that she takes for tension headaches. Her last meal was "five-alarm chili" for supper. What condition could she be experiencing? a. Gastroenteritis b. Gastritis c. Upper GI bleed d. Esophagitis	*Answer: b* Her risk factors for gastritis are intake of spicy foods and NSAIDs. Gastric pain often returns as the gastric contents empty. Since gastric emptying also occurs during sleep, the gastric pain can be severe enough to wake a person. Typically fever, vomiting, and diarrhea accompany gastroenteritis, which she is not experiencing. She does not have any sign of hematemesis or other signs of bleeding associated with upper GI bleeding. With esophagitis, there is frequent belching (eructations) and a burning pain associated with swallowing.

Question	Rationale
13. A pale 75-year-old man with severe osteoarthritis comes to the emergency department reporting having black tarry stools for the past week. This morning, he "…vomited blood." He takes 600 mg of ibuprofen three times a day to control his arthritis pain, drinks 2 to 3 beers at night and lives alone. Current vital signs: T-98.6°F (37°C) orally; P-116, BP-100/66, R-20, SpO_2-92% on room air. Epigastric tenderness is noted. An IV is established and lab results are pending. He is nauseated and vomits bright red blood. The emergency nurse anticipates the next intervention as a priority a. Prepare for a hospital admission b. Obtain a stat GI consult and prepare for endoscopy c. Insert gastric tube and gently lavage with water d. Start a vasoactive infusion such as Dopamine	*Answer: c* Gastric lavage, with room temperature water or saline, allows assessment of the aspirate and improves visualization with an endoscopy for suspected bleeding. Endoscopies can be diagnostic and therapeutic. Diagnosis of bleeding sources as well as administration of hemostatic agents can be accomplished with endoscopies. A hospital admission is warranted after stabilizing treatment. Dopamine is not indicated since his vomiting and tachycardia suggest that he is most likely hypovolemic.
14. The following symptoms are all indicative of possible cirrhosis of the liver *except* a. Palmar erythema b. Hypersplenism c. Spider angiomas d. Rebound tenderness	*Answer: d* Depressing the abdomen slowly downward and then quickly releasing is the test for rebound tenderness. A patient with rebound tenderness will feel greater pain with the release and this can raise the suspicion of an acute peritoneal irritation, such as peritonitis or appendicitis. Palmar erythema is seen in the patient with alcoholic cirrhosis and has the appearance of a centralized pallor on the palms surrounded by erythema. Hypersplenism occurs from portal hypertension that results from the changes in blood flow surrounding the cirrhotic liver. Spider angiomas can be seen in normal skin conditions, but typically they are seen more frequently in patients who have liver disease. The central arteriole surrounded by thin-wall capillaries has a resemblance of a spider.
15. A patient tells the nurse that he has just been diagnosed with Hepatitis D. What classification of viral hepatitis did he have prior to contracting this? a. Hepatitis A b. Hepatitis B c. Hepatitis C d. Hepatitis E	*Answer: b* The hepatitis B virus is a carrying portal for the hepatitis D virus to enter the liver. Since hepatitis B can convert to a chronic form of hepatitis, hepatitis D can invade the liver much later. Hepatitis A and E are transmitted via the oral-fecal route, and Hepatitis B and C are transmitted through blood and body fluids.

Question	Rationale
16. A 28-year-old female arrives to the emergency department complaining of nausea, vomiting, diarrhea, and RUQ abdominal pain for a week. After arriving from Mexico with her 4-year-old daughter, the patient (mother) appears dehydrated and weak. Her color is pale. Her serology tests confirm hepatitis A (HAV-Ab/IgM is present). She insists her child is fine and does not need testing for hepatitis since she is "not sick." An important teaching point to the mother would be a. Symptoms for hepatitis A to watch for with her daughter b. Hepatitis A is not contagious with young children since they are not symptomatic c. Avoid sexual contact while being treated d. Young children who are infected with hepatitis A are usually not symptomatic despite being contagious	*Answer: d* Hepatitis A is transmitted via the oral-fecal route and children less than 6 years of age rarely have symptoms despite being contagious. Hepatitis A is not transmitted through sexual contact. Hepatitis serology tests are important to determine if the child is positive and would be considered contagious.
17. Which of the following symptoms are *not* associated with Hepatitis B? a. Clay-colored stools b. Jaundice c. Right lower quadrant pain d. Pruritus	*Answer: c* Generally, right lower quadrant pain may indicate an inflammatory process such as appendicitis or diverticulitis. Since hepatitis B involves the liver, often the patient has abdominal pain localized to the right upper quadrant. Clay-colored stools, jaundice, and pruritus are all signs of liver dysfunction associated with fulminant hepatitis B.
18. A 41-year-old man appears at the emergency department. He states that he lives "on the street," and while riding the bus to the hospital, he swallowed an object that he found on the bus. He will not state what the object is. The nurse knows all of the following conditions would indicate an emergent upper endoscopy *except* a. Clear lung sounds and is smiling while freely conversing b. A button battery is ingested c. Ingestion of a razor blade confirmed d. Shortness of breath, respiratory stridor, and SpO$_2$ is 86% on room air	*Answer: a* For various reasons including age or mental illness, a patient's history may be vague regarding the ingested foreign object. Diagnostic imaging such as radiographic films are helpful; however, CT imaging is more useful to identify the object, location, and any potential damage from the foreign body, such as perforation. A patient exhibiting no signs of respiratory distress on admission but providing a vague history would probably need diagnostic imaging to determine the presence of a foreign body. If the foreign body were believed to be corrosive, sharp, and/or harmful, an emergency upper endoscopy would be indicated. Respiratory compromise requires airway management and upper endoscopy.

Question	Rationale
19. The emergency nurse is discharging a 20-month-old boy after receiving oral fluids and a PO antiemetic. He was diagnosed with gastroenteritis following a 2-day history of nausea and vomiting. Evaluating his condition, the nurse reassess for what cues that signal his ED treatment was effective and he can be safely discharged home? a. Makes eye contact and smiles with the nurse while his mom holds him b. Consumed prescribed oral rehydration solution during last 3 hours without vomiting c. Mother plans to begin feeding him the BRAT diet at home d. Playing with his toy train on the floor and is more active	*Answer: b* Rehydration is essential for the patient with gastroenteritis. Nausea and vomiting impede consuming adequate oral hydration therapy, and dehydration ensues. Once nausea and vomiting have subsided, oral fluids are indicated and can effectively hydrate in mild to moderate dehydration. Although a child's increased activity and interaction are good signs, ensuring he can tolerate oral rehydration is imperative before discharge home. The BRAT diet, consisting of bananas, rice, applesauce, and toast, is believed to be bland enough when the child or adult is ready to return to solid foods. Although the BRAT diet is not strongly supported with evidence or as popular, it occasionally is recommended for patients with gastroenteritis.
20. A 20-year-old presents to the emergency department with complaints of abdominal cramping and non-bloody, liquid diarrhea. She denies foreign travel, dietary changes, alcohol or drug use. Vital signs are T-98.2°F. (36.8°C), P-108, R-18, BP-98/58, SpO_2-99% on room air. She is weak, pale and tenderness with palpation is noted in her RLQ. Initial labs are within normal limits except an increased Erythrocyte sedimentation rate (ESR) and decreased serum potassium. The emergency nurse suspects Crohn's disease rather than ulcerative colitis because of her a. History of non-bloody diarrhea b. Elevated Erythrocyte sedimentation rate (ESR) c. Weakness and dehydration d. Cramping abdominal pain	*Answer: a* Ulcerative colitis (UC) and Crohn's disease (CD) can have similar signs and symptoms in the early stages. The patient exhibits inflammatory bowel disease characterized by abdominal cramping, diarrhea, elevated markers of inflammation such as ESR and C-reactive protein (CRP), and possible electrolyte imbalances secondary to diarrhea. Typically, UC has visible bloody diarrhea and CD is characterized by non-bloody diarrhea. A fecal occult blood test may be positive with CD due to the inflammation and irritation from the GI tract.
21. A 80-year-old female arrives via EMS from an assisted living facility with abdominal pain and constipation for 12 hours. Her past medical history includes hypertension, dementia, and abdominal hysterectomy. Vital signs are stable. She is moaning and holding her abdomen. Bowel sounds are high-pitched; abdomen is rigid and tender upon palpation. Her pain is diffuse and worse in her periumbilical area. Abdominal series radiography demonstrates multiple dilated fluid-filled loops of bowel. What is her primary risk factor for a small bowel obstruction? a. Dementia b. Hypertension c. Older age d. Abdominal hysterectomy	*Answer: d* A history of abdominal surgery can lead to adhesions (scar tissue formation), which can subsequently lead to a mechanical blockage causing a bowel obstruction. Pain is usually severe and often localized to a specific area of the abdomen. Bowel motility continues with an obstruction, hence bowel sounds are high-pitched and hyperactive, especially with an early obstruction. Age and dementia alone are not risk factors; however, constipation and fecal impactions are potential risk factors for bowel obstructions. Hypertension is not a risk factor for bowel obstructions.

Question	Rationale
22. A 61-year-old female arrived to the emergency department via EMS following a 2-day history of fever, nausea, and epigastric pain radiating to her back. Serum amylase, lipase, and WBC count are elevated. Past medical history includes intermittent urinary tract infections. Her work of breathing is labored and she is not responding to verbal stimuli. She is intubated and placed on mechanical ventilation. Current vital signs: 102°F (38.9°C), P-128, R-16 assisted on vent, BP-86/52, SpO$_2$-90% and ETCO$_2$ is 42. The nurse's next intervention will focus on a. Fluid resuscitation b. Administering an albuterol nebulizer treatment c. Obtaining blood cultures and administering an acetaminophen suppository d. Inserting an indwelling urinary catheter	*Answer: a* Cholelithiasis is a leading cause of pancreatitis. Epigastric pain that radiates to the back and right shoulder with fever are signs of possible cholelithiasis. Gallstones can create a blocked duct causing the pancreas to become inflamed from the autodigestive process as digestive enzymes release into the pancreas. Fluid shifts occur with acute pancreatitis and can lead to hypotension and hypovolemic shock. Fluid resuscitation takes priority following airway stabilization. Her history and presentation do not suggest asthma or other symptoms needing a bronchodilator. Blood cultures, acetaminophen administration and indwelling catheter insertion may be part of treatment and can be implemented after fluid resuscitation is started.
23. A 37-year-old male arrived by EMS following an MVC at highway speeds. He was a restrained passenger, and the car was t-boned with intrusion on his side. After a short extrication, he was intubated and an IV was started at the scene. Lung sounds equal and bilateral. A FAST exam reveals intra-abdominal fluid, and a liver injury is suspected. His abdomen is distended and rigid. Facial grimacing with palpating his RUQ and LUQ. Vital signs: T-97.4°F (36.3°C); P-127; R-16 assisted on vent; BP-88/56; SpO$_2$–98%. Plan is emergent surgery. Packed red blood cells are infusing. What intervention is needed before his CT scan? a. Administer warmed crystalloids such as Lactated Ringers solution b. Administer the prescribed antibiotic c. Administer fresh frozen plasma using a fluid warmer d. Prepare for a chest tube insertion	*Answer: c* Depending on the extent of liver injury or other abdominal organ, blood loss, and hemorrhage are of concern. Clotting factors will be depleted quickly; therefore, replacing clotting factors and circulating blood volume are equally important. Injury and hypothermia can create more complications in trauma such as coagulopathy and acidosis. Hence, warming fluids during administration is important. Blood products are superior to crystalloids for replacing blood loss. Although antibiotic administration is important, hemodynamic stabilization takes priority over administering a prophylactic antibiotic. Breath sounds are equal and a chest tube is not indicated at this point.
24. In the pediatric patient with a seatbelt sign and no other signs of injury, the emergency nurse knows a priority intervention is to a. Prepare for intubation b. Administer high-flow oxygen c. Calculate a weight-based fluid bolus d. Assist with a FAST exam	*Answer: d* The seatbelt sign, ecchymosis across the abdomen in the shape of a seatbelt, can be correlated with hollow abdominal organ injuries, underlying spinal and chest injuries. A FAST exam (focused assessment with sonography for trauma) can detect intra-abdominal fluid with ultrasound examination and be performed at the stretcher side. The exam is not as sensitive as an abdominal CT and is dependent on the operator's skill. If peritoneal fluid is suspected, a stat CT should follow to assess for injuries. This scenario does not describe a patient in respiratory distress; therefore airway management is not indicated. If signs of hypovolemic shock exist, a fluid bolus would be indicated.

Genitourinary, Gynecology, and Obstetrical Emergencies

7

Geraldine M. Maurer, DNP, CRNP, FNP-C, RNC-OB, MPM and Lorna Woodhall, Ed.D(c), MSN, RN, CEN, EMT-P

Genitourinary

Foreign Bodies

The placement of foreign bodies in or around the male or female urethra may occur intentionally or accidently. Some examples of intentionally placed objects include safety pins, a screwdriver, marbles, writing instruments, straws, cocaine, wire, and metal rods. Foreign bodies accidentally lodged in the urethra include urinary incontinence devices or part of a urinary catheter.

Consider the possibility of urethral injury from a variety of practices including the injection of ink in the process of tattooing the skin of the penis, implanting plastic spheres under the skin of the penis to enhance sexual stimulation of the partner, injecting olive oil, Vaseline™, or paraffin into the penis to enlarge the organ, and the insertion of sharp or penetrating objects into the urethra and/or bladder for self-stimulation.[1]

Smaller noninjurious objects may be removed cystoscopically or at the bedside; larger objects or objects associated with trauma to the urethra require open and reconstructive operations. Death secondary to perforation of the urethra and resulting sepsis has occurred.[1]

Assessment/Analysis[1,2]
- Evaluation of urethral pain
  - Constant or only with voiding
- Foul odor: may be initial sign in child with foreign body
- Change in urinary patterns
  - Inability to urinate or dysuria
  - Oliguria
  - Hematuria

Intervention
- Establish IV access for crystalloid fluids and medications as needed
  - Broad-spectrum antibiotics may be required as most inserted foreign objects are not sterile nor are most non-operative removal techniques
- Pain management
- Procedural sedation may be required for removal
- Tetanus immunization
- Anticipate need for endoscopy/urological consult
- Surgical intervention may be required
- Consider psychiatric evaluation and treatment

Evaluation
- Successful retrieval of foreign object from the urinary tract
- Management of pain
- No signs of infection

Infection

Urinary Tract Infection: Male and Female

Urinary tract infections (UTI) occur more frequently in females than in males. The incidence with females is seen in all age groups and increases to half of all women reporting UTIs by age 35. Age groups affected includes neonates, women throughout the lifespan, and men older than 50 years of age with prostatic hypertrophy.[3,4] The most common UTI is cystitis.[4]

Cystitis

Cystitis is an uncomplicated bacterial infection of the bladder.[3] Most of the time, properly functioning urethral valves keep bacteria confined to the bladder to prevent bacteria advancing to the kidneys. Cystitis is identified as uncomplicated when there is no existence of pyelonephritis.[3]

Assessment/Analysis[4–6]
- Dysuria (painful urination)
- Nocturia (waking up to urinate during the night)
- Urinary frequency or urgency
- Fever and malaise which may or may not be present
- Abdominal pain
- Suprapubic tenderness on palpation
- Prostate tenderness
- Urinary retention in male patients
- Pregnancy test: any female patient of childbearing age with abdominal pain
- Check urine for presence of nitrites, leukocytes, or blood
- Urine culture for sensitivity: to ensure appropriate antibiotic treatment has been ordered

Interventions
- Encourage increased oral fluids
- Treat with appropriate antibiotic
- May offer medication, phenazopyridine (Pyridium™) to decrease frequency, urgency, and dysuria symptoms
    - Patient education: will turn urine orange or reddish orange color[5,6]

Evaluation
- Subsiding symptoms
- Absence of nitrites, leukocytes, or blood in follow-up urinalysis

Pyelonephritis

Pyelonephritis is an infection of the kidney and renal structures including tubules, glomeruli, and renal pelvis and is caused by an ascending bacterial infection of the lower urinary tract.[3-6] Pyelonephritis during pregnancy can cause serious complications including prenatal infections, preterm labor, and hypertension, including preeclampsia.[6]

Assessment/Analysis[3-6]
- Dysuria
- Nocturia
- Urinary urgency
- Urinary frequency
- Fever and chills may be present
- Nausea and vomiting may be present
- Flank pain: may be unilateral or bilateral
- Costovertebral angle (CVA) pain: may be unilateral or bilateral
- Hematuria
- Pregnancy test in women of childbearing age
- Labs
    - CBC with differential
    - Serum chemistries
    - Blood cultures
    - Urinalysis (presence of leukocytes, blood and/or nitrites)
    - Urine culture and sensitivity
    - Urine pregnancy test if female of childbearing age
- Renal ultrasound
- Renal CT scan

Interventions
- Establish IV access for crystalloids/medications as needed
- Appropriate antibiotic treatment
- Analgesia
- Anticipate hospitalization
    - Pregnant
    - Severely ill and/or nausea and vomiting and/or fever

Evaluation
- Resolving symptoms
- Follow-up urine culture for effective treatment of infection[5,6]

Epididymitis

Epididymitis is an infection of the epididymis, which is on the posterior surface of the testicle, and most commonly affects men in the age group from 19 to 40 years of age.[6] Potential causes of epididymitis include infection from sexual contact, cystoscopic exams, prostate surgery, and bladder catheterization. The most common cause of epididymitis infection is caused by exposure to Chlamydia or Gonorrhea through sexual contact. It is rarely seen in prepubescent boys. In elderly men, it may follow urologic manipulation.[5-7]

Assessment/Analysis[5,6]
- Dysuria
- Urinary frequency or urgency
- Ureteral discharge: more associated with sexual contact infection
- Scrotal warmth and tenderness
- Scrotal swelling
- Mild to moderate testicular or scrotal pain
    - With a gradual onset, may begin as a dull ache
    - Discomfort increases with sexual activity and may decrease with scrotal elevation
- Fever and chills
    - Severe cases may become septic
- Nausea
- Urinalysis: presence of nitrites, leukocytes, or blood
- Urine culture and sensitivity
- Culture urethral discharge
- CBC with differential
- Scrotal ultrasound: differentiate from testicular torsion

Interventions
- Appropriate antibiotic therapy
- Encourage patient to increase oral fluid intake
- Scrotal elevation may decrease scrotal pain—(positive Prehn's sign)
- Patient education[5]
    - Scrotal support/elevation when ambulating
    - Complete course of prescribed antibiotics
    - Safe sexual practices

Evaluation
- Resolving symptoms
- Follow-up evaluation with provider
- Analgesia for relief of discomfort[5-7]

Orchitis

Orchitis is the inflammation of the testicle, is quite rare, and usually occurs in conjunction with other systemic, frequently viral infections, such as mumps, coxsackie virus, Epstein-Barr, varicella, or echovirus.[8] Orchitis is most often seen as a complication of the mumps infection and although rare, can be seen with other viruses, as mentioned.[7,8] Orchitis from a bacterial cause is almost always associated with epididymitis. Orchitis presents with testicular swelling and tenderness over a few days. Ultrasound can differentiate orchitis from testicular torsion.[8]

Assessment/Analysis[7,8]
- Testicular tenderness: varies in severity
- Testicular swelling with a gradual onset over a few days
- Scrotal skin reddened
- Lower abdominal pain
- Nausea and vomiting
- Fever, headache, malaise, and myalgias
- Doppler ultrasound: to rule out testicular torsion

Interventions
- Bed rest
- Scrotal elevation
- Ice packs
- Analgesia medications for pain relief
- Bacterial orchitis is treated as epididymitis
- Isolation precautions if communicable disease (mumps) associated

Evaluation
- Decreased pain
- Resolving symptoms

Priapism

Priapism is a prolonged, painful erection persisting beyond or unrelated to sexual stimulation. There are three major types of priapism: ischemic, nonischemic (self-limiting), and stuttering (recurrent self-limiting episodes of ischemic priapism). Identifying the type of priapism is vital to the effective treatment. Ischemic priapism, also referred to as venoocclusive or low-flow priapism, is a urological emergency affecting the corpus cavernosa, while the corpus spongiosum of the glans penis remains flaccid. The imbalance of vasoregulatory mechanisms, trapped mixed-venous blood, and venous congestion create an ischemic environment causing pain and rigidity of the penis. Scarring and fibrosis in this cavernous space can lead to impotence and is directly related to the length of time the penis was ischemic.[9]

Physiologic causes of priapism include several disease states, such as sickle cell disease/crisis, spinal cord injuries, spinal anesthesia, and cancers such as leukemia or multiple myeloma. Several medications, including some antipsychotics and those used in the treatment for impotence, are associated with ischemic priapism such as sildenafil citrate (Viagra™) and tadalafil (Cialis™). Other substances associated with priapism are cocaine, marijuana, and ethanol abuse.[6,9]

Assessment/Analysis
- History of chief complaint
  - Duration of priapism
  - Any clinical treatments used
  - Previous priapism episodes
  - Presence of pain
  - Erectile function status prior to the priapism
- Past medical history
  - Presence of associated pathophysiologic diseases previously listed
- Physical exam
  - Degree of pain
  - Bladder distention
  - Ability to urinate

Intervention[5,9]
- Pain control: analgesics, narcotics, or sedation if needed
- Manage underlying medical conditions
- Assist with medical interventions
  - Insertion of urinary catheter
  - Assist with aspiration/irrigation of corpus cavernosa
  - Assist with sympathomimetic injections
    - Epinephrine, phenylephrine, or terbutaline injected into the penis to help reverse engorgement
- Anticipate urology consult
- Patient education[6]
  - Signs of infection-fever, drainage
  - Restrictions on physical and sexual activity per physician's instructions
- Anticipate possible hospital admission after surgical intervention

Evaluation
- Relief of pain
- Reduced penile congestion and swelling[5,9]

Renal Calculi

Renal calculi is the presence of renal stone(s).[6] Calculi vary with composition and size, and can be located anywhere along the genitourinary tract.[6] Renal colic is pain caused by the ureteral distention when passing a renal stone from the renal pelvis through the ureter. The level of pain is dependent on the amount of ureteral obstruction and ureteral spasm as the stone is passed.[5] Renal colic pain usually radiates from the flank to the lower quadrant.[5] Pain can continue down to the groin and even to the leg.[5,6]

Assessment/Analysis[5,6]
- Sudden onset of pain
  - Severe, colicky, radiating, flank pain, with a dull underlying pain
  - Pain may radiate to the abdomen, scrotum, groin, or labia
- Dysuria: painful urination
- Urinary urgency

- Urinary frequency
- Nausea and vomiting
- Fever
- Hematuria
- Diaphoresis, pallor
- Costovertebral angle (CVA) tenderness on palpation
- Restlessness and irritable
  - Unable to find a comfortable position
- History of renal calculi
- Urinalysis for blood and potential infection
- Urine culture and sensitivity
- Ultrasound to reveal calculi
- Strain urine samples for any calculi
  - May be very small resembling a range from white stones to flecks of black pepper
- Abdominal KUB (kidney, ureter, and bladder) X-ray
- CT scan

Interventions
- Establish IV access for crystalloid fluids and medications as needed
  - IV fluid bolus
- Analgesia for severe pain
- Antiemetic for nausea and vomiting
- Possible hospitalization for pain control
- Potential lithotripsy if stones do not pass without intervention
- Patient/family education
  - Straining urine
  - Dietary restrictions (dependent on stone analysis)
    - Limiting foods with high calcium content
    - Uric acid (avoiding sardines, herring, and liver)[6]

Evaluation
- Adequate fluid intake, IV and PO
- Monitor intake and output
- Pain relief with analgesia

Testicular Torsion

A true urologic emergency is a testicular torsion caused by the twisting of the spermatic cord structures resulting in strangulation of the testicular blood supply on the affected side.[5,6] Any diagnostic studies should not delay operative procedure. Testicular torsion may occur at any age, but is frequently seen between the ages of 12 and 18 years, often in puberty with maximal hormone stimulation, which causes profound growth spurts of different tissues, all of which might not be at the same pace.[5,6] If surgical repair is completed within 6 hours, testicular salvage rate improves, but after 12 hours following torsion, the salvage rate drops.[6]

Assessment/Analysis[5,6]
- Young men complaining of the rapid onset of severe pain in one testicle
  - Can occur during exertion or during sleep
  - Can be trauma related
- Radiating pain to lower abdomen and to inguinal canal which is not relieved by elevation or ice
- Nausea and vomiting
- Fever
- Scrotal swelling and erythema
- Tense scrotal mass
- Elevated testicle on the affected side, as pictured in Figure 7-1
- Doppler ultrasound[7]

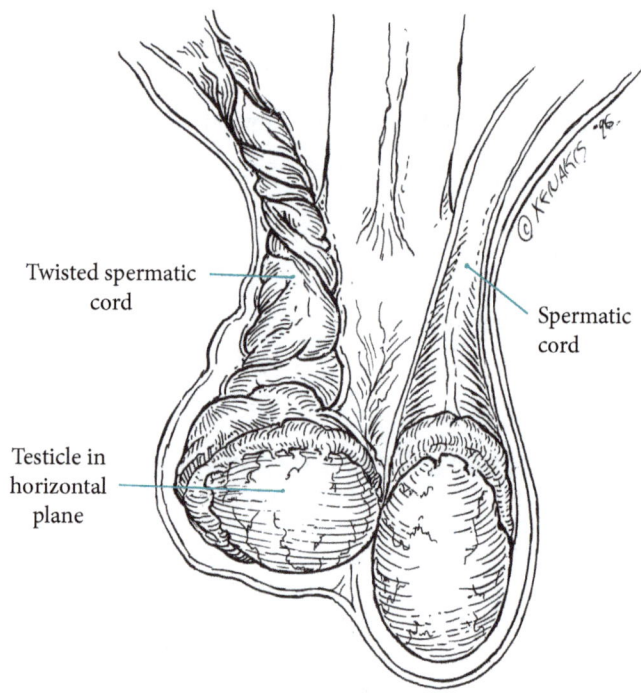

FIGURE 7-1 Elevated testicle "Bell-Clapper Deformity". Twisting of the spermatic cord causes the testicle to be elevated with a horizontal lie. Lack of fixation to the posterior scrotum predisposes the freely movable testicles to rotation and subsequent torsion. Asymptomatic patients with bell-clapper deformity are at risk for torsion
Reproduced with permission from Knoop KJ, Stack LB, Storrow AB, et al: The Atlas of Emergency Medicine, 4th ed. New York: McGraw-Hill Education; 2016.

Interventions
- Analgesia for pain management
- Urology consult
- Anticipate prompt operative intervention
- Supportive measures for the patient

Evaluation
- Relief of pain

Genitourinary Trauma

Injury to the genitourinary (GU) system should be suspected in any patient presenting with an injury to the chest, abdomen, or back. Falls, assaults, motor vehicle crashes (MVC), and sports injuries are the most common mechanisms causing blunt GU injuries. Gunshot wounds and stab wounds are the most common causes for penetrating injuries.[10]

Blunt injury to the GU organs may be subtle and are often not evident on initial physical exam. Frequent reassessment is essential to detect these types of injuries.[11] Children are more susceptible to GU injury due to lack of periadipose tissue and a large kidney size relative to overall body size.[10]

Renal

The kidneys are injured in nearly 10% of patients who sustain trauma to the abdomen.[11] Lacerations, contusions, and injury to the vasculature perfusing the kidney are the most common types of renal injuries. Renal trauma should be suspected in patients with a history of a sudden deceleration or lateral force injuries, such as with MVC and contact sports, and those with fractures of the posterior lower ribs or lower spine injuries.[2]

Assessment/Analysis
- Mechanism of injury/chief complaint
- Costovertebral angle (CVA) pain and/or bruising over the flank area (Grey-Turner sign)
- Hematuria[2] or blood at the meatus or on underwear[10]

Intervention
- Assist with stabilizing and medical interventions
- Pharmacologic therapy as ordered
  - Pain medications
  - Antibiotics
  - Tetanus

Evaluation
- Stable hemodynamic status
- Relief of pain
- Minimum urine output
  - Adults: 0.5 mL/kg/hr[12]
  - Pediatrics: 1 mL/kg/hr
  - <1 year: 2 mL/kg/hr

Bladder

Bladder trauma may be caused by penetrating or blunt injury to the lower abdomen. Stabbing, gunshot wounds, or any object piercing the abdominal wall should cause suspicion of injury to the bladder. Blunt trauma to the bladder may occur with any major compression of the abdominal wall, such as by a seat belt during a motor vehicle collision (MVC), especially when the bladder is full or distended. Pelvic fractures are the most common cause of bladder trauma.[13]

Assessment/Analysis
- Hematuria
- Inability to void
- Inspect urinary meatus for blood

Intervention
- Preparation for surgical intervention
- Anticipate inpatient hospitalization
- Closely monitor hourly urine output

Evaluation
- Stable hemodynamic status
- Relief of pain
- Minimum urine output
  - Adults: 0.5 mL/kg/hr[12]
  - Pediatrics: 1 mL/kg/hr
  - <1 year: 2 mL/kg/hr

Ureters

Because the ureters are well protected in the retroperitoneum, ureteral injuries are rare in trauma patients.[10] The majority of ureteral injuries occur from inadvertent injury during abdominal/pelvic surgical procedures. Ureteral injuries from external trauma are almost always a result of penetrating trauma. Only 10% of ureteral injuries are associated with external blunt trauma.

Ureteral injuries are easily missed due to the lack of specific associated assessment findings. Only 70% of patients with ureteral injuries have either gross or microscopic hematuria. Therefore, the absence of hematuria does not rule out ureteral injury.[10]

Assessment/Analysis
- Hematuria
- Inability to void
- Inspect urinary meatus for blood

Intervention
- Establish IV access for crystalloid fluids and medications as needed
- Possible diagnostic tests
  - Assess allergy to IV contrast dye
  - IV urography
  - Retrograde pyelography[10]
- Preparation for surgical intervention
- Anticipate hospital admission

Evaluation
- Stable hemodynamic status
- Relief of pain
- Minimum urine output
  - Adults: 0.5 mL/kg/hr[12]
  - Pediatrics: 1 mL/kg/hr
  - <1 year: 2 mL/kg/hr

Urethral

Urethral injuries are classified as *posterior* or *anterior* based on anatomic site. Urethral injuries occur in 5 to 10% of pelvic fractures. Untreated injuries can have a delayed presentation, appearing years later as a stricture. Penile fracture and urethral injury can result from rupture of the corpus cavernosum if the penis is forcibly bent during sexual activity. A cracking sound is heard, followed by penile pain, immediate detumescence, rapid swelling, discoloration, and visible deformity. Penetrating trauma to the urethra usually occurs to the penile urethra.[10]

Assessment/Analysis
- Mechanism of injury
  - Pelvic fracture
  - Traumatic catheterization
  - Straddle injury
  - Recent abdominal surgical procedure
  - Penetrating injury to the perineum
- Hematuria, dysuria, or inability to void
- Inspect urinary meatus for blood

Intervention
- Assist with insertion of a suprapubic catheter for male patients with posterior urethral injury secondary to pelvic fracture[10]
- Preparation for surgical intervention
- Anticipate hospital admission

Evaluation
- Stable hemodynamic status
- Relief of pain
- Minimum urine output (adult): 0.5 mL/kg per hour for >6 hours[12]

Urinary Retention

Urinary retention occurs when the bladder is not able to empty of urine. This condition can be chronic or acute.[6] Causes can be gender specific or classified as obstructive, pharmacologic, traumatic, neurogenic, psychogenic, childhood, and extraurinary.[14] Urinary retention in men, especially elderly men, is most commonly caused by benign prostatic hypertrophy (BPH). Urinary retention in females is usually caused by gynecologic problems.[14]

Assessment/Analysis[6,14]
- History of urinary problems
- Lower abdominal discomfort
- Bladder distention
- Ultrasound of the bladder
  - Confirm retention or identify mass or other obstruction
  - Bladder scan can help quantify amount of urinary retention
- Urinalysis

Interventions
- Insert indwelling urinary catheter for relief bladder distention
- Possible urology consult for follow-up

Evaluation
- Urination with complete bladder emptying
- No bladder distention or discomfort

Gynecology

Perform a pregnancy test on females of childbearing age to guide treatment options. Consider having a chaperone present whenever breast, genital, or rectal examinations are performed. Case-specific specimens may include urinary, vaginal, rectal, and urethral samples for diagnostic testing.[15]

Vaginal Bleeding: Abnormal and Dysfunctional

Vaginal bleeding (VB) with a non-pregnant patient occurs for a variety of reasons.[17] The term abnormal uterine bleeding (AVB) includes all causes of abnormal bleeding in non-pregnant patients.[15] Causes of AVB include structural and non-structural problems.[15] These may include fibroids or trauma, hormone level imbalance, menstrual cycle irregularities, infections from sexually transmitted disease STDs, coagulopathy problems, or even a malignancy.[15,17] Dysfunctional uterine bleeding (DUB), a form of AVB, has a hormonal relation and may be seen at the beginning or near the end of childbearing years. DUB can be described as painless VB without clots or tissue present.[16,17]

With VB, cause, volume, time, and frequency of bleeding can vary with individuals and identifying these characteristics is important to determine treatment. Knowing the last menstrual period (LMP) is necessary in women who are in childbearing years.[18] The amount of bleeding can range from spotting to very significant amounts of blood loss. Treating life-threatening symptoms is most important since the specific cause of a VB episode may need to be addressed by a gynecologist. Much of the assessment will be done by interviewing the patient. Any patient with postmenopausal bleeding should have a prompt gynecologic referral for evaluation of bleeding where the goal is to diagnose the reason for the AVB.[15-18]

Vaginal Hemorrhage

VB in a non-pregnant patient can reach significant levels and may require treatment for hemodynamic instability. Gynecologic abnormal bleeding usually presents with a chronic history and is commonly non-life-threatening, but VB can range from spotting to life-threatening. In the case of a patient with a coagulation problem, bleeding can be excessive and occur abruptly with no warning to the patient. Bleeding severity can range from chronic spotting to life-threatening situations. In the case of a life-threatening situation, maintaining the patient's well-being and hemodynamic status is the most important treatment.[15-17]

Assessment/ Analysis[15-17]
- Vital sign evaluation and pulse oximetry, level of consciousness
- Estimated amount of blood loss
  - Number of pads or tampons used
    - Are pads saturated
    - How often is the patient changing pads or tampons
    - Bleeding amounts in relation to a normal menstrual cycle bleed
- Other characteristics of the bleeding episode
  - Color of the blood (bright, darker)
  - Onset
  - Activity when it began
  - How often bleeding occurs
  - How long bleeding lasts
  - Presence of clots or tissue
- Pain level
- Fever, chills, body aches, or fatigue
- Headache, dizziness
- Pregnancy status: LMP
- Birth control method
- Sexual history
- Menstrual cycle history
- History of pregnancy(s)
- History previous gynecological infections
- History of bowel or bladder problems
- History of bleeding problems, past medical history
- Laboratory studies
  - CBC with differential
  - Coagulation studies
  - Thyroid-stimulating hormone (TSH)
  - Follicle-stimulating hormone (FSH)
  - Luteinizing hormone (LH)
  - Liver function tests
  - Pregnancy test and urinalysis
  - Type and screen
  - Sexually transmitted disease (STD) screening[16,17]

Interventions
- Supplemental oxygen if needed (maintain pulse oximetry ≥94%)
- Assist with pelvic exam
- Ultrasound evaluation
- Possible surgical preparation to stop the bleeding
- Dilation and curettage (D&C) procedure
- In the case of vaginal hemorrhage
  - Establish IV access for crystalloids, blood products, and medications as needed
  - Administer packed blood cells and clotting factors (plasma and platelets) as needed
  - Anticipate and prepare for surgical intervention

Evaluation
- Volume loss from blood: current hemodynamic status
- Pain decreased
- Cessation of bleeding
- Activity tolerated
- Appropriate gynecological follow-up for further evaluation

Foreign Bodies

Objects not intended for vaginal placement may be inserted accidentally or intentionally and may or may not cause symptoms. Objects larger than the vaginal introitus may cause pain due to tissue distention. Vaginal foreign bodies are commonly seen in children and may include a variety of objects, such as crayons or beads.[19] Young women may seek emergency medical care due to foreign body concerns such as inability to remove tampons or broken portions of condoms. Medical attention may be required for removal of vaginal foreign objects which may have been inserted intentionally for sexual purposes or placed during an episode of abuse.

Assessment/Analysis
- Vaginal bleeding and/or itching
- Foul-smelling vaginal discharge in a variety of colors
- Vulvar rash, erythema, and/or swelling due to vaginal discharge
- Dysuria and/or pain with intercourse
- Pelvic pressure
- Vaginal tears or perforation
- Systemic infection
- Development of fistulas between the vagina and the bladder, rectum, or perineum

Interventions
- Prepare for pelvic exam
  - Assist with inspection of vagina for foreign object(s), with or without speculum
  - Removal of the foreign object(s) using forceps or warm saline irrigation[1,19]
- Possible procedural sedation or anesthesia required for removal of large or unusual objects
- Patient/family education
  - Monitor for vaginal bleeding or discharge, abnormal odor, or burning/pain with urination
  - If any abnormal symptoms occur after an object has been removed from the vagina, the patient should be reevaluated

Evaluation[1,19]
- Successful removal of foreign object

Infection

Vaginal Discharge

Female vaginal discharge is largely composed of secretions from the endocervical glands and is normally clear or milky-white. The amount and character of vaginal discharge varies depending on where a woman is in her menstrual cycle. The quantity of vaginal discharge before menarche and after menopause is generally less than during a woman's reproductive years.[20] Normal vaginal bacteria interact with vaginal secretions to maintain an acidic pH (3.5 to 5), which helps prevent infections in the vagina.[13] Any disruption to the balance of normal bacteria in the vagina can affect the smell, color, or texture of vaginal discharge. A change in vaginal discharge, or the presence of vaginal discharge associated with irritation or other uncomfortable symptoms, may indicate an infection is present.[21] Common causes of abnormal vaginal discharge include Candidiasis (often from antibiotic use), birth control pills, sexually transmitted diseases (STD), diabetes, douches/fragranced soaps/bubble baths, and vaginitis.[16,17,22]

Assessment/Analysis
- Color, odor, duration, and quantity of vaginal discharge
- Vaginal itching, edema, redness, or irritation
- Pain/burning with urination; urinary frequency
- Dyspareunia or bleeding with intercourse[17]

Interventions/Treatment
- Assist with pelvic examination
  - Collection of vaginal cultures to test for antimicrobial susceptibility before initiation of therapy
- Antibiotic prescription for infectious organisms[16]
- Patient education
  - Medication
  - Personal hygiene
    - Wipe perineum from front to back after urination and defecation
    - Use only mild soap and water to cleanse perineum
    - Avoid feminine sprays and douches
    - Wear cotton underwear
    - Avoid tight-fitting clothing
  - Prevention of reoccurrence of STD
    - No sexual activity until treatment is complete and patient is asymptomatic; assessment and treatment of sexual partner(s) if applicable; methods to prevent transmission of sexually transmitted diseases[16]

Evaluation
- Successful resolution of abnormal vaginal discharge and associated symptoms
- Follow-up with medical professional as applicable to confirm resolution of infectious disease

Pelvic Inflammatory Disease

Pelvic inflammatory disease (PID) is any inflammatory condition of the female pelvic organs, especially one caused by bacterial infection.[13] The upper genital tract structures (fallopian tubes, ovaries, or pelvic peritoneum) become infected by the upward migration of bacteria from the lower reproductive tract.[16] Many different types of bacteria can cause PID, including those normally found in the lower genital tract. Common bacteria causing PID include *N. gonorrhoeae* (gonorrhea) and *C. trachomatis* (chlamydia). Women at risk for PID include those with an intrauterine device (IUD), sexually transmitted infection, history of unprotected sex with a new or multiple sexual partners, recent abortion, and a history of douching. Complications of untreated PID include infertility, ectopic pregnancy, and chronic abdominal pain.[16,23]

Assessment/Analysis
- May be asymptomatic or experience only mild symptoms
- Pain in lower abdomen
  - Dull, aching, or cramping
  - Pain and/or bleeding during intercourse
  - Pain/burning with urination
  - Pain noted soon after the onset of the last menstrual period
  - Pain exacerbated by ambulation or movement of pelvic area[16,17,24]
- Fever >38.3°C (101°F)
- Nausea or vomiting
- Vaginal discharge, often malodorous
- Bleeding between periods

Interventions/Treatment
- Physical exam, including pelvic exam
- Pain management
- Broad-spectrum antibiotics
- Treatment of associated sexual partners[16]
- Hospitalization is indicated when
  - Pregnant
  - Severely ill, nausea/vomiting, or high fever
  - Unable to follow outpatient treatment or tolerate oral medications
  - No clinical response to the oral antibiotic treatment[24]
- Patient education
  - Abstain from sexual intercourse until antibiotic treatment is complete, symptoms have resolved, and sexual partners have been adequately treated

Evaluation
- Improvement of symptoms (decreased pelvic pain, afebrile, etc.) within 3 days of initiation of treatment[24]
- Reevaluated if no clinical improvement after 72 hours
  - Inpatient IV treatment and additional diagnostics may be indicated[24]
- Associated diagnosis of chlamydia or gonorrhea retested 3 months after treatment[25]
- HIV counseling and testing for high-risk patients[17]

Sexually Transmitted Disease

In all societies, sexually transmitted diseases (STDs) rank among the most common of all infectious diseases, with over 30 infections now classified as predominantly sexually transmitted or as frequently sexually transmissible.[22] The terms sexually transmitted infections (STIs) or sexually transmitted diseases (STDs) refer to a variety of clinical syndromes and infections caused by pathogens acquired and transmitted through sexual activity.[27]

General patient education and treatment procedures

- ❖ Use a barrier method to prevent transmission of STD
- ❖ Abstain from sexual activity until treatment completed
- ❖ Sexual partner(s) also need treatment
- ❖ Avoid contact with any lesions, both initially and any that reoccur
- ❖ Follow-up care required within 7 to 10 days[17]

Assessment/Analysis
- Clinical features, characteristics, treatments, and patient education for STDs as shown in Table 7-1

Interventions/Treatment
- See www.cdc.gov/std for the most up-to-date recommended antibiotic treatment regimen[27]

Evaluation
- Treatment of infection
- Education regarding prevention of spread
- Relief of symptoms

Ovarian Cyst

A globular sac filled with fluid or semifluid material that develops in or on an ovary is an ovarian cyst.[20] Ovarian cysts occur more frequently in menstruating women due to the associated cyclic changes of the ovaries.[16] Most ovarian cysts do not cause symptoms and will resolve without treatment. However, complications such as ovarian torsion (painful twisting of the ovary) or rupture of the cyst may result in severe pain and internal bleeding, requiring emergency medical treatment.[28,29]

Assessment/Analysis
- Pain or discomfort in the lower abdomen
- Severe pelvic or abdominal pain characterized by sudden, unilateral, sharp pelvic pain associated with trauma, exercise, or intercourse
- Pain accompanied by fever or vomiting
- Rupture of a cyst may lead to abdominal distention, guarding, and rebound tenderness
- Vaginal bleeding may or may not be present
- Hemorrhagic shock if accompanied with substantial bleeding[16,28,29]
- Laboratory studies for initial management and pre-operative screening
    - CBS with differential
    - Blood bank analysis (type and screen/cross), if transfusion likely
    - Pregnancy test to rule out ectopic pregnancy
- Pelvic ultrasound or CT scan to confirm diagnosis of ovarian cyst

Interventions/Treatment
- Establish IV access for crystalloid fluids, blood products, and medications as needed
- Pain medication administration
- Antibiotics may be ordered for administration
- If hemodynamically unstable, prepare for emergency surgery[16]

Evaluation
- Pain relief
- Hemodynamically stable
- Gynecology consult and/or management

Sexual Assault or Battery

Sexual assault is a crime of violence, not an act of sexual gratification. Defined by forcible, inappropriate sexual behavior and lack of consent.[30] Sexual assault is dissimilar from other assaults in that the absence of observable physical injury does not mean an assault did not occur. Sexual assault survivors feel helpless, violated, and disempowered and present with a wide range of physical and psychological needs. Males and females of all ages have been victims of sexual assault.[31] Approximately half of all victims have genital or rectal trauma and about two-thirds have some evidence of bruising elsewhere on the body.[32]

Care of the sexual assault victim is complex and can be time-consuming for emergency department staff. Nursing responsibilities may include obtaining and documenting a medical and forensic history, assisting with the medical examination, treating acute medical problems or injuries, collecting forensic evidence, ensuring the evidence carefully follows a chain of custody, arranging referral for crisis intervention and sexual assault advocates, and testifying in court if required.

Substance related/drug induced sexual assault is a crime according to Public Law (H.R.4137/104-305) and is punishable by law. Medications identified in connection with sexual assault include but are not limited to GHB (gamma hydroxybutyrate), ketamine (Ketalar™), and flunitrazepam (Rohypnol™). If drug induced sexual assault is suspected, a urine specimen should be collected. If the incident has occurred within 48 hours, blood specimens should be collected in addition to urine.

Assessment/Analysis
- Care is delivered in a nonjudgmental, caring, and safe atmosphere to aid the patient in psychological trauma recovery

TABLE 7-1 **Clinical Features, Characteristics, Treatments and Patient Education for Sexually Transmitted Diseases**[8,22-28]

	Clinical Features	Incubation Period	Pain
Bacterial Vaginosis (BV)	White or grey; malodorous; moderate amount		
Chlamydia	Mucopurulent	5–10 days	Males = burning on urination, urethral itching; females = usually asymptomatic
Chancroid	Multiple painful, irregular, purulent ulcers with potential exudative base	3–14 days	Very painful; increased pain on urination
Gonorrhea	Yellow, mucopurulent discharge	3–5 days	Males = dysuria; Females = s/s of PID
Herpes, Genital	Multiple small, grouped vesicles coalescing and forming shallow ulcers; vulvovaginitis	2–12 days	Very painful dysuria
Human Papillomavirus (HPV)		3–6 months	No
Syphilis	Indurated, relatively clean base; heals spontaneously	3 weeks	No
Trichomoniasis	White, yellow, green or grey; thin, frothy; profuse; malodorous	1 week	Worse immediately after menses; most acute during pregnancy

- Assess and respond to safety concerns upon arrival of the patient, such as threats to patient or staff
- Respond to acute injury, trauma care, and safety needs of patients before collecting evidence
- Consider utilizing the expertise of a Sexual Assault Nurse Examiner (SANE), Sexual Assault Forensic Examiner (SAFE), or Sexual Assault Examiners (SAEs)
- Consent is explained and obtained for medical evaluation and/or release of information and evidence to law enforcement agency following sexual assault
- A victim of drug-induced sexual assault may present with some of the following symptoms
  - Appearance of intoxication disproportionate to the amount of alcohol consumed or lack of alcohol consumption

Lesions; Other Signs & Symptoms	Treatment	Patient Education/Special Instructions
No; Amine ("fishy") odor when 10% KOH solution (potassium hydroxide) applied to microscope slide smear	Metronidazole PO OR gel intravaginally OR Clindamycin cream intravaginally	
No	Azithromycin OR Doxycycline OR Erythromycin OR Ofloxacin	Abstain from sex during treatment, use condoms, and inform sexual partners to seek treatment
Yes; Multiple painful, irregular, purulent ulcers with potential exudative base. Non-indurated	Ceftriaxone OR Azithromycin OR Erythromycin	Lesions heal within weeks but are infectious during that time
No; Urinary frequency, abnormal vaginal bleeding	Ceftriaxone OR Cefixime OR Ciprofloxacin OR Ofloxacin	Abstain from sex during treatment, use condoms, and inform sex partners to seek treatment
Yes; May have inguinal lymphadenopathy, urinary retention related to pain, fever, headache, malaise, myalgias, pain with ambulation	Famciclovir OR Vancyclovir	May reoccur every 2 months; local hyperesthesia usually occurs 24 hours before eruption of vesicular lesions. Abstain from sex during treatment, to use condoms, and inform sex partners to seek treatment
Pink-grey soft lesions, taller than they are wide, occur singly or in clusters, may bleed	Topically: 10%–25% podophyllin in tincture of benzoin (not for use in pregnancy); or 50% trichloroacetic acid or liquid nitrogen	Abstain from sex during treatment, to use condoms, and inform sex partners to seek treatment
Primary: chancre; May have fever, lymphadenopathy Secondary: rash, mucocutaneous lesions, lymphadenopathy Tertiary: cardiac, ophthalmic, auditory, central nervous system lesions	Benzathine penicillin G IM	Abstain from sex during treatment, to use condoms, and inform sex partners to seek treatment
No; Severe pruritus; genital edema; erythema of vaginal vault; Amine ("fishy") odor when 10% KOH solution (potassium hydroxide) applied to microscope slide smear	Metronidazole	Avoid the concurrent use of alcohol when taking metronidazole; inform all being treated to abstain from sex during treatment, to use condoms, and inform sex partners to seek treatment

- Unexplained drowsiness
- Impaired motor coordination
- Dizziness, confusion, impaired judgment, and loss of inhibition
- Impaired ability to remember details
- Decreased respiratory effort
- Seizure-like activity
- Coma[33]

Interventions
- Consider digital photographs of injuries for evidence with permission of the patient
- Patients should not wash, change clothes, urinate, defecate, smoke, drink, or eat until initially evaluated by forensic

examiners, unless necessary for treating acute medical needs
- Scrapes, abrasions, and human bite wounds are swabbed with a cotton swab moistened with sterile water (not saline) before the wounds are cleaned. Retain the air-dried cotton swabs of these areas as evidence by placing in an envelope. Label the envelope with the body location collected. This same procedure should be used to take samples of dried body fluids or blood found on the victim
- All specimens collected are air-dried for 30 minutes and packaged separately in paper bags (never use plastic
- bags)
- Each item collected is labeled according to facility procedure
- Medical treatment for sexual assault victims includes prevention of unwanted pregnancy and STIs
  - See www.cdc.gov for STI treatment guidelines for victims of sexual assault.[27] Expect medical treatment to include pregnancy prophylaxis (offered if the patient's pregnancy test results are negative), tetanus booster when applicable, and administration of hepatitis B vaccine if the patient has not previously been vaccinated
- An advocate may be offered to the patient
  - Center for Victims of Violent Crimes: 412-392-8582 (hotline)
  - National Sexual Assault Hotline: 800-656-HOPE (4673)
- If child abuse is suspected, consult Social Services to aid in filing a Child Abuse report
  - Childline: 800-932-0313[30–32,34,35]

Evaluation
- Resolution of emergency medical conditions
- Patient safety
- Decreased patient anxiety

Gynecological Trauma

Consider any abrasion, laceration, or bruising of the female genital or perineal area as gynecological trauma. Injury to external structures are easily identified, but must be examined carefully to evaluate deeper extension. Trauma to the internal gynecological structures are more difficult to assess. Any female child, adolescent, or adult complaining of genital or perineal area pain, bleeding, or swelling should be examined for vulvar or vaginal trauma. Patients with vulvar or vaginal trauma may also complain of abdominal or low back pain.

Genital trauma may be accidental or may be the result of sexual abuse. The examination and care of the vulvovaginal area injury may cause significant anxiety for the patient, especially pediatric patients and caregivers. Ensure a safe, private atmosphere during the examination of a patient of any age.

Accidental genital trauma may be the result of motor vehicle accidents, animal bites, burns, falls, or penetrating injuries. The most common accidental genital trauma is the straddle injury, resulting in lacerations or hematoma formation due to blunt force trauma. Vaginal insufflation injuries (rapid distension of the vagina resulting in a tearing of the vaginal walls with resultant bleeding) are associated with water slides and falls while water or jet skiing. Genital trauma may also occur as a result of sexual assault. Burns, human bites, ecchymosis, or lacerations of the genital area all warrant careful evaluation and care.[36,37,38]

Assessment/Analysis

- Injury may be classified based on the TEARS pneumonic[34]
  - T (tears)
  - E (ecchymosis)
  - A (abrasions)
  - R (redness)
  - S (swelling)

- Consider mechanism of injury
- Evaluate details of the events causing the traumatic injury
- Ensure history is consistent with physical findings and report any discrepancies (consider sexual abuse or assault)[39]

Interventions/Treatment
- Control bleeding
- Nonexpanding hematomas can be managed with cold compresses, analgesia, and rest
- Expanding hematomas can occlude the flow of urine from the urethra
  - A urinary catheter should be placed until the hematoma decreases in size
- Rapid expansion of a hematoma or hemodynamic instability requires surgical intervention
- Lacerations generally heal within 2 to 3 days without medical intervention
  - Moderate lacerations may be sutured using local anesthesia in the ED
  - Large lacerations with persistent bleeding involving the urethra, vagina, or anal area require surgical exploration and management[40]

Evaluation
- Hemodynamically stable
- Relief of pain
- Adequate urinary output
- Emotional status
- Follow-up medical management with gynecology and/or pediatric trauma specialty

Obstetrical

Threatened/Spontaneous Abortion

Spontaneous abortion of a fetus occurs when the pregnancy products are expelled from the uterus resulting in death of the fetus and termination of the pregnancy before 20 weeks gestation.[41] Spontaneous abortion should be considered for any female of childbearing age who presents to the emergency department with vaginal bleeding.[17] The types or classifications of spontaneous abortions are described as threatened, inevitable, incomplete, complete, missed, and septic.[17,41,42]

In Table 7-2, the varying types of abortion are identified with assessment considerations and the nursing interventions described.

Additional Interventions for Any Abortion Type[17,41]
- Compassionate care for the patient following pregnancy loss is indicated, including offering contact information for support groups; avoid using the term "abortion"
- Educating the patient about potential causes of pregnancy loss is important; referral from physician for counseling as advised, including social services, genetics, or psychological
- Assess pain level and pain medication as needed

TABLE 7-2 **Spontaneous Abortion Types/Classifications with Assessment and Interventions**[17,41,42]

Abortion Type	Description of Symptoms	Interventions
Threatened	• Painless bright red bleeding • May have menstrual-like cramping. • Cervical os closed	• Vital signs, assess bleeding based on amount of bleeding, i.e., spotting versus pad saturation • Ultrasound to identify presence of pregnancy • Speculum exam of cervix • Activity – bed rest • Pelvic rest – patient education on pelvic rest, i.e., no tampons, douche or sexual intercourse • Pain assessment – analgesia medication
Inevitable	• Increasing pain with cramping and bleeding increases • Cervical os dilates to 3 cm or more • May have gush of fluid – gross rupture of membranes	Same as Threatened Abortion, also including • Establish IV access for crystalloids/blood products/medications • May require uterine dilation and curettage Administer Rho(D) immune globulin (Rhogam™, Rhophylac™) if patient Rh negative blood type
Incomplete	• Pain from cramping is severe and bleeding is heavy • Cervical os is dilated open • Some of the products of pregnancy have passed, but some may be retained	• Same as Inevitable abortion, also including • Administer Pitocin IV, per order • May require uterine dilation and curettage (D & C)
Complete	• Some bleeding occurs with mild cramps • The product of conception is passed and cervical os is closed	Same as incomplete abortion, also including • Ultrasound to assess contents of uterus
Missed	• Symptoms range from none to slight bleeding and no cramping to mild cramping • Products of conception demise but are not passed	Same as complete abortion
Septic—Infection following abortion of a pregnancy	• Monitor vital signs for fever with chills • Vaginal discharge will have a foul odor • Uterine tenderness with pelvic pain • Closed cervical os • Condition can occur with complete or incomplete abortions, or after an elective abortion	Same as complete abortion, also including • Antibiotic therapy according to suspected microorganism • Culture and Sensitivity of vaginal discharge • Ultrasound to assess for uterine contents • Schedule uterine D & C if indicated, and prepare patient for procedure • Monitor for signs of toxic shock syndrome including tachycardia, hypotension and signs of renal failure

Evaluation

- Patient/Family Education[17,41]
  - Bleeding may last up to two weeks but amount will decrease and color become lighter gradually
  - Cramping may continue intermittently for a few days and then subside
  - Do not put anything into the vagina for two weeks or until re-evaluated by a gynecologist
  - Monitor for signs and symptoms of infection including
    - Temperature elevation
    - Chills
    - Nausea or vomiting
    - Return of cramps and/or bleeding after they had subsided[17,42]

Hyperemesis Gravidarum

Hyperemesis gravidarum occurs when symptoms include persistent severe nausea and vomiting due to pregnancy. This usually occurs in the first trimester and in severe cases can continue to the 20th week of the pregnancy. Symptoms include sustained vomiting lasting 4 to 8 weeks and can be severe resulting in dehydration due to the inability to tolerate any oral fluids.[17] Also, because patients continue to vomit, adequate nutrition cannot be maintained. After a period of time, this condition can be severe enough to cause problems for maternal and fetal well-being and may require hospitalization. The cause is unclear and is suggested to occur in about 2% of pregnancies.[17,43]

Assessment/Analysis[17,43]

- Severe nausea and vomiting during pregnancy
- No weight gain and possibly weight loss
- Weakness and dizziness
- Possible oliguria
- Laboratory studies for initial management
  - Serum chemistries
  - CBC with differential
  - Serum ketones
  - Urinalysis, include specific gravity and ketones
  - Pregnancy test: urine or serum

Interventions

- Establish IV access for fluids and medications as needed
- Antiemetic
  - Appropriate meds for pregnancy (i.e., Vitamin B_6 and doxylamine)[43]
- Admission for inpatient therapy as indicated

Evaluation

- Relief of nausea symptoms
- Retention of fluids
- Serum electrolytes

Ectopic Pregnancy

An ectopic pregnancy occurs when the fertilized ovum implants other than in the uterine cavity, usually along the fallopian tubes.[17,44] Nearly 95% of ectopic pregnancies are implanted in the various segments of the fallopian tubes as illustrated in Figure 7-2.[17,44] It is important to diagnose an ectopic pregnancy early to avoid a potential rupture of the fallopian tubes. To achieve early diagnosis, ectopic pregnancies should be considered in all women of childbearing age who present with abdominal or pelvic complaints or with unexplained signs or symptoms of hypovolemia.[17,45] Some risk factors include abnormal fallopian tube anatomy, previous

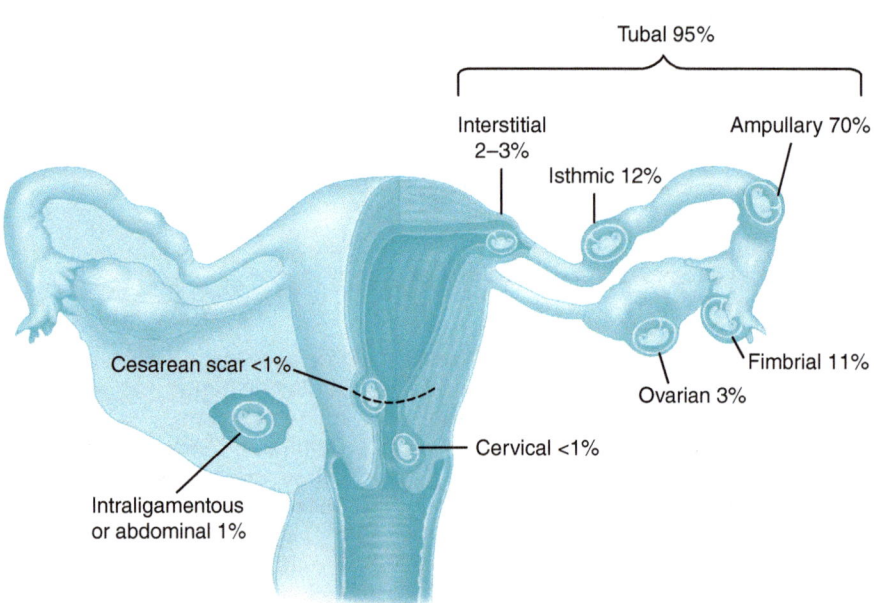

FIGURE 7-2 Sites of implantation of 1800 ectopic pregnancies from a 10-year population-based study
Data from Callen, 2000; Bouyer, 2003.

ectopic pregnancy, or history of tubal surgery. The chance for a subsequent successful pregnancy is reduced after an ectopic pregnancy.[44]

Assessment/Analysis[17,44,45]
- Pelvic pain
  - In the adnexal area or across the lower abdomen
- Abnormal bleeding
  - Vaginal bleeding or spotting in a woman with amenorrhea
- Abdominal or pelvic tenderness
- Adnexal mass by clinical exam or no uterine pregnancy by ultrasound
- Uterine changes
  - Appropriate for gestational age
- Vital signs
  - Prior to rupture: normal
  - Following rupture of an ectopic pregnancy with moderate hemorrhage: remain normal with slight rise in blood pressure
  - Values indicating hypovolemic hemorrhagic shock with severe bleeding (tachycardia and hypotension)
- Laboratory studies
  - CBC with differential
  - Type and crossmatch
  - Coagulation studies
  - Serum chemistries
- Positive pregnancy test
- May have cervical motion tenderness
- No uterine pregnancy on ultrasound

Interventions
- Establish IV access for crystalloids/blood products/medications, as needed
- Administer methotrexate as ordered
  - Patient education: expected effects including bleeding and discomfort
- Assisted with uterine evacuation according to facility policy/procedure
- Prepare for surgical intervention

Evaluation
- Patient with stable hemodynamic status
- Pain relief[17]

Preterm Labor

Preterm labor is diagnosed when consistent contractions of the uterus occur in a pattern of regular intervals causing cervical changes (up to 2 cm) before 37 weeks gestation.[46,48] When possible, attempts are made to delay preterm delivery. Clinical signs of preterm labor may include contractions approximately every 10 minutes, possible vaginal discharge, pelvic pressure, low dull back pain, menstrual like cramps, abdominal cramps with or without diarrhea, and spotting or leaking of fluid.[48,49] Cause of preterm labor is not known, but some factors associated with preterm labor may include previous preterm delivery, smoking, poor nutrition, infection, and multiple gestation.[48]

Assessment/Analysis[48]
- Screening through history: previous preterm labor or delivery including cause
- Assess fetal heart tones and fetal activity (fetal monitor)
- Identify presence of contractions
- Laboratory studies
  - CBC with differential
  - Coagulation studies
  - Serum chemistries
  - Blood bank analysis in preparation for transfusion
  - Kleihauer–Betke test: test for presence of fetal hemoglobin (blood) presence in the mother's blood[17]
- Sterile speculum vaginal exam to
  - Assess cervical dilation
  - Assess for rupture of membranes: if fluid is leaking during the sterile speculum exam, test fluid for fetal fibronectin (fFN). Positive test has a ferning or fern-like pattern on the slide when dry
  - Cervical length assessment
- Pelvic ultrasound

Interventions
- Establish IV access for crystalloid fluids/blood products/medications as needed

Evaluation
- Cessation of contractions
- Patient may be hospitalized if decision to add tocolytic medication (for prolongation of pregnancy up to 48 hours), to allow for administration of steroids and/or magnesium sulfate for preterm neonate treatment in the event delivery is imminent[50]

Placenta Previa

Placenta previa is defined as a condition when the placenta is abnormally implanted in the lower uterine segment and partially or completely covers the internal cervical os, as shown in Figure 7-3.[17,42] If the placenta covers any portion of the cervical os, it is called previa and when the placenta is near but not covering the os, it is called low-lying placenta.[50] It is suspected when a patient experiences symptoms of painless vaginal bleeding during pregnancy in amounts ranging from spotting to life threatening hemorrhage. Symptoms of placenta previa include vaginal bleeding, usually occur in the second and third trimester, and are based on the location of the implanted placenta.[50] When the placenta implants in the lower uterine segment of the posterior uterine wall early in the pregnancy, it usually will move up the uterine wall (placental migration) due to the stretching of the lower segment uterine wall occurring with the fetal growth.[17,46,50,52] As the uterine wall contracts or cervical changes

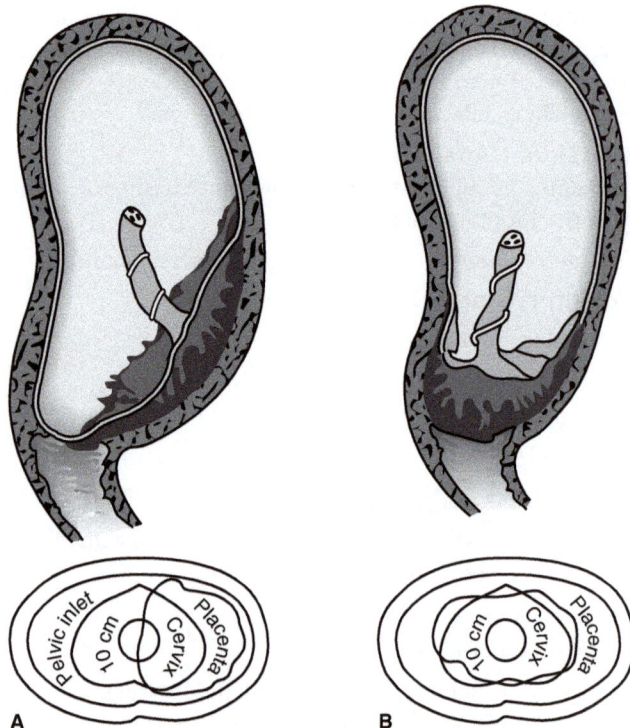

FIGURE 7-3 **Placenta previa. A: Partial. B: Complete**
Reproduced with permission from Benson RC: Handbook of Obstetrics & Gynecology, 8th ed. New York: McGraw-Hill Education; 1983.

occur during the second or third trimesters of pregnancy, bright red bleeding may occur. In most cases of placenta previa, surgical delivery is indicated, but in some cases of low-lying placenta, vaginal delivery may be possible.[17,45,46,52,53]

Assessment/Analysis[17,42,46,52,53]
- Painless vaginal bleeding: 2nd or 3rd trimester of pregnancy
- Note if color is bright red or dark bleeding, possibly with clots
- Maternal vital signs
- Fetal monitor pattern of fetus
- Assess hemodynamic status
- Symptoms of hypovolemic shock
- Presence of contractions
- Ultrasound exam to assess placenta edge and location

Interventions
- Establish IV access for fluids/blood products/medications as needed
- Oxygen therapy if needed (for pulse oximetry <94%)
- Fetal monitoring
- Laboratory studies[17]
  - CBC with differential
  - Coagulation studies
  - Kleihauer–Betke test
  - Blood bank analysis preparing for transfusion
  - Serum chemistries
- Caution during vaginal exam until ultrasound identification of placenta location

Evaluation
- Bleeding decrease or cessation
- Location of placenta
- Hemodynamic status of patient and fetus
- Fetal heart rate pattern of fetus and contractions pattern (if present)
- Cervical dilation (if present)
- Presence of abdominal pain

Abruptio Placenta

Abruptio placenta is an emergent obstetric condition occurring when the placenta partially or completely separates from the uterine wall before delivery of the fetus.[17,52,53] Damage due to this separation can cause significant blood loss to the mother and diminished perfusion to the fetus. Bleeding may be noted vaginally, but may also be concealed behind the placenta with bleeding occurring behind the placenta.[17] With significant blood loss, there may be an associated maternal hypotension and hypovolemic shock. Due to placental separation, there will be a decrease in perfusion from the placenta to the fetus, eventually causing fetal distress.[17,52] Traumatic abruption is distinguished when an external trauma has caused a placental separation, such as in the case of a motor vehicle crash (MVC) or assault.[52]

A classic symptom of abruptio placenta is a tender or painful and firm uterus, with varying amounts of vaginal bleeding.[17,42] Disseminated intravascular coagulopathy (DIC) is a potential complication with patient who has abruptio placenta.[17,42]

Assessment/Analysis[17,42]
- Mechanism of injury
- Presence of associated risk factors previously listed
- Painful uterine irritability or contractions
  - Most sensitive finding in abruption associated with trauma
  - Signs: extreme uterine tenderness and rigidity
- Vaginal bleeding may or may not be present, usually dark red
- Increasing fundal height of uterus
- Complaint of abdominal or back pain
- Maternal hypotension or tachycardia
- Fetal bradycardia[54]
- Decreased or increased fetal activity
- Laboratory studies[17]
  - CBC with differential
  - Coagulation studies
  - Kleihauer–Betke test
  - Blood bank analysis in preparation for transfusion
  - Serum chemistries

Intervention
- Administer high-flow oxygen
- Establish IV access for fluids, blood products, and medications as needed

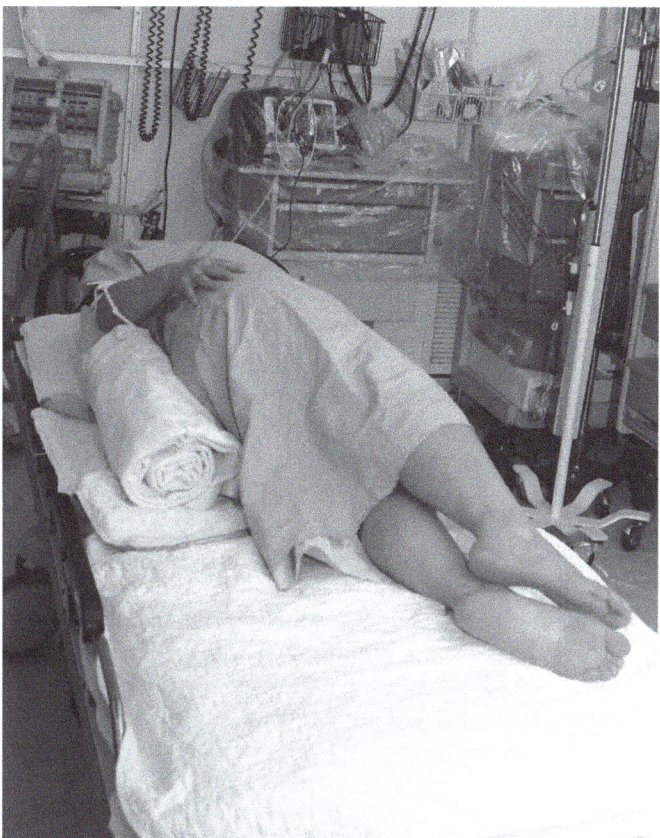

FIGURE 7-4 Left lateral recumbent or left lateral tilt position used to displace the weight of the uterus away from the inferior vena cava

Reproduced with permission from Tintinalli J, Stapcyzynski J, Ma OJ, et al: Tintinalli's Emergency Medicine: A Comprehensive Study Guide, 8th ed. New York: McGraw-Hill Education; 2015.

- ○ Place mother in left lateral recumbent position (Figure 7-4)
- ○ Turn patient on her left side or manually displace the uterus to the left, which relieves the weight of the uterus on the aorta and inferior vena cava (aorta-vena cava syndrome)[55]
- Anticipate transport to an obstetrical capable facility or emergent delivery by cesarean

Evaluation
- Stable maternal hemodynamic status
- Relief of pain
- Stabilization of associated illness/injury(ies)
- Fetal heart rate within normal limits[17,42,56]

Complications in Pregnancy: Preeclampsia, Eclampsia, and HEELP Syndrome

Preeclampsia is a serious complication of pregnancy. It is an immune mediated, systemic, and vasospastic condition of the endothelium of the mother's vasculature. The actual cause of preeclampsia is unknown but the disease process relates to a problem with placental dysfunction that leads to inadequate placental vessel development and maternal systemic vasospasms, which increase peripheral vasculature resistance.[17] The vasospasms also decrease circulation to the placenta and consequently perfusion to the fetus; therefore, there is a decrease in oxygen and nutrients delivered to the fetus. Edema was once believed to be a distinctive sign of preeclampsia; however, because swelling and edema often occur in normal pregnancy, these signs are no longer used for diagnosing preeclampsia.[57] Eclampsia begins with seizure onset in the presence of preeclampsia.[46] Preeclampsia is more common with first pregnancies, and some potential risk factors include chronic hypertension, multiple gestation, diabetes, and history of eclampsia.[17] The American College of Obstetricians and Gynecologists recommend that preeclampsia no longer be referred to as mild or severe preeclampsia but rather preeclampsia with severe features or without the severe features.[58]

In addition to the new onset of hypertension and proteinuria, as seen in preeclampsia, preeclampsia with severe features involves end-organ damage.[58] These severe features may include:[58]

- ❖ Severe hypertension (>160/110 mm Hg)
- ❖ Central nervous dysfunction (i.e., headaches, blurred vision, seizures, and/or coma)
- ❖ Renal dysfunction
- ❖ Pulmonary edema
- ❖ HELLP syndrome is a distinct subtype of preeclampsia with severe features: HELLP syndrome (**H**emolysis, **E**levated **L**iver enzymes, and **L**ow **P**latelets)

Platelet dysfunction and coagulopathy increase the risk for stroke.[58] The only cure for preeclampsia, eclampsia, and HELLP syndrome is delivery of the baby.[59] Following delivery of the placenta, symptoms usually diminish and resolve. However, always be mindful that preeclampsia, eclampsia, and HELLP syndrome can be seen following delivery of the fetus and during the postpartum period.[17,42]

Assessment/Analysis[17,42]
- Fetal heart rate within normal limits
- BP elevated; remainder of vital signs within normal limits
- Level of consciousness
  - ○ Varies from alert and oriented to confusion
- Presence of headache
- Nausea, epigastric pain, or upper right quadrant tenderness
- RUQ or abdominal pain possibly indicating a hemorrhaging liver hematoma due to the necrotic liver along with the coagulopathies
- Visual disturbances, such as blurred vision
- Non-dependent edema
  - ○ Various areas including facial or periorbital edema
- Hyperreflexia
- Proteinuria
- Decreased urine output
- Fetal status: monitor placental perfusion through fetal heart rate

- Laboratory studies
  - CBC with differential
  - Serum chemistries
  - Urinalysis for proteinuria
  - Renal function studies: creatinine and GFR
  - Lab values specific for HELLP Syndrome include[46]
    - Liver function studies: elevated
    - Platelet count is <100,000
    - Renal function: normal or elevated BUN and creatinine levels
    - Coagulation profile: abnormal

Interventions
- Establish IV access for crystalloid fluids/blood products/medications as needed
- Vital signs including pulse oximetry and fetal heart rate monitoring
- Monitor ABC's and pulse ox levels: supplemental oxygen, if indicated (pulse oximetry <94%)
- Decrease stimuli in room
- Position patient on left lateral recumbent position
- Prepare for inpatient admission to Obstetrical unit
- Patient/family education about potential pharmacology therapy
  - Antihypertensive medications: hydralazine or labetalol[46] (is more effective with reducing maternal cerebral perfusion pressure without compromising uteroplacental perfusion)
  - Anticonvulsant—Magnesium sulfate (Mag): IV infusion
    - Monitor BP, respiratory rate, and deep tendon reflexes (DTR) every hour while on Mag and as indicated
    - With eclampsia, treat seizures with magnesium sulfate 4 to 6 grams in an IV 100 mL over 20 to 30 minutes. Then a continuous infusion of 2 grams/hour for at least 24 hours[46]
    - Reduce Mag infusion to 2 grams for women in reduced renal function
- Patient/family education about potential interventions
  - Urinary catheter
  - Seizure precautions
  - Possible emergency delivery
  - Possible inpatient admission for monitoring
  - Possible cesarean delivery
- Interventions following initial assessment and continuous monitoring during admission[17,42]
  - Admit to high-risk antepartum care unit or ICU if postpartum[46]

Evaluation
- Maternal hemodynamic stability
- Fetal heart tones
- Serum magnesium levels, if mag administered
- Signs of magnesium toxicity[17]: absent patellar reflex, respiratory depression, and cardiac depression (antidote is calcium gluconate)

Obstetrical Trauma

Trauma is the leading non-obstetric related cause of death among pregnant women, with blunt trauma more common than penetrating injuries. Motor vehicle crashes are the most common cause of serious, life-threatening, or fatal blunt-trauma during pregnancy,[60] followed by falls and assault.[61] Approximately 80% of trauma-related fetal deaths were a result of motor vehicle crashes, with injury to the placenta the cause in about half.[60] Penetrating injuries commonly seen in pregnant women include gunshot wounds and stab wounds.[62]

It is imperative to remember that even a seemingly minor traumatic event may not adequately predict the health of the fetus and healthcare providers must take care to avoid 'tunnel vision' when caring for the obviously pregnant trauma patient. Trauma during pregnancy is associated with an increased risk of preterm labor, feto-maternal hemorrhage, placental abruption, and pregnancy loss.[61]

Maternal stability and survival offer the best chance for fetal survival. Initial resuscitation efforts must be directed toward the mother prior to evaluation of the fetus. No critical interventions or diagnostic procedures should be withheld from the treatment of pregnant trauma patients out of concern for potential adverse fetal consequences.[61] The initial sequence of trauma resuscitation should remain unchanged, but with some important obstetric-related caveats as the following discusses.

Assessment and Interventions
- Assess fetal gestational age by palpating the height of the uterine fundus
  - At 12 weeks gestation, the uterine fundus may be palpated at or about the level of the pubic symphysis
  - At approximately 20 weeks gestation, it may be felt at about the level of the maternal umbilicus. Add 1 cm beyond the umbilicus per additional week of gestation. Fetal viability is generally ≥24 weeks gestation
- Obstetric-related caveats of trauma care assessment considerations and interventions as described in Table 7-3

Evaluation
- Stable maternal hemodynamic status
- Relief of pain
- Fetal heart rate within normal limits[61–65]

Emergent Delivery

Childbirth in an emergency department is an emergent condition. Although a natural process, associated complications can place both the mother and her infant(s) at risk. Transport of the woman in labor to a facility with obstetric and neonatal capabilities and resources is ideal, but precipitous childbirth during transport adds to the risk of harm to both patients.[17,42] If delivery of a pregnant woman is imminent, it is essential to obtain a rapid obstetric history and physical exam.

Assessment/Analysis

- Signs of imminent childbirth
  - Obvious pregnancy with frequent, painful contractions
  - Mother has a desire to push, bear down, or have a bowel movement
  - Mother states "the baby is coming"
  - Perineal bulging is visible
  - Presentation of a fetal head in the vagina[17,42]
  - Widening of the vulvovaginal area
- Four key questions if delivery is imminent
  - How pregnant are you? (weeks gestation if known, or LMP)
  - How many babies are you expecting?
  - Is anything coming out of your vagina?
    - A head, large amounts of blood, hands, feet, cord, greenish fluid, etc
  - Have you used any illicit drugs in the past 24 hours?
- If time permits, additional assessment questions should include
  - Frequency, intensity, and duration of contractions
  - If spontaneous rupture of amniotic membranes has occurred
    - "Water broke"
    - Time, color, and odor
  - Bloody show or vaginal bleeding
  - Maternal past medical history, including medications taken routinely and any allergies
  - Reproductive history
    - Gravidity (# of pregnancies, including current)
    - Parity (# of live babies born)
    - Estimated gestational age/date of confinement (EDC, i.e., "due date")
    - Previous cesarean section delivery(ies)
    - Complications during delivery(ies)
  - Prenatal care (yes/no)
  - Known complications of this pregnancy
    - Multiple infants
    - Placenta previa
    - Preeclampsia
    - HELLP syndrome
    - Diabetes

Intervention

- Establish IV access for crystalloid fluids/blood products/medications as needed
- Assist mother to deliver her infant(s)
  - Place mother on stretcher, or in exam room when possible, into a low Fowler's position lying slightly on her left side; maintain patient safety and privacy
  - Call for assistance with delivery and care of neonate if time permits, and if qualified personnel are available within the facility[42,54,66–68]
  - Have an emergency birthing pack available
  - If delivery is precipitous, at a minimum don gloves and have a clean towel or other clean, dry material available
    - Protective eyewear, gowns, masks, and sterile gloves should be used if time permits
- Confirm to mother that baby is going to be delivered in the present location. Direct the mother to "pant like a puppy" to prevent an uncontrolled delivery and encourage slow, controlled pushes. Have a support person stay with mother and assist with breathing technique
- Communicate with the mother as the infant is being delivered, explaining each step of the process, giving the mother positive feedback and encouragement for her efforts
- Support the perineum and the fetal head with a sterile gloved hand or sterile towel, but do not exert pressure on the head
- As the head delivers: if membranes are intact at delivery, rupture membranes at nape of neck, then sweep over back of head towards front to clear face
- After delivery of head, assess for breathing or crying. If present, no suctioning or clearing of the airway is required. If the baby is cyanotic or has labored breathing, suction the baby's mouth, and then nose with a bulb syringe to prevent aspiration. (Baby is obligate nose breather so if the nose is suctioned first, the baby will take a deep breath and aspirate the secretions and debris that is in their mouth.) If meconium is present and/or suspected but the neonate is vigorous with good respiratory effort and muscle tone, no suctioning is needed. Gentle clearing of the meconium from the mouth and nose with a bulb syringe may be done if needed[66,67]
- Check if the cord is wrapped around the neonate's neck by sliding fingers around the head and neck. If present, try to slide cord around the baby's head. Unwind if necessary. Do not exert force. If tight, carefully clamp the cord in two places and cut between the clamps before delivering the remainder of infant
- Allow the natural alignment and external rotation of the fetal head to occur. Support the neonates head and deliver the anterior shoulder by applying gentle, downward traction with the neonate's head
- When the anterior shoulder is delivered (visible under the pubic arch of the mother), the posterior shoulder may be delivered by applying gentle upward traction with the neonate's head. The rest of the body almost always follows without difficulty
- As the body delivers, slide the upper hand along the baby's back to grasp the legs and feet. Use caution; newly delivered neonates are very slippery. Ideally, allow the mother to deliver her infant directly onto the surface of the stretcher she is laying on to minimize any inadvertent mishandling of the infant. If this is not possible, use the lower hand and forearm to maintain control of the delivery and support the head and chest. Attempt to keep the infant's head slightly lower than the trunk to minimize the possibility of aspiration

TABLE 7-3 **Obstetric-Related Caveats of Trauma Care**[61-65]

	Maternal Physiologic Changes
CV; Utero-placental unit	• Cardiac output increased 30%–50% • Peripheral resistance decreased 20% • Blood pressure decreases 10–15 mm Hg systolic in first half of pregnancy, then returns back to baseline • Blood volume 100 mL/kg or 6–7 Liters • Central venous pressure increased up to 10 mm Hg • Central venous oxygen saturation increased as high as 80% • Plasma volume increased 30%–50% • 25% of blood flow directed to uteroplacental unit • No autoregulation of blood flow • Beginning at approximately 18 to 20 weeks gestation, the enlarging uterus can compress the aorta and the inferior vena cava and vessels below the diaphragm, mother is at risk of "supine hypotension syndrome," (aorta-vena cava syndrome) when lying in the supine position
Respiratory	• Upper airway edema, increased capillary friability can result in bleeding and swelling, creating difficult airway management • Diaphragm elevated up to 4 cm due to displacement by gravid uterus • Fetal hemoglobin has greater affinity for oxygen than maternal hemoglobin—Fetal oxygen maintained at expense of maternal oxygenation • Respiratory rate remains 12–20/min with increased tidal volume, minute ventilation • Normal blood gas values are different. The "normal" state is compensated respiratory alkalosis due to the increased minute ventilation | Arterial blood gases	Non-pregnancy	Pregnancy
---	---	---
pH	7.35–7.45	7.40–7.45
$PaCO_2$	35–45 mm Hg	25–30 mm Hg
PaO_2	80–100 mm Hg	101–104 mm Hg
Base excess or deficit	−2 to +2 mEq/L	3–4 mEq/L
Bicarbonate	22–26 mEq/L	22–26 mEq/L	
Hematologic	• Increased fibrinogen or increased factors V, VII, VIII, X, von Willebrand factor during second half of pregnancy
GI	• Decreased lower esophageal sphincter tone • Increased intra-abdominal pressure, delayed gastric emptying. Increased likelihood of aspiration of gastric contents • Diaphragm elevated up to 4 cm due to displacement by gravid uterus • The most common cause of abdominal hemorrhage in pregnancy is splenic injury • Bowel and liver injuries are less frequent because of the protective effect of a large uterus, unless mechanism is penetrating over those areas
Orthopedic	• Orthopedic injuries such as pelvic and acetabular fractures cause increased risk for placental abruption, preterm delivery, and perinatal mortality • The incidence of falls increases with the progression of pregnancy due to changing center of gravity and ligamentous laxity

	Trauma-care
CV; Utero-placental unit	• Place patient in left lateral tilt position (approximately 30 degrees) and/or provide manual displacement of the uterus during third trimester to prevent hypotension from aorta-vena cava compression by the gravid uterus. Maintain spinal alignment if suspected cervical injury • A pregnant patient may lose 30% to 35% of circulating blood volume before showing signs of hypotension or shock • Establish IV access for crystalloids/blood products/medications, as needed 　○ Avoid femoral and lower extremity access sites for blood and volume delivery in second half of pregnancy due to increased risk for DVT • Identify and control sources of hemorrhage—maternal blood loss and hypovolemia will worsen fetal hypoperfusion • Adequately replace volume before considering vasopressors (uterine arteries are maximally dilated and blood flow is pressure dependent)
Respiratory	• Preoxygenate to 95% oxygen saturation to prevent hypoxia during intubation • Provide high-flow supplemental oxygenation set to deliver 15 L/min during intubation, even after chemical paralysis, to continue passive apneic oxygen delivery to the alveoli • Place the patient in the supine position and manually displace the uterus to the left during intubation. Elevate the head and shoulders with a pillow or folded sheets to achieve the sniffing position, especially in obese patients • Use of a laryngeal mask airway (LMA) should be considered, especially after failed intubation • All pregnant trauma patients should receive supplemental oxygen, because the pregnant patient is less able to compensate for hypoxia • Keep maternal pulse oximetry readings >95% to maintain a PaO_2 of >70 mm Hg to optimize maternal oxygenation and oxygen delivery to the placenta • Do not dismiss tachypnea as a normal part of pregnancy • The $CO_0 - PaCO_2$ is a sensitive indicator of respiratory failure. Because a pregnant woman's baseline $PaCO_2$ is lower than a non-pregnant woman's, even a "high normal" $PaCO_2$ might indicate significant respiratory compromise this shows the pregnant patient is moving toward acidosis. If the results already show an acidotic state, the pregnant patient is even more acidotic than you think
Hematologic	• Heightened risk for venous thromboembolism • Include blood typing and Rh status in laboratory studies
GI	• Place a nasogastric tube early in the resuscitation sequence to prevent aspiration of gastric contents • Assess for diaphragmatic, splenic, liver, and kidney injuries • Bedside ultrasound: FAST may be used to determine fetal heart rate and estimate fetal gestation/viability (normal fetal heart rate is 120 to 160 beats/min) • Administer Rho(D) immunoglobulin (Rhogam™, Rhophylac™) to Rh-negative pregnant women with abdominal trauma within 72 hours of injury
Orthopedic	• Shield fetus during maternal radiation exposure when possible Diagnostic imaging for any injury should not be delayed • Provide tetanus prophylaxis as needed (Category C for all trimesters of pregnancy but commonly accepted as safe) Tetanus antibody crosses the placenta, so it can also reduce the incidence of neonatal tetanus
Other considerations	• Laboratory studies[17] 　○ CBC with differential 　○ Coagulation studies 　○ Kleihauer–betke test 　○ Blood bank analysis preparing for transfusion 　○ Serum chemistries • Obstetrics consultation • Anticipate hospital admission for external monitoring for uterine contractions (tocodynamometric monitoring) for potentially viable fetus • Screen for potential intimate partner violence

- Note and record the time of delivery
- Place the baby on mother's abdomen or keep the neonate at the level of the uterus. Clamping and cutting the umbilical cord may be delayed up to 3 minutes for infants who do not require medical intervention[69]
- Vigorously dry the neonate and replace any wet material with warm, dry towels or blankets
- Encourage crying by tactile stimulation and assess the infant's respiratory effort
- Use the bulb syringe to aspirate mucous from infant's nose and mouth ONLY if needed. There is no evidence that routine bulb suctioning for clear or meconium-stained fluid is beneficial[54]
- Assess/score APGAR criteria at one and five minutes and record (see Table 7-4)[54,66]
- Identify mother, infant, and significant other per the facility policy on patient identification. Identification and banding should take place before the mother and baby are separated
- Promote bonding by allowing the mother/father to hold the infant skin-to-skin when possible and as the patient/infant condition warrants
- Clamp the umbilical cord in 2 places, approximately 12 inches from the umbilicus of the neonate and cut the cord using sterile scissors[42,66-68]

Delivery of the Placenta

The placenta should separate from the uterine wall to be expelled spontaneously after delivery, generally occuring 5 to 30 minutes after delivery of the infant. Never pull on the umbilical cord and avoid uterine massage until the placenta is completely delivered.

Interventions to Assist in Delivery of the Placenta
- The umbilical cord will advance 2 to 3 inches further out of the vagina
- The fundus will bulge upward into the abdomen
- Anticipate a large gush of blood from the vagina (normal finding)
- Allow the placenta to be spontaneously expelled
- Examine the placenta and note any missing sections
- Place the placenta and attached umbilical cord in a bag or basin and transport with the mother and infant
- Massage the fundus (should feel firm and be approximately the size of a grapefruit) to encourage uterine contraction and prevent postpartum hemorrhage. Breastfeeding or nipple stimulation may also be utilized to contract the uterus and prevent excessive bleeding

Placenta Accreta

If the placenta has not delivered spontaneously within 30 minutes, consider placenta accreta. This is an abnormal adherence of the placenta to the uterine wall, and occurs at varying degrees.

- ❖ Placenta increta: adheared through the uterine wall into the utuerine muscle
- ❖ Placenta percreta: adheared through the muscle and may attach to the bladder or other pelvic structures

It is not possible to manage this type of obstetrical complication in the emergency department. Surgical intervention is required to remove the placenta from the uterus. Monitor the hemodynamic status of the mother and closely assess for postpartum hemorrhage. Anticipate transport to the operating room.[68]

Meconium Aspiration

Meconium is a thick, pasty, greenish black substance present in the fetal bowel. If the infant is stressed in utero, this substance may be expelled into the amniotic fluid. The infant may aspirate this substance with the first breath after birth. Meconium can irritate the airway or cause a blockage resulting in respiratory distress.[68] Amniotic fluid may be green or dark yellow and have a "pea soup" consistency.[62] For the infant born limp, poorly responsive, and with meconium-stained fluid, anticipate the need for endotracheal intubation with direct tracheal suction.[68]

Umbilical Cord Prolapse

Umbilical cord prolapse occurs when the umbilical cord is positioned in front of the presenting part. Circulation to the infant is occluded when the fetal presenting part compresses the umbilical cord against the bony pelvis. Incidence of cord prolapse is increased in breech presentations, multiple gestations,

TABLE 7-4 **APGAR Criteria to Score Infant at One and Five Minutes of Life**

Sign	0 Points	1 Point	2 Points
Heart rate	Absent	<100 bpm	≥100 bpm
Respiratory effort	Absent	Slow, irregular	Good, crying
Muscle tone	Flaccid	Some extremity flexion	Active motion
Reflex irritability	No response	Grimace	Vigorous cry
Color	Blue, pale	Body pink, extremities blue	Completely pink

bpm = beats per minute.
Data from Apgar, 1953.

and if the infant is delivering prematurely and not yet 'head first'. Umbilical cord prolapse is rare in full term, head first presentations and will likely be noted after the spontaneous rupture of membranes. Ask or assess the mother for "something coming out" of the vagina. Unless pressure is relieved immediately, the fetus will die or experience permanent brain damage from a lack of oxygen. Along with the potential for cord compression decreasing perfusion to the fetus, just the actual temperature change from the cord coming out of the uterus can cause the cord to vasospasm, again decreasing perfusion. An emergent, immediate cesarean delivery is required.[62,66,68]

Interventions to Relieve Pressure From the Exposed Cord During Vaginal Delivery
- Place gloved hand against the presenting part and push it away from the cord
- Place the mother in the Trendelenburg position
- Administer the mother high-flow oxygen
- Keep the mother warm
- Maintain this position until vaginal delivery is complete or until emergent cesarean delivery occurs
- Do not try to return the prolapsed cord to the vagina
- Do not handle the cord to prevent vessel spasm
- Emptying the bladder with an indwelling catheter may temporarily relieve cord compression but do not delay delivery or cesarean delivery

Evaluation
- Successful delivery of one or multiple infant(s) and placenta(s)
- Stable maternal and infant respiratory status
- Stable maternal and infant hemodynamics
- Minimal vaginal bleeding[62,66,68]

Neonatal Resuscitation

Most newly born infants transition to extrauterine life without complications requiring only maintenance of temperature, mild stimulation, and minimal airway suctioning. Approximately 10% of all newborns require some medical intervention immediately after birth, and only 1% require extensive resuscitation. Assessment and intervention should occur concurrently when a newborn is in distress. Resuscitation of the newborn is required when born with any cardiovascular or respiratory compromise.[66,67] Apgar scores of less than 6 as assessed at 1 or 5 minutes are indicative of such compromise and resuscitation should be implemented immediately.

Assessment/Analysis
- Signs of respiratory distress
- Heart rate >100 bpm
- Calculate an Apgar score

Intervention
- Dry, warm, position, suction, and stimulate
  - Immediately after delivery, place the infant on its back in a warmed environment
  - Stimulate and dry the infant with a warm towel while assessing the need to resuscitate
  - If the infant is crying, pink, has spontaneous respirations, and has a heart rate (HR) faster than 100 beats/min, further medical intervention is likely not required
  - If the Apgar score is less than 6 at either 1 or 5 minutes, immediately proceed to the next step in the resuscitation process[64,66,67]
- Oxygen
  - Open the airway by positioning the head in the sniffing position
  - If the infant is breathing/crying, no suctioning or clearing of the airway is required. If the baby is cyanotic or has labored breathing, suction the baby's mouth, and then nose with a bulb syringe to prevent aspiration. Alternately, mechanical suction with an 8F suction catheter may be used
  - If apneic and/or bradycardic (<100 beats/min), provide blow-by oxygen[64,66,67]
- Ventilation
  - Bag-mask device
  - If suctioning and blow-by oxygen administration do not improve the infant's condition, initiate positive pressure ventilation with bag-mask ventilation
  - Use an appropriately sized mask, maintain a tight seal, and ventilate at 40 to 60 breaths/min. Ventilate and visually check for adequate chest rise
  - Do not hyperinflate the infant's lungs
  - Successful resuscitation with bag-mask ventilation is indicated by an increase in HR to >100 beats/min and improved color and muscle tone[64,66,67]
- Endotracheal Intubation
  - Assist with endotracheal intubation
  - Pre-oxygenate the newborn using bag-mask ventilation with 100% oxygen and place the infant's head in the "sniffing position," with the neck slightly extended
  - During the procedure, maintain continuous blow-by oxygen
- To calculate correct endotracheal tube placement depth (centimeter marker) add 6 to the weight of the infant (in kilograms). For example, a 3-kg infant is 9 cm (6 + 3) at the lips[67]
- Confirm proper endotracheal tube placement through observation, auscultation of lung sounds bilaterally and exhaled carbon dioxide detection (capnography)[67]
- Chest Compressions
  - If the newborn remains severely bradycardic (HR <60 beats/min) after assisted ventilation, start chest compressions
    - Use either the "two-thumb" or "two-finger" technique in a cycle of three chest compressions to one breath (90 compressions to 30 breaths/min)

- **Medications**
  - If bradycardia continues despite bag-mask ventilation, endotracheal intubation, ventilation, and chest compressions, fluids and medications should be administered
  - The intravenous route is preferred, but the intraosseous or umbilical venous route may be used
  - Epinephrine can be given via endotracheal route in the absence of vascular access[66,67]

Evaluation
- Patent newborn airway and adequate respiratory effort
- Adequate cardiovascular status, HR >100 beats/minute
- Newborn with pink mucous membranes, warm skin[64]

Postpartum Hemorrhage

Postpartum hemorrhage (PPH) defined as excessive vaginal bleeding can occur following the placental release after delivery of a baby up to 6 weeks postpartum, and can occur in patients with vaginal or post op cesarean deliveries.[17] Although PPH can occur up to 6 weeks postpartum, late PPH usually occurs around 6 to 10 days post delivery.[17,42] Primary PPH can occur anytime starting immediately following delivery, referred to as primary if within the first 24 hours. PPH occurring after 24 hours up to 6 weeks postpartum is called secondary PPH.[17,46] PPH occurring immediately following the delivery of the baby is usually due to uterine atony.[46] Additional causes of PPH may include lacerations of the vagina or the cervix, retained placenta, uterine inversion, and maternal coagulopathy problems.[17,46] Postpartum patients do have an excess amount of blood supply due to a naturally hypervolemic state (plasma volume increases by 40% and red blood cell volume by 25% at the end of the third trimester[46]); a loss >500 mL is considered PPH.[42,71] Fundal massage followed by administration of oxytocin usually controls mild uterine atony, but when bleeding is significant enough to change hemodynamic status, PPH protocols are implemented.[17,42,46,71]

Excessive blood loss in the postpartum period is defined as a 10% drop in the hematocrit, a need for transfusion of packed red blood cells, or volume loss that causes symptoms of hypovolemia.[46] Due to the hypervolemic status at the end of the third trimester, the hematologic changes of pregnancy can mask the typical symptoms of hemorrhage, and the first sign may be only a mild increase in pulse rate. Up to a 30% loss in total blood volume may be required before blood pressure drops.[46]

Assessment/ Analysis[17,42,46,70]
- Date of delivery and pregnancy complications
  - High-risk pregnancy, multiple fetus, and type of delivery
- Vaginal bleeding
  - When did bleeding begin
  - Location of origin of bleeding
  - Color of blood: bright or dark
  - Describe amount of bleeding: number of pads saturated per hour to steady stream of blood
  - Clots or tissue present
  - Odor present
- Painful or painless bleeding
- Palpate uterus and identify location: midline and firm versus displaced and boggy
- Symptoms of shock present
- Pale and clammy skin
- Nausea
- Laboratory studies for initial management
  - CBC with differential
  - Type and screen/crossmatch if transfusion likely

Interventions
- Uterine massage
- Establish IV access for fluids, blood products, and medications as needed
  - Fluid bolus (IV crystalloids); may need blood products
  - Oxytocin agents
- Oxygen via facemask

Evaluation
- Patient may be admitted for observation and support care for hemorrhage (to monitor for continued bleeding)
- Monitor vaginal bleeding and evidence of clots or tissue
- Monitor maternal hemodynamic status[17,42,46,70]

Postpartum Infection

A postpartum patient presenting with a fever is assumed to have a postpartum infection until proven otherwise.[46,71] The term puerperal infection describes any bacterial infection of the genital tract after delivery, but a number of factors can cause fever, a temperature of 38.0°C (100.4°F) or higher, in the puerperium. Postpartum infection can present as an infection of the uterus, such as endometritis, renal infection such as pyelonephritis or UTI, wound infection such as vaginal laceration, episiotomy, cesarean surgical wound, mastitis, deep vein thrombophlebitis (DVT), or appendicitis.[46] However, most persistent fevers after childbirth are caused by genital tract infection.[70]

Assessment/Analysis[49,71,72]
- Maternal fever: 38.0°C (100.4°F) or higher
- Foul smelling lochia
  - Decreased vaginal discharge, paste-like salmon colored discharge, or purulent discharge
- Back or flank pain
- Uterine tenderness
- Surgical site tenderness
  - Possible purulent exudates from surgical site
- Leukocytosis
- Tachycardia
- Watch for signs of sepsis

- Laboratory studies for initial management
  - CBC w/ differential, evaluation for leukocytosis
  - Blood cultures
  - Suspected site culture
  - Urinalysis

Interventions
- Establish IV access for crystalloid fluids, blood products, and medications as needed
  - Fluid bolus with continuous infusion
- Anti-pyretic
- Pain medication
- Antibiotic therapy
- Possible inpatient hospitalization for IV antibiotics

Evaluation
- Fever within normal range
- Pain management under control
- Appropriate antibiotic treatment[49,70]

REFERENCES

1. Rieder J, Brusky J, Tran V, et al. Review of intentionally self-inflicted, accidental and iatrogetic foreign objects in the genitourinary tract. *Urol Int.* 2010;84(4):471–475. Epub 2010 Mar 12.
2. Campbell M. Abdominal and urologic trauma. In: Hoyt KS, Selfridge-Thomas J, eds. *Emergency Nursing Core Curriculum.* 6th ed. St. Louis, Mo: Saunders Elsevier, 2007:781–800.
3. Askew K. Urinary tract infections and hematuria. In: Tintinalli JE, Stapczynski J, Ma O, et al, eds. *Tintinalli's Emergency Medicine: A Comprehensive Study Guide.* 8th ed. New York, NY: McGraw-Hill; 2016.
4. Gupta K, Trautner BW. Urinary tract infections, pyelonephritis, and prostatitis. In: Kasper D, Fauci A, Hauser S, et al, eds. *Harrison's Principles of Internal Medicine.* 19th ed. New York, NY: McGraw-Hill; 2015.
5. Quallich S. Genitourinary emergencies. In: Hammond BB, Zimmermann PG, eds. *Sheehy's Manual of Emergency Care.* 7th ed. Des Plaines, IL: Elsevier. 2013:353–360.
6. Jordan KS. Genitourinary emergencies. In: Hoyt KS, Selfridge-Thomas J, eds. *Emergency Nursing Core Curriculum.* 6th ed. St. Louis, Mo: Saunders Elsevier, 2007:387–408.
7. Davis JE. Male genital problems. In: Tintinalli JE, Stapczynski J, Ma O, et al, eds. *Tintinalli's Emergency Medicine: A Comprehensive Study Guide.* 8th ed. New York, NY: McGraw-Hill; 2016.
8. Peard AS. Communicable and infectious disease. In: Hoyt KS, Selfridge-Thomas J, eds. *Emergency Nursing Core Curriculum.* 6th ed. St. Louis, Mo: Saunders Elsevier, 2007:438–477.
9. Levey H, Segal R, Bivalacqua T. Management of priapism: an update for clinicians. *Ther Adv Urol.* 2014;6(6):230–244. doi: 10.1177/1756287214542096
10. Gratton MC, French LK. Genitourinary trauma. In: Tintinalli JE, Stapczynski J, Ma O, et al, eds. *Tintinalli's Emergency Medicine: A Comprehensive Study Guide.* 8th ed. New York, NY: McGraw-Hill; 2016.
11. Harris C. Abdominal trauma. In: Hammond BB, Zimmermann PG, eds. *Sheehy's Manual of Emergency Care.* 7th ed. Des Plaines, IL: Elsevier; 2013.
12. Hannon C, Murray PT. Acute kidney injury. In: Hall JB, Schmidt GA, Kress JP, eds. *Principles of Critical Care.* 4th ed. New York, NY: McGraw-Hill; 2015.
13. Ignatavicius DD, Workman ML. *Medical-Surgical Nursing: Patient Centered Collaborative Care.* 7th ed. St. Louis, MO: Elsevier; 2013:1620–1621.
14. Yen D, Lee C. Acute urinary retention. In: Tintinalli JE, Stapczynski J, Ma O, et al, eds. *Tintinalli's Emergency Medicine: A Comprehensive Study Guide.* 8th ed. New York, NY: McGraw-Hill; 2016.
15. Hang B. Abnormal uterine bleeding. In: Tintinalli JE, Stapczynski J, Ma O, et al, eds. *Tintinalli's Emergency Medicine: A Comprehensive Study Guide.* 8th ed. New York, NY: McGraw-Hill; 2016.
16. Kelly L. Gynecologic emergencies. In: Hammond BB, Zimmermann PG, eds. *Sheehy's Manual of Emergency Care.* 7th ed. Des Plaines, IL: Elsevier; 2013:497–503.
17. Jordan KS. Obstetric and gynecologic emergencies. In: Hoyt KS, Selfridge-Thomas J, eds. *Emergency Nursing Core Curriculum.* 6th ed. St. Louis, Mo: Saunders Elsevier; 2007:536–570.
18. Hoffman BL, Schorge JO, Bradshaw KD, et al. Abnormal uterine bleeding. In: Hoffman BL, Schorge JO, Bradshaw KD, et al, eds. *Williams Gynecology.* 3rd ed. New York, NY: McGraw-Hill; 2016.
19. Bauman D. Pediatric and adolescent gynecology. In: DeCherney AH, Nathan L, Laufer N, et al, eds. *CURRENT Diagnosis & Treatment: Obstetrics & Gynecology.* 11th ed. New York, NY: McGraw-Hill; 2013.
20. Myers T. *Mosby's Dictionary of Medicine, Nursing, and Health Professions.* 8th ed. 2009:1410.
21. LeBlond RF, Brown DD, Suneja M, et al. The female genitalia and reproductive system. In: LeBlond RF, Brown DD, Suneja M, et al, eds. *DeGowin's Diagnostic Examination.* 10th ed. New York, NY: McGraw-Hill; 2015.
22. Marrazzo JM, Holmes KK. Sexually transmitted infections: overview and clinical approach. In: Kasper D, Fauci A, Hauser S, et al, eds. *Harrison's Principles of Internal Medicine.* 19th ed. New York, NY: McGraw-Hill; 2015.
23. Health Resources and Services Administration. Pelvic inflammatory disease fact sheet. *U.S. Department of Health and Human Services* Barclift S. https://www.womenshealth.gov/publications/our-publications/fact-sheet/pelvic-inflammatory-disease.html#a. Accessed April 12, 2015.
24. CDC. Pelvic Inflammatory Disease (PID). Atlanta, GA: Department of Health and Human Services; May 4, 2015. http://www.cdc.gov/std/pid/stdfact-pid.htm. Accessed April 12, 2015.
25. Hosenfeld CB, Workowski KA, Berman S, et al. Repeat infection with chlamydia and gonorrhea among females: a systematic review of the literature. *Sex Transm Dis.* 2009;36:478–89.
26. Nobay F, Promes SB. Sexually transmitted diseases. In: Tintinalli JE, Stapczynski J, Ma O, et al, eds. *Tintinalli's Emergency Medicine: A Comprehensive Study Guide.* 8th ed. New York, NY: McGraw-Hill; 2016.
27. CDC. Sexually transmitted diseases treatment guidelines, 2015. Atlanta, GA: Department of Health and Human Services; June 5, 2015. http://www.cdc.gov/mmwr/preview/mmwrhtml/rr6403a1.htm. Accessed August 12, 2015.
28. Qaseem A, Humphrey LL, Harris R, et al. Screening pelvic examination in adult women: a clinical practice guideline from the American College of Physicians. *Ann Intern Med.* 2014;161(1):67–72.
29. Bottomley C, Bourne T. Diagnosis and management of ovarian cyst accidents. *Best Pract Res Clin Obstet Gynaecol.* 2009;23(5):711–24.
30. Weintraub B. Sexual assault. In: Hammond BB, Zimmermann PG, eds. *Sheehy's Manual of Emergency Care.* 7th ed. Des Plaines, IL: Elsevier; 2013:497–503.
31. Moreno-Walton L. Female and male sexual assault. In: Tintinalli JE, Stapczynski J, Ma O, et al, eds. *Tintinalli's Emergency Medicine: A Comprehensive Study Guide.* 8th ed. New York, NY: McGraw-Hill; 2016.
32. Ruiz-Contreras A. Abuse and neglect/sexual assault. In: Hoyt KS, Selfridge-Thomas J, eds. *Emergency Nursing Core Curriculum.* 6th ed. St. Louis, Mo: Saunders Elsevier; 2007:51–68.
33. Office on Violence Against Women. National Protocol for Sexual Assault Medical Forensic Examinations (Adults/Adolescents), 2nd ed. *US Dept of Justice.* Apr 2013. Available at https://www.ncjrs.gov/pdffiles1/ovw/241903.pdf. Accessed: May 8 2013 taken from https://www.gpo.gov/fdsys/pkg/PLAW-104publ305/pdf/PLAW-104publ305.pdf.
34. Sommers MS, Brown, KM, Buschur C, et al. Injuries from intimate partner and sexual violence: significance and classification systems. *J Forensic Leg Med.* 2012;19:250–263. doi:10.1016/j.jflm.2012.02.014
35. Cunningham N. Sexual assault consultations—from high risk to high reliability. *J Forensic Leg Med.* 2012;(2):53–59.
36. Bui PV, Sachs C, Wheeler M. Correlates of anogenital injuries in adolescent females. *Intl J of Clin Med.* 2014;(5):63–71.

37. Larsen ML, Hilden M, Lidegaard Ø. Sexual assault: a descriptive study of 2500 female victims over a 10-year period. *BJOG.* 2015;122(4):577–584. doi: 10.1111/1471-0528.13093
38. Cohen S. Abuse and neglect In: Hammond BB, Zimmermann PG, eds. *Sheehy's Manual of Emergency Care.* 7th ed. Des Plaines, IL: Elsevier; 2013:521–530.
39. Merrit DF. Genital trauma. In: Emans SJ, Laufer MR, eds. *Pediatric & Adolescent Gynecology.* 6th ed. Philadelphia, PA: Wolters Kluwer Lippincott Williams & Wilkins; 2012:293.
40. Karjane NW. A seven year old girl with vaginal bleeding. In: Chelmow D, Issacs CR, Carrol A, eds. *Acute Care and Emergency Gynecology: A Case-Based Approach.* 2014:220–227.
41. Umbreen IM, Ortman MJ, Mando-Vandrick J, et al. Management of first trimester complications in the emergency department. *Am J Health-Syst Pharm.* 2013;70:90–111.
42. Poole JH, Thompson JE. Obstetric emergencies. In: Hammond BB, Zimmermann PG, eds. *Sheehy's Manual of Emergency Care.* 7th ed. Des Plaines, IL: Elsevier; 2013:483–495.
43. American College of Obstetrics and Gynecology. Clinical Management for obstetricians and gynecologists, Practice Bulletin no. 154 – Nausea and vomiting of pregnancy. *Obstet and Gynecol.* 2015;126(3):e12–e24.
44. Cunningham F, Leveno KJ, Bloom SL, et al. Ectopic pregnancy. In: Cunningham F, Leveno KJ, Bloom SL, et al, eds. *Williams Obstetrics.* 24th ed. New York, NY: McGraw-Hill; 2013.
45. Buckley RG, Knoop KJ. Gynecologic and obstetric conditions. In: Knoop KJ, Stack LB, Storrow AB, et al, eds. *The Atlas of Emergency Medicine.* 3rd ed. New York, NY: McGraw-Hill; 2010.
46. Young J. Maternal emergencies after 20 weeks of pregnancy and in the postpartum period. In: Tintinalli JE, Stapczynski J, Ma O, et al, eds. *Tintinalli's Emergency Medicine: A Comprehensive Study Guide.* 8th ed. New York, NY: McGraw-Hill; 2016.
47. Cunningham F, Leveno KJ, Bloom SL, et al. Preterm labor. In: Cunningham F, Leveno KJ, Bloom SL, et al, eds. *Williams Obstetrics.* 24th ed. New York, NY: McGraw-Hill; 2013.
48. Doyle J, Silber A. Preterm labor: role of the nurse practitioner. *The Nurse Practitioner.* 2015;40(3):49–50.
49. Rogers VL, Worley KC. Obstetrics and obstetric disorders. In: Papadakis MA, McPhee SJ, Rabow MW, eds. *Current Medical Diagnosis & Treatment 2016.* New York, NY: McGraw-Hill; 2016.
50. American College of Obstetricians and Gynecologists. Practice bulletin No. 159 summary: management of preterm labor. *Obstet Gynecol.* 2016;127(1):190–191. doi: 10.1097/AOG.0000000000001260
51. Silver RM. The American College of Obstetricians and Gynecologists. Abnormal placentation: placenta previa, vasa previa, and placenta accreta. *Obstet Gynecol.* 2015;126(3):654–668. doi: 10.1097/AOG.0000000000001005
52. Cunningham F, Leveno KJ, Bloom SL, et al. Obstetrical hemorrhage. In: Cunningham F, Leveno KJ, Bloom SL, et al, eds. *Williams Obstetrics.* 24th ed. New York, NY: McGraw-Hill; 2013.
53. Wagner SA. Third-trimester vaginal bleeding. In: DeCherney AH, Nathan L, Laufer N, et al, eds. *CURRENT Diagnosis & Treatment: Obstetrics & Gynecology.* 11th ed. New York, NY: McGraw-Hill; 2013.
54. Cunningham F, Leveno KJ, Bloom SL, et al. The newborn. In: Cunningham F, Leveno KJ, Bloom SL, et al, eds. *Williams Obstetrics.* 24th ed. New York, NY: McGraw-Hill; 2013.
55. Kither H, Moneghan S. Intrauterine fetal resuscitation. *Anaesthesia & Intensive Care Medicine.* 2013:14:287–290.
56. Fox NS, Goldberg J, Smith RS. Critical care obstetrics. In: DeCherney AH, Nathan L, Laufer N, et al, eds. *CURRENT Diagnosis & Treatment: Obstetrics & Gynecology.* 11th ed. New York, NY: McGraw-Hill; 2013.
57. Miller DA. Hypertension in pregnancy. In: DeCherney AH, Nathan L, Laufer N, et al, eds. *CURRENT Diagnosis & Treatment: Obstetrics & Gynecology.* 11th ed. New York, NY: McGraw-Hill; 2013.
58. Barbieri RL, Repke JT. Medical disorders during pregnancy. In: Kasper D, Fauci A, Hauser S, et al, eds. *Harrison's Principles of Internal Medicine.* 19th ed. New York, NY: McGraw-Hill; 2015.
59. Cunningham F, Leveno KJ, Bloom SL, et al, Hypertensive disorders. In: Cunningham F, Leveno KJ, Bloom SL, et al, eds. *Williams Obstetrics.* 24th ed. New York, NY: McGraw-Hill; 2013.
60. Tucker R, Platt M. Obstetric and gynecological emergencies and rape. In: Stone C, Humphries RL, eds. *CURRENT Diagnosis & Treatment Emergency Medicine.* 7th ed. New York, NY: McGraw-Hill; 2011.
61. Burns B. Resuscitation in pregnancy. In: Tintinalli JE, Stapczynski J, Ma O, et al, eds. *Tintinalli's Emergency Medicine: A Comprehensive Study Guide.* 8th ed. New York, NY: McGraw-Hill; 2016.
62. Criddle L. Obstetric trauma. In: Hammond BB, Zimmermann PG, eds. *Sheehy's Manual of Emergency Care.* 7th ed. Des Plaines, IL: Elsevier; 2013:463–468.
63. DeIorio NM. Trauma in pregnancy. In: Tintinalli JE, Stapczynski J, Ma O, et al, eds. *Tintinalli's Emergency Medicine: A Comprehensive Study Guide.* 8th ed. New York, NY: McGraw-Hill; 2016.
64. Cunningham F, Leveno KJ, Bloom SL, et al. Critical care and trauma. In: Cunningham F, Leveno KJ, Bloom SL, et al, eds. *Williams Obstetrics.* 24th ed. New York, NY: McGraw-Hill; 2013.
65. Repasky T. Obstetric trauma. In: Hoyt KS, Selfridge-Thomas J, eds. *Emergency Nursing Core Curriculum.* 6th ed. St. Louis, Mo: Saunders Elsevier, 2007:879–890.
66. Frasure S. Emergency delivery. In: Tintinalli JE, Stapczynski J, Ma O, et al, eds. *Tintinalli's Emergency Medicine: A Comprehensive Study Guide.* 8th ed. New York, NY: McGraw-Hill; 2016.
67. Collin MF. Resuscitation of neonates. In: Tintinalli JE, Stapczynski J, Ma O, et al, eds. *Tintinalli's Emergency Medicine: A Comprehensive Study Guide.* 8th ed. New York, NY: McGraw-Hill; 2016.
68. Hatfield N. *Introductory Maternity and Pediatric Nursing.* Baltimore, MD: Wolters Kluwer; 2014:428.
69. Hutton EK, Hassen ES. Late vs early clamping of the umbilical cord in fullterm neonates: systematic review and meta-analysis of controlled trials. *JAMA.* 2007;297:1241–52.
70. Cunningham F, Leveno KJ, Bloom SL, et al. Puerperal complications. In: Cunningham F, Leveno KJ, Bloom SL, et al, eds. *Williams Obstetrics.* 24th ed. New York, NY: McGraw-Hill; 2013. http://accessmedicine.mhmedical.com/content.aspx?bookid=1057&Sectionid=59789180. Accessed March 31, 2016.
71. Poggi SH. Postpartum hemorrhage and the abnormal puerperium. In: DeCherney AH, Nathan L, Laufer N, et al, eds. *CURRENT Diagnosis & Treatment: Obstetrics & Gynecology.* 11th ed. New York, NY: McGraw-Hill; 2013. http://accessmedicine.mhmedical.com/content.aspx?bookid=498&Sectionid=41008611. Accessed April 11, 2016.
72. Burke, C. Perinatal sepsis. *J. Perinat Neonat Nurs.* 2008:23(1):42–51.

Practice Questions

Question	Rationale
1. A male patient presents to the emergency department with genitourinary complaints. What specific complaint leads the ED nurse to suspect a possible STD? a. Burning pain with blood in his urine b. Right flank pain that radiates to his groin c. Left testicular pain that he awoke with d. Penile mucopurulent discharge	*Answer: d* Mucopurulent discharge and painful urination are two common symptoms that often cause male patients to seek treatment for a STD. Burning pain and hematuria can be signs of renal colic or a UTI. Flank pain radiating to the groin is a sign of possible renal colic. Unilateral testicular pain, often following physical activity or sleeping, can indicate testicular torsion.
2. A 41-year-old male patient arrives to the emergency department with his wife. As he is assisted into a wheelchair, the nurse notices he is diaphoretic and pale. He is complaining of severe pain in his right lower back radiating to his groin. He writhes in pain, and states he has had blood in his urine for the past two days. A top priority is a. A stat CBC and type and crossmatch b. IV analgesia c. IV bolus of crystalloid fluids d. Abdominal CT scan	*Answer: b* This patient is exhibiting signs of a renal calculus. Pain management is a top priority. IV analgesia provides faster relief and often narcotic analgesics are needed for effective pain management. Crystalloid fluids will assist with rehydrating the patient and diagnostic testing may include an abdominal CT as this often provides more detailed information about the kidney stone's size and location. A CBC may be indicated if an infection or blood loss was suspected. Typically hematuria with renal calculi is not severe enough to warrant requiring blood products.
3. The waiting room is full with no available rooms or treatment spaces. An 18-year-old arrives with fever, weakness, tachypnea, and pale mucous membranes. She tells the triage nurse she has had a fever and chills following an abortion at a nearby clinic last week. The triage nurse should a. Send her to the urgent care clinic adjacent to the emergency department b. Find available treatment space so she can be seen and treated c. Give her a blanket and have her wait until a room becomes available d. Assess her vital signs to determine if she needs to come back right away	*Answer: b* This patient has signs suggesting early septic shock. Finding a treatment space for her to be assessed and treated are priorities. Her ED course of care will require many resources, including IV access, lab studies, ultrasound, antibiotics, and a potential surgical admission. Even though the urgent care clinic may be part of the emergency department, this patient requires too many resources to be managed in an urgent care setting. Although her vital signs may be within normal limits, given her history and current symptoms, she is at risk for deteriorating and should not wait.

Question	Rationale

4. Which of the following symptoms suggest a patient may have a ruptured ovarian cyst?
  a. Yellow, mucopurulent discharge
  b. Vaginal bleeding
  c. Sharp abdominal pain
  d. Intermittent abdominal cramping
	Answer: c
	The rupture of an ovarian cyst results in constant, severe pain and internal bleeding, rather than intermittent cramping or vaginal bleeding. Yellow, mucopurulent discharge is characteristic of gonorrhea.

5. A 52-year-old male presents to the emergency department with a complaint of a prolonged, painful erection (priapism) after taking sildenafil citrate (Viagra™). The emergency nurse should first assess
  a. If he has any sexual feelings associated with the erection
  b. How long he has had the erection
  c. If he has a history of sexually transmitted disease
  d. When his last episode of sexual activity occurred
	Answer: b
	Priapism is a prolonged, painful erection that persists beyond or is unrelated to sexual stimulation. Medications used in the treatment of impotence, such as sildenafil citrate (Viagra™), are associated with priapism. Damage to the penis is directly related to the length of time the penis was ischemic and can lead to impotence. History of sexually transmitted diseases are unrelated to priapism. Assessing when the last episode of sexual activity is only applicable if it assists in determining the length of time the patient has had the erection.

6. A 20-year-old female college student walks into the emergency department for treatment following an MVC the day before. The nurse notes bruising over the right flank area and costovertebral angle (CVA) pain. These findings are most indicative of what type of injury?
  a. Kidney injury
  b. Ruptured bladder
  c. Detached urethra
  d. Ureter stricture
	Answer: a
	Renal trauma should be suspected in patients with a history of a sudden deceleration or lateral force injuries. Costovertebral angle (CVA) pain and/or bruising over the flank area (Grey-Turner sign) is most likely seen with an injury to the kidney. A ruptured bladder or a detached urethra would likely result in symptoms such as inability to void, suprapubic area pain, and blood at the meatus. A ureter stricture does not occur as a result of such a traumatic injury.

7. A 30-year-old woman presents to the emergency department complaining of pain during intercourse, pelvic pressure, and a foul-smelling vaginal discharge. Her last menstrual period was 1 week ago. The most likely cause of her symptoms would be
  a. Toxic-shock syndrome
  b. Herpes
  c. Retained tampon
  d. Gynecological trauma
	Answer: c
	Young women may seek emergency medical care due to foreign body issues such as inability to remove tampons or broken portions of condoms. Foul-smelling vaginal discharge and pelvic pressure are due to the retained tampon. Small, painful ulcers in the perineal area are characteristic of a herpes infection. Toxic-shock syndrome is characterized by a high fever, rash, hypotension, and multisystem organ failure. Abrasions, lacerations, or bruising of the female genital/perineal area would be noted with gynecological trauma.

Question	Rationale
8. The emergency nurse has just delivered an infant in a car in the emergency department parking lot. After drying and stimulating, additional intervention is necessary if the infant has 　a. Dusky hands and feet 　b. A heart rate of 75 beats/minute 　c. A respiratory rate of 48 breaths/minute 　d. A surface temperature of 98.6°F (37°C)	*Answer: b* If the infant is crying, pink, has spontaneous respirations, and has a heart rate (HR) faster than 100 beats/min, further medical intervention is likely not required. A heart rate of 75 beats/minute requires intervention. Successful resuscitation with bag-mask ventilation is indicated by an increase in HR to >100 beats/min and improved color and muscle tone. Dusky hands and feet (acrocyanosis) is an expected finding in a newborn and generally resolves spontaneously. A respiratory rate of 48 breaths per minute does not require any intervention. A temperature of 98.6°F (37°C) and warming of the infant should not take precedence over the slow heart rate.
9. The emergency nurse is reviewing discharge instructions with a patient diagnosed with a sexually transmitted infection (STI/STD). Which of the following is essential information to be reviewed with this patient? 　a. Abstain from sexual activity until treatment is complete 　b. Abstain from swimming in pools or using hot tubs 　c. Do not place tampons into the vagina for 7 to 10 days 　d. Expect vaginal bleeding for the next few days	*Answer: a* Patient education regarding an STD must include abstaining from sexual activity until treatment is completed. Abstaining from submersion in water or the use of tampons are not contraindicated in women with an STD. Vaginal bleeding is not associated with sexually transmitted infections.
10. The emergency nurse is caring for a 19-year-old female victim of rape. Before beginning the evidence collection process, the nurse should do which of the following 　a. Screen her for recreational drug use 　b. Obtain a clean catch urine specimen 　c. Treat her physical injuries 　d. Call the police	*Answer: c* The nurse should respond to acute injury, trauma care, and safety needs of patients before collecting evidence. The patient may decline police involvement at the time of evidence collection in the emergency department. Obtaining a history of recreational drug use may be obtained after any physical injuries are addressed. A urine specimen should not be obtained before beginning the forensic evidence collection unless necessary for treating acute medical needs. A clean catch urine specimen would not be obtained as the cleaning process would disrupt potential evidence.
11. The ED nurse is collecting and packaging evidence collected from a victim of rape. It is essential that the nurse package the evidence separately in 　a. Plastic only 　b. Paper only 　c. Office supply folders 　d. ED nurses do not collect this type of evidence	*Answer: b* All specimens collected should be packaged separately in paper bags. The use of plastic bags will hold moisture and ruin the evidence. A folder would not securely contain the evidence. ED nurses are often involved in the collecting and packaging of forensic evidence of various types.

Question	Rationale
12. The emergency nurse is caring for a female trauma patient who was physically assaulted by her boyfriend. When cutting off the patient's clothing in order to care for her physical injuries, the nurse should a. Avoid cutting through any existing tears or stains in the clothing b. Obtain a physician order before packaging the clothing for evidence c. Provide radiant warming with heat lamps d. Pause the video recording of the trauma resuscitation	*Answer: a* If it is necessary to cut clothing off of the patient, avoid cutting through any existing fabric tears or stains since these may be valuable evidence and should remain intact as found. A physician order is not required for packaging clothing for evidence. The use of heat lamps is not applicable in this situation, and if a trauma resuscitation is video recorded by a facility, the recording is forensic evidence and should never be interrupted for any reason.
13. The parents of a 9-year-old girl present to triage and report the child is complaining of pain in her 'private area', vaginal bleeding, and having difficulty walking after being at a water park earlier that day. The child states the pain started after she rode a water slide. The emergency nurse should suspect a. Sexual assault b. The onset of puberty c. Child abuse d. An insufflation injury	*Answer: d* Vaginal insufflation injuries (rapid distension of the vagina resulting in a tearing of the vaginal walls with resultant bleeding) can result from the force of water enerting the vagina, such as when riding down a water slide. There is no suspicion of any sexual assault or child abuse provided by the child or parents that would explain the symptoms. The child's symptoms are consistent with the insufflation injury. The onset of puberty does not cause pain in the perineal area.
14. The emergency nurse is caring for a patient who delivered a healthy, full-term infant 45 minutes ago while enroute via ambulance. She has not yet delivered the placenta and is having brisk vaginal bleeding not decreasing despite uterine massage and oxytocin IV. What is the next appropriate intervention the emergency nurse should consider? a. Titrate oxytocin per protocol b. Assess for feelings safety at home c. Prepare for surgical intervention d. Obtain hourly orthostatic vital signs	*Answer: c* If the placenta has not delivered spontaneously within 30 minutes, the nurse should consider placenta accreta. This abnormal adherence of the placenta to the uterine wall is not manageable in an emergency department, and surgical intervention is required to remove the placenta from the uterus. The nurse should continuously monitor the hemodynamic status of the mother, closely assess for postpartum hemorrage and anticipate transport to the operating room. An increased use of oxytocin IV, which is administered to vasoconstrict bloodvessels in the uterus and minimize bleeding, would be contraindicated in this situation. It is the retained placenta that is likely causing the brisk vaginal bleeding in this situation. Orthostatic vital signs are not indicated for this patient and assessment for safety at home is not appropriate at this time.

Question	Rationale
15. The emergency nurse is having difficulty inserting a urinary drainage catheter into a patient with no contraindications following a traumatic pelvic injury. This most likely indicates a. The catheter is an inappropriate size b. The urethra has been injured c. The bladder has been injured d. The patient is in pain	*Answer: b* Urethral injuries occur in 5% to 10% of pelvic fractures. When resistance to insertion of a urinary drainage catheter occurs with a patient with a traumatic pelvic injury, injury to the urethra should be suspected. Further insertion attempts should cease so as not to cause further damage. While a large urinary catheter and pain could hinder insertion, the mechanism of injury should cause suspicion that the insertion problem is an injured urethra. An injury to the bladder, situated well above the urethra, would not result in difficulty inserting a urinary drainage catheter.
16. A patient is rushed to the ED via EMS after experiencing blunt force trauma to her abdomen. The EMT states she is 27 1/7 weeks gestation. Upon arrival, she is guarding her abdomen due to pain and fetal heart rate is 140 bpm. No vaginal fluid discharge or bleeding is present, but her abdomen is hard and board-like. What pregnancy-related bleeding problem does this nurse suspect? a. Cystitis b. Placenta previa c. Abruptio placentae d. Dysfunctional vaginal bleeding of pregnancy	*Answer: c* Pain in the abdomen could be cystitis but cystitis is not a bleeding problem related to pregnancy. Placenta previa is a bleeding problem of pregnancy with bright bleeding but not painful. Painful board-like abdomen should be assessed for abruptio placentae; bleeding may not be present if the rupture is concealed or occult with the edges of the placenta intact with the uterine wall; the placenta may be partially detached with hemorrhaging next to the uterine wall causing the uterus to be irritated and start contracting. Sudden blunt force trauma to the abdomen can cause the placenta to become detached from the uterine wall.
17. A 72-year-old male arrives to the ED via EMS following flu-like symptoms with fever for the past five days. He is talking but confused. His vital signs are T-102°F (38.9°C); P-112, R-20; BP-92/58; SpO_2-91% on room air. His urine is foul smelling. The emergency nurse anticipates the immediate interventions a. Assist with securing an airway with endotracheal intubation b. Obtain a clean catch urine specimen and other ordered labs c. Insert an indwelling Foley catheter and measure an accurate output d. Obtain IV access, labs and administer prescribed antibiotics following collection of blood cultures	*Answer: d* This patient's flu-like symptoms, fever and foul smelling urine suggest a urinary tract infection and possibly pyelonephritis. Pyelonephritis is a serious infection of the urinary tract that involves the kidney and renal structures. IV fluids and antibiotics are indicted. This patient is also exhibiting signs of possible sepsis with a fever, tachycardia and hypotension, warranting a set blood cultures before antibiotic administration. A clean catch urine specimen and other labs such as a CBC with differential and serum chemistries are also indicated; however, antibiotic administration is equally a high priority. Supplemental oxygen for his lower pulse oximetry may be needed; however, he is not exhibiting respiratory failure.

Question	Rationale
18. A patient at 26 weeks gestation is brought to the emergency department. She was watching television with her husband and son when she felt something warm and wet. Concerned that she may have ruptured her membranes, she ran to the bathroom and discovered she was bleeding. She saturated a mini pad but the bleeding stopped after the initial gush. She has had no bleeding since but she came in to the ED because she is scared the baby may have been bleeding. The ED nurse suspect a. Ruptured ovarian cyst b. Vasa previa c. Placenta abruptio d. Placenta Previa	*Answer: d* Painless bright bleeding during pregnancy is usually caused by the placenta becoming separated either completely or sometimes partially. It is due to the placenta implantation being close or over the cervical os. Rupture ovarian cyst will not cause painless bleeding; placenta abruptio is related to painful bleeding or board-like abdomen; vasa previa is much more serious and if ruptured the bleeding would not stop.
19. A woman who is pregnant comes in the emergency department with irregular contractions that began 2 hours ago and are occurring more frequently. She is 31 2/7 weeks gestation. Baby is active and fetal heart tones are ranging 150 to 155 bpm. Her contractions are palpable and occurring every 10 minutes. What symptom will suggest preterm labor? a. Patient feels like she needs to void b. There is evidence of cervical change and dilation c. Regular contractions at 5 minutes apart d. Patient feels better sitting up	*Answer: b* Pre-term labor is defined as: contractions that become regular (begin and end in a rhythmic regular pattern of timed intervals) and cause cervical changes which is considered preterm labor (up to 2 cm change). Regular contractions could be associated to Braxton-Hicks contractions that can present in a regular pattern but do not change cervical dilation. In some cases pre-term labor can be associated to urinary tract infections (UTI), but the need to void is not specific to a UTI; bedrest and positioning do not affect pre-term labor.
20. While shopping, Jane notices a dull headache beginning. Jane is 35 weeks pregnancy and has noticed additional swelling and heartburn over the past two weeks. Upon arrival to the emergency department, Jane begins to have a seizure. The nurse knows to expect what treatment to be ordered a. Oxytocin b. D_{50} c. Magnesium sulfate d. Phenytoin	*Answer: c* In a pregnant patient experiencing seizures, preeclampsia should be suspected. Magnesium sulfate reduces seizure activity through an unknown mechanism, but has been shown to be more effective than other seizure medications, such as phenytoin. Oxytocin and D_{50} are not indicated at this time.
21. The emergency nurse is discharging an otherwise healthy 75-year-old male patient diagnosed with cystitis. He is prescribed Bactrim™ and Pyridium™. All of the following statements demonstrate his understanding of his discharge instructions *except* a. "I need to drink at least 8 glass of water a day" b. "I need to take all of my Bactrim as it is prescribed" c. "If my urine turns a rusty orange color I should come back here" d. "I need to follow up with my doctor next week"	*Answer: c* Pyridium™ may be prescribed for dysuria and urinary frequency and can turn the urine orange or a reddish orange color. Patients should be informed of this and not to be alarmed if they observe this. Increasing oral fluid intake and completing the prescribed antibiotic are essential teaching points for the patient to understand. Follow-up with their primary care physician may be prescribed if the infection's etiology may need further study.

Question	Rationale
22. A young professional woman has delayed pregnancy until timing is more appropriate with her lifestyle. She had a positive pregnancy test at 9 weeks gestation and has seen the nurse practitioner in her obstetrician's office for her first prenatal visit at 11 weeks gestation. She is currently 12 4/7 weeks gestation and is having spotting of bright red bleeding. Terrified that something is going wrong with the pregnancy, she comes to your ED. She has no pain with the bleeding but did have some menstrual like cramping earlier that has gone away. FHT are 135 bpm. After checking her cervix, it is closed. There is a small amount of darker blood in her vagina but no active bleeding is seen. Patient is suspected of having a. Threatened abortion b. Inevitable abortion c. Missed abortion d. Complete abortion	*Answer: a* Threatened abortion: cervix remains closed; inevitable abortion: cervix dilates to 3 cm; missed abortion: no bleeding or cramping are present; complete abortion: some bleeding, mild contractions and product of conception is passed and cervical os is closed. You may confuse the somewhat similar symptoms of threatened abortion and complete abortion but this patient still has FHTs.
23. A 28-year-old male patient is being discharged from the emergency department following a diagnosis of epididymitis. The ED nurse knows the patient understands his discharge instructions when he makes the following statement a. I may not ever be able to have kids b. I need to wear support, like a jock strap, when I am up walking c. I can keep running in preparation for the marathon I'm in next month d. My antibiotic is only needed if the pain doesn't get better	*Answer: b* Epididymitis can be from a sexually transmitted infection. Other causes can be from urological procedures such as a cystoscopy. Pain is a hallmark of the illness, and elevating and supporting the penis especially during physical activity decreases the pain. Often, the patient may be advised not to resume vigorous physical activity until they have followed up with their primary care physician or urologist. Infertility typically is not related to epididymitis. Antibiotics may be prescribed if a STD is suspected, and the patient should complete the entire course of antibiotics.

Psychosocial Emergencies

8

Nathan Whitman, DNP, RN, PMHNP-BC, PMHCNS-BC

Psychosocial emergencies are multi-faceted conditions of acute or acute-on-chronic emergencies with or without physical findings. In all cases, an environment should be provided where the patient feels safe and secure before assessment occurs and caregivers should strive to build a trusting relationship with patients and their social support system, as appropriate. As with any other emergency, primary survey assessment and related intervention take priority over specialized psychosocial emergency care.

Abuse and Neglect

The emergency department is often the contact point where patients reporting or suspected of abuse or neglect enter the health care system. The ability to identify and address abuse and neglect in the emergency department may prevent future incidents.[1] Abuse and neglect can occur across the lifespan. Abuse is characterized by treatment of an individual with violence or cruelty leading to physical and/or psychological harm. Physical abuse may include punching, kicking, shaking, hitting with objects, choking, and other means to physically harm someone in a non-accidental manner.

Neglect is characterized by the failure to provide proper attention or care for someone. In the health care setting, medical neglect (not providing appropriate medical attention) and physical neglect (not meeting basic physical needs) are the most common types of neglect encountered.

Populations at higher risk for abuse and neglect include the elderly, children below age 4, and children with special needs who increase the burden of caregivers.[2,3] Assessment should include an understanding and evaluation of any cultural and financial factors which may contribute to the perception of abuse or neglect. When encountering possible neglect or abuse, the nurse should use real time case discussion with other staff to aid in detection and problem solving. Using child abuse screening mechanisms for high risk injuries in children can also aid in detection.[4] There are many barriers to detecting abuse or neglect, including the nurse's personal bias, inability to recognize abuse or neglect, a perceived burden of reporting, and belief in the caregivers' stories.[4]

Assessment/Analysis
- Abuse indicators raising the suspicion of abuse
  - Refusal to allow the patient to be interviewed alone
  - Injuries not matching described mechanism of injury
  - A vague description of events or mechanism of injury
  - Description of events changes (with children, repeated questions may lead to answers the child believes the nurse wants to hear)
  - Injuries matching the shape of an object (hand, belt, or cord)
  - Bruising in non-cruising (walking) children
  - Old bruising or injuries are present
  - Immersion burns in children
- Neglect indicators raising the suspicion of neglect
  - Inadequate clothing or hygiene
  - Failure to thrive
  - Inadequate nutrition
  - Lack of medical care for an individual
  - Not providing reasonable safety for an individual (such as access to weapons or an absent caregiver)

Intervention
- Provide immediate safety
- Treat medical issues
- Case discussion with other staff
- Provide a safe disposition
- Mandatory reporting
  - Reporting varies state to state; however, in all states a nurse must report child abuse[5]
- Involvement of social worker if available or provide resources available in the community
- Child protective services may need to be involved

Evaluation
- Safety of the patient is the primary concern
- Reporting is completed if required
- Documentation is clear in the medical record
- Safe disposition plan is in place

Aggressive Violent Behavior

Violence in the health care setting is common. The emergency department is one of the highest risk areas for the potential for violence.[6] Certain symptoms and diagnoses may place the patient at increased risk for violence in the ED setting. Individuals at greater risk of violence may be intoxicated, withdrawing from substances, confused, experiencing pain, frustrated, experiencing trauma, or living with mental illness. The best violence prevention programs are comprehensive in nature and include environmental factors, personal training for nurses, and identifying early warning signs of violence.[7] Prevention of violent behaviors should occur before the patient arrives. Nurses should be aware of cues indicating impending violence and act to mitigate escalation.

Assessment/Analysis
- Patient characteristics increasing potential for violence[8]
  - Male gender
  - History of violence: recent violence places the patient at high risk
  - Intoxication or withdrawal from substances
  - Altered mental status
  - Psychosis: active hallucinations or delusions
  - Agitated behaviors (verbal and non-verbal)
  - Body language: pacing, wringing hands, and clenching fists
  - Aggressive behaviors: destruction of property
  - Threatening behaviors: physical or verbal

Intervention
- Staff safety
  - Always maintain an easy exit[9]
  - Ensure safety for the staff, visitors, and other patients
  - Ensure safety for the patient including use of restraints if indicated to prevent violence
  - Training including techniques to de-escalate and safely manage aggressive patients
  - Beware of weapons or items that could be utilized as weapons; ideally a patient should be searched
  - Treat the underlying cause of the aggression
  - Medications: antipsychotics (such as haloperidol) and benzodiazepines (lorazepam) are the mainstay of treatment to address aggressive or violent behaviors,[8] but the most likely underlying cause of agitation must be considered[10,11]
- Environmental factors: structural[11]
  - Increased presence of security or police
  - Metal detectors
  - Limiting access for non-patients
  - Secure patient rooms (non-moveable furniture)
  - Securing potential items that could be used as weapons
  - Barriers for cars to prevent driving into the emergency department/hospital building

Evaluation
- Safety is maintained
- Decrease or cessation of aggressive behaviors
- Treatment and resolution of the cause of behaviors
- Decreased agitation/anxiety with pharmacological treatments

Anxiety/Panic

Anxiety is a normal human emotion experienced in response to a real or perceived threat. Anxiety is often associated with an autonomic response, emotional, cognitive, or physical symptoms. The level of anxiety can vary for individuals from mild to severe including panic attacks. Anxiety disorders are characterized by anxiety interfering with the individual's life in a persistent manner and includes the anticipatory fear of a future threat. Panic disorders are common in the ED setting due to the somatic and autonomic responses accompanying the disorder. A key feature of panic disorders is the fear of reoccurrence.[12]

Panic

Panic attacks are intense, short-lived episodes of anxiety or fear commonly associated with symptoms including tachycardia, dyspnea, chest pain, paresthesia, dizziness, agitation, and impending doom. Panic attacks are more common in women than men.[12]

> Differential diagnoses: an individual may exhibit symptoms of anxiety/panic with the use of amphetamines, caffeine, energy drinks, marijuana, cold medications, or withdrawal from alcohol, benzodiazepines, or hypnotics. Medical conditions should be considered and addressed when assessing a patient with anxiety/panic.

Assessment/Analysis
- Explore the events preceding the patient's presentation to the emergency department; traumatic events can trigger acute anxiety[13]
- History of panic attacks or anxiety, including prior episodes, treatments, and effective interventions
- Gather additional assessment information from friends, family or someone who knows the patient
- Suicide screening (see Suicide)
- Panic attacks begin abruptly and can last 10 to 60 minutes
- Signs/Symptoms
  - Trembling
  - Dizziness, light headedness
  - Nausea
  - Shortness of breath
  - Chest pain
  - Tachycardia, possible hypertension
  - Intense anxiety and fear
  - Fear of dying
  - Subjective loss of control
  - Fear of recurrent attacks
  - Often associated with agoraphobia: fear of crowded or enclosed places

Interventions

- Ensure safety
- Reassure the patient that panic attacks can be treated[14]
- Address and treat somatic and physical symptomology such as shortness of breath or tachycardia
    - Focused or guided breathing may reduce anxiety
- Rule out and treat differential diagnoses causing symptoms
- Antianxiety agents may be used for panic attacks or acute anxiety; benzodiazepines are the recommended treatment[15]
- Discuss recognition of signs/symptoms of anxiety or panic attacks and educate about coping mechanism to prevent future attacks
- Assist patient in problem solving activities and option identification
- Long term: antidepressants are used to treat anxiety and panic attacks with benzodiazepines used sparingly as needed[15]

Evaluation

- Subjective decrease in anxiety or panic
- Safety maintained
- Decrease in physical symptoms such as increased heart rate, blood pressure, and respirations
- Verbalization of strategies to recognize and cope with future anxiety or panic attacks

Bipolar Disorder

Bipolar disorder is a chronic, treatable mental illness with onset of symptoms typically in the early 20s but may present into the 40s or 50s. It is characterized by episodic shifts of mood from depression, mania, hypomania, or mixed states. The key characteristic feature of bipolar is mania or hypomania.[12] Mania is characterized by an abnormally elevated mood, expansive, or irritable. Hypomania is a lesser form of mania. Mixed states are characterized by rapid alternating moods of depression and mania.[12]

The treatment for bipolar disorders is mood stabilizers, such as lithium or valproic acid. Undiagnosed bipolar disorder may be unmasked by antidepressant medication treatment for depression resulting in the first episodes of hypomania or mania.[15]

Mania

Patients presenting to the emergency department during a manic episode can be challenging to manage. The primary goal is to ensure safety for the patient and the staff. Mania must be evaluated in the context of possible other illnesses or injuries, including substance-induced mania (amphetamines or cocaine), hyperthyroidism, personality disorders, and medication-induced mania.[13] Manic episodes can occur quickly or have a slower onset. Characteristics to assess when evaluating a patient with possible bipolar disorder are described as follows.

Assessment/Analysis[12,13]

- History of bipolar, manic, or hypomanic episodes
- Mood disturbances from elevated mood to irritability
- Agitation, increased psychomotor activity, or hyper-verbal
- Increased goal directed activities, such as projects at work or home
- Early mania or hypomania can lead to increased productivity, which may be subjectively enjoyed by the individual
- Thought process: flight of ideas, disorganized thinking, grandiose thinking, or distractibility
- Loud, disruptive, flamboyant, and exaggerated behaviors
- Sleep disturbance: long periods of not needing sleep (patient may report feeling rested after a few hours of sleep)
- Excessive spending, sexual activities, and impulsive life decisions. These occur due to the mania and may be regretted after the episode has passed
- Interference with social, academic, and/or vocational activities
- Patients may lack insight into their illness/state and are often brought to the ED by someone else
- Seek history from other individuals who know the patient such as family or friends
- Suicide screening (see Suicide)
- History of suicidal ideation or attempts: patients in a mixed or depressive state of bipolar are at increased risk for suicide[16]
- Medications: mood stabilizers such as lithium or valproic acid
- Labs: serum levels for both lithium and/or valproic acid if applicable

Interventions

- Ensure immediate safety of the patient, staff, and other patients
- Treat agitation: may present as irritability or hyperactivity
- Psychopharmacological treatments may include medication to manage acute agitation such as antipsychotics (olanzapine, quetiapine, or aripiprazole)[15]
- Benzodiazepines (lorazepam) may decrease the anxiety and agitation[13]
- Psychiatric consultation may be indicated
- Psychiatric hospitalization may be needed if the patient presents as a risk to self or others
- Plan of care should address risky behaviors which place the patient at risk of serious occupational or financial disruption
- Patients with bipolar disorder are often followed by a psychiatrist due to the complex nature of this disorder
- Long-term treatment for bipolar disorder
    - Psychopharmacological treatments include mood stabilizers, such as lithium or valproic acid. Atypical antipsychotics such as quetiapine, aripiprazole, and

olanzapine are also approved for maintenance of bipolar disorders[15]

- Antidepressants are not used alone in bipolar disorder. The patient should have a mood stabilizer prescribed due to the risk of causing manic episodes when antidepressants are used alone[15]

Evaluation
- Patient and staff safety is maintained
- Decreased agitation, irritability, or anxiety
- Decreased agitation/anxiety with pharmacological treatments
- Plan for safe disposition

Depression (in Bipolar Disorder)

Depressive episodes are characterized by the same diagnostic criteria as depression, without manic or hypomanic symptoms. Depression is the more common presentation of bipolar. When encountering depressive symptoms assessing for a history of manic or hypomanic symptoms can help identify bipolar disorder.[17]

Depression

Depression is characterized by changes in mood, affect, cognition, and functional impairment. Depression does not include normal sadness related to grief or bereavement. Patients with depression have a higher risk for suicide, and this is often the primary concern for patients or family members. Patients may have multiple ED visits and present with somatic complaints, such as anxiety, chronic pain, weakness, or fatigue.[17] Depression is a chronic, treatable mental illness and recurrent episodes are common.

Some medications, substance abuse, and/or medical conditions may cause the patient to present with depression-like symptoms. These different causes need to be considered and ruled out before a diagnosis of depression is made. Examples of depression due to a medical condition may include stroke, recent MI, Parkinson's disease, Huntington's disease, hypothyroidism, Cushing's disease, or a traumatic brain injury.[12] Depressive symptoms may also occur in the context of intoxication such as with alcohol. Additionally, some medications such as steroids, some antihypertensives, CNS drugs, chemotherapeutic agents, or antibiotics can all lead to depressive-like symptomology.[12]

Assessment/Analysis[12]
- History of depression: prior episodes, medications, and suicidal ideation or past attempts
- Depressed mood occurring most of the day, almost every day, for at least two weeks
- Mood can be a subjective sense of feeling sad, depressed, and hopeless or observed by others
- Decreased interest or pleasure in activities
- Statements of hopelessness
- Changes in appetite; significant weight gain or loss
- Sleep disturbances: insomnia or hypersomnia
- Guilt, feelings of worthlessness, or burdensomeness
- Low energy, low volition
- Cognitive changes: indecisive, poor decisional making capacity
- Suicide screening (see Suicide)
- History: depression is a recurrent mental illness
- Self-harm or suicide attempts increase risk for future attempts[12]

Interventions
- Provide safety as needed
- Provide reassurance and build therapeutic alliance
- Labs for screening: toxicology screen and thyroid panel
- Consider referral to psychiatric services
- Psychiatric hospitalization may be indicated if the patient presents as a danger to themselves
- Psychopharmacology
  - Antidepressants are the mainstay of treatment for depression
    - Due to lengthy onset of action, discharge teaching includes safety plans and coping strategies
  - Several second generation antipsychotics are commonly used as adjunct treatment for depression including aripiprazole and quetiapine[15]

Evaluation
- Patient safety is maintained
- Family is reassured and educated
- Plan for safe disposition is established

Homicidal Ideation

Homicidal ideation may be encountered in the emergency department. Homicidal ideation includes the patient expressing the thought or intention to kill or seriously harm an individual or group of people. All homicidal ideation should be taken seriously.

Assessment/Analysis[18]
- Homicidal threats should be taken seriously
- Assess for immediate dangers especially access to weapons
- Assess for indicators of intoxication including behaviors or blood alcohol level
- History of violent behaviors
- History of mental illness
- Symptoms or verbalizations of paranoia or persecution
- Hallucinations: assess for command hallucinations (telling the individual to harm others)
- Determine plausibility of threat
- Suicide screening (see Suicide)

Interventions[9]
- Homicidal threats should be reported and taken seriously
- Ensure immediate safety of patients and staff

- Remove any potential weapons, may include metal detection of the patient
- Secure area for interview with easy exits
- Nurses should not be alone in the room with patient and always maintain an easy exit
- Psychiatric consultation
- Develop plan to ensure safety including security, police, and mental health evaluation for dangerous behavior, as indicated
- HIPAA privacy act allows personal health information disclosure when there is a good faith belief the disclosure is necessary to prevent or reduce a serious imminent threat to the patient or any known individual[19]
- Report to authorities to ensure safety of any third parties threatened by the patient[9]

Evaluation
- Provide safety for individual and community
- Reporting may be indicated[9]
- Decrease or cessation of homicidal ideation
- Plan to ensure safety is in place

Psychosis

Psychosis is characterized by a loss of contact with reality as evidenced by delusions (fixed false beliefs), visual, auditory, or tactile hallucinations, and disorganized speech. Psychosis is seen in conjunction with medical illness, mental illness, and when induced by substances including medications, intoxicating chemicals, or "street drugs." Psychosis due to mental illness may occur with a wide range of mental disorders including personality disorders, bipolar disorders, depression, and schizophrenia. Psychosis is associated with increased risk for violence; risk factors include paranoia, hostile behaviors, poor impulse control, substance misuse, and non-adherence with medications.[20]

Assessment/Analysis
- Medical, substance use, or medication-induced psychosis should be ruled out before primary psychiatric diagnosis is considered
- Current symptoms including type of delusion or hallucination, onset, duration, and severity
- History of psychosis can help determine the cause
- Psychiatric onset: auditory hallucinations are the most common presentation in mental illness, characteristics include
  - Gradual onset starting in late teens to 30s[12]
  - Family history of mental illness is often present
- Medical or drug induced psychosis. Psychosis in the context of substance use should be ruled out. Characteristics include
  - Rapid onset
  - Mental illness history may not be present
  - Non-auditory hallucinations
- Safety: loss of reality can lead to risk for self-injury or dangerous behaviors, delusions, homicidal ideations, and paranoid behaviors
- Suicide screening (see Suicide)
- Alcohol withdrawal hallucinations or delirium tremens often present with visual and tactile hallucinations[9]
- Loss of reality can lead to making dangerous judgments or self-care inability
- Delusional content may be associated with increased safety risk. Common delusions include paranoia, grandiosity, persecutory, delusions of control by others[13]
- Psychosis with paranoia, command hallucinations, or hostility is associated with increased risk for violence[13]
- Hallucinations
  - Auditory: most common type in mental illness such as schizophrenia[12]
  - Visual: suspect medical illness, chemical exposure, or substance use
- Psychiatric consultation
- Serum toxicology screen may indicate substances underlying psychosis

Interventions
- Ensure a safe, low stimulation environment
- Limit external stimulation such as televisions which may be interpreted into the content of delusions or hallucinations
- Antipsychotics are the treatment of choice for acute psychosis[15]
- First generation or typical antipsychotics such as haloperidol carry an increased risk for extrapyramidal side effects, but are commonly used in acute emergencies[15]
- Second generation or atypical antipsychotics such as olanzapine, carry less extrapyramidal side effects than typical antipsychotics[15]
- Medication
  - Psychosis: antipsychotic
  - Substance use/misuse/abuse: benzodiazepines,[10] alcohol, etc.

Evaluation
- Patient and staff safety is maintained
- Family education and referral to supportive community resources
- Referral to psychiatric services if indicated
- Safety plan in place, including after discharge

Situational Crisis

Situational crisis may be caused by traumatic injuries, unexpected deaths, job loss, divorce, relationship issues, or hospitalization.

An unexpected crisis arising suddenly in response to an external event or circumstance results in a situational crisis. Crisis can be defined as a breakdown of an individual's problem-solving and ability to cope with a situation. Normal coping mechanisms used by the individual fail and lead to a state of crisis.[21] The nurse's role is to recognize a patient or family in crisis and support the individual or family's coping. Bereavement is an experience in which someone close to the patient dies. Grief is the normal human reaction to the bereavement. The emergency department is the setting where many unexpected deaths occur which can lead to the possibility of abnormal and prolonged grief responses in the bereaved. ED staff can influence the reactions of the bereaved through their interactions and responses to the bereaved.

Assessment/Analysis
- Determine the level of distress
- People with preexisting mental health disorders are at risk for increased reactions
- Safety should be established
- Suicide screening (see Suicide) may be indicated
- Grief and reactions to crisis vary by individual and culture

Interventions
- Use an empathetic supportive therapeutic approach; enlist the help of resources such as social work or chaplains if available
- Establish rapport
- Maintain control of the situation: provide safety and security for patients and staff
- Lower stimulation: provide a quiet, calm area
- Calm the individual or family
- Provide support
- Death: ideally family should be present before someone dies
- Inform family of the death, provide condolences, and offer to answer questions[22]
- Provide resources including support such as friends, family, spiritual care, or clergy
- Most people have normal bereavement reactions

Evaluation
- Ideal is a return to normal pre-crisis state
- Resources are provided for additional support

Suicidal Ideation

Assessment of suicide is complex and should consider both short-term and long-term safety for the patient. The emergency department is a common place suicidal individuals will present for care. It is estimated for every completed suicide, 25 people attempt suicide.[23] Due to the unpredictable nature of suicide, all reports of suicidal ideation or plans should be taken seriously. The primary role of the nurse is to ensure safety for the patient. Developing initial rapport with the patient is important to establish trust. Patients who present with a suicide attempt should be assessed for the lethality of their attempt and the likelihood of rescue from the attempt.[24] Asking about suicide does not increase suicide risk.[25]

Assessment/Analysis

> Before assessment, the nurse must ensure immediate safety: begin by placing the individual with suicidal ideation in a secure area free of items with potential to be used for self-harm or suicide. This includes items the individuals may have on their person possibly presenting a risk of self-harm or suicide.

- Risk factors for suicide[23,26]
  - Health factors
    - Mental illness: 90% of people in the United States who die by suicide have a diagnosable mental illness[27]
    - Depression or history of depression
    - Chronic health problems or chronic pain
    - Substance use disorder/intoxication
  - Behavioral factors
    - Talking about suicide
    - Researching how to die by suicide
    - Change in behaviors, such as isolating, withdrawing, increased sleep, or aggression
    - Giving away possessions
    - Impulsive and reckless behaviors: high risk behaviors
  - History
    - History of self-harm or suicide attempts
    - Family history of suicide
    - Recent loss, especially suicidal loss
  - Demographics
    - Middle aged people and older men (over 75) have the highest rates of suicide[23,28,29]
    - Men die by suicide 3.5 times more than women[23]
    - Women attempt suicide more than men
  - Environmental Factors
    - Access to firearms: 50% of suicides involve firearms[23]
    - Access to lethal means as described in the patient's plan
    - Lack of social support
    - Stressful life events: suicide, separation/divorce, breakups, and death of a loved one
    - Bullying
  - Mood
    - Hopelessness: reluctance to talk about the future; lack of belief things will get better
    - Depressive symptoms
  - Protective Factors
    - Religious or cultural beliefs prohibiting suicide
    - Strong social support
    - Future oriented behaviors or verbalizations

Interventions

- Ensure safety including safety from self-harm behaviors. This includes both environmental factors and possible medication or restraints to prevent self-harm[17]
- Remove items possibly posing a danger for injury, including hanging or strangulation
- Maintain dignity
- Develop rapport with the patient
- Use an evidence-based suicide screening tool such as: the Behavioral Health Screening–ED (BHS-ED); Mental Health Triage Scale (MHTS); Manchester Self-Harm Rule (MASH); P4; or Re-ACT Self-Harm Rule[30] which are all recommended by Emergency Nurses Association
- Additional evidence-based screening tools commonly used include Columbia Suicide Severity Rating Scale (C-SSRS) and Patient Health Questionnaire (PHQ-9)[29]
- Psychiatric evaluation if available
- Determination of involuntary legal hold; process differs by state
- Medical clearance if psychiatric treatment is indicated
- Removal of access to lethal means from home if indicated (firearms, stockpiled medications, etc.)
- "No harm contracts" or "contracting for safety" has not shown to reduce suicidal behaviors and has no legal status[17,31]
- Suicide information is provided such as crisis lines and resources[32]
- Development of a safety plan in collaboration with the patient

Evaluation

- Plan is in place to ensure safety, including after discharge
- Involuntary hospitalization may be considered if risk is high
- Referral as indicated

Post-Traumatic Stress Disorder (PTSD)

PTSD can occur after someone experiences a traumatic event such as sexual trauma, violent assault, terrorist attacks, military combat, and death of a significant other or other events. The event exposure can be direct experience or witnessing others experiencing the event. Symptoms of PTSD include recurrent distressing re-experiencing of the event; this can include intrusive thoughts, dreams, flashbacks, and physiological reactions when re-experiencing the event.[12]

Assessment/Analysis

Patients may experience the following symptoms including[12]

- Irritable behavior or anger
- Hypervigilance
- Self-destructive behaviors/suicide
- Difficulties with sleep
- Difficulties with concentration
- Increased risk for alcohol use disorders[33]
- Negative emotional states
- Detachment from others
- Decreased interest in other activities
- Comorbid mental health disorders[33]
- PTSD is associated with an increased risk for suicide[34]

Intervention

- Ensure immediate safety of the patient, staff and other patients
- PTSD may be associated with acute anxiety or panic attacks.[12] Antianxiety agents (benzodiazepines) may be used for panic attacks or acute anxiety[15]
- PTSD is typically treated in an outpatient setting with cognitive behavioral therapy or other therapies and may also include psychopharmacological treatments, such as antidepressants or benzodiazepines for acute symptoms[15]
- Psychiatric consultation may be indicated

Evaluation

- Patient and staff safety is maintained
- Decrease in subjective or physiological symptoms
- Decreased agitation, irritability, or anxiety
- Decreased agitation/anxiety with pharmacological treatments
- Plan for safe disposition

Telepsychiatry

Virtual health is a growing field improving access to specialists, such as mental health experts who can provide assessment and recommendations otherwise limited in some rural, urban, and suburban areas. This resource limitation can lead to difficulties in management, diagnosis, and treatment of patients with mental health issues. Telepsychiatry utilizes technology to connect an ED patient to a team of mental health providers at a centralized location.[35] The technological connection allows for both consultation and assessment if needed through the use of mental health experts. Assessments can be provided via telephone consultation with the ED staff or through direct video with the patients themselves. Implications for the nursing staff to ensure a safe environment and follow the organizational policies related to confidentiality, safety, and documentation are unchanged, regardless of the method of providing care.

REFERENCES

1. King AJ, Farst KJ, Jaeger MW, et al. Maltreatment-related emergency department visits among children 0 to 3 years old in the United States. *Child Maltreat*. 2015;20(3):151–161.
2. Centers for Disease Control and Prevention. *Child Maltreatment: Risk and Protective Factors*. http://www.cdc.gov/violenceprevention/childmaltreatment/riskprotectivefactors.html CDC. Published 2016. Accessed May 31, 2016.
3. Hall J, Karch D, Crosby A. Elder Abuse Surveillance: Uniform Definitions and Recommended Core Data Elements For Use In Elder Abuse Surveillance, Version 1.0. Atlanta, GA: National Center for Injury Prevention and Control, Centers for Disease Control and Prevention. http://www.cdc.gov/violenceprevention/pdf/ea_book_revised_2016.pdf. Published 2016. Accessed May 31, 2016.

4. Tiyyagura G, Gawel M, Koziel JR, et al. Barriers and facilitators to detecting child abuse and neglect in general emergency departments. *Ann Emerg Med.* 2015;66(5):447–454.
5. Children's Bureau. *Mandatory Reporters of Child Abuse and Neglect: U.S. Department of Health and Human Services Administration for Children and Families.* https://www.childwelfare.gov/pubPDFs/manda.pdf. Published, 2015. Accessed May 31, 2016.
6. Kowalenko T, Gates D, Gillespie GL, et al. Prospective study of violence against ED workers. *Am J Emerg Med.* 2013;31(1):197–205.
7. Gillespie GL, Gates DM, Kowalenko T, et al. Implementation of a comprehensive intervention to reduce physical assaults and threats in the emergency department. *J Emerg Nurs.* 2014;40(6):586–591.
8. Moore G, Pfaff J. *Assessment and Emergency Management of the Acutely Agitated or Violent Adult.* http://www.uptodate.com/contents/assessment-and-emergency-management-of-the-acutely-agitated-or-violent-adult?source=search_result&search=acutely+agitated&selectedTitle=1~150. Published July 2015. Accessed May 31, 2016.
9. Stone K, Humphries R. *Current Diagnosis and Treatment, Emergency Medicine.* 7th ed. New York, NY: McGraw-Hill Companies Inc; 2011.
10. Wilson MP, Pepper D, Currier GW, et al. The psychopharmacology of agitation: consensus statement of the American association for emergency psychiatry project, beta psychopharmacology workgroup. *West J Emerg Med.* 2012;13(1):26–34.
11. Henson B. Preventing interpersonal violence in emergency departments: practical applications of criminology theory. *Violence Vict.* 2010;25(4):553–565.
12. American Psychiatric Association. *Diagnostic and Statistical Manual of Mental Disorders.* 5th ed. Arlington, VA: American Psychiatric Association; 2013.
13. Ebert M, Loosen P, Nurcombe B, et al. *Current Diagnosis & Treatment: Psychiatry.* 2nd ed. New York, NY: The McGraw-Hill Companies, Inc; 2008.
14. Zun, L. Mental health disorders: ED evaluation and disposition. In: Tintinalli J, Stapczynski S, Ma J, et al, eds. *Tintinalli's Emergency Medicine: A Comprehensive Study Guide.* 7th ed. New York, NY: The McGraw-Hill Companies, Inc.; 2011.
15. Stahl S. *Essential Psychopharmacology, Neuroscientific Basis and Practical Applications.* 4th ed. New York, NY: Cambridge University Press; 2013.
16. Beyer JL, Weisler RH. Suicide behaviors in bipolar disorder: a review and update for the clinician. *Psychiatr Clin North Am.* 2016;39(1):111–123.
17. Kuo DC, Tran M, Shah AA, et al. Depression and the suicidal patient. *Emerg Med Clin North Am.* 2015;33(4):765–778.
18. Sood TR, Mcstay CM. Evaluation of the psychiatric patient. *Emerg Med Clin North Am.* 2009;27(4):669–683, ix.
19. U.S. Department of Heath and Human Services. *Health Information Privacy: FAQ. U.S. Department of Health and Human Services.* http://www.hhs.gov/hipaa/for-professionals/faq/520/does-hipaa-permit-a-health-care-provider-to-disclose-information-if-the-patient-is-a-danger/. Published 2016. Accessed May 31, 2016.
20. Witt K, van Dorn R, Fazel S. Risk factors for violence in psychosis: systematic review and meta-regression analysis of 110 studies. *PLoS ONE.* 2013;8(2):e55942.
21. Mosby's Dictionary. Situation Crisis. Mosby. http://medical-dictionary.thefreedictionary.com/situational+crisis. Published 2015. Accessed May 31, 2016.
22. Zisook S, Simon NM, Reynolds CF, et al. Bereavement, complicated grief, and DSM, part 2: complicated grief. *J Clin Psychiatry.* 2010;71(8):1097–1098.
23. American Foundation for Suicide Prevention. *Risk Factors and Warning Signs.* http://afsp.org/about-suicide/risk-factors-and-warning-signs/. Published 2015. Accessed May 31, 2016.
24. Bolton JM, Gunnell D, Turecki G. Suicide risk assessment and intervention in people with mental illness. *BMJ.* 2015;351:h4978.
25. Dazzi T, Gribble R, Wessely S, et al. Does asking about suicide and related behaviours induce suicidal ideation? What is the evidence? *Psychol Med.* 2014;44(16):3361–3363.
26. Amore M, Menchetti M, Tonti C, et al. Predictors of violent behavior among acute psychiatric patients: clinical study. *Psychiatry and Clinical Neurosciences.* 2008;62(3):247–255.
27. National Alliance of Mental Illness. *Risk of Suicide.* https://www.nami.org/Learn-More/Mental-Health-Conditions/Related-Conditions/Suicide. Published 2015. Accessed May 31, 2016.
28. Centers for Disease Control. *National Suicide Statistics.* http://www.cdc.gov/violenceprevention/suicide/statistics/index.html. Updated August 28, 2015. Accessed May 31, 2016.
29. Substance Abuse and Mental Health Services Association (SAMHSA). *Suicide Prevention.* http://www.samhsa.gov/suicide-prevention. Published 2016. Accessed May 31, 2016.
30. Brim C, Lindauer C, Halpern J, et al. *Clinical Practice Guideline: Suicide Risk Assessment.* Des Plaines, IL: Emergency Nurses Association; 2012.
31. Lewis LM. No-harm contracts: a review of what we know. *Suicide Life Threat Behav.* 2007;37(1):50–57.
32. The Joint Commission. Detecting and treating suicide ideation in all settings. *Sentinel Event Alert The Joint Commission.* http://www.jointcommission.org/assets/1/18/SEA_56_Suicide.pdf. Published February 26, 2016. Accessed May 31, 2016.
33. Department of Veterns Affairs. *PTSD and Problems with Alcohol Use.* http://www.ptsd.va.gov/public/problems/ptsd-alcohol-use.asp. Updated 2015. Accessed May 31, 2016.
34. Department of Veterns Affairs. *Suicide and PTSD.* http://www.ptsd.va.gov/professional/co-occurring/ptsd-suicide.asp. Updated 2015. Accessed May 31, 2016.
35. Saurman E, Johnston J, Hindman J, et al. A transferable telepsychiatry model for improving access to emergency mental health care. *J Telemed Telecare.* 2014;20(7):391–399.

Practice Questions

Question	Rationale
1. A patient presents to the emergency department with a primary concern of suicidal ideation. He has attempted suicide four times before, overdosing on medications each time. Which of the following statements is *not* true? a. It is important to realize someone who has overdosed four times in the past is at decreased risk for suicide b. Suicidal "contracts" made with patients have not been shown to decrease suicide c. Firearms are used in the United States more than any other means to die by suicide d. Mental illness is a risk factor which is important to consider	*Answer: a* A past history of suicide attempts is a strong indicator of future suicidal risk. Although suicide contracts are still sometimes used, there is a lack of evidence to support the efficacy of contracts and contracts are not considered legally binding documents. Always consider the individual in front of you and their risk factors. Firearms should always be considered when assessing an individual for suicide. Access to lethal means has been shown to be an important factor which is modifiable. Firearms should be removed and access should be restricted if an individual expresses suicidal ideation. Any mental illness diagnosis should be considered a risk factor for suicide. Both bipolar disorder and depression are two of the most common mental illnesses increasing suicide risk.
2. You are working the evening shift and are concerned several of the patients in the emergency department currently are at risk for violence. You know the patient with the highest risk for violence is a. An 88-year-old male who is confused and is using a loud voice to get his point across b. A 40-year-old woman coming in on the ambulance who has been violent in the ambulance c. A 24-year-old male who is intoxicated and has a laceration to his foot d. A 23-year-old patient with a diagnosis of schizophrenia who has hallucinations	*Answer: b* Although each of these patients present with risk factors, the best predictor of violent behavior is a history of violent behavior. The woman who is violent in the ambulance has demonstrated recent violence and is at the highest risk. The 88-year-old male demonstrates risks of being male, confusion, and using a loud voice, which may indicate an escalation of behaviors. An intoxicated male in his twenties demonstrates a risk for violence related to the intoxication and being male. A patient with schizophrenia who has hallucinations may be at risk if the hallucinations are causing paranoia. In this case, we do not know the content of the hallucinations.
3. The most common presentation for a patient with bipolar in a manic state is a. Suicidal ideation b. Depressed mood and irritability c. Elevated mood and psychomotor agitation d. Both depressed mood and elevated mood	*Answer: c* Patients who are experiencing a bipolar manic state often present with an elevated mood frequently accompanied by irritability and psychomotor agitation. Bipolar disorder does convey an increased risk for suicide but the risk is greater during the depressive episodes of bipolar. Episodes of bipolar include mania or hypomania and depression. In the manic state, someone would not have a depressed mood.

Question	Rationale

4. Which of the following would not be an indicator of potential abuse?
  a. Elderly dementia patient with patterned bruising
  b. Toddler who has bruising in various stages of healing
  c. Husband refuses to let the nurse interview his wife alone
  d. Stories of a child's injuries change
	Answer: b
	Patients who have patterned bruising, especially in the shape of objects, should be investigated for abuse. Care providers who refuse to allow the patient to be interviewed alone may raise suspicion of abuse. When stories are inconsistent or if the descriptions of the events do not match the injury, the nurse should discuss these findings with his or her team and report as local laws mandate. It is not unusual for toddlers at the cruising age to have bruising from falls.

5. One key characteristic of panic attacks which is often most difficult for patients is
  a. Embarrassment over the attacks
  b. Fear of recurrent attacks
  c. Associated nausea
  d. That they are not taken seriously
	Answer: b
	Panic attacks are associated with a fear of reoccurrence. This fear may be debilitating to patients. The panic attacks may be associated with a wide range of physiological systems and sometimes social impact such as embarrassment. Panic attacks are often taken seriously due to the associated physical symptomology.

6. The priority in the assessment of a patient with homicidal ideation is
  a. Ensuring the individual that they are targeting is informed
  b. Assessing for immediate danger
  c. Developing a plan to ensure the patient and others are safe
  d. Calling the police to inform them of the risk
	Answer: b
	During the assessment phase, the nurse should ensure immediate safety is ensured. The other answers represent appropriate interventions which do not represent the priority.

7. A patient has just been in a traumatic MVC in which a passenger is killed. The patient does not appear injured, but is visibly distressed. The emergency nurse enters the room and understands the patient may have all of the following characteristics of a situational crisis *except*
  a. The nurse may need to take control of the situation
  b. Reactions can differ based on individuals
  c. Culture can often play a role in the way someone responds to situational crisis
  d. People with preexisting mental health diagnosis react better to crisis situations
	Answer: d
	Patient with mental illness often present with increased reactions to situational crisis. During a situational crisis, a nurse may need to take control to ensure safety of the individual. Reactions to situational crisis can vary based on past experiences, mental health, culture, and an individual's coping mechanisms.

Question	Rationale
8. A 65-year-old patient presents to the emergency department with a new onset of psychosis. He has no history of mental illness per his and his wife's report. The nurse begins the assessment. All of the following statements are true *except* a. This is unlikely a new onset of mental illness b. Toxicology screen would be important to assess c. Sudden cessation of alcohol use could be a factor d. Medication such as steroids could be a factor	*Answer: a* It would be unlikely this presentation would be a new onset of mental illness. If the patient has a history of mental illness, this could be causing the psychosis. Toxicology and medication review could reveal a cause for the psychosis. Cessation of alcohol use could lead to alcohol withdrawal which can present with psychosis.
9. Environmental factors contributing to reducing the risk for violence include all of the following *except* a. Use of metal detectors b. Training for staff in de-escalation techniques c. Rooms free of potential weapons d. Limiting access for non-patients	*Answer: b* The training of staff in de-escalation would not be considered an environmental factor reducing the risk for violence. It is important to keep rooms free of items that could be used as weapons and to maintain an easy exit at all times.
10. You enter the room of a 2-year-old child who arrived in cardiac arrest after being hit by a car. Trauma resuscitation efforts are discontinued 90 minutes later and the child is pronounced dead. The grieving parents remain with their child. One of the most important nursing interventions is a. Assist with funeral arrangements b. Remind them the death was not their fault c. Call the Coroner/Medical Examiner and organ donation service d. Support their bereavement and provide a quiet calm area for them	*Answer: d* The ED nurse often encounters situational crises that occur suddenly and are often catastrophic. The nurse's role is to support the individual or family's coping. Allowing open communication and providing a calm atmosphere can encourage their grieving. Funeral arrangements can be made later. Suggesting fault should not be assigned may be perceived that someone is to blame. Notifying other agencies may be required, but can be delegated or prioritized once the family is provided immediate support.
11. An ED nurse enters a patient's room to collect a patient history. The patient's chief complaint is "hearing voices" and has a history of psychosis. Currently, he is quiet and calm. To ensure safety, the nurse should a. Turn the television on to provide a distraction for the patient b. Offer a meal to the patient if he answers all of the questions c. Confirm an escape route by positioning between the door and patient d. Place the patient in 4-point restraints	*Answer: c* Delusions, hallucinations and/or a loss of reality may lead to dangerous judgments made by the patient suffering from psychosis. The ED nurse must provide safety. One way to assist with this safety is not to become trapped in a patient's room. The nurse should always have an escape route in case the patient becomes threatening or violent. Turning a TV on would not ensure a low stimulating environment, which is more therapeutic for the patient with psychosis. Bribing the patient is not therapeutic and would not be effective since the patient's rational reasoning skills are not intact. 4-point restraints are not indicated if the patient presents no imminent danger to self or others.

Question	Rationale
12. The ED nurse is in the hall when they hear screaming from a room down the hall. The nurse responds and finds a patient's wife yelling and screaming. She is standing in the corner, appears red in the face, and is breathing rapidly. Her husband is hiding under the covers. The nurse attempts to de-escalate the situation. The first action of the nurse is to a. Approach the patient with arms extended b. Yell at the patient's wife to calm herself or Security will be called c. Manage personal reactions d. Ask for PRN lorazepam to calm the wife	*Answer: c* The first step to manage a disruptive situation is for the nurse to calm himself or herself. Approaching the patient at this time would not be indicated; first establish safety and maintain a safe distance. Yelling is rarely effective when attempting to calm someone. Calling for Security may be an intervention but threatening is rarely an effective means to de-escalate someone. Family members would only be treated if the family member was also a patient.
13. A wife brings her husband to the emergency department reporting he has not been sleeping and has been up all night every night working on new business plans for over a week. The patient states nothing is wrong. The ED nurse suspects he may be experiencing a manic episode. During the assessment the nurse should a. Offer a PRN of an antidepressant to stabilize his mood b. Assess if he is hearing or seeing things c. Ask the wife to leave the room to determine if her reports are valid d. Tell the patient that in order to complete his project, he will need to provide a urine sample	*Answer: b* Assessing if the patient is hallucinating (hearing or seeing things) is an important question. Due to his lack of sleep, it would not be an unusual finding. Offering a PRN of an antidepressant is not indicated. Antidepressants are not used alone in bipolar disorder and during a manic phase would not be the treatment of choice. Asking the wife to leave may not be necessary; typically in mania, the patient presents with little insight into his/her mental illness or current functioning. Using someone's illness as a means to get him to do something should not be done in practice. In this case, using his "project" as a means to get a urine sample would not be appropriate.
14. The ED nurse is in the room alone assessing a patient when he discloses that he wants to kill his neighbor. He appears anxious. He has a detailed plan and explains he is going to kill him after he leaves the emergency department. The nurse's next actions include all of the following actions *except* a. Informing the authorities about the threat to the neighbor b. Walking the patient to the secure room c. Asking the patient if they have a weapon d. Leave the patient alone while the nurse obtains a PRN antianxiety medication for him	*Answer: d* The nurse should consider and consult with other team members about the threats. The nurse may call the police if there is a good faith belief that the disclosure is necessary to prevent or lessen a serious imminent threat to the patient or other. Walking the patient to a secure room is appropriate. The nurse should ask for additional staff to complete the interview. Asking if the patient has a weapon should be done as soon as additional staff is available. A patient should not be left alone if they have stated a credible threat to kill someone.

Question	Rationale
15. A female patient presents to the emergency department with psychological concerns. During the suicide assessment, she admits that she is considering suicide by firearm. Which of the following risk factors is most important to consider? a. She recently broke up with her boyfriend b. She has a diagnosis of depression c. She has a detailed plan to die by suicide d. She comes into the emergency department alone	*Answer: c* All of these items could be risk factors for suicide. However, the one that is most concerning and increases the risk is a detailed plan to die by suicide. Patients who have a plan and means (such as access to a firearm) to follow through with the plan are at highest risk. Additionally, firearms are used in more suicides than any other means, so access to a firearm is an alarming risk factor. Situational stressors often contribute to suicidal ideation and depression conveys an increased risk for suicide. Presenting to the emergency department alone could be for a variety of reasons. However, social isolation is a risk factor.
16. A patient's wife is concerned that her husband is at risk for suicide. Her husband has a diagnosis of bipolar disorder. When educating her about the diagnosis and suicide risk, the ED nurse should include the following statement a. The risk for suicide is highest for patients in the depressive state of bipolar b. The risk for suicide is highest during the impulsive manic state of bipolar c. The risk for suicide is not significantly higher than the general public d. The risk for suicide is the same in the depressive and manic states	*Answer: a* During the depressive state of bipolar disorder, the patient is at higher risk for suicide. Bipolar disorder, carries an increased risk for suicide. During the manic state, patient may engage in risky and dangerous behaviors. However, the suicide risk is lower during manic states.

Medical Emergencies and Communicable Diseases

9

Carla Brim, MN, RN, PHCNS-BC, CEN, FAEN and Tami Wheeldon, BSN, RN, CEN

Medical Emergencies

Medical emergencies are common in the emergency department. The ED nurse must be aware of common presentations for medical emergency in order to triage and intervene appropriately.

Allergic Reactions and Anaphylaxis

Allergic reactions range from minor to life threatening. Minor reactions generally begin with skin reactions of urticarial rash such as urticaria and pruritus. The reaction is self-limiting based on exposure to the allergen. Allergens include medications, food, and environmental particles. Serious reaction of anaphylaxis refers to a life-threatening condition in which prominent dermal and systemic signs and symptoms manifest. Signs of anaphylaxis may include: stridor, swelling of the tongue and airway, hoarse or rasping voice, urticaria and/or angioedema with hypotension and bronchospasm.[1] See Figure 9-1. Rapid assessment and intervention to maintain and secure the airway is the priority of care. The patient may exhibit signs of distributive shock. See the Shock chapter (chapter 5) for a review of distributive shock.

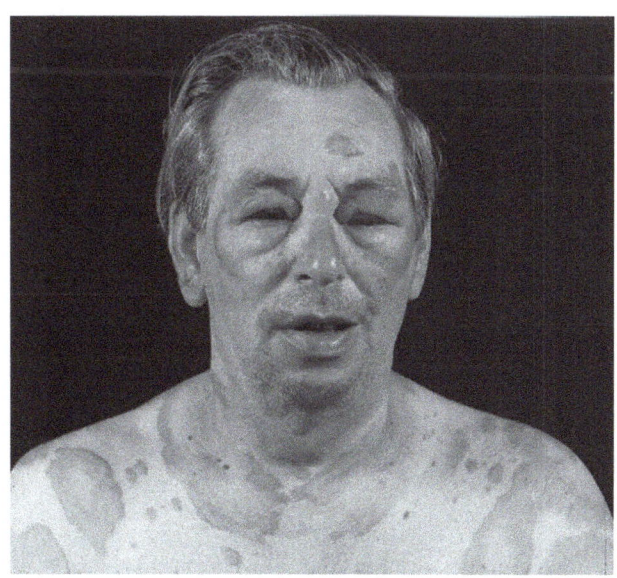

FIGURE 9-1 Urticaria and angioedema
Reproduced with permission from Goldsmith L, Katz S, Gilchrest B, et al: Fitzpatrick's Dermatology in General Medicine, 8th ed. New York: McGraw-Hill Education; 2012.

Assessment/Analysis
- Airway narrowing
- Increased work of breathing
- Wheezes auscultated on lung sounds
- Possible respiratory stridor
- Onset of symptoms
- Suspected allergen exposure
- Skin, observe for any changes or reactions

Interventions
- Triage and immediate placement or treatment in cases of severe reaction
- Minor allergic reaction
  - Oral diphenhydramine
  - Topical hydrocortisone for pruritus
- Severe allergic reaction[2]
  - Place on cardiac and pulse oximetry monitoring devices; consider capnography monitoring
  - Airway management to include possible endotracheal intubation or emergency cricothyrotomy for severe symptoms
  - Place in position of comfort
  - Administration of IM epinephrine
    - Administer 0.01 mg/kg to max dose of 0.5 mg, of 1 mg/mL concentration
    - Dose can be repeated every 5 to 15 minutes, depending upon the response, for three to four doses
    - For severe cases, an IV infusion may be needed
  - Establish IV access for crystalloid/medications as needed
    - Fluids administered at a rapid rate
  - Administer corticosteroid
  - Administer β_2 bronchodilator for bronchospasm
  - Administer (histamine) H1 blocker (diphenhydramine) and H2 blocker (ranitidine or famotidine)
  - Patient/family instruction on use of epinephrine auto-injector (EpiPen™)
  - In patients on β-blockers consider administration of glucagon for possible refractory reaction

Evaluation
- Monitor the patient response to interventions.
- Patient should be observed for 4 to 8 hours to monitor for possible rebound reaction[2]
- Patient/family instruction to avoid future exposures

Blood Dyscrasias

Blood dyscrasia is a nonspecific term referring to a disorder of a blood component. Alterations to blood cells or platelets are known by specific terms, and in general are referred to as blood dyscrasias. Similar elements of assessment, intervention, and evaluation are common to all blood dyscrasias.

Assessment/Analysis
- Tachycardia, fever, and/or possible orthostatic hypotension[3]
- Fatigue
- Weakness or dizziness
- Nausea, vomiting, or diarrhea
- Skin alterations, such as excessive bruising or rashes
- Unusual bleeding
- Medical history, including current treatment

Interventions
- Lab studies for initial management
  - CBC with differential
  - Liver Function tests
  - Coagulation studies
  - Consider blood bank analysis (Type and Screen/Cross)
- Patient and family teaching
- Pain or anxiety management

Evaluation
- Symptoms and plan of care
- Instruct patient to monitor signs of bleeding such as epistaxis, bleeding gums or easy bruising
- Provide instructions to avoid contact sports and medications that may illicit bleeding complications such as NSAIDs

Anemia

Anemia is defined as low levels of hemoglobin/hematocrit through loss, destruction, or decreased production resulting in decreased oxygen carrying capacity.

Assessment/Analysis
- CBC with red blood cell indices
- Decreased reticulocyte count
- Respiratory compromise
- Altered level of consciousness
- Pale skin or mucus membranes
- Weakness or dizziness

Interventions
- Based on cause
  - Loss: red blood cell transfusion
  - Destruction: treatment for Hemolytic anemia
    - Cold Antibody/Cold Agglutinin: pharmacologic or supportive[3]
    - Warm Antibody/Warm Agglutinin: pharmacologic, Surgical, or Plasma replacement[4]
  - Decreased production: Iron, Vitamin B12, or Folic Acid deficiency
- Patient and family teaching

Evaluation
- Resolution of symptoms
- Patient and family understanding of diagnosis and treatment

Thrombocytopenia

- ❖ Idiopathic Thrombocytopenia Purpura (ITP) is caused by decreased production or increased destruction of platelets leading to a decrease in the body's ability to clot
- ❖ Thrombotic Thrombocytopenia Purpura (TTP) is a condition in which microclots form in small blood vessels throughout the body and impede normal blood flow. Since platelets are used in the formation of clots, there is a general lack of platelets throughout the body leading to increased bleeding and bruising

Assessment/Analysis
- Acute following pediatric viral illness[5] (ITP)
- Chronic in women 20 to 40 years old[5] (ITP)
- Ecchymosis
- Petechial rash, as pictured in Figure 9-2

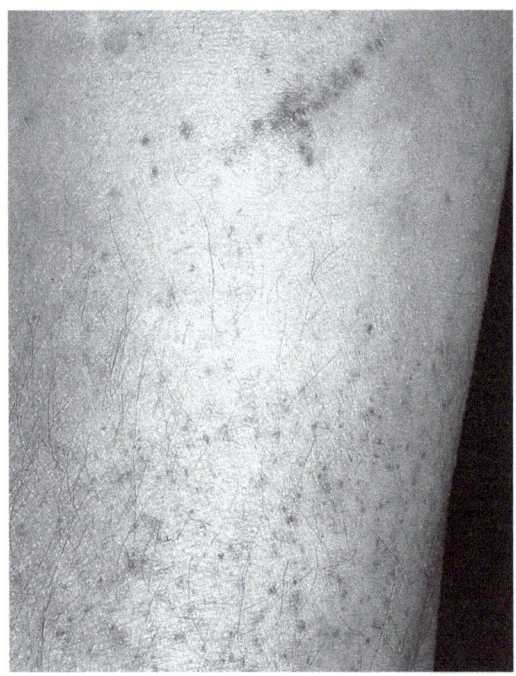

FIGURE 9-2 Thrombocytopenic purpura Multiple petechiae on the upper arm of an HIV-infected 25-year-old male were the presenting manifestation of his disease. The linear arrangement of petechiae at the site of minor trauma is called vibices

Reproduced with permission from Wolff K, Johnson R, Saavedra A: Fitzpatrick's Color Atlas and Synopsis of Clinical Dermatology, 7th ed. New York: McGraw-Hill Education; 2013.

- Bleeding gums
- Hematuria
- Gastrointestinal Bleeding

Intervention
- CBC and coagulation studies to determine cause
- Limit invasive procedures
- Ice to injuries for comfort
- Platelet transfusion (TTP)
- Corticosteroid therapy (ITP)
- Immune Globulin treatment
  - Quickly increases platelet levels[5]
- Consider surgical splenectomy

Evaluation
- Bleeding sites
- Consider admission for platelet transfusion or plasmapheresis

Hemophilia

Hemophilia is a genetic disorder occurring most commonly in males, though women may carry the recessive gene. The four types of hemophilia are von Willebrand's disease due to deficient Factor VIII, hemophilia A due to variation in Factor VIII, hemophilia B due to deficient Factor IX, and hemophilia C due to deficient Factor XI.[5]

Assessment/Analysis
- Unusual bleeding from any site, with or without a known cause
- Excessive bruising
- Pain
- X-ray of affected joint if hemarthrosis suspected

Interventions
- Laboratory studies for initial management
  - CBC with differential
  - Coagulation studies
- Factor replacement
- Medication for pain
  - No Aspirin or NSAIDs
- Diagnostic imaging for joint concerns
  - Ultrasound or MRI
  - Head imaging such as CT or MRI
- Assist with arthrocentesis
  - Rule out infection
  - Bloody appearance highly suggestive of hemarthrosis

Evaluation
- Hemodynamic status and level of consciousness
- Resolution or reduction of symptoms

Leukemia[6]

Leukemia is a malignancy resulting in abnormal production of leukocytes. This results in alterations in bleeding and transport oxygen as well as immune response. Leukemias are classified as acute (composed of blasts) or chronic (composed of more mature precursor cells), and further defined as lymphoid or myeloid in origin. This results in four types of leukemia: acute myeloid (AML), acute lymphoid (ALL), chronic myeloid (CML), and chronic lymphoid (CLL). About 90% of cases of adult acute leukemia are AML, and 90% of cases of childhood acute leukemia are ALL.

Assessment/Analysis[7]
- Fatigue
- Pallor, purpura, and petechiae
- Hepatosplenomegaly and lymphadenopathy are variable
- Bone tenderness, particularly in the sternum, tibia, and femur
- Signs of bleeding; gums, epistaxis, easy bruising
- In some cases acute leukemia may result in disseminated intravascular coagulation (DIC)

Interventions
- Protective isolation as needed
- CBC with differential and platelet count
- Consider blood bank analysis (Type and Screen/Cross), if transfusion likely

Evaluation
- Symptom management
- Referral for oncology

Sickle Cell Crisis

Sickle cell disease is an inherited genetic disorder primarily affecting the African American population. When Hemoglobin S becomes deoxygenated due to cold exposure, low hemoglobin levels, infection, or dehydration, a sickling crisis may occur. Sickling occurs from deoxygenated red blood cells changing from biconcave discs to a rigid crescent shape. Crescent shaped cells are not able to pass through microcirculation and cause obstructed capillary blood flow. See Figure 9-3. Since obstruction causes tissue hypoxia, the sickling cycle continues and can worsen leading to complications such as myocardial infarction or stroke. Patients in sickle cell crisis are critically ill requiring rapid assessment, fluid administration, and pain control.

Assessment/Analysis
- Pain
  - Location and time frame
  - Factors triggering crisis
  - Chest pain or abdominal pain can be red flags
- Hypoxia
- Lung sounds
- Fever
- Capillary refill: possibly delayed
- Laboratory studies
  - CBC with differential and platelet count
  - Increased reticulocyte count
  - Urinalysis

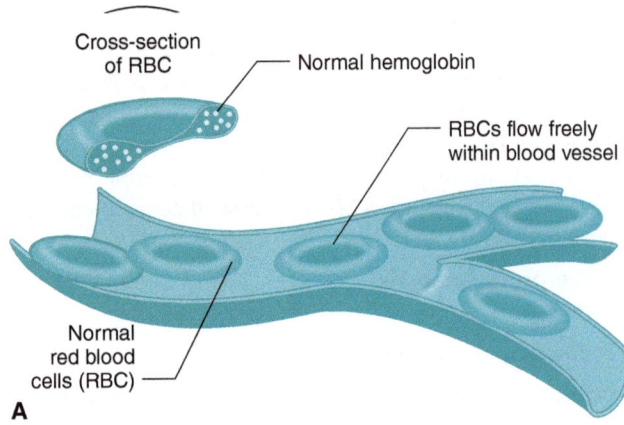

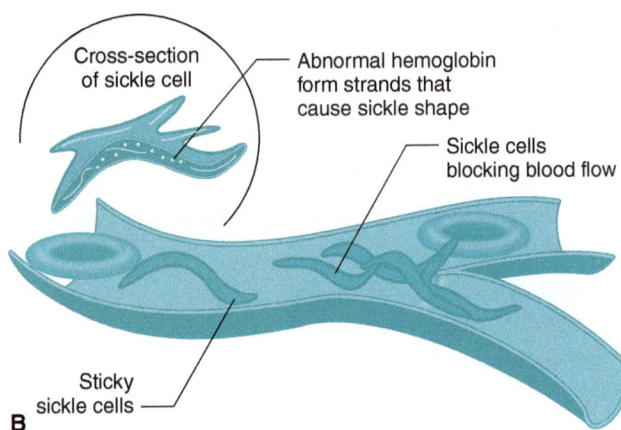

FIGURE 9-3 Intravascular blood flow of normal and sickle red blood cells (RBCs). A. Normal RBCs flowing freely in a blood vessel. B. Abnormal, sickled RBCs clumping and blocking blood flow in a blood vessel. Other cells also may play a role in this clumping process

Reproduced with permission from Tintinalli J, Stapcyzynski J, Ma OJ, et al: Tintinalli's Emergency Medicine: A Comprehensive Study Guide, 8th ed. New York: McGraw-Hill Education; 2015.

Interventions
- Oxygen, if hypoxic
- Establish IV access for crystalloid fluids, blood products, and medications as needed
- Medications for condition
  - Antiemetic
  - Antimetabolites (hydroxyurea)
  - Pain medications: OTC (such as ibuprofen) and opioids for severe pain
- Warm packs or blankets

Evaluation
- Patient tolerating oral fluids
- Pain symptoms managed
- Consider admission for transfusion, plasmapheresis, or pain control

Disseminated Intravascular Coagulation (DIC)

Disseminated intravascular coagulation (DIC) is an acquired thromboembolic disorder characterized by generalized activation of the clotting mechanism, which results in the intravascular formation of fibrin and ultimately thrombotic occlusion of small and midsize vessels.[8] The result of this clotting cascade activation is the blood's clotting factors are depleted causing abnormal bleeding. The overall management goal is to locate and treat the underlying disorder. Common conditions associated with DIC include sepsis, trauma, obstetric complications, envenomation, neoplasms, hepatic disease, acute respiratory disease, and transfusion reactions.[9] Mortality rate in severe DIC exceeds 75%.[8] Death generally results from progression of the underlying disease and complications such as acute renal failure, intracerebral hematoma, shock, or cardiac tamponade.[8]

Assessment/Analysis
- Airway management, effective breathing
- Assess for source of blood loss
- Observe for signs of hypovolemic shock: hypotension, tachycardia, cool pale skin, and altered mental status
- Laboratory studies for initial management
  - CBC with differential
  - Blood bank analysis (Type and Screen/Cross)
  - Coagulation studies
  - Serum chemistries and liver function tests
  - Fibrinogen
  - Fibrin split products
  - D-dimer
  - ABGs

Interventions
- Cardiac monitor with continual pulse oximetry; consider capnography monitoring
- Correct and eliminate underlying cause
- Establish IV access for crystalloids/blood products/medications, as needed
  - Initiate IV crystalloid fluids followed by
  - Administration of blood products (packed cells, FFP, platelets, cryoprecipitate)
    - Anticipate implementation of massive transfusion protocol

Evaluation
- Patient response to blood administration
- Anticipate admission to ICU

Electrolyte/Fluid Imbalance

Fluid imbalance: water is the most abundant constituent in the body. Total body water (TBW), which accounts for approximately 60% of total body weight, can be divided into intracellular fluid (ICF) and extracellular fluid (ECF) compartments.[10-12] The ECF is comprised of intravascular fluid and extravascular, or interstitial fluid.

Dehydration and Hypovolemia

Fluid deficit leads to conditions known as dehydration and hypovolemia. Dehydration is a disorder of water loss with or without loss of sodium.[10] Fluid balance is maintained by water intake as well as fluid losses via renal excretion, respiratory, skin and gastrointestinal sources. Symptoms of hypovolemia are nonspecific and include fatigue, weakness, thirst, and postural dizziness; more severe symptoms and signs include oliguria, cyanosis, abdominal and chest pain, and confusion or coma.[10,11]

Evaluation of the degree of dehydration is an important consideration for the emergency nurse in order to triage for appropriate care. The degree of dehydration is rated as follows.[13]

- ❖ **Early dehydration:** asymptomatic
- ❖ **Moderate dehydration:** thirst, restless or irritable behavior, decreased skin elasticity, and sunken eyes
- ❖ **Severe dehydration:** symptoms become more severe including signs of shock, with diminished consciousness, lack of urine output, cool, moist extremities, a rapid and feeble pulse, low or undetectable blood pressure, and pale skin

The treatment goal is to restore homeostasis and replace ongoing fluid losses. Mild hypovolemia can usually be treated with oral hydration and resumption of normal diet. More severe hypovolemia requires intravenous hydration. Patients with severe hemorrhage or anemia should receive red cell transfusions, without increasing the hematocrit beyond 35%.[13]

Assessment/Analysis
- History of present illness
- Source of fluid loss: inadequate fluid intake, diaphoresis, vomiting, diarrhea, and blood loss
- Vital signs: tachycardia, hypotension, and orthostatic changes, possibly febrile, and oliguria
- Level of consciousness: confusion or lethargy
- Skin assessment: turgor, tenting, or depressed fontanels in infants
- Laboratory studies for initial management
    - Serum chemistries with possible liver function tests
    - CBC with differential
- Urinalysis to include electrolytes

Interventions
- Consider oral rehydration in mild to moderate dehydration
- Establish IV access for crystalloids and medications as needed
    - Especially needed in severe dehydration
- Administer antiemetics as indicated
- Monitor intake and output (I/O)

Evaluation
- Vital signs
- Serum electrolytes
- I/O
- Patient response to interventions
- Hemodynamic status
- Symptoms and plan of care

Electrolyte Disorders

Electrolyte imbalance is assessed by abnormal levels. Increased concentration (hyper-) of an electrolyte is a result of excess total body amount, shift between compartments, and/or a relative fluid loss. Similarly, decreased concentrations (hypo-) are a result of depleted total body amount, shift among compartments, and/or relative fluid gain.[10] The rate of change for electrolyte concentrations rather than absolute concentrations usually determines the severity of symptoms. Correction of the electrolyte disturbance should occur over a time frame similar to the course during which the abnormality developed.[11]

Sodium

Sodium is the major extracellular cation and maintains normal water balance, acid-base balance, and impulse conduction (normal is 135 to 145 mEq/L).[10]

<u>Hyponatremia</u> may result from either actual sodium deficits or dilutional causes. Symptoms related to hyponatremia usually do not occur unless the sodium level is less than 120 to 125 mEq/L.[10] Symptoms of hyponatremia begin as a headache, nausea, disorientation, confusion, agitation and may progress to seizure and/or coma with risk for brain herniation.[11] Antidiuretic hormone (ADH) is secreted in response to hypovolemia and hyperosmolality. Syndrome of inappropriate ADH secretion (SIADH) is the release of ADH without physiologic causes. The major causes of SIADH are disorders affecting the central nervous system (structural, metabolic, psychiatric, or pharmacologic processes) or the lungs (infectious, mechanical, or oncologic). Medications commonly cause SIADH by increasing ADH or its action. Some carcinomas, especially small cell lung carcinoma, can autonomously secrete ADH.[11]

Assessment/Analysis[11]
- History of present illness
- Sources of sodium decrease
    - Inadequate fluid intake
    - Diaphoresis
    - Vomiting
    - Diarrhea
    - Excessive water intake
    - Inappropriate water intake, such as tap water to infants
    - Trauma or burns
- Other possible causes include metabolic imbalances, hyperglycemia, and SIADH
- Assess for lethargy, confusion, and seizure or decreased level of consciousness (LOC) with possible coma
- Vital signs
    - Tachycardia
    - Hypotension or orthostatic changes
    - Febrile, possibly
- Oliguria
- Skin assessment: turgor, tenting, or depressed fontanels in infants

- Laboratory studies for initial management
  - Serum chemistries, possible liver function tests
  - Urinalysis including electrolytes and specific gravity
  - CBC with differential

Interventions[11]
- Establish IV access for crystalloids/medications as needed
  - 3% hypertonic saline when symptomatic and sodium is <120 mEq/L
- Anticipate possible free water restriction
- Monitor I/O
- Seizure precautions if seizures present
- Safety for confused patient

Evaluation
- Hemodynamic status
- Mental status
- Serum electrolytes
- Hydration status
- Patient response to interventions

Hypernatremia presents similar to signs of hypovolemia. A careful assessment of medication history and medical history should be obtained for possible causes.[11] Diabetes insipidus (DI) may lead to hypernatremia. The result is the inability of the kidney to reabsorb free water. The disorder is characterized by polyuria, polydipsia, and an increased volume of hypo-osmolar urine. Hypernatremia is present only when the thirst center is impaired or water intake is reduced.[11]

Assessment/Analysis
- History of present illness
- Focused assessment to identify neurologic, renal, and GI symptoms
- Medication history[11]
  - Lactulose
  - Loop diuretics
  - Lithium
  - Nonsteroidal anti-inflammatory drugs (NSAID)
- Assess for lethargy, confusion, or altered mental status
- Vital signs: tachycardia, hypotension, and orthostatic changes, possibly febrile, and oliguria
- Skin assessment: turgor, tenting, or depressed fontanels in infants
- Laboratory studies for initial management
  - Serum chemistries, possible liver function tests
  - CBC with differential
  - Urine electrolytes

Interventions
- Establish IV access for crystalloids/medications as needed
- Monitor intake and output

Evaluation
- Hemodynamic status
- Mental status
- Serum electrolytes
- Hydration status
- Patient response to interventions

Calcium

Calcium has several major roles in electrolyte balance and is crucial for muscle and cardiac contraction, nerve conduction, cell growth, enzyme activation, and coagulation (Normal 8.5 to 10.2 mg/dL).[10] Consequently, any hypo- or hypercalcemia leads to severe dysfunctions.[11] Calcium imbalance results predominately in neuromuscular and cardiovascular disturbances.[12]

Hypocalcemia: as serum calcium decreases, neuronal membranes become increasingly more permeable to sodium, thereby enhancing excitation, causing smooth and skeletal muscle contractions. Irritability, confusion, dementia, extrapyramidal symptoms, seizures, and hallucination may occur. Decreased calcium leads to a reduction in strength of myocardial contraction primarily by inhibiting relaxation.[11,12] Causes of hypocalcemia include alkalosis, hypoparathyroidism, and massive transfusions. Treatment of hypocalcemia is tailored to the individual patient's severity of symptoms and directed toward correcting the underlying cause.

Assessment/Analysis[11]
- History of present illness
- Assess for lethargy, confusion, or altered mental status
- Assess Chvostek sign (facial twitch elicited by tapping facial nerve)
- Assess Trousseau sign (carpopedal spasm with paresthesia elicited by BP cuff pressure to exceed systolic blood pressure for 2 to 3 minutes)
- EKG changes: prolonged QT interval, wide T wave, and prolonged ST segments
- Laboratory studies for initial management
  - Serum chemistries
  - Ionized calcium: unaffected by a low albumin level
  - Albumin level: if the albumin level is low (such as in malnourished patients), generally, the serum calcium level will also be low
  - Parathyroid Hormone (PTH)

Interventions
- Cardiac monitor
- 12-lead ECG
- Establish IV access for crystalloids and medications as needed
- Minor hypocalcaemia: administer oral calcium replacement[11,12]
- Severe hypocalcemia: administer IV calcium gluconate[11,12]
  - Observe for signs of infiltration and/or extravasation
- Monitor mental status

Evaluation
- Hemodynamic status
- Serum electrolytes
- Hydration status
- Neurological status
- Symptoms and plan of care

Hypercalcemia: symptoms vary depending upon the level of calcium. Patients may experience neurologic changes ranging from mild confusion to coma. Renal symptoms include polyuria or renal calculi. Cardiac symptoms are the most worrisome, as elevations may lead to cardiac arrest.[11,12]

Common causes are hyperparathyroidism, malignancy, renal failure, Addison's disease, and hyperthyroidism.[11]

Assessment/Analysis
- History of present illness
- Focused assessment to identify neurologic, renal, and GI symptoms
- EKG changes: bradycardia, ST changes, widened, flattened, or inverted T-wave, shortened QT segment
- Laboratory studies for initial management
  - Serum chemistries
  - Ionized calcium
  - Serum creatinine

Interventions
- Establish IV access for crystalloids and medications as needed
- Possible corticosteroid if associated with Addison's disease
- Management of cardiac dysrhythmias
- Possible hemodialysis in severe cases

Evaluation
- Monitor mental status
- Hemodynamic status
- Serum electrolytes
- Cardiac rhythm
- Neurological status

Potassium

Potassium is the major intracellular cation which maintains electrical membrane excitability, acid-base balance, and regulates intracellular osmolarity (Normal 3.5 to 5.0 mEq/L).[10,11] Homeostasis is maintained through distribution between the ICF and ECF spaces with excretion occurring primarily by the renal system. In critically ill patients, there is significant and rapid intracellular to extracellular shifting in response to severe injury, acid-base imbalance, catabolic states, increased extracellular osmolality, or insulin deficiency. Duration of imbalance influences the clinical response; chronic potassium depletion or surplus allows adaptation through shifts in intra-/extracellular potassium concentration to maintain the resting membrane potential, thus mitigating neuromuscular and cardiac electrophysiologic effects.[11]

Hypokalemia is defined as serum potassium less than 3.5 mEq/L. Hypokalemia causes include insufficient dietary intake, shifts due to medications such as insulin, and increased losses from vomiting, diarrhea, or diuretics. Moderate hypokalemia may be treated with oral replacement. Severe (<2.5 mEq/L) hypokalemia and in symptomatic patients with moderate (2.5 to 3 mEq/L) hypokalemia should receive intravenous replacement.[9] Commonly, hypokalemic patients are also hypomagnesemic therefore, an assessment of magnesium level and a possible addition to the infusion may be required.[1]

Assessment/Analysis
- History of present illness
- Medication history
  - Diuretics
  - Corticosteroids
- Assess for lethargy, confusion, or altered mental status
- EKG changes: T-wave depression, PVCs, PACs, heart blocks, and ventricular fibrillation
- Muscle tenderness, hyporeflexia
- Nausea or vomiting
- Leg cramps
- Laboratory studies for initial management
  - Serum chemistries, including magnesium level

Interventions
- Monitor mental status
- Cardiac monitor
- 12-lead ECG
- Treat cardiac dysrhythmias
- For minor hypokalemia and if able to tolerate oral intake, administer oral potassium chloride
- Establish IV access for crystalloids/medications as needed
  - Administer IV potassium chloride using an IV pump (with a controlled rate) at maximum of 20 to 40 mEq/hour[10,11]
- Antiemetic
- Pain management

Evaluation
- Hemodynamic status
- Hydration status
- Serum electrolytes
- Cardiac rhythm
- Neurological status

Hyperkalemia is serum levels greater than 5.5 mEq/L. Common causes of elevated potassium include medications such as angiotensin-converting enzyme inhibitors, angiotensin receptor blockers, potassium sparing diuretics, renal disease, and Addison's disease. The most significant effects of elevated potassium are cardiac dysrhythmias due to hyperpolarization impacting the ability of cardiac cells to repolarize and causing ventricular asystole.[10]

Assessment/Analysis
- History of present illness
- Medication history

- Assess for irritability, anxiety, or confusion
- ECG changes: tachycardia, widened QRS, prolonged PR intervals, ventricular dysrhythmias, and elevated, or peaked T waves
- Muscle irritability and weakness of lower extremities
- Laboratory studies for initial management
  - Serum chemistries

Interventions
- Monitor mental status
- Cardiac monitor
- 12-lead ECG
- Establish IV access for crystalloid fluids/medications as needed
  - Administer 50% dextrose with 5 to 10 units of regular insulin[12]
  - Administer calcium gluconate[10]
- Kayexalate orally or rectal enema[10]
- Anticipate possible emergent dialysis for severe hyperkalemia
- Treat cardiac dysrhythmias

Evaluation
- Hemodynamic status
- Hydration status
- Serum electrolytes
- Cardiac rhythm
- Neurological status
- Anticipate possible admission to ICU

Endocrine Conditions

Adrenal

Primary adrenal insufficiency, Addison's disease, is most commonly an autoimmune disease due to an intrinsic adrenal gland dysfunction and subsequent decrease in cortisol and aldosterone production.[14] Secondary adrenal insufficiency commonly is a result of long-term use of glucocorticoids. Acute adrenal insufficiency or adrenal crisis occurs in response to an acute stressor, such as infection, hemorrhage, trauma, surgery, burns, pregnancy, or abrupt cessation of long-term steroid use.[13] Adrenal crisis should be suspected in patients who have hypotension unresponsive to fluid resuscitation and vasopressor medications.[14,16] Death occurs because of circulatory collapse and hyperkalemia-induced dysrhythmia.

Assessment/Analysis
- Vital signs, in particular BP unresponsive to interventions[14-16]
- Signs of dehydration
- New onset confusion, disorientation, or lethargy
- Abdominal pain, nausea/vomiting

Interventions
- Establish IV access for crystalloids and medications as needed
  - Consider fluids containing glucose
  - IV hydrocortisone
  - Vasopressors only after steroid therapy in patients unresponsive to fluid resuscitation

Evaluation
- Monitor vital signs
- Patient response to treatments
- Anticipate admission to ICU

Glucose-Related Conditions

In general, glucose-related emergencies occur as a result of decreased or increased blood glucose levels.

Hypoglycemia: decreased blood glucose level <60 mg/dL is often a result of adverse drug events related to insulin or oral hypoglycemic medications. Other more rare cause may include tumor of the pancreas called an insulinoma.

Hyperglycemia: elevated blood glucose levels are categorized in three events: undiagnosed or untreated diabetes, diabetic ketoacidosis (DKA), or hyperosmolar hyperglycemic state (HHS). See Table 9-1 for expected lab values.[15] The goal of therapy is a gradual return to normal metabolic balance. Complications of therapy such as cerebral edema, hypoglycemia, and electrolyte imbalance may contribute to death during treatment.[12,15-17]

Assessment/Analysis
- Airway patency, effective breathing
- Level of consciousness
- Bedside glucose testing
- Diabetic ketoacidosis
  - Type I diabetic and Type II diabetic on insulin
  - Insulin deficiency
  - Excess stress hormone
  - Hyperglycemia
  - Hyperosmolality
  - Dehydration
  - Electrolyte depletion
  - Metabolic ketoacidosis
- Hyperosmolar hyperglycemic state (HHS)
  - Type II diabetic
  - Presence of endogenous insulin
  - Hyperglycemia
  - Hyperosmolarity
  - Dehydration
- Medication history
- Oral intake and diet history
- GI symptoms: nausea, vomiting, or abdominal distension

TABLE 9-1 **Laboratory Values in Diabetic Ketoacidosis (DKA) and Hyperglycemic Hyperosmolar State (HHS) (Representative Ranges at Presentation)**

	DKA	HHS
Glucose,[a] mmol/L (mg/dL)	13.9–33.3 (250–600)	33.3–66.6 (600–1200)
Sodium, meq/L	125–135	135–145
Potassium[a,b]	Normal to ↑	Normal
Magnesium[a]	Normal	Normal
Chloride[a]	Normal	Normal
Phosphate[a,b]	Normal	Normal
Creatinine	Slightly ↑	Moderately ↑
Osmolality (mOsm/mL)	300–320	330–380
Plasma ketones[a]	++++	+/−
Serum bicarbonate,[a] meq/L	<15	Normal to slightly ↓
Arterial pH	6.8–7.3	>7.3
Arterial Pco_2,[a] mm Hg	20–30	Normal
Anion gap[a] (Na − [Cl + HCO_3])	↑	Normal to slightly ↑

[a]Large changes occur during treatment of DKA.
[b]Although plasma levels may be normal or high at presentation, total-body stores are usually depleted.
Reproduced with permission from Kasper DL, Fauci AS, Hauser S, et al: Harrison's Principles of Internal Medicine, 19th ed. New York: McGraw-Hill Education; 2015.

- Additional laboratory studies for hyperglycemia
  - Serum chemistries with liver function studies
  - Blood Gases
  - Hemoglobin A1c (HbA_{1c})

Interventions
Hypoglycemia[16]
- Provide 15 grams of oral carbohydrate, if the patient is alert and able to safely ingest juice or a sandwich
- Establish IV access for crystalloid and medications as needed
  - Especially important if altered level of consciousness
  - For patients with decreased LOC, administer 12.5 gms (25 mL)-25 gms (50 mL) dextrose 50% IV push.
- If intravenous access is delayed, 1 mg of glucagon can be administered intramuscularly

Hyperglycemia[15,17]
- Establish IV access for crystalloids and medications as needed
  - Crystalloid fluids followed by fluids including dextrose and potassium as determined by lab values
- Electrolyte replacement
- Insulin replacement after adequate hydration and potassium level stablized[15,17]

Evaluation
- Hemodynamic status
- Mental status
- Glucose-point of care testing
- I & O
- Serum chemistries including glucose and potassium
- Symptoms and plan of care
- Anticipate hospital admission

Thyroid Disorders

Myxedema Coma: hypothyroidism is called myxedema coma (MC) when severe. Though rare, myxedema coma causes central nervous system impairment and cardiovascular decompensation. Often proceeded by stroke, cold exposure, recent use of sedatives, infective illness such as pneumonia, or discontinuation of thyroid hormone replacement medications. Myxedema coma has a high rate of mortality, if not identified early.[16,18]

Assessment/Analysis
- Abnormally low vital signs
  - Bradycardia
  - Hypoventilation
  - Hypotension
  - Mild Hypothermia: generally above 95°F (35°C)[16]
- Altered, decreased mental status, possible new onset depression
- Dry, cool, and pale skin
- Hair loss or thinning, also known as alopecia areata
- Anorexia
- Recent weight gain

Interventions
- Airway management, possible intubation
- Laboratory studies for initial management
  - CBC with differential for anemia or leukopenia
  - Serum chemistry studies for hyponatremia, hypochloremia, and elevated renal tests
  - Thyroid studies for low T_4 and elevated TSH[17]
- Active or passive warming

- Establish IV access for crystalloid fluids, blood products, and medications as needed
  - Including hypertonic saline or blood products, if indicated
- Medications
  - Thyroid hormone replacement (levothyroxine)
  - Adrenal glucocorticoids
  - Vasopressors

Evaluation
- Hemodynamic status and level of consciousness
- Resolution or reduction of symptoms

Thyroid Storm (or Thyrotoxic Crisis), also a rare condition with a high mortality rate, is caused by hyperthyroidism. Thyroid storm (TS) is characterized by a hypermetabolic state. Stressors similar to myxedema coma and including DKA, pregnancy, or thyroid treatment using radioactive isotopes can cause thyroid storm. GI disorders, neurological impairment, and cardiac decompensation with often-fatal heart failure are symptoms of thyroid storm. Graves' disease is a form of thyrotoxicosis with hyperthyroidism. Initial presentation may include weight loss in spite of increased appetite, hyperthermia, hypertension, tachycardia, diarrhea, polyuria, hyperactivity, irritability, dysphoria, heat intolerance, and sweating.[19] The initial treatment includes administration of beta blockers and/or propylthiouracil (PTU) followed by chronic thyroid hormone replacement.

Assessment/Analysis
- Elevated vital signs
  - Tachycardia of 100 to 120 bpm
  - Hypertension: systolic elevation and widening pulse pressure
  - Hyperthermia, possibly over 104°F (40°C)
- Anxiety or restlessness
- Lung sounds: possible crackles with auscultation related to heart failure
- Changes in vision such as blurred vision
- Enlarged
- Nausea, vomiting, and diarrhea
- Weakness or fatigue
- Sweating
- Cardiac arrhythmias: tachycardia, atrial fibrillation
- Exophthalmos (see Figure 9-4)
- Weight loss

Interventions
- Patent airway, effective breathing
- Cardiac monitor with continuous oximetry
- Supplemental oxygen as needed
- Establish IV access for crystalloid fluids and medications as needed
  - Consider dextrose related to high metabolic rate[17]

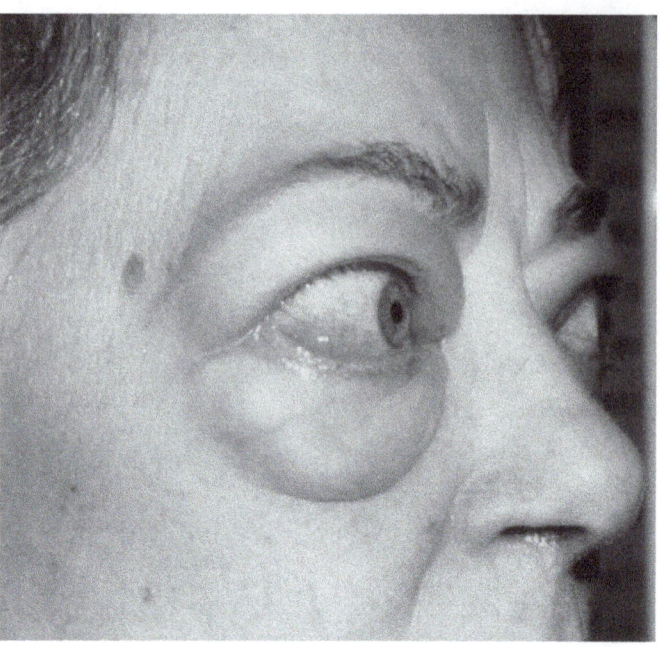

FIGURE 9-4 **The patient pictured exhibits exophthalmos with periorbital and conjunctival swelling**
Reproduced with permission from Brunicardi F, Andersen D, Billiar T, et al: Schwartz's Principles of Surgery, 10th ed. New York: McGraw-Hill Education; 2014.

- Laboratory studies for initial management
  - CBC with differential
    - Leukocytosis indicating bacterial infection
  - Serum chemistries with liver function tests
    - Elevated liver function studies often observed
  - Thyroid studies for elevated T_4 and T_3, decreased TSH
  - Cholesterol studies: total cholesterol decreased[16]
- Active or passive cooling measures
- Medications
  - Antiadrenergic medications for heart rate and blood pressure
    - Beta-blockers
  - Antipyretics, avoiding Aspirin
  - Antithyroid agent (propylthiouracil [PTU]) blocks thyroid hormone synthesis
  - Hydrocortisone to block conversion of T_4 to T_3

Evaluation
- Hemodynamic status and level of consciousness
- Resolution or reduction of symptoms
- Anticipate hospital admission

Fever

Fever is a symptom of possible infection. Causes of fever vary and can include bacterial, viral, and parasitic infections as well as non-infectious sources such as connective tissue disease, malignancies, or certain pharmacologic agents including medications and illicit drugs. Tissue inflammation in response to bacteria causes release of histamine, bradykinin, and serotonin, which increases the local blood flow and permeability of capillaries.[1] Rectal or bladder core temperatures are recommended in cases of sepsis or critically ill patients. Rectal temperatures are the standard for detecting fever in infants less than three months of age or critically ill children,[20] unless the child is immunocompromised or a history of rectal surgery.

Fever greater than 38°C (100.4°F) in elderly, infants under age 28 days, or immunocompromised patients should be considered emergent and a sign of a serious infection.[21] Patients in these populations should be assigned a high priority acuity level at triage in order for the provider to evaluate the patient immediately. See Table 9-2 for fever evaluation and treatment guidelines.

Febrile Seizure
Seizures may occur in responses to rapid changes of temperature in children ages 5 months to 5 years, with the greatest incidence between 8 to 20 months.[1] Febrile seizures may be very frightening to parents, but often is self-limiting and not diagnostic of epilepsy. Care of immunocompromised patients with a fever is discussed later in this chapter.

Assessment/Analysis
- Pediatric population: prioritization utilizing the Pediatric Assessment Triage (PAT)[22]
  - General impression
    - Appearance
    - Work of breathing
    - Circulation to skin
- History of present illness, including any possible exposures
- Travel history
- Assess immunization status
- Focused assessment to include suspected source of infection, such as respiratory or skin
- Laboratory studies for initial management
  - CBC with differential
    - Increased in immature production (bands or stab cells) can indicate bacterial infection
  - Serum chemistries with liver function studies
  - Erythrocyte sedimentation (ESR)
- Urinalysis
- Culture of suspected source(s): blood, sputum, or urine
- Possible lumbar puncture
- Chest X-ray

Interventions
- Identify possible source of infection
- Establish IV access for crystalloids and medications as needed
  - Fluid administration when signs of dehydration are present
- Administer antipyretic (acetaminophen or ibuprofen)
- Antibiotic administration either oral or parental as indicated
- Implement sepsis interventions as indicated

Evaluation
- Vital signs, especially temperature
- Symptoms and plan of care
- Educate parents of pediatric patients about fever management

Immunocompromise/Oncological
Disease, drugs, or nutritional deficits may adversely affect the immune system. Typically, the patient with immune compromise seen in the emergency department is receiving treatment for cancer or immunosuppressive therapy following organ transplantation.[3] The patient with immune compromise experiences neutropenia. Neutropenia, defined as a low absolute neutrophil count <500 cells/mm[3], places the patient at risk for infection from normal body flora, as well as from opportunistic organisms.[23] Classic signs of infection do not occur because of an impaired systemic immune response. Consequently, the most significant indicator of infection in the patient with neutropenia is fever. The patient is instructed to call the medical provider any time the temperature is greater than 100°F (38°C). Care of the patient with immune compromise in the emergency department focuses on placing the patient in protective isolation, identifying the source of infection, and initiating antibiotic therapy immediately.[3]

Assessment/Analysis
- Vital signs
  - Fever >100.4°F (38°C), rectal temps should be avoided
  - Possible tachycardia, tachypnea, and hypotension
- History of present illness
- Medication history to include chemotherapy or immunosuppressive therapy
  - Determine date of last chemotherapy therapy
  - Depending on the chemotherapy agent, neutropenia may not develop for a few weeks following therapy
- Focused assessment to include suspected source of infection such as respiratory, skin, or other organ
- Inspect any implanted venous access device (VAD) or peripheral inserted central line (PICC) for signs of infection
- Laboratory studies for initial management
  - CBC with differential
  - Absolute neutrophil count (ANC)
  - Serum chemistries with liver function tests
  - Urinalysis
  - Culture: blood, urine, sputum, VAD if present
- Urinalysis
- Blood cultures

Interventions
- Identify possible source of infection
- Establish IV access for crystalloids and medications as needed
- Administer appropriate antibiotic

TABLE 9-2 **Suggested Guidelines for the Evaluation and Management of Neonates, Infants, and Children with Fever Who Are Well Appearing, Have Had All Relevant Immunizations, and Have No Clinical Source for Fever**

Age Group	Evaluation	Treatment
Neonate, 0–28 d[a] of age, ≥38°C (100.4°F) SBI incidence of ill appearing: 13%–21%; if not ill appearing: <5%	CBC and blood culture and Urinalysis and urine culture and CSF cell count, Gram stain, and culture. Chest x-ray is optional, if no respiratory symptoms. Stool culture if diarrhea is present.	*Admit and treat with:* Parenteral antibiotic therapy with ampicillin, 50 milligrams/kg, and either cefotaxime, 50 milligrams/kg, or gentamicin, 2.5 milligrams/kg
Infant 29–56 d[a] of age, ≥38.2°C (100.8°F) (Philadelphia Protocol) SBI incidence of ill appearing: 13%–21%; if not ill appearing: <5%	Same as for neonates.	*Discharge if:* • WBC ≤15,000/mm^3 and ≥5000/mm^3 and <20% band forms • Urinalysis negative • CSF WBC <10 cells/mm^3 • Negative chest x-ray or fecal leukocytes if applicable *Admit if:* Any of above criteria are not met and treat with parenteral ceftriaxone, 50 milligrams/kg with normal CSF, 100 milligrams/kg with signs of meningitis.
Infants 57 d[a] to 6 mo[a] of age, ≥38°C (100.4°F) Non-UTI SBI incidence is estimated to be negligible UTI is 3%–8%.	Urinalysis and urine culture alone. or For conservative management, treat infants 57–90 d using Philadelphia Protocol.	*Discharge if negative.* *Treat for UTI* with cefixime, 8 milligrams/kg/dose daily, or cefpodoxime, 5 milligrams/kg/dose twice a day, or cefdinir, 7 milligrams/kg/dose twice daily for 10 d as outpatient. *Admit and treat* with parenteral ceftriaxone if fails conservative criteria for discharge.
Infants 57 d to 6 mo[a] of age ≥39°C (102.2°F) SBI incidence is estimated as <1%; non-UTI SBI incidence is estimated to be negligible. UTI is 3%–8%.	Urinalysis and urine culture alone. or Urinalysis and urine culture in addition to CBC and blood culture.	*Discharge if negative.* *Treat for UTI.* If WBC ≥15,000/mm^3, consider treatment with ceftriaxone, 50 milligrams/kg IV/IM, and follow-up in 24 h. If WBC ≥20,000/mm^3, consider chest x-ray and CSF testing.[b]
Infants/children 6–36 mo of age Non-UTI SBI incidence is <0.4% UTI in girls ≤8% UTI in boys (<12 mo) ≤2% Uncircumcised boys (1–2 y) remains 2%	Urinalysis and urine culture. Girls 6–24 mo Boys 6–12 mo Uncircumcised boys 12–24 mo	*Discharge if negative.* *Treat for UTI* as outpatient.
Children >36 mo and older	No workup is routinely necessary.	*Discharge and treat with antipyretics:* acetaminophen, 15 milligrams/kg PO/PR every 4 h, or ibuprofen, 10 milligrams/kg PO every 6 h as needed.

Abbreviations: CSF = cerebrospinal fluid; SBI = serious bacterial illness; UTI = urinary tract infection.
[a]For preterm infants, count age by estimated postconception date and not by actual delivery date for the first 90 days of life.
[b]Meningismus is difficult to discern in infants <6 months of age, and especially in infants <2 months of age. Therefore, we recommend routine CSF testing in infants <2 months of age, but selective CSF testing in infants 2 to 6 months of age. There is no absolute cutoff point for prediction of meningitis with a peripheral WBC count.
Reproduced with permission from Tintinalli J, Stapcyzynski J, Ma OJ, et al: Tintinalli's Emergency Medicine: A Comprehensive Study Guide, 8th ed. New York: McGraw-Hill Education; 2015.

- Implement sepsis interventions as indicated
- Provide protective isolation

Evaluation
- Vital signs
- Symptoms and plan of care
- Anticipate possible admission

Human Immunodeficiency Virus (HIV) and Acquired Immunodeficiency Syndrome (AIDS)

The diagnosis of HIV and AIDS is complex and comprehensive. For this reason, HIV disease should be viewed as a spectrum ranging from primary infection, with or without the acute syndrome, to the asymptomatic stage, and to the advanced stages associated with opportunistic diseases.[24]

Primary HIV infection is rarely diagnosed in the ED. In approximately, two-thirds of patient illness is associated with primary HIV infection. Symptoms occur approximately 10 to 20 days after exposure, with average symptom duration of 1.5 to 2 weeks. The most common symptoms include fever, swollen lymph nodes, sore throat, myalgias/arthralgias, diarrhea, nausea/vomiting, weight loss, headache, mucocutaneous lesions, and a generalized maculopapular rash located over the face, neck, and trunk (see Figure 9-5). This rash is seen in over 50% of persons with symptomatic primary HIV infection. The lesions are typically small, well circumscribed, erythematous, non-pruritic, and non-tender.

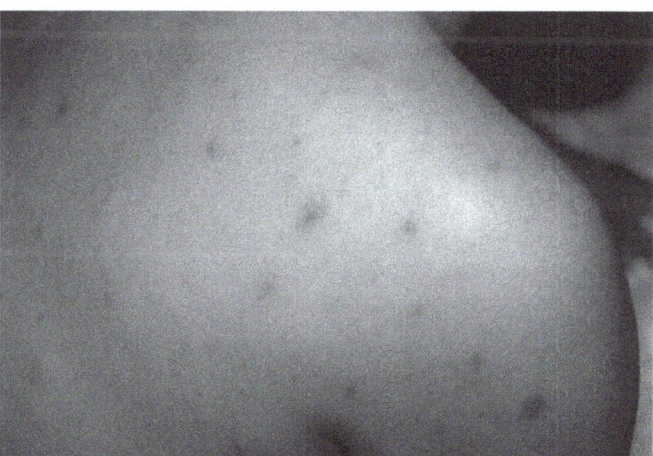

FIGURE 9-5 Primary HIV Infection. A maculopapular rash is seen in over half of persons with symptomatic acute HIV infection. This less typical papular/vesicular rash was present in a patient with primary HIV infection
Reproduced with permission from Knoop KJ, Stack LB, Storrow AB, et al: The Atlas of Emergency Medicine, 4th ed. New York: McGraw-Hill Education; 2016: Photo contributor: Gregory K. Robbins, MD, MPH.

Less frequently, patients may demonstrate neurologic signs and symptoms consistent with meningoencephalitis, myelopathy, and peripheral neuropathy. Laboratory studies may show lymphopenia and thrombocytopenia.[25] The current U.S. CDC classification system for HIV infection and AIDS categorizes people on the basis of clinical conditions associated with HIV infection and CD4+ T lymphocyte measurement.[24] HIV is staged according to lab values.

Assessment/Analysis
- Fever
- Fatigue
- Lymph node
- Opportunistic infections such as Kaposi sarcoma, Candidiasis, and Cytomegalovirus infections
- Laboratory studies for initial management
  - CBC with differential
  - T-cell count

Interventions
- Possible protective isolation
- Symptom management: nausea, diarrhea, fever, pain etc.
- Implement sepsis interventions as indicated

Evaluation
- Patient response to intervention
- Education and counseling on "safe practice" during sex and when using needles, etc.
- Referral to outpatient immunologist for disease management

Renal Failure

Patients with kidney disease may have a variety of different clinical presentations. Symptoms are dependent upon area of damage, such as gross hematuria with direct kidney involvement compared to edema, hypertension, or signs of uremia with extrarenal damage. Patients may also be asymptomatic. Specific disorders are more likely to be either acute or chronic in duration. Acute renal failure (ARF) has been replaced by the term, acute kidney injury (AKI). Chronic kidney disease (CKD) has replaced older terms such as chronic renal failure or chronic renal insufficiency. Patients may develop AKI as a result of traumatic injury, hypovolemia, or sepsis. Consensus panels have defined AKI and CKD.[26]

- ❖ Acute[26]
  - ◆ Serum creatinine concentration can typically increase by 1.0 to 1.5 mg/dL daily
  - ◆ Stage 1: 1.5- to 1.9-fold increase in serum creatinine or a decline in urinary output to 0.5 mL/kg/h over 6 to 12 hours
  - ◆ Stage 2: 2.0 to 2.9 increase in serum creatinine or a decline in urinary output to 0.5 mL/kg/h over >12 hours
  - ◆ Stage 3: 3-fold or greater increase in serum creatinine or a decline in urinary output to <0.3 mL/kg/h for ≥24 hours or anuria for ≥12 hours
- ❖ Chronic
  - ◆ Abnormal GFR (<60 mL/min) persisting for at least 3 months
  - ◆ Renal abnormalities, kidney size and or perfusion

Assessment/Analysis
- Possible jugular vein distension (JVD)
- Urine volume, characteristic (hematuria)
- History of present illness
- Medication history
- Laboratory studies for initial management
  - CBC with differential
  - Serum chemistries with serum creatinine and liver function tests
  - Urinalysis
- Possible renal ultrasound
- Abdominal CT scan

Interventions
- Identify possible source of AKI
- Establish IV access for crystalloids and medications as needed
  - Volume replacement in trauma or sepsis
  - Use caution with IV and oral fluid to avoid overload
- Consider possible alterations in drug dosing, as appropriate related to creatinine clearance
- Consider electrolyte management
- Possible emergent dialysis in acute failure may be required to correct electrolyte imbalance, especially hyperkalemia

Evaluation
- Vital signs
- Patient response to intervention
- Patient education on disease process, diet, and fluid intake

Sepsis

Septic shock is also reviewed in the Shock chapter (chapter 5) of this book. The focus of this chapter is the initial recognition and treatment of early sepsis, severe sepsis, and septic shock.

Early recognition of signs and symptoms of sepsis is essential for timely implementation of interventions to improve patient outcomes. In the emergency care setting screening for sepsis should occur during triage and with any change in patient condition.

Sepsis has a high mortality rate increasing linearly according to the disease severity of sepsis.[21] Sepsis is the clinical syndrome resulting from an inflammatory response to an infection and often leads to organ dysfunction. Sepsis has been represented as a spectrum ranging from systemic inflammatory response syndrome (SIRS) to septic shock.[27-29]

SIRS Criteria
- ❖ Temperature >38°C or <36°C
- ❖ Heart rate >90 beats/min
- ❖ Respiratory rate >20 breaths/min or $Paco_2$ <32 mm Hg
- ❖ WBC count >12,000 cells/μL or <4,000 cells/μL or >10% immature forms (bands)

Sepsis is ≥2 SIRS criteria with known or suspected infection.
Severe sepsis is sepsis with organ dysfunction. Cardiovascular failure is typically manifested by hypotension, respiratory failure by hypoxemia, renal failure by oliguria and/or azotemia, and hematologic failure by coagulopathy.
Septic shock is sepsis with refractory hypotension and impaired end organ perfusion (hemodynamic instability) despite adequate fluid resuscitation.[27] Sepsis bundle interventions from 2015, with time frame are discussed in chapter 5.[29] Reassessment criteria is also detailed in chapter 5.

Assessment/Analysis
- History of present illness including presence of suspected infection (urinary, respiratory, integumentary, etc.)
- Evaluate for ≥2 SIRS criteria
- Laboratory studies for initial management
  - CBC with differential
  - Lactate
  - Serum chemistries
  - Blood gases
  - Urinalysis
  - Culture areas of suspected infection
    - Blood
    - Urine
    - Sputum
    - Wound

Interventions[29]
- Early screening during triage to assign acuity appropriately
- Initiate isolation precautions, as indicated
- Initiate sepsis alert, if applicable at your facility
- Begin sepsis bundle
  - Obtain appropriate cultures
  - Establish IV access for crystalloid fluids and medications as needed
    - Administer crystalloid fluids at controlled rate
    - Fluid bolus at 30 mL/kg with hypotension or MAP <65
    - Administer broad spectrum antibiotics after blood cultures obtained
    - Administer vasopressors for hypotension not responding to fluid bolus
  - Anticipate intubation for respiratory distress
  - Anticipate possible insertion of urinary catheter in septic shock
  - Anticipate possible central venous access in septic shock

Evaluation
- Hemodynamic status
- Patient response to interventions
- Volume status
- Obtain repeat lactate level in septic shock
- Anticipate critical care admission

Communicable Diseases

The emergency department is a common location for patients seeking treatment of conditions related to communicable diseases. Communicable disease, also referred to as infectious or contagious disease, is spread between humans, as well as from animal to human. It is important for emergency nurses to recognize common signs and symptoms for a variety of these illnesses including the mode of transmission, incubation period, and the appropriate isolation precautions needed to aid in reducing the spread of infectious disease.

Isolation precautions are established by The Center for Disease Control and Prevention (CDC) to protect healthcare workers and patients. Precautions can be further divided into Standard Precautions and Transmission-based Precautions. Standard Precautions should be used for all patient care. Additional measures to ensure patient safety include respiratory hygiene/cough etiquette, safe injection practices, and use of masks for invasive procedures. Transmission-based precautions are added when Standard Precautions are not sufficient to interrupt the cycle of the disease. Transmission-based precautions are further divided into three categories: contact Precautions, Droplet Precautions, and Airborne Precautions depending on the mode of transmission associated with a specific disease.[30] Personal protective equipment (PPE) may include gloves, gown, and eye protection while providing care to patients with added transmission-based precautions. The emergency nurse must be aware of presenting complaints, quickly assess and determine appropriate care, and implement isolation precautions necessary to protect patients and ED staff.

Clostridium Difficile (C. difficile)

C. difficile infection (CDI) is a spore-forming, Gram–Positive Anaerobic Bacillus that produces two exotoxins: toxin A and toxin B,[30] which cause inflammation and mucosal damage to the GI tract. CDI develops through an antibiotic-acquired or community-acquired diarrhea. CDI is shed in feces and can be transmitted via any surface, material, or equipment in contact with the infection. The infection is typically spread via caregiver hands touching a contaminated surface or item without using proper hand hygiene between the infected patient and the newly contaminated surface.

Common characteristics of patients on antibiotic therapy at risk for contracting CDI.[30]

- Prolonged length of stay in a healthcare setting
- Immunocompromised
- Elderly
- Serious underlying illness
- Proton pump inhibitor medications
- Gastrointestinal surgery/manipulation

Assessment/Analysis
- History of present illness
- Medication history
- Observe for signs of dehydration
- Assess for common symptoms of CDI including
  - Watery diarrhea
  - Fever
  - Loss of appetite
  - Nausea
  - Abdominal pain/tenderness

Interventions[30]
- Place patient in private room. If private rooms are not available, these patients can be placed in rooms with other patients (a cohort) with *Clostridium difficile* infection
- Isolation cart/supplies with instructions outside of room
- Implement contact precautions
  - Adhere to strict hand washing practice
  - No gel-based sanitizer as alcohol will not eliminate *C. difficile*
- Discontinue the potential causative antibiotic
- Laboratory studies
  - Stool culture
  - CBC with differential
- Initiate appropriate antibiotic therapy aimed at eliminating the causative bacteria
  - Example: metronidazole, vancomycin, or fidaxomicin
- Provide patient and visitor education regarding proper hand hygiene, isolation needs, and disease management
- Intake and output

Evaluation
- Monitor intake and output, especially fecal elimination
- Patient response to interventions
- Educate patient, family about isolation therapy, hand washing, and transmission precautions

Childhood Diseases

Measles

Measles is a highly contagious, acute viral respiratory illness. There are two types of measles: rubeola and rubella (German measles). Transmission of the measles virus is through nasal secretions, either directly or by respiratory droplet, and the incubation period is from 7 to 21 days. Approximately 14 days post exposure, a maculopapular rash occurs that spreads from the head, as in Figure 9-6, to the trunk and distally to the lower extremities. A person is considered contagious four days before a rash is present and continues to be contagious up to four days after the rash appears.[31] The majority of cases are diagnosed in under-vaccinated or non-vaccinated individuals and related to international travel.

Assessment/Analysis
- Pediatric population: prioritization utilizing the Pediatric Assessment Triage (PAT)[22]
  - General impression
    - Appearance

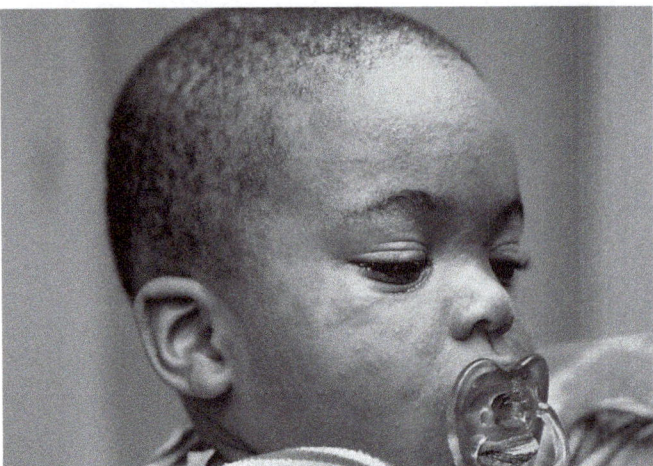

FIGURE 9-6   Measles. School-age child with a morbilliform rash on his face consistent with measles
Reproduced with permission from Knoop KJ, Stack LB, Storrow AB, et al: The Atlas of Emergency Medicine, 4th ed. New York: McGraw-Hill Education; 2016: Photo contributor: Javier A. Gonzalez del Rey, MD.

- Work of breathing
- Circulation to skin
- History of present illness
- Observe for signs of dehydration
- Assess for symptoms including
  - Rash
  - Fever
  - Malaise
  - Cough
  - Runny nose
  - Conjunctivitis
  - Koplik's spots
    - Tiny white spots inside the mouth that may occur 2 to 3 days after symptoms begin
    - Specific to rubeola
- Skin inspection
- Consider consultation with an infectious disease specialist
- Common complications
  - Otitis media, hearing loss
  - Diarrhea
- Severe Complications
  - Pneumonia, the most common cause of death from measles in immunosuppressed populations or young children[31]
  - Encephalitis
  - Death
- Immunization status

Interventions[31]
- Place patient in private, negative airflow room
- Implement airborne precautions
- Supportive care, hydration and nutrition
- Establish IV access for crystalloids and medications as needed
  - IV fluids for symptomatic treatment
- Antipyretics
- Analgesics
- Diphenhydramine for itching
- Maintain oxygen saturation with supplemental oxygen as needed
- I/O
- Provide patient, family and caregiver education
  - Ensure adequate rest, nutrition
  - Provide increased fluid intake
  - Administer antipyretics for fever control (no aspirin in pediatrics)
  - Diphenhydramine for itching
  - Seek medical attention for respiratory, cardiac or neurologic complications
  - Provide vaccination information

Evaluation
- Vital signs
- Monitor I/O
- Patient response to interventions

Mumps

Mumps is a viral illness caused by a paramyxovirus.[32] Mumps has an average incubation period of 16 to 18 days, with a range of 12 to 25 days. Mumps is transmitted through direct contact with respiratory secretions or saliva.

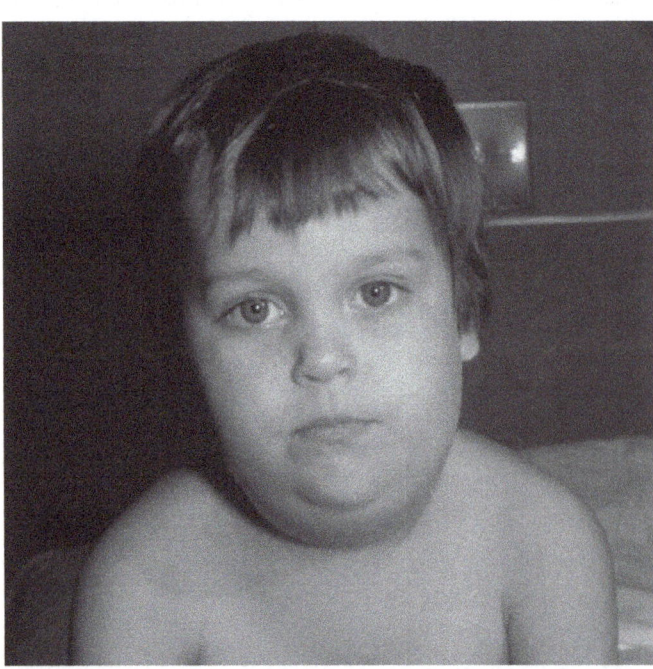

FIGURE 9-7   Parotitis, commonly seen in patients with mumps
Reproduced with permission from Public Health Image Library, CDC.

Assessment/Analysis
- Pediatric population: prioritization utilizing the Pediatric Assessment Triage (PAT)[22]
  - General impression
    - Appearance
    - Work of breathing
    - Circulation to skin
- Monitor for airway compromise
- Assess for symptoms including[32]
  - Fever
  - Parotitis: involves pain, tenderness, and swelling in one or both parotid salivary glands as pictured in Figure 9-7
  - Non-specific upper respiratory tract infection
- History of present illness
- Consider consultation with an infectious disease specialist
- Complications[32]
  - Orchitis: 20 to 50% of post-pubertal males with mumps develop orchitis, which means swollen and painful testicles[1]
  - Deafness
  - Encephalitis: inflammation of the brain
  - Meningitis: inflammation of the tissue covering the brain and spinal cord
  - Oophoritis: inflammation of the ovaries
  - Pancreatitis
- Immunization status
- Observe for signs of dehydration

Interventions[32]
- Maintain patent airway
- Place patient in a private room and implement droplet precautions
- Head of bed elevated
- Maintain oxygen saturation with supplemental oxygen as needed
- Suction as needed related to parotitis and airway management
- Analgesics
- Antipyretics
- Scrotal support and/or ice packs
- Supportive care
- Hydration
- Nutrition
- Provide patient education
  - Ensure adequate rest
  - Nutrition: soft diet to avoid excessive chewing
  - Warm or cold compresses for facial and neck swelling
  - Elevate testes, wear scrotal support, and cold packs to testes
  - Provide increased fluid intake
  - Administer antipyretics for fever control
  - Administer analgesics for pain control
  - Seek medical attention for symptoms related to complications such as orchitis, pancreatitis, encephalitis, or meningitis
  - Provide vaccination education

Evaluation
- Airway patency
- Vital signs
- Patient response to interventions

Pertussis

Pertussis, also known as "whooping cough," is a respiratory illness caused by a gram-negative bacteria, *Bordetella pertussis*.[33] Pertussis is a very contagious bacterium, which attacks the cilia of the upper respiratory system. The bacteria releases toxins causing airway edema, which can be fatal in infants less than a year old. Children are more frequently infected than adults.

The incubation period is 7 to 10 days and is characterized by 3 phases as shown in Figure 9-8: stage I—catarrhal stage, Stage II—paroxysmal stage, and Stage III—convalescent stage.[33] A person with active pertussis is most contagious approximately 2 weeks after the cough begins. Even with vaccination, Pertussis may be contracted if exposure has occurred.

Assessment/Analysis
- Paroxysmal cough
- Pediatric population: prioritization utilizing the Pediatric Assessment Triage (PAT)[22]
  - General impression
    - Appearance
    - Work of breathing
    - Circulation to skin
- Focused assessment including
  - Patent airway management for all ages
  - Effective breathing including auscultation of lung sounds, cough and pediatric assessment for stridor, retractions, or nasal flaring
  - Capillary refill time to assess perfusion in pediatrics
- Vital signs including continual pulse oximetry
- History of present illness
- Immunization status
- Complications[32]
  - Infants <12 months
    - Apnea
    - Pneumonia
    - Seizures
    - Death
  - Adolescents and Adults
    - Weight loss
    - Urinary incontinence

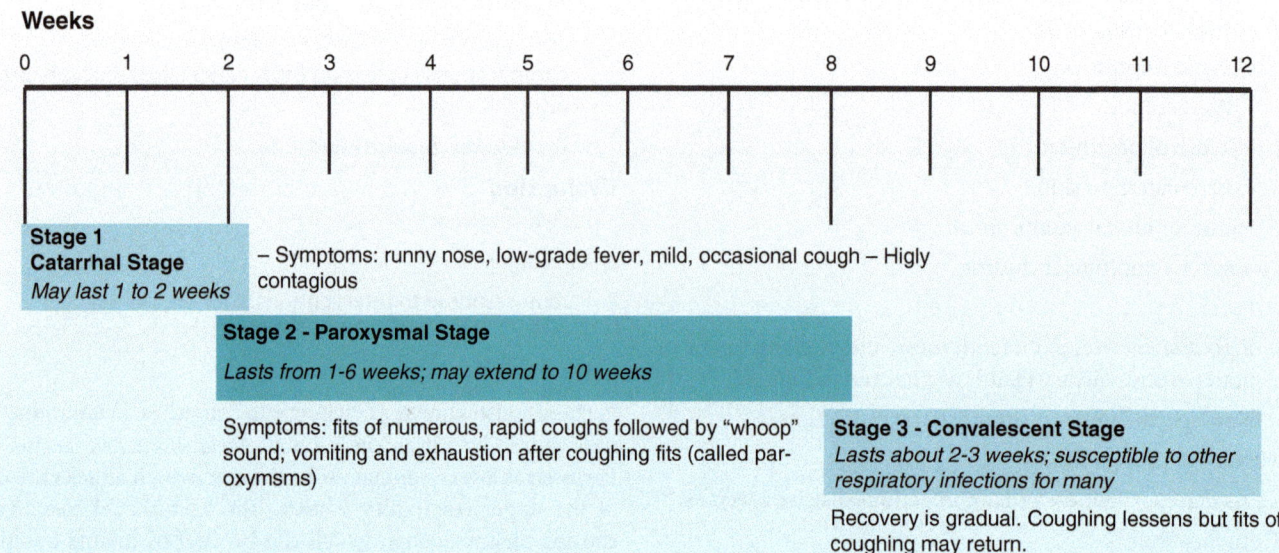

FIGURE 9-8 **Stages of Pertussis with Associated Symptoms**
Reproduced with permission from Centers for Disease Control http://www.cdc.gov/pertussis/about/signs-symptoms.html

- Syncope
- Rib fractures
- Anorexia
- Dehydration
- Encephalopathy
- Pneumothorax

Interventions
- Place patient in private room
- Implement droplet precautions
- Monitor for airway compromise
- Maintain oxygen saturation with supplemental oxygen as needed
- Suction as needed to maintain a patient airway
- Establish IV access for crystalloid fluids and medications as needed
- Hydration
- Nutrition
- Consider consultation with an infectious disease specialist
- Prophylactic antibiotic treatment post contact exposure, as recommended by the CDC[33]
  - Household contacts with infected patient (even if current with immunizations)
  - Infants and pregnant women in their third trimester
  - Immunocompromised persons
  - Persons with chronic health conditions
- Provide patient, family, and caregiver education
  - Adequate rest
  - Fluid intake
  - Transmission of disease
  - Vaccine information
  - When to seek medical treatment related to complications

Evaluation
- Airway patency and effective breathing pattern
- Vital signs
- Patient response to interventions

Chicken Pox

Chickenpox is caused by the varicella-zoster virus (VZV), a member of the herpes virus group, and is very contagious. VZV is spread through the air when an infected person coughs or sneezes. It is also spread by touching or breathing the virus particles released by chickenpox blisters.[34] A person may develop a mild fever and is contagious from 1 to 2 days before the outbreak of the chickenpox rash and is contagious until all the blisters have formed scabs. Chicken pox may develop 10 to 21 days post exposure. A rash develops that is generalized and rapidly progresses from macules, to papules, to vesicular lesions before the blisters crust and scab over. Typically, the rash appears on the head, chest and back, then spreads to the rest of the body. After a primary infection, VZV stays in the sensory nerve ganglia as a latent infection. Reactivation of the latent infection then causes herpes zoster (shingles).[34]

Assessment/Analysis
- Pediatric population: prioritization utilizing the Pediatric Assessment Triage (PAT)[22]
  - General impression
    - Appearance
    - Work of breathing
    - Circulation to skin

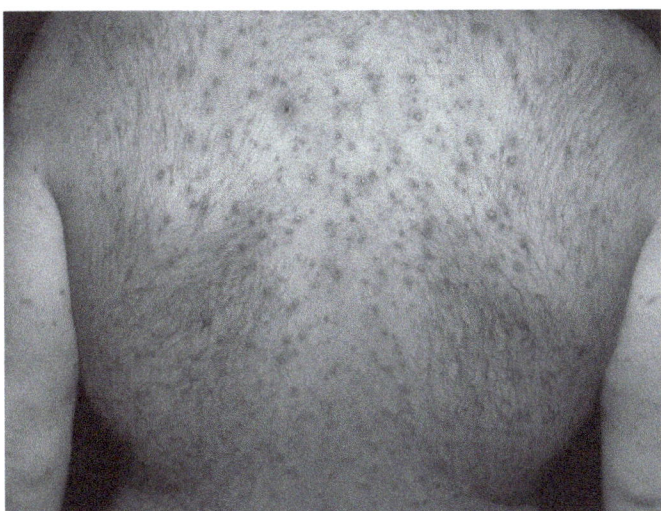

FIGURE 9-9 Characteristic rash associated with VZV
Used with permission from VisualDx.

- Assess for common symptoms associated with VZV including
  - Recent exposure to VZV
  - Fever
  - Malaise
  - Rash including characteristics, onset, and location. See Figure 9-9 for an example of VZV rash
- History of present illness
- Immunization status
- Complications[34]
  - Bacterial infection of the skin and soft tissue in children
  - Pneumonia in adults
  - Immunocompromised patients are at risk for developing
    - VZV dissemination to the visceral organs
    - Pneumonia
    - Hepatitis
    - Encephalitis
    - Disseminated intravascular coagulopathy (DIC)
  - Pregnant women are at risk for developing[34]
    - Pneumonia
    - Increased risk of mortality
    - First or Second trimester fetal risk of congenital varicella syndrome
    - Delivery with VZV, the infant is at risk for neonatal varicella

Interventions
- Place patient in private, negative airflow room
- Implement airborne precautions
- Caregiver should have evidence of immunity
- Support patent airway and effective breathing as needed
- Continual pulse oximetry
- Antipyretics
- Diphenhydramine for itching
- May consider antiviral agents for complicated cases
- Hydration
- Nutrition
- Supportive care
- Provide patient, family, and caregiver education
  - Adequate rest
  - Fever control
  - Diphenhydramine for itching
  - Fluid intake
  - Transmission of disease
  - Vaccine information
  - When to seek medical treatment related to complications

Evaluation
- Vital signs
- Patient response to interventions

Herpes Zoster

Herpes zoster, also known as shingles, is caused by the reactivation of the varicella-zoster virus (VZV). This is the same virus that causes chickenpox. Once a person has had chickenpox, the virus becomes dormant in the dorsal root ganglia. VZV can reactivate later in life, causing a very painful and itchy maculopapular rash. The outbreak commonly appears on the trunk and follows a unilateral dermatome. Within 48 hours of the onset of pain, the tiny blisters erupt along the affected dermatome.[26] Transmission is caused by direct contact with the lesions. The lesions are infectious until dry and crusted over.[35]

Assessment/Analysis
- History of present illness including history of chicken pox
- Immunization status
- Assess for common symptoms associated with herpes zoster including[35]

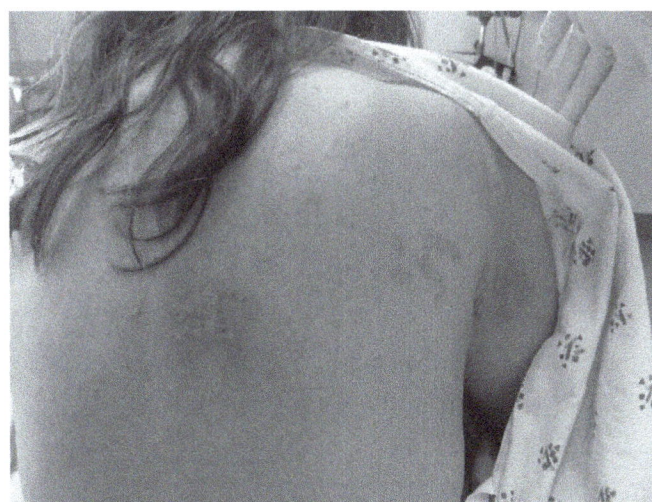

FIGURE 9-10 Characteristic rash associated with Herpes zoster
Used with permission from the University of North Carolina Department of Dermatology.

- A unilateral rash in one or two adjacent dermatomes commonly appears on the trunk. The rash does not cross the body's midline and is usually painful, itchy, or tingly. The rash develops into clusters of clear vesicles as pictured in Figure 9-10. New vesicles continue to form over three to five days and progressively dry and crust over. These symptoms may precede the rash onset by days or weeks. Healing may take up to four weeks and can leave permanent pigment changes and scarring
  - Headache
  - Photophobia
  - Malaise
- Complications[35]
  - Herpes zoster ophthalmicus, includes involvement of the eye and trigeminal nerve
  - Bacterial superinfections of the lesions
  - Cranial and peripheral nerve palsies
  - Visceral involvement
    - Meningoencephalitis
    - Pneumonitis
    - Hepatitis
    - Acute retinal necrosis
  - High risk population includes
    - Immunocompromised
    - Post transplantation patients
    - Age > 50 years

Interventions
- Place patient in private room with airborne precautions
- Implement airborne and contact precautions
  - Until all blisters are "dried and crusted"[35]
- Antipyretics
- Antiviral medications
- Hydration
- Nutrition
- Supportive care
- Provide patient, family, and caregiver education
  - Adequate rest
  - Fever control
  - Pain management
  - Diphenhydramine for itching
  - Transmission of disease
  - Vaccine information
  - When to seek medical treatment related to complications

Evaluation
- Vital signs
- Patient response to interventions

Diphtheria

Diphtheria is caused by the pathogen *Corynbacterium diphtheriae* and is an infection of the mucous membranes. Before vaccinations in the US, diphtheria was a major cause of illness and death among children. Currently, diphtheria cases are still reported globally in countries lacking immunization resources. The incubation period of diphtheria ranges from 1 to 10 days and transmission occurs through respiratory droplets.[36]

Assessment/Analysis
- Pediatric population: prioritization utilizing the Pediatric Assessment Triage (PAT)[22]
  - General impression
    - Appearance
    - Work of breathing
    - Circulation to skin
- History of present illness
- Assess for common symptoms association with diphtheria including[36]
  - Low grade fever
  - Sore throat
  - Airway obstruction related to a membranous covering of the mucous membranes, which may affect the tonsils, pharynx and/or larynx
- Complications from diphtheria may include[36]
  - Airway obstruction
  - Myocarditis
  - Polyneuropathy
  - Paralysis
  - Respiratory failure
  - Pneumonia
- Immunization status
- Consider consultation with an infectious disease specialist

Interventions
- Place patient in private room
- Implement droplet precautions
- Maintain a patent airway
- Supplemental oxygen to maintain oxygen saturation
- Suction as needed
- Supportive care
- Establish IV access for crystalloid fluids and medications as needed
- Hydration
- Nutrition
- Administer medications as ordered
  - Diphtheria antitoxin: consult Centers for Disease Control (CDC) if administering
  - Erythromycin[36]
- Administer vaccination if indicated

- Provide patient, family, and caregiver education
  - Adequate rest
  - Fever control
  - Fluid intake
  - Transmission of disease
  - Vaccine information
  - When to seek medical treatment related to complications

Evaluation
- Airway and ventilation status
- Vital signs
- Patient response to interventions

Multi-Drug Resistant Organisms (MDROs)

MRSA

Methicillin-resistant Staphylococcus aureus (MRSA) is a type of bacteria resistant to many antibiotics. MRSA in the community setting (CA-MRSA) is typically associated with skin infections, such as pimples or boils.[37]

However, in a medical setting, the infection known as health care-associated MRSA (HA-MRSA) may cause life threatening bloodstream infections, pneumonia, and surgical site infections. Skin infection caused by MRSA usually starts as swollen and sometimes painful red bumps. They may be warm to touch, have pus or other drainage, and the patient may be febrile. The infection may spread into bones, joints, surgical wounds, bloodstream, heart valves, and lungs.[37]

Both healthcare-acquired and community-acquired MRSA respond to specific antibiotic therapy when treatment is indicated. Prevention is key to controlling the spread of MRSA.

Assessment/Analysis
- History of present illness
- Increased index of suspicion with presenting complaint of "spider bite"[37]
- Exposure to known infection
- Assess for risk factors
  - Patients at risk for CA-MRSA are those participating in contact sports and people living in crowded or unsanitary conditions
  - Patients most at risk of HA-MRSA are those being hospitalized, having an invasive procedure, or residing in a long-term care facility
- Common symptoms of MRSA include
  - Previous documented history of MRSA
  - Known exposure to MRSA
  - Known high risk situation
  - Lesion with redness, swelling, warmth, purulence or visible drainage
- Past medical history
- Consider consultation with an infectious disease specialist

Interventions
- Implement contact precautions
- Additional isolation precautions based on source of infection
- Incise and drain the lesion if purulent[38]
  - Presence of fluctuant or palpable fluid filled cavity
  - Yellow or white center
  - Central point or "head" draining pus
- Laboratory studies
  - Wound culture
- Antibiotic Therapy[38]
  - Antibiotic treatment is recommended for severe or extensive disease, multiple site involvement, cellulitis, or systemic involvement
  - Antibiotic treatment as recommended by the CDC may include clindamycin, trimethoprim-sulfamethoxazole (TMP-SMX), doxycycline, or vancomycin depending on the circumstances and severity of the infection
- Provide patient, family, and caregiver education
  - Hand hygiene
  - Environmental cleaning
  - Education regarding transmission of the disease
  - Emphasis on prevention
  - Keep wounds covered
- Management is aimed at prevention
  - Hand hygiene
  - Prudent use of antibiotics by clinicians
  - Early detection and prompt reporting of MRSA via hospital developed infection control plan

Evaluation
- Patient response to interventions
- Patient verbalizes understanding of treatment plan

Vancomycin-Resistant Enterococci (VRE)

Enterococci bacteria is normally present in the human intestines and in the female genital tract. The bacteria can sometimes be colonized in these environments, causing infection of the urinary tract, bloodstream, or from wounds associated with catheters or surgical procedures. In some cases, the enterococci have become resistant to standard treatment, such as the drug vancomycin, hence the name vancomycin-resistant enterococci. VRE mostly occurs in the hospital setting, known as a hospital acquired infection (HAI). Contaminated hands of caregivers and contaminated surfaces are the culprits for spreading VRE.

Assessment/Analysis
- History of present illness
- Assess for VRE based on known patient risk factors including[39,40]
  - Patients who have had surgical procedures such as abdominal or chest surgery
  - Patients who have invasive devices such as indwelling catheters or central venous catheters

- Past Medical History
  - Patient who have tested positive with VRE
  - Patients previously treated with vancomycin or other long-term antibiotics, especially when hospitalized

Interventions[39,40]

- Immediate and strict implementation of infection control measures
- Contact precautions
- Medication treatment with antibiotics other than vancomycin
  - Patients with colonized VRE, but have no symptoms do not need treatment
- Specimen culture to determine susceptibility
- Removal of indwelling catheter for bladder/urine VRE
- Management is aimed at prevention including
  - Hand hygiene
  - Prudent use of vancomycin by clinicians
  - Early detection and prompt reporting of VRE via hospital developed infection control plan
- Consider consultation with an infectious disease specialist
- Provide patient, family, and caregiver education
  - Hand hygiene
  - Environmental cleaning
  - Education regarding transmission of the disease
- Emphasis on prevention
  - Hand hygiene
  - Prudent use of vancomycin by clinicians
  - Early detection and prompt reporting of VRE via hospital developed infection control plan

Evaluation

- Patient response to interventions
- Patient verbalizes understanding of treatment plan

Tuberculosis

Tuberculosis (TB) is a respiratory disease caused by *Mycobacterium tuberculosis*.[41] However, TB can also attack any part of the body, such as the kidney, spine, or brain. TB is spread through the air via respiratory droplets from one person to another. It is classified as either active, also known as "infectious," or inactive, also known as "latent." TB in the latent form does not cause the person to appear sick. Patients with latent TB are not infectious and do not spread the bacteria to others. However, if or when the TB bacteria becomes active, the patient becomes sick and infectious. Only persons with active TB can spread the disease. Persons at risk for developing the disease include anyone who has recently been infected with the TB bacteria and anyone immunocompromised. TB is prevalent among the homeless, and people living in overcrowded conditions, such as shelters and jails.

Assessment/Analysis

- History of present illness
  - Including recent travel to TB endemic areas
- Assess for common symptoms of TB including
  - Cough with hemoptysis or sputum
  - Chest pain
  - Fever
  - Chills
  - Night sweats
  - Weight loss
  - Decreased appetite
  - Weakness/fatigue
- Past Medical History

Interventions[41]

- Place patient in private, negative airflow room
- Implement airborne precautions
- Laboratory studies
  - CBC with differential
  - Serum chemistries with liver function tests
  - Sputum for acid-fast bacillus (AFB) smear and culture
  - Nasopharyngeal swab
  - Mantoux skin test
- Chest X-ray
- Establish IV access for crystalloid fluids and medications as needed
- Antitubercular Medications[41]
  - Rifampin
  - Isoniazid
  - Ethambutol
  - Pyrazinamide, for active TB disease
  - Rifapentine
- Consider consultation with an infectious disease specialist
- Patient/family and caregiver education
  - Symptoms of TB
  - Transmission of TB
  - Importance of medication compliance (course of antibiotics may be 3 to 6 months)
- Anticipate hospital admission

Evaluation

- Patient response to interventions
- Patient verbalizes understanding of treatment plan

REFERENCES

1. Lazear SE, Medical emergencies. In: Hoyt KS, Selfridge-Thomas J, eds. *Emergency Nursing Core Curriculum*. 6th ed. Philadelphia, PA: Elsevier Saunders; 2007:483–509.
2. Campbell RL, Li JT, Nicklas RA, et al. Emergency department diagnosis and treatment of anaphylaxis: a practice parameter. *Annals of Allergy, Asthma & Immunology*. 2014:599–608. doi:10.1016/j.anai.2014.10.007
3. Hunt S. Hematologic/oncologic emergencies. In: Hoyt KS, Selfridge-Thomas J, eds. *Emergency Nursing Core Curriculum*. 6th ed. Philadelphia, PA: Elsevier Saunders; 2007:409–437.

4. Crowther M, Chan YL, Garbett IK, et al. Evidence-based focused review of the treatment of idiopathic warm immune hemolytic anemia in adults. *Blood.* 2011;118(15):4036–4040. doi:http://dx.doi.org/10.1182/blood-2011-05-347708

5. Berentsen S, Tjønnfjord GE. Diagnosis and treatment of cold agglutinin mediated autoimmune hemolytic anemia. *Blood reviews.* 2012;26(3): 107–115. doi: 10.1016/j.blre.2012.01.002

6. Kemp WL, Burns DK, Brown TG. Hematopathology. In: Kemp WL, Burns DK, Brown TG, eds. *Pathology: The Big Picture.* New York, NY: McGraw-Hill; 2008.

7. Papadakis MA, McPhee SJ. Leukemia, acute. In: Papadakis MA, McPhee SJ, eds. *Quick Medical Diagnosis & Treatment 2016.* New York, NY: McGraw-Hill; 2016.

8. Ferri FF. Ferri's Clinical Advisor 2016, 5 Books In 1. Elsevier; 2015.

9. Shaffer RW, Santen SA. Acquired bleeding disorders. In: Tintinalli JE, Stapczynski J, Ma OJ, et al. *Tintinalli's Emergency Medicine: A Comprehensive Study Guide.* 8th ed. (Book and DVD). New York, NY: McGraw-Hill; 2016.

10. Kuiper BL. Fluid and electrolyte abnormalities. In: Hoyt KS, Selfridge-Thomas J, eds. *Emergency Nursing Core Curriculum.* 6th ed. Philadelphia, PA: Elsevier Saunders; 2007:361–387.

11. Petrino R, Marino R. Fluids and electrolytes. In: Tintinalli JE, Stapczynski J, Ma OJ, et al, eds. *Tintinalli's Emergency Medicine: A Comprehensive Study Guide.* 8th ed. (Book and DVD). New York, NY: McGraw-Hill; 2016.

12. Mount DB. Fluid and electrolyte disturbances. In: Kasper D, Fauci A, Hauser S, et al., eds. *Harrison's Principles of Internal Medicine.* 19th ed. New York, NY: McGraw-Hill; 2015.

13. World Health Organization (WHO). *Diarrhoeal Disease Fact Sheet N330.* www.who.int/entity/mediacentre/factsheets/fs330/en/. Published April 2013. Accessed May 28, 2016.

14. Idrose A. Adrenal insufficiency. In: Tintinalli JE, Stapczynski J, Ma OJ, et al. *Tintinalli's Emergency Medicine: A Comprehensive Study Guide.* 8th ed. (Book and DVD). New York, NY: McGraw-Hill; 2016.

15. Jalili M, Niroomand M. Type 2 diabetes mellitus. In: Tintinalli JE, Stapczynski J, Ma OJ, et al. *Tintinalli's Emergency Medicine: A Comprehensive Study Guide.* 8th ed. (Book and DVD). New York, NY: McGraw-Hill; 2016.

16. Wall SM. Endocrine emergencies In: Hoyt KS, Selfridge-Thomas J, eds. *Emergency Nursing Core Curriculum.* 6th ed. Philadelphia, PA: Elsevier Saunders; 2007:290–309.

17. Powers AC. Diabetes mellitus: management and therapies. In: Kasper D, Fauci A, Hauser S, et al, eds. *Harrison's Principles of Internal Medicine.* 19th ed. New York, NY: McGraw-Hill; 2015.

18. Mathew V, Misgar RA, Ghosh S, et al. Myxedema coma: a new look into an old crisis. *J Thyroid Res.* 2011;2011:493462. doi: http://dx.doi.org/10.4061/2011/493462

19. Jameson J, Mandel SJ, Weetman AP. Disorders of the thyroid gland. In: Kasper D, Fauci A, Hauser S, et al, eds. *Harrison's Principles of Internal Medicine.* 19th ed. New York, NY: McGraw-Hill; 2015.

20. Barnason S, Williams J, Proehl J, et al. Emergency nursing resource: non-invasive temperature measurement in the emergency department. *J Emerg Nurs.* 2012;38(6):523–30.

21. Wang VF. Fever and serious bacterial illness in infants and children. In: Tintinalli JE, Stapczynski J, Ma O, et al, eds. *Tintinalli's Emergency Medicine: A Comprehensive Study Guide.* 8th ed. New York, NY: McGraw-Hill; 2016.

22. Hohenhaus SM. Prioritization: Focused assessment, triage, and decision making. In: Emergency Nurses Association. *Emergency Nurse Pediatric Course (ENPC) Provider Manual.* 4th ed. Park Ridge, IL: Emergency Nurses Association; 2012:51–62.

23. Gucalp R, Dutcher JP. Oncologic emergencies. In: Kasper D, Fauci A, Hauser S, et al, eds. *Harrison's Principles of Internal Medicine.* 19th ed. New York, NY: McGraw-Hill; 2015.

24. Fauci AS, Lane H. Human immunodeficiency virus disease: AIDS and related disorders. In: Kasper D, Fauci A, Hauser S, et al, eds. *Harrison's Principles of Internal Medicine.* 19th ed. New York, NY: McGraw-Hill; 2015.

25. Ballester J, Morrison R. HIV conditions. In: Knoop KJ, Stack LB, Storrow AB, et al, eds. *The Atlas of Emergency Medicine.* 3rd ed. New York, NY: McGraw-Hill; 2010.

26. Papadakis MA, McPhee SJ. Kidney injury, acute. In: Papadakis MA, McPhee SJ, eds. *Quick Medical Diagnosis & Treatment 2016.* New York, NY: McGraw-Hill; 2016.

27. Munford RS. Severe sepsis and septic shock. In: Longo DL, Fauci AS, Kasper DL, et al, eds. *Harrison's Principles of Internal Medicine.* 18th ed. New York, NY: McGraw-Hill; 2012.

28. Merck Manuals Professional Edition. *Sepsis and Septic Shock—Critical Care Medicine.* http://www.merckmanuals.com/professional/critical-care-medicine/sepsis-and-septic-shock/sepsis-and-septic-shock. Published 2015. Accessed May 28, 2016.

29. Survivingsepsis.org. *Surviving Sepsis Campaign Bundles.* 2015. http://www.survivingsepsis.org/Bundles/Pages/default.aspx. Published 2015. Accessed May 28, 2016.

30. Frequently Asked Questions about Clostridium difficile for Healthcare Providers. *Centers for Disease Control and Prevention.* http://www.cdc.gov/hai/organisms/cdiff/cdiff_faqs_hcp.html#a1. Published 2012. Accessed May 28, 2016.

31. For Healthcare Professionals. *Centers for Disease Control and Prevention.* http://www.cdc.gov/measles/hcp/index.html. Published 2015. Accessed May 28, 2016.

32. For Healthcare Providers. Centers for Disease Control and Prevention. http://www.cdc.gov/mumps/index.html. Published 2015. Accessed May 28, 2016.

33. Pertussis (Whooping Cough). Centers for Disease Control and Prevention. http://www.cdc.gov/pertussis/index.html. Published 2016. Accessed May 28, 2016.

34. For Healthcare Professionals. *Centers for Disease Control and Prevention.* http://www.cdc.gov/chickenpox/index.html. Published 2015. Accessed May 28, 2016.

35. Clinical Overview. *Centers for Disease Control and Prevention.* http://www.cdc.gov/shingles/hcp/clinical-overview.html. Published 2014. Accessed May 28, 2016.

36. Clinicians. *Centers for Disease Control and Prevention.* http://www.cdc.gov/diphtheria/clinicians.html. Published 2014. Accessed May 28, 2016.

37. Methicillin-resistant Staphylococcus aureus (MRSA) Infections. *Centers for Disease Control and Prevention.* http://www.cdc.gov/mrsa/healthcare/index.html. Published 2014. Accessed May 28, 2016.

38. MRSA infection—*Mayo Clinic.* http://www.mayoclinic.org/diseases-conditions/mrsa/basics/definition/con-20024479. Accessed May 28, 2016.

39. Healthcare-associated Infections (HAI). *Centers for Disease Control and Prevention.* http://www.cdc.gov/hai/organisms/vre/vre.html#a1. Published 2011. Accessed May 28, 2016.

40. Vancomycin-Resistant Enterococci (VRE). *Vancomycin-Resistant Enterococci (VRE).* http://www.niaid.nih.gov/topics/antimicrobialresistance/examples/vre/pages/default.aspx. Accessed May 28, 2016.

41. Tuberculosis (TB) in Healthcare Settings. *Centers for Disease Control and Prevention.* http://www.cdc.gov/hai/organisms/tb.html. Published 2011. Accessed May 28, 2016.

Practice Questions

Question	Rationale
1. A patient presents to triage with skin reactions of urticarial rash and pruritus after consuming crab cakes. After assessing stable ABCs, what is the priority of care? a. IV Access b. Administer epinephrine 0.01 mL/kg to max dose of 0.5 mg c. Administer oral diphenhydramine d. Set up for anticipated intubation	*Answer: c* This is a minor allergic reaction. Oral Diphenhydramine should be administered to reduce the skin reaction. The patient should be instructed to avoid shellfish in the future and to carry an *epinephrine* auto-injector for future reactions. The other options are reserved for severe reactions or anaphylaxis.
2. A patient presents with headache, nausea and irritability. She has recently started to drink 2 gallons of water daily to "wash out" toxins. What electrolyte imbalance is suspected? a. Hyperkalemia b. Hypernatremia c. Hypokalemia d. Hyponatremia	*Answer: d* The patient is exhibiting signs of low sodium and the excessive water intake would add to the concern. For this reason it is unlikely that she would have an elevated sodium level. Potassium imbalances are not generally impacted by water intake, rather food has more of an influence on this electrolyte.
3. A patient presents with complaints of easy bruising, fatigue, and dizziness with positional changes. What lab tests would would require particular review? a. CBC, chemistry panel, and coagulation studies b. CBC, liver function tests, and coagulation studies c. CBC and chemistry panel d. CBC, troponin, CK-MB	*Answer: b* The patient is demonstrating signs of blood dyscrasia. CBC, liver function tests, and coagulation studies are required to review the imbalance in order to help make a definitive diagnosis and treatment plan.
4. Discharge instructions are being provided to a patient with a new diagnosis of von Willebrand's disease. What statement indicates understanding of discharge instructions? a. "I will take Ibuprofen for pain as needed" b. "I will take a daily baby aspirin to avoid further complications" c. "I cannot take any over the counter medications for discomfort; I must call the provider to get narcotics for any pain I have" d. "I will take acetaminophen for discomfort and contact my provider if I need additional medications"	*Answer: d* The patient has a bleeding disorder and should not take OTC NSAIDs. The only OTC pain medication appropriate for this patient is acetaminophen.

Question	Rationale
5. A homeless patient presents with Hemoglobin S complications. He is experiencing dehydration with significant pain. What is the priority of care? a. Provide warming measures, oxygen, IV fluids, and pain management b. Get a stat CBC and type and cross for blood product administration c. Institute universal precautions and monitor for signs of bleeding d. Provide warming measures, cardiac monitoring, and antibiotics	*Answer: a* This patient is in sickle cell crisis requiring rewarming, adequate oxygenations, rehydration, and pain control. Sickle cell disease results in Hemoglobin S deoxygenation due to cold exposure, low hemoglobin levels, infection, or dehydration, a sickling crisis may occur. Sickling occurs from deoxygenated red blood cells changing from biconcave discs to a rigid crescent shape. Crescent shaped cells are not able to pass through microcirculation and cause obstructed capillary blood flow.
6. The trauma patient with multiple injuries is hypotensive, tachycardic, with cool pale skin despite 2000 mL bolus of isotonic fluids. He is suspected of being in early DIC. What actions should be taken? a. Send him to CT to determine the source of bleeding b. Administer blood products (FFP, Platelets, cryoprecipitate) anticipate implementation of massive transfusion protocol c. Administer additional fluids until his VS improve d. Send him to the OR to correct source of bleeding	*Answer: b* This patient requires replacement of clotting factors and blood components. Disseminated intravascular coagulation (DIC) is an acquired thromboembolic disorder characterized by generalized activation of the clotting mechanism, which results in the intravascular formation of fibrin and ultimately thrombotic occlusion of small and midsize vessels. The activation of the clotting cascade is the blood's clotting factors is depleted causing abnormal bleeding. The overall management goal is to locate and treat the underlying disorder. However, this patient is showing signs of hypovolemia and requires blood products prior to sending to CT or the OR. Additional fluids will only further dilute the volume in circulation.
7. A mother presents to triage with her 9-month-old son who has had diarrhea and poor feeding for the past 24 hours. The vital signs are T-98.6°F (37°C) rectally; P-120; R-30. His skin is warm and pink with slight tenting and mildly depressed fontanels. His capillary refill is >2 seconds. He has had 10 diaper changes, including 3 bowel movements, in the past 24 hours. What is his level of dehydration based upon this information? a. No signs of dehydration b. Early dehydration c. Mild/Moderate dehydration d. Severe dehydration	*Answer: c* This child is showing signs of mild/moderate dehydration. His VS are within normal parameters for his age. He is showing skin signs of dehydration: tenting and depressed fontanel. The following are WHO guidelines for evaluation of degree of dehydration. **Early dehydration:** Aysmtomatic. **Moderate dehydration:** Thirst, restless or irritable behavior, decreased skin elasticity, and sunken eyes. **Severe dehydration:** Symptoms become more severe including signs of shock, with diminished consciousness, lack of urine output, cool, moist extremities, a rapid and feeble pulse, low or undetectable blood pressure, and pale skin.

Question	Rationale
8. What would be the priority of care for a pediatric patient showing signs of mild to moderate dehydration? a. Triage as level 3 (on a 5-level triage scale) and ask the mother to keep the infant NPO until seen by the provider b. Triage as level 3 (on a 5-level triage scale) and ask the mother to feed the child small volumes of oral electrolyte solution until seen by the provider c. Triage as level 4 (on a 5-level triage scale), place in a room immediately to start IV fluids d. Triage to an urgent care center	*Answer: b* Oral replacement is the best option for rehydration if the child tolerates fluids. Since the child is dehydrated you would not want to make NPO. The child is not severely dehydrated so IV access may be avoided if the child is able to maintain oral intake.
9. A patient presents with mild confusion and GI upset. Vital signs are within normal parameters. The cardiac monitor shows sinus rhythm without ectopy. While reviewing her labs, a calcium level of 8.3 mg/dL is noted. After notifying the provider, what medication regimen can be anticipated to be ordered? a. Oral calcium replacement b. IV calcium gluconate c. PO/PR Sodium polystyrene sulfonate (Kayexalate™) d. Fluid bolus	*Answer: a* This patient has mild hypocalcaemia. Oral replacement would be the most appropriate medication regimen. IV calcium gluconate would be for severe hypocalcaemia. Sodium polystyrene sulfonate (Kayexalate™) is the medication of choice for elevated potassium level. Fluid bolusing is not needed at this time, as her vital signs are stable.
10. EMS arrives with a patient experiencing new onset of confusion and muscle weakness. Her medications include ACE inhibitor and furosemide, potassium replacement and tamoxifen. The cardiac monitor shows tall peaked T waves. What electrolyte imbalance is suspected? a. Hypocalcemia b. Hypercalcemia c. Hypokalemia d. Hyperkalemia	*Answer: d* This patient is showing signs of hyperkalemia, or elevated potassium. The tall peaked T wave is the hallmark cardiac arrhythmia associated with this electrolyte imbalance. Common causes of elevated potassium include medications such as ACE- inhibitors, angiotensin receptor blockers, potassium sparing diuretics, renal disease, and Addison's disease. The most significant effects of elevated potassium are cardiac dysrhythmias. EKG changes associated with low calcium include; prolonged QT, Wide T wave, prolonged ST segments. ECG changes associated with high calcium include; bradycardia, ST changes, widened T, shortened QT. ECG changes associated with low potassium include; T wave depression, PVC, PAC, heart blocks, V fib.
11. A patient has a three day history of new confusion, nausea and vomiting. He is tachycardic, hypotensive, and showing signs of dehydration. His BP is unresponsive to several fluid boluses or to a dopamine infusion. What disease process is suspected? a. Renal failure b. Thyroid storm c. Adrenal crisis d. Graves' Disease	*Answer: c* This person is in adrenal crisis. Adrenal crisis should be suspected in patients who have hypotension unresponsive to fluid resuscitation and vasopressor medications. Thyroid storm or Graves' Disease may have similar presentations. However, the BP is usually responsive to adequate fluid replacement. Renal failure commonly presents with signs of fluid overload.

Question	Rationale
12. A 68-year-old patient with type 2 diabetes recently started on Lantus® to manage her blood sugars. The emergency nurse knows the patient has understood discharge teaching when she makes this statement a. "This is a fast acting medicine, so I should eat right after my injection so my sugar doesn't drop too low. If I become shaky, dizzy or have a headache I should eat a candy bar" b. "This is a fast acting medicine, so I should eat right after my injection so my sugar doesn't drop too low. If I become shaky, dizzy or have a headache I should eat a peanut butter sandwich" c. "This is a slow acting medicine, so I should eat right after my injection so my sugar doesn't drop too low. If I become shaky, dizzy or have a headache I should eat a candy bar" d. "This is a slow acting medicine, so I should take my medicine at bedtime. If I become shaky, dizzy or have a headache I should check my sugar level and eat a sandwich if it is lower than 70"	*Answer: d* Lantus is a long-acting or basal insulin that is administered once daily. So the patient would not need to eat immediately after administration nor would eating a candy bar be the correct action for hypoglycemia.
13. A 13-year-old girl with Type 1 Diabetes is being treated for diabetic ketoacidosis (DKA). The priority of care is to a. Confirm her insulin pump is functioning correctly b. Administer IV insulin c. Administer IV isotonic fluids d. Administer IV potassium chloride at a controlled rate maximum of 40 mEq/hour	*Answer: c* The first priority of care is rehydration. Hyperglycemia leads to osmotic diuresis with dehydration, hyperosmolality, and electrolyte depletion. Initial fluid replacement should be with isotonic solution, followed by fluids containing potassium based upon electrolyte level. Insulin replacement is appropriate after adequate hydration and potassium level is stabilized. While you may be concerned with the insulin pump, the priority of care is to stabilize the patient.
14. A patient presents to the ED with myxedema when they stopped taking thyroid medicine. What vital sign changes are anticipated? a. Bradycardia, hypotension, hypothermia b. Tachycardia, hypertension, hyperthermia c. Tachycardia, BP unresponsive to fluids, normothermia d. Tachycardia, hypotension and hyperthermia	*Answer: a* The vital signs are symptomatic for myxedema related to the lack of thyroid replacement. Hyperthyroid symptoms include tachycardia, hypertension, and hyperthermia. Tachycardia, BP unresponsive to fluids, normothermia describe symptoms of adrenal crisis. Tachycardia, hypotension and hyperthermia describe symptoms of sepsis.
15. A patient consumed a bottle of ibuprofen in an attempted suicide. She is now in renal failure with severe acidosis. What is the most definitive treatment? a. Syrup of ipecac b. Oral lavage with activated charcoal c. Massive IV fluid replacement d. Anticipate arrangement for dialysis	*Answer: d* Ibuprofen is nephrotoxic. The most definitive treatment is dialysis. Syrup of ipecac and activated charcoal are not recommended. She is in renal failure so you would not want to overload her with massive fluid replacement.

Question	Rationale

16. A 2-week-old presents to be triaged with fever of 100.6°F (38.1°C). What actions are most appropriate?
  a. Triage as level 4 (on a 5-level triage scale)
  b. Triage as level 4 (on a 5-level triage scale) and give Tylenol
  c. Triage as level 2 (on a 5-level triage scale), give Tylenol and Motrin
  d. Triage as level 2 (on a 5-level triage scale), room immediately and suspect sepsis
	Answer: d
	Fever greater than 38°C or 100.4°F in infants under age 28 days should be considered emergent and a sign of a serious bacterial infection. This patient should be assigned a high acuity 2 at triage in order for the provider to evaluate the patient immediately. Infants under age 6 months should not receive Motrin.

17. A breast cancer patient receiving chemotherapy presents to the triage desk with a temperature of 100.2°F (37.9°C). She has no complaints or distress other than the fever. What interventions should be initiated?
  a. Have her take a seat in the waiting room. She is stable
  b. Provide protective isolation, obtain orders for blood cultures and antibiotics
  c. Call a sepsis alert and place her in a room
  d. Call her oncologist for advice
	Answer: b
	The patient with immune compromise experiences neutropenia, a decrease in total white cell count and neutrophils. The patient at risk for infection from normal body flora as well as from opportunistic organisms. Classic signs of infection do not occur because the body's immune response is impaired. Consequently, the most significant indicator of infection in the patient with neutropenia is fever. Care of the patient with immune compromise in the emergency department focuses on protecting the patient, identifying the source of infection, and initiating antibiotic therapy immediately.
	Even though she appears stable, a full evaluation is needed. Although she may be septic, she should be placed in isolation for her protection. The oncologist may be consulted but that is not an immediate priority.

18. A patient with hypokalemia is likely to have this dysrhythmia
  a. Torsades de pointes
  b. Atrial fibrillation
  c. Supraventricular tachycardia (SVT)
  d. Junctional
	Answer: d
	Hypokalemia causes conduction delays and decreased automaticity in the myocardium leading to slowed heart rates, including Junctional rhythms. Electrolyte disturbance leading to Torsades is hypomagnesemia. Hypokalemia typically does not lead to atrial fibrillation or SVT.

19. A post-operative bariatric patient arrives to the emergency department reporting 3 days of vomiting. The patient and family also report unsteady gait, double vision, and confusion. The emergency nurse anticipates what intravenous treatment will be ordered?
  a. Dextrose
  b. Fluid resuscitation
  c. Sodium bicarbonate
  d. Vitamin replacement, also known as a "Banana bag"
	Answer: d
	Post-operative patients recovering from bariatric surgery are at risk for malnutrition. Prolonged vomiting increases that risk. The patient is exhibiting symptoms of Wernicke encephalopathy, which is treated with Thiamine (Vitamin B1), a common component of a "banana bag." While dextrose, fluids, and sodium bicarbonate might be needed for the patient, delay of treatment for Wernicke encephalopathy could be life-threatening.

Question	Rationale
20. A patient arrives to the emergency department unable to effectively communicate with ED staff due to generalized, extreme pain. The emergency nurse notices a healing surgical wound on the patient's anterior neck and anticipates replacement of which electrolyte? a. Sodium b. Potassium c. Calcium d. Magnesium	*Answer: c* Hypocalcemia, in this scenario resulted from a parathyroidectomy, can present with paresthesias around the mouth and in hands and feet. More significant hypocalcemia may present with generalized tetany (muscle spasms) in the hands, feet, and large muscles of the body. Calcium replacement is a priority before life-threatening cardiac arrhythmias appear. Sodium, potassium, and magnesium are generally not abnormal following a parathyroidectomy.
21. Family members bring their elderly mother to the emergency department for decreased mental status and refusal to eat. They mention their mother was discharged from the hospital two weeks prior following treatment for pneumonia. The patient's vital signs are T-95.6°F (35.3°C); P-56; R-12; BP-96/56; SpO_2 94% on room air. Following airway management, the priority intervention is a. Hypertonic saline b. Active or Passive rewarming c. Thyroid hormone replacement d. Antibiotics	*Answer: c* Frequently preceded by infectious illness, myxedema coma symptoms include bradycardia, hypotension, hypothermia, and decreased respiratory effort. Treatment priority for this life-threatening disease is airway management followed by replacement of thyroid hormone. While passive rewarming is recommended, active rewarming may increase vasodilation causing further hypotension. Hypertonic saline and antibiotics are not indicated from the information in the scenario.
22. Proper isolation precautions for the nurse performing phlebotomy for a patient with mumps includes a. Gown and gloves b. Gown, gloves, and mask c. Gown, gloves, N-95 (or equivalent) mask d. Gown, gloves, N-95 (or equivalent) mask, and negative airflow	*Answer: b* Mumps is transmitted via coughing, sneezing, or direct contact with infected saliva. Proper isolation precaution type for mumps is droplet isolation, consisting of gown, gloves, and a standard surgical-type or procedure mask. Goggles or other eye protection should be considered for interventions resulting in exposure to respiratory fluids, such as during intubation or a bronchoscopy. Airborne precautions would require an N-95 level mask, which is not indicated for treatment of a patient with mumps.

Question	Rationale
23. An elderly female patient arrives via ambulance with complaints of multiple episodes of watery diarrhea and abdominal tenderness. While assessing the patient and placing her in a gown, her clothing is noted to be grossly contaminated with feces. While reviewing records sent from a long-term care facility, additional information stating she has had a recent, lengthy hospitalization and has been taking prescribed antibiotics for the past week is noted. The patient is alert and oriented with stable vital signs. The patient becomes anxious, tearful and is incontinent of stool. What measures are implemented while caring for the patient? a. Assist the patient to the bedside commode, instruct the patient to use the call light when further assistance is needed and use hand sanitizer as you leave the patient room b. Provide support while acknowledging the patient's concern and provide peri-care placing an incontinent brief on the patient c. Instruct the patient to calm down and clean the patient will maintaining standard precautions d. Provide support to the patient while acknowledging her anxiety. Provide peri-care while maintaining contact precautions. Assure all caregivers follow strict hand washing practice while caring for the patient	*Answer: d* This patient is at risk for potential *C. difficile* as noted by her complaint of watery diarrhea, abdominal pain, recent hospitalization, and antibiotic therapy. It is important to provide support, maintain standard and contact precautions, and follow strict hand washing practice. *C. difficile* is shed in feces, spread via caregiver hands who have touched a contaminated surface or item. Use of alcohol gel-based hand sanitizer does not kill the bacteria.
24. A mother presents to triage with her 4-year-old son and reports the child may have measles. The only noted symptoms are a cough and runny nose over the past 3 days. The child attends a large daycare. As a triage nurse, what history and symptoms increase suspicion of measles? a. Fever, malaise, and rash noted to the child's face. The child is up to date with immunizations b. Cough, fever, weight loss, and diarrhea c. Nausea, vomiting, and diarrhea with a rash noted to the patient's lower extremities. No history of immunizations d. Fever, malaise, cough, and runny nose. No history of immunizations. A rash noted on a child's face and trunk spreading distally onto the lower extremities	*Answer: d* Fever, malaise, cough, runny nose, and conjunctivitis are symptoms of Measles. Since the child has not received his immunizations, the child is at risk. A maculopapular rash occurs; typically about 14 days post exposure and spreads from the head to the trunk and distally to the lower extremities.

Question	Rationale
25. Three young children in the same family are diagnosed with chicken pox. Discharge instructions noted for this family include all of the information *except* a. Chicken pox is caused by the varicella zoster virus (VZV) and is very contagious b. The rash which develops, is pruritic in nature c. A person may develop a mild fever and is contagious from 1 to 2 days before the outbreak of the chicken pox rash d. There is no risk of exposure to immunocompromised individuals	*Answer: d* An immunocompromised individual diagnosed with chicken pox is at risk for developing complications such as VZV dissemination to the visceral organs, pneumonia, hepatitis, encephalitis, and DIC.
26. A triage nurse would anticipate a diagnosis of shingles with a patient presenting with complaints of a. Painful, bilateral flank pain b. A generalized, urticarial rash; with a history of exposure to chickenpox c. A painful, itchy rash appearing with tiny blisters along a unilateral dermatome of the trunk d. A generalized, pruritic rash that appears to have small blisters	*Answer: c* Herpes Zoster, also known as shingles, is characterized by a maculopapular rash, which is very painful and itchy, and commonly appears on the trunk and follows a unilateral dermatome.
27. A patient presents with urticarial rash, angioedema, and hoarse voice after consuming crab cakes. His airway is patent; what is the priority of care? a. Administer 0.01 mL/kg epinephrine (1 mg/mL concentration) IM to max dose of 0.5 mg b. Administer H1/H2 blockers c. Administer corticosteroid d. Administer oral Diphenhydramine	*Answer: a* The patient is displaying symptoms of anaphylaxis. Once airway patency is established immediate administration of epinephrine is the first priority. Epinephrine in the 1 mg/mL should primarily be given via intramuscular or subcutaneous routes for patient safety. The patient should be instructed to avoid shellfish in the future and to carry an *epinephrine* autoinjector for future reactions. The other options would be the next interventions.
28. A patient presents with a maculopapular rash on his trunk, fever, fatigue, and diarrhea. He states, he is an IV drug user sex worker. What is the likely cause of his symptoms? a. Measles b. MRSA c. HIV d. Herpes Zoster virus	*Answer: c* Given his history and symptoms, he likely has primary HIV infection. MRSA and measles have similar rashes however, the history is highly suspicious for HIV. Herpes Zoster rash has vesicles. This patient should be tested and provided counseling on follow up community resources. He should also be counseled and provided with measures for safe sex practices as well as needle exchange information.

Maxillofacial and Ocular Emergencies

10

Jayne McGrath, MS, RN, CEN, CCRN, CNS-BC and Andi Foley, DNP, RN, ACCNS-AG, CEN

Maxillofacial

Facial injuries may threaten airway patency and ocular emergencies may lead to vision loss. Most of the following content pertains to the secondary survey *after* airway, breathing, and circulation requirements are identified and managed in the primary survey. Although airway, breathing, and circulation (ABCs) are not listed for each illness/injury, they are always the first priority.

Abscesses (Oral and Pharyngeal)

Peritonsillar Abscess

Peritonsillar abscess is a collection of pus adjacent to a tonsil which penetrates the capsule of the tonsil and superior constrictor muscle of the throat. The illness usually presents as progressive pharyngitis with severe throat pain. Peritonsillar abscess is one of the more common soft tissue infections of the neck and accounts for 30% of all abscesses of the head and neck.[1]

Assessment/Analysis
- Drooling, neck swelling
- Trismus (inability to open mouth due to muscle spasm)

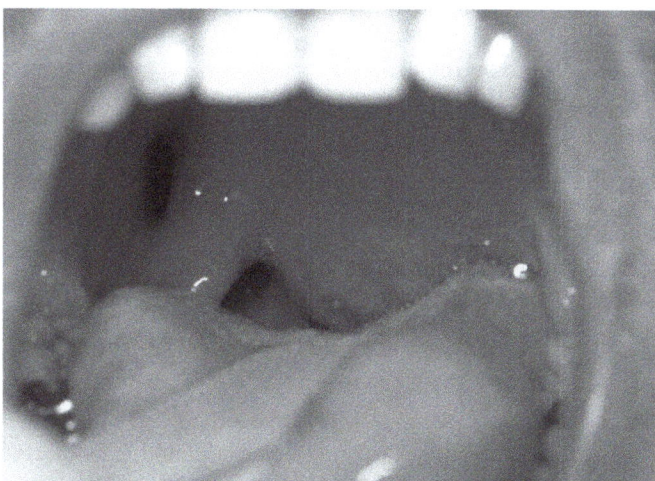

FIGURE 10-1 Peritonsillar abscess with a displaced uvula
Reproduced with permission from Knoop KJ, Stack LB, Storrow AB, et al: The Atlas of Emergency Medicine, 4th ed. New York: McGraw-Hill Education; 2016: Photo contributor: Kevin J. Knoop, MD, MS.

- Dysphagia (difficulty swallowing) or odynophagia (pain with swallowing)
- Throat pain, unilateral
- Ipsilateral otalgia (earache)
- Muffled sounding voice
- Foul breath
- Inspection reveals tonsils enlarged with purulent exudate. Uvula may appear displaced as pictured in Figure 10-1.
- Fever, chills and general malaise, elevated WBC
- Laboratory studies
  - Rapid strep test
  - Throat culture; possible culture of abscess
  - CBC with differential
- Possible CT scan of neck

Interventions
- Establish IV access for crystalloids and medications as needed
- Antibiotics, steroids, and antipyretics
- Pain management
  - Nonsteroidal anti-inflammatory drugs (NSAIDs): may need liquid form
  - Warm water or warm saline rinses
  - Ice pack to neck
- Assist with needle aspiration of abscess

Evaluation
- Patent airway and effective breathing
- Normal hemodynamic status
- Decreased pain

Retropharyngeal Abscess

A retropharyngeal abscess occupies the space posterior to the pharynx and can expand into the mediastinum. It occurs more frequently in children but the incidence in adults has increased in recent years.[2] Adults with a greater risk for developing a retropharyngeal abscess include those who are immunocompromised or have chronic illnesses such as diabetes or alcoholism. This abscess can also occur after ingestion of a foreign body such as a chicken bone or following a pharyngeal procedure such as intubation. Dyspnea and stridor can signal impending airway obstruction.

Assessment/Analysis
- Sore throat often with limited range of neck motion
- Fever
- Dysphagia
- Drooling
- Edema and erythema may be observed upon inspection of the pharynx
- Decreased oral intake
- CBC with differential
  - Increased neutrophils suggests an acute bacterial infection
- Lateral soft tissue X-ray of neck
- CT scan of neck, contrast-enhanced

Interventions
- Monitor for signs of airway occlusion and breathing distress
- Pulse oximetry, cardiac monitor, and supplemental oxygen as needed
- Head of bed elevated
- Establish IV access for crystalloids and medications as needed
- IV antibiotics
- Analgesia
- Anticipate potential need for immediate interventions to restore airway: oral or nasal intubation, or surgical airway (cricothyrotomy)

Evaluation
- Patent airway and effective breathing
- Normal hemodynamic status
- Decreased pain

Dental Conditions and Dental Abscesses

The outer surface of the tooth is enamel, the hardest substance found in the human body. A buildup of dental plaque fosters bacteria growth that can destroy tooth enamel leading to dental caries, also known as cavities.

Under the enamel is dentin, a porous layer surrounding core area, which is the pulp. The pulp contains the neurovascular supply of the tooth. When the pulp is exposed through dental caries or trauma, pain and infection commonly occur.

Pulpitis

Pulpitis, an inflammation of the dental pulp, often arising from dental caries. If left untreated, pulpitis extends through the dentin and can lead to necrosis.

Assessment/Analysis
- Pain assessment
  - Determine duration of symptoms[3]
    - If pain is short duration (lasting seconds) and intermittent, inflammation may be reversible
    - If painful symptoms last minutes to hours, inflammation may be irreversible resulting in pulpal necrosis
- Facial edema
- Foul breath odor
- Inspect of teeth and gums: condition of teeth, erythema, and edema of soft tissue

Interventions
- Establish IV access for crystalloids and medications as needed
- Assist with an anesthetic dental nerve block if indicated
- Analgesics: NSAIDS and narcotics
- Antibiotics
- Follow-up should include dental care referral

Evaluation
- Patent airway and effective breathing
- Decreased pain

Post Tooth Extraction

The inflammation, of the periosteum, often causes pain and swelling for about 24 to 48 hours following a tooth extraction. In addition to pain, bleeding may follow a tooth extraction.

Pain that persists and intensifies following an extraction may be caused by alveolar osteitis or dry socket wherein the alveolar bone is exposed when the clot is dislodged from the socket. This may result in local osteomyelitis.[3]

Assessment/Analysis
- Recent tooth extraction and history
  - Bleeding may occur post extraction
  - If alveolar osteitis occurs, this will typically occur 2 to 3 days post-procedure[3]
- Pain-may be severe
- Presence of bleeding
- History of any tobacco, alcohol, or drug use
- Observe for presence of trismus
  - Can occur directly following extraction[3]
  - From nerve block, perioperative inflammation, or injury to the temporomandibular joint and surrounding muscles
  - Peaks around 24 hours and should subside afterward
  - If trismus does not subside, infection may be present
- Inspect oral mucosa and gums for edema, erythema, and bleeding

Intervention
- Control bleeding
  - Apply folded 2 × 2 gauze pad over the extraction site
  - Instruct patient to clench their teeth, and the pressure from the opposing teeth should provide hemostasis[3]
  - Assist with other procedures designed to control bleeding such as suturing and/or injection of lidocaine with epinephrine
- Establish IV access for crystalloids, blood products, and medications as needed
- Antibiotics
- Pain management: dental block, NSAIDs, and narcotic analgesics
- Refer to dentist or endodontist for follow-up
- Patient education: signs and symptoms of infection, avoidance of spicy, hot or hard foods, follow-up

Evaluation
- Hemostasis
- Decreased pain

Periapical Abscess

When dental caries, also known as a cavity, is left untreated, the cavity can extend down into the pulp of the tooth. With a periapical abscess, the infection extends into the alveolar bone and supporting dental structures.

Periodontal Abscess

Abscesses can form in the gingival tissue (gums) around the tooth with advancing periodontitis. Periodontitis, characterized by inflammation, is a progressive loss of the bone and supporting tooth structures. The gum tissue surrounding the tooth is erythematous and painful. Unlike a periapical abscess, the tooth may be healthy with no dental caries.[4]

Assessment/Analysis
- Pain
- Edema
  - Unilateral neck edema: infection may involve the surrounding soft tissues
- Oral cavity with localized swelling, erythema, and purulence
- Note foul breath
- Fever, chills and general malaise
- Laboratory studies
  - CBC with differential
  - Culture drainage for both aerobic and anaerobic bacteria
- Mandibular panoramic x-ray
- Soft tissue neck X-ray

Interventions
- Establish IV access for crystalloids and medications
- Pain management
  - NSAIDs provide better pain management than narcotics and reduce narcotic use[4]
  - Dental block may also be performed by the provider
- Antibiotics
- Follow-up care to include referral to a dentist or endodontist

Evaluation
- Patent airway and effective breathing
- Normal hemodynamic status
- Decreased pain

Epistaxis

Anterior epistaxis occurs more frequently than posterior epistaxis. The most common site of bleeding occurs at the Kiesselbach's plexus, a group of superficial arteries and veins, located in the anterior area of the nasal septum. Posterior epistaxis often involves the sphenopalatine artery. See Figure 10-2 for nasal arterial anatomic locations. Posterior epistaxis has a higher risk for hemorrhage and/or airway compromise.

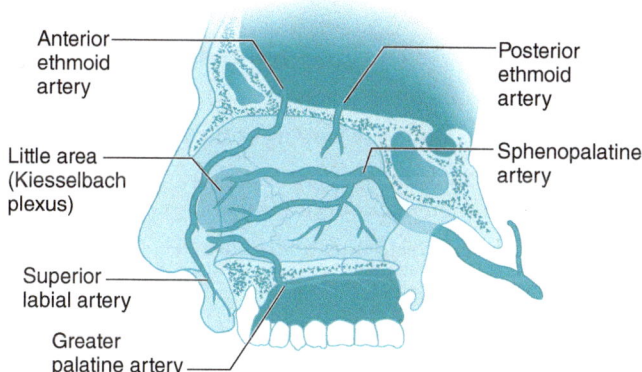

FIGURE 10-2 Nasal arterial blood supply
Reproduced with permission from Tintinalli J, Stapczynski J, Ma OJ, et al: Tintinalli's Emergency Medicine: A Comprehensive Study Guide, 8th ed. New York: McGraw-Hill Education; 2015.

Assessment/Analysis
- Estimated blood loss: onset of bleeding, intermittent versus continuous, saturation of tissues or a towel
- Common risk factors
  - History of anticoagulants
  - Herbal supplements containing anticoagulation properties such as garlic and ginseng[5]
  - Trauma
  - History of intranasal drug abuse (i.e., cocaine)
  - Nose picking
  - Neoplasm

- Common concomitant illnesses
  - Hypertension-poorly controlled[6]
  - Coagulopathy
  - Liver and/or renal dysfunction
  - Thrombocytopenia: primary or drug induced
- Inspect anterior nares and oropharyngeal area for bleeding, edema and erythema
- Laboratory studies
  - CBC
  - Coagulation studies
  - Consider blood bank analysis (Type and Screen/Cross), if bleeding is significant

Intervention
- Uninterrupted manual pressure or nasal clamp for 15 minutes
- High Fowler's position
- Encourage patient to lean forward to help prevent swallowing of blood which may induce nausea and vomiting
- Establish IV access for crystalloids, blood products, medications as needed
- Pulse oximetry; cardiac monitor if cardiac history or significant blood loss
- Suction readily available
- Oxygen, as indicated
- Assist with interventions to control bleeding
  - Procedural sedation and anesthesia as indicated
  - Remove clots with nose blowing or suction
  - Topical vasoconstrictors (oxymetazoline, phenylephrine, cocaine) and anesthetic agents (lidocaine)
  - Chemical cauterization with silver nitrate
  - Nasal packing
    - Petroleum jelly impregnated gauze
    - Nasal tampons which expand with hydration
    - Gelfoam™ and Surgicel™ contain hemostatic properties[7]
- Electrocautery (usually performed in the operating room)
- Antibiotics. After nasal packing, broad-spectrum antibiotic may be prescribed for the prevention of toxic shock syndrome[5]
- Otolaryngology consultation if indicated
- Anticipate hospitalization for airway and cardiac monitoring if posterior packing is inserted
- Instruct patient to avoid things that increase the risk of recurrent bleeding: nose blowing, sneezing, heavy lifting, bearing down, hot or spicy foods

Evaluation
- Patent airway and effective breathing
- Hemostasis
- Hemodynamically stable
- Pain control

Facial Nerve Disorders

Bell's Palsy (Facial Nerve Palsy)

Bell's palsy is unilateral facial muscle weakness or paralysis resulting from dysfunction of the seventh cranial nerve. It is often idiopathic but may be related to a viral infection, inflammation, trauma, or illnesses or medical conditions such as diabetes. The onset is usually sudden although some symptoms, such as decreased tearing and posterior ear pain, may present before facial paralysis.[8] The symptoms are not usually permanent but may take months to completely resolve.

Assessment/Analysis
- Acute onset of unilateral facial weakness and/or paralysis[8]
  - Asymmetrical facial expression
  - Lagging eyelid which does not close completely
  - Drooping of mouth and asymmetrical smile
- Pain-headache, facial discomfort
- Decreased ability to taste
- Drooling

Interventions
- Protect the affected eye
  - Lubricating topical eye drops (artificial tears)
  - Patch to keep eyelid closed for protection
- Analgesics
- Steroids: greater likelihood of recovery if administered within 72 hours of onset of symptoms[8]
- Antiviral medications, as indicated
- Follow-up ophthalmology referral

Evaluation
- Decreased pain
- Intact cornea and visual acuity in affected eye

Trigeminal Neuralgia

Trigeminal neuralgia (Tic Douloureux) is characterized by sudden bursts of severe electric-shock type pain along the pathway of the fifth cranial nerve. The paroxysms of pain usually subside abruptly and alternate with pain free intervals.

Assessment/Analysis
- Pain-intermittent, sudden onset of electric-shock like pain with intervals of no pain
- Pain may be triggered by chewing, lightly touching the face, or slight breeze blowing across the face[8]
- Possible MRI

Interventions
- Carbamazepine can be effective for decreasing pain[8]
- Regional anesthetic block
- Referral treatment may include surgical intervention

Evaluation
- Decreased pain

Foreign Body

Laryngeal Foreign Body

Foreign bodies of the airway can cause a partial or complete obstruction and are more common in children. If the person is able to speak or cough and is moving air, he/she should be encouraged to use their efforts to relieve the partial obstruction. If the person's efforts do not relieve the obstruction, and their efforts for air exchange are ineffective, immediate assistance such as the abdominal or chest thrusts are required to relieve the airway obstruction.

Radiographic imaging may help locate the object. Treatment decisions are made based on what is causing the obstruction and where it is located. Direct laryngoscopy and Magill forceps are frequently used to remove foreign objects from the upper airway.[9]

Assessment/Analysis
- Onset of symptoms while eating
- Coughing: sudden onset
- Wheezing: unilateral or bilateral
- Difficulty in swallowing
- Shortness of breath or difficulty breathing
- Changes in voice and/or difficulty speaking
- Aphonia
- Inspect airway and mouth for debris, signs of trauma, and foreign body
- Breathing pattern: labored, tachypnea, increased work of breathing, retractions
- Pulse oximetry
- Tachycardia
- Skin color and temperature: pale, cyanotic
- Skin temperature: cool, diaphoretic
- Laryngoscopy
- X-ray, possible CT scan

Interventions
- Perform or assist with removal of the foreign body
  - Finger sweep only if you can see and reach the object
  - Abdominal or chest thrusts
- Assist with procedures to visualize/remove foreign body
- Assist with insertion of airway or surgical airway, if required
- Supplemental oxygen if indicated
- Establish IV access for crystalloids and medications as needed

Evaluation
- Patent airway and effective breathing
- Decreased pain

Otic Foreign Bodies

Foreign bodies of the ear are more common in young children[10] but can also occur in adults. Objects vary and can range from organic matter such as sand to inanimate objects such as a toy part or insects. The object can lead to inflammation and edema possibly obstructing the cerumen and sebaceous glands.[10]

Assessment/Analysis
- Otorrhea-drainage from ear
- Pain
- Decreased hearing
- Foul odor from affected ear[9]
- Children may display increased irritability, crying, and pulling on the affected ear
- Otoscopic exam: presence of foreign body, possibly erythema, drainage and edema[10]

Interventions
- Irrigation (contraindicated with ruptured tympanic membrane)
- Type of foreign body will impact method of removal
  - Vegetable matter—do not irrigate—cause more swelling of the matter which can lead to further occlusion
  - Insect
    - Should be killed before removing by instilling alcohol or mineral oil[10]
    - Extract with forceps or irrigate
- Analgesia
- Antibiotics
- Possible referral to otolaryngology for failed removal[10]

Evaluation
- Decreased pain
- Improvement of any hearing loss, foul odor, and/or irritability
- Removed foreign body

Infection

Parotitis

Parotitis is inflammation of the parotid glands, the largest of the salivary glands. The etiology may be viral (mumps) or bacterial. Parotitis can also occur when the flow of saliva through the parotid (Stensen) duct is decreased or obstructed. Bacteria may flow retrograde through the parotid duct. Some causes of restricted salivary flow are sialolithiasis (one or more salivary calculus), dehydration, and certain medications such as anticholinergics and diuretics. Other conditions that may predispose one to parotitis are human immunodeficiency virus, diabetes, and malnutrition.

Assessment/Analysis
- Facial edema: unilateral or bilateral
- Mass that is tender with palpation
- Pain
- Erythema
- Trismus
- Fever

- Laboratory studies
  - Culture and sensitivity[8] of purulent parotid duct drainage
  - CBC with differential
- Possible imaging: ultrasound, CT scan

Interventions
- Establish IV access for crystalloids and medications as needed
- Antibiotics
- Analgesics for pain
- Patient education to promote increasing saliva production: increase fluid intake

Necrotizing Ulcerative Gingivitis (NUG)

Necrotizing Ulcerative Gingivitis (NUG), also referred to as Vincent disease or trench mouth, is an aggressive oral infection that is varied but it can be associated with human immunodeficiency virus (HIV) infection, poor hygiene, malnutrition, alcohol, or tobacco use.[3] The infection may be contained to the gingiva or spread through the mouth and lips and facial bones

Assessment/Analysis
- A triad of characteristics are present with this condition: pain, interdental ulceration or necrosis, and bleeding[4]
- Inspection of mouth reveals erythema, bleeding, and possible loose teeth
- Fever and lethargy may be present

Intervention
- Oral rinses of chlorhexidine 0.12% mouthwash or half-strength hydrogen peroxide twice daily help reduce bacteria[4]
- Antibiotics may be prescribed
- Patient education
  - Reinforce good oral hygiene
  - Adequate nutritional intake
  - Importance of follow-up with provider

Evaluation
- Hemostasis
- Decreased pain

Epiglottitis

Epiglottis is an airway emergency historically more common in children than in adults. A common pathogen associated with epiglottis is *Haemophilus influenzae* type b. With the advent of *H. influenzae* type b (Hib) vaccine, the incidence of pediatric epiglottis has significantly decreased. This condition is also noted in adults. *H. influenzae* continues to be the leading pathogen but other bacterial causes include *H. parinfluenzae*, *Streptococcus pneumonia* and *Staphylococcus aureus* (methicillin susceptible and methicillin resistant).[11] Less common causes are viral infections and thermal injuries. There is a high risk of rapidly progressing airway obstruction with epiglottitis.

Assessment/Analysis
- Pharyngitis
- Odynophagia
- Fever
- Tachycardia
- Voice changes
- Drooling
- Respiratory stridor
- Dyspnea when lying supine (Patients may assume a "tripod position," (sitting and leaning forward at the waist)
- Cervical adenopathy with tenderness
- Lateral neck radiograph with swollen epiglottis, also known as the "thumb sign" as pictured in Figure 10-3

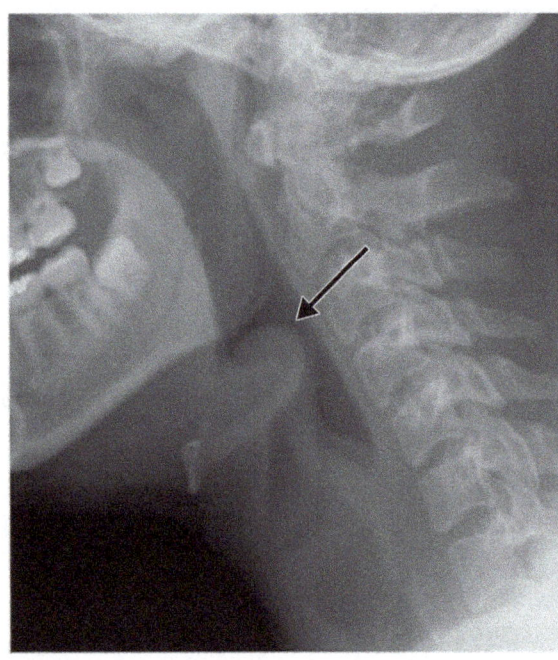

FIGURE 10-3 "Thumb sign" of epiglottitis viewed on lateral neck radiograph
Reproduced with permission from Elsayes KM, Oldham SAA: Introduction to Diagnostic Radiology. New York: McGraw-Hill Education; 2014.

Interventions
- If the patient is a young child, it is essential to keep the child calm and try to avoid precipitating crying. This may mean delaying invasive maneuvers (e.g., rectal temperature, IV access, etc.) until all preparations are in place to intubate or in the operating room for a surgical airway
- When respiratory stridor and other signs of respiratory distress are present, early intubation is indicated[1]
- Cardiac and pulse oximetry monitoring
- Supplemental oxygen if indicated
- Establish IV access for crystalloids and medications
- Antibiotics
- Anticipate need for surgical airway (cricothyrotomy) if intubation fails

Evaluation
- Airway patency and effective breathing pattern
- Decreased pain

Ludwig's Angina (Submandibular Cellulitis)

Typical causes of Ludwig's Angina are dental infections, such as a periapical abscess involving the second and third mandibular molars and extending airway infections such as a peritonsillar abscess. Causative organisms can be aerobic and anaerobic.

The infection spreads bilaterally into the submental (below the chin), submandibular and sublingual areas causing diffuse swelling and tongue elevation. The displaced tongue can lead to dysphagia and dysphasia (difficulty speaking). Since this space is not naturally distensible, the edema can lead to rapid airway deterioration and collapse.[4]

Assessment/Analysis
- Submandibular swelling
- Erythema of submandibular area that can vary from mild to extensive
- Dysphagia
- Dysphasia
- Fever
- Hoarse voice
- Neck pain
- Drooling
- Choking sensation
- Trismus
- Inspect facial and neck area for edema and/or erythema
- Restless and agitation may be signs of airway compromise
- CT scan
- Laboratory studies
  - CBC with differential
  - Erythrocyte sedimentation rate (ESR)
  - ABGs if indicated
  - Culture and sensitivity of exudate
- Soft tissue X-ray of neck and/or CT scan

Intervention
- Assure intubation and surgical airway supplies are readily accessible
- Pulse oximetry and cardiac monitoring
- Establish IV access for crystalloids and medications as needed
  - IV antibiotics
- Assist with hospital admission and/or transfer to operating room for management of a definitive airway

Evaluation
- Patent airway and effective breathing
- Hemodynamic stability
- Decreased pain

Acute Otitis Externa (AOE) "Swimmers Ear"

AOE involves inflammation of the external auditory canal or auricle (pinna) of the ear. More prevalent in warmer weather, AOE has variable causes ranging from allergy, bacteria, viral, fungal, and trauma. Some of the noninfectious causes can involve a contact dermatitis from hearing aids or psoriasis.[12] With proper treatment, AOE usually resolves within a week. Malignant otitis externa is when the infection has extended into the soft tissues around the pinna and possibly into the bone. This rare and serious form of otitis externa is seen primarily in the patient who is immunocompromised or may have diabetes.

Assessment/Analysis
- Pruritus
- Tenderness of the external outer ear[12]
- Pain upon palpation of outer ear, lymph node area, and tragus
- Erythema and swelling of external auditory canal[12]
- Possible decreased hearing
- External auditory canal may have encrustation[12]
- Hearing assessment
- Increased pressure in ear or feeling of fullness
- Otorrhea may be clear or purulent
- Tympanic membrane is usually intact and appears normal with otoscopy

Interventions
- Topical antimicrobials
- Ear wick may be applied: placed in the external canal and facilitates delivery of ear drops
- Topical steroids (if allergic etiology)
- Analgesia
- Patient education
  - Application of prescribed drops to ear(s)
  - Keeping ear canal dry and wearing of ear plugs
  - Avoid use of cotton tipped applicators in ear

Evaluation
- Decreased pain
- Demonstrates knowledge on prescribed home care

Acute Otitis Media (AOM)

More common illness in pediatric patients; however, diagnosis and treatment for AOM is similar for children and adults.[12] Often AOM accompanies upper respiratory infections. As the eustachian tube swells, fluid accumulates within the tube creating a reservoir for bacteria to collect causing an infection that can spread to the middle ear. Pediatric eustachian tubes are shorter and oriented more horizontally which creates a more favorable pathway for bacteria to gain entry into the middle ear.

Assessment/Analysis
- Otalgia (ear pain)
- Fever
- Otorrhea (may be purulent)
- Hearing loss
- Possible tinnitus and/or dizziness
- Erythema of pharynx, and tympanic membrane (TM)
- TM may be red (inflamed) or white or yellow in color
- TM may be bulging or retracted
- Pneumatic otoscopy reveals impaired TM mobility

Interventions
- Analgesics
- Possible antibiotics (if believed to be bacterial origin)
- Follow-up with provider or otolaryngologist specialist

Evaluation
- Decreased pain
- Verbalizes understanding of any prescribed follow-up with provider

Sinusitis

This acute inflammation involves the paranasal sinuses. Since the inflammation usually includes the nasal mucosa, the term "rhinosinusitis" is more accurate.[13] The paranasal sinuses contain a mucociliary lining, and with inflammation sinus secretions accumulate leading to clinical symptoms. Often rhinosinusitis is viral in nature. Leading pathogens that cause bacterial rhinosinusitis are *Haemophilus influenzae* and *Streptococcus pneumonia*. Acute rhinosinusitis typically does not last beyond 4 weeks and if it lasts longer, it may be characterized as chronic rhinosinusitis.

Complications occur when the infection extends into other areas outside the paranasal sinuses. Although rare, meningitis, cavernous sinus thrombosis and intracranial abscess are serious complications of rhinosinusitis. Other serious complications include orbital and periorbital cellulitis, which can lead to blindness.

Assessment/Analysis
- Nasal congestion
- Facial pain usually increases with postural changes, especially bending forward
- Sinus pressure
- Hyposmia (diminished sense of smell)
- Fever
- Cough
- Nausea
- Decreased appetite
- Foul breath
- Erythema and swelling in nasal mucosa
- Nasal drainage-possibly purulent
- Tenderness upon palpation over involved sinus area
- Sinus X-rays
- Sinus cultures rarely collected in the emergency department but may be collected in outpatient if chronic rhinosinusitis is suspected
- CT Scan if complications are suspected

Interventions
- Comfort measures are directed at relieving pain and congestion
- Analgesics
- Nasal and systemic decongestants
- Antihistamines
- Saline irrigation
- Warm packs to face
- Head of bed elevated
- Intranasal steroids
- Mucolytics
- Antibiotics for rhinosinusitis accompanied by fever and lasting more than 7 to 10 days
- Establish IV access for crystalloids and medications as needed for rhinosinusitis with complications

Evaluation
- Airway patency
- Effective breathing pattern

Labyrinthitis

Labyrinthitis typically follows an inner ear infection but can also develop from other causes such as trauma, cardiovascular or neurological disease, drug or alcohol use, allergies, or certain medications. The inflammation can lead to dizziness, vertigo (sensation that the room is spinning) of sudden onset, copious vomiting, and ataxia (unsteady gait).

Assessment/Analysis
- Pressure or fullness in the ear
- Vertigo: may be sudden onset[14]
- Tinnitus
- Disequilibrium: may be debilitating and could last weeks
- Diminished hearing
- Otorrhea
- Nystagmus
- Nausea and vomiting
- If suspected infectious etiology, laboratory studies
  - CBC with differential
  - Blood cultures
  - Possible lumbar puncture
- MRI or CT scan

Interventions
- Establish IV access for crystalloids/medications as needed
- Anxiolytics/Sedatives: benzodiazepines such as diazepam[14]

- Anticholinergic such as meclizine (indicated for vertigo and nausea)[14]
- Antiemetics
- Antibiotics if suspected bacterial origin[14]
- Safety measures to prevent falling from disequilibrium and resting during exacerbation of symptoms
- May need follow-up with otolaryngology[14]

Evaluation
- Increased balance and equilibrium
- Resolution of nausea and vomiting

Meniere's Disease (Endolymphatic Hydrops)

The exact cause of Meniere's disease is unknown but believed to be as a result of excess endolymph (fluid within the cochlea and labyrinth) causing a disturbance in the vestibular system. Typically, Meniere's disease occurs in older men and women.[14] The vestibular disturbance leads to symptoms including severe vertigo, nausea, vomiting diaphoresis, tinnitus, and hearing loss. The symptoms can last for hours or longer and is characterized by exacerbations and remissions.

Assessment/Analysis
- Severe debilitating vertigo during acute exacerbations and difficulty ambulating without falling
- Nausea, vomiting, or diaphoresis
- Headache
- Diaphoresis
- Feeling of fullness or pressure in ear (s)
- Tinnitus

Interventions
- Anticholinergic such as meclizine (antiemetic and antivertiginous properties)
- Antiemetic
- Antihistamine
- Diuretics
- Patient education: safety and fall prevention strategies
- Referral to specialist for follow-up

Evaluation
- Increased balance and equilibrium
- Relief of nausea and vomiting

Ruptured Tympanic Membrane

TM perforations are typically caused by infection. However, other causes including barotrauma can occur with scuba diving, a blast injury or blunt trauma such as a blow to the head. Usually the ruptured TM will heal spontaneously.

Assessment/Analysis
- Pain (The rupture may relieve the middle ear pressure caused by the infection, with the patient reporting a decrease in pain)
- Otorrhea (purulent, clear, or bloody)
- Hemotympanum (blood seen behind intact TM): may be observed with barotrauma or blunt trauma[9]
- History of illness, previous illness, and/or fever
- Tinnitus
- Dizziness
- Hearing loss
- Possible ataxia
- Otoscopy shows a tear, defect, or slit in the TM
- Signs of trauma around ear, depending on cause
- X-rays: skull and spine, if suspected or actual trauma

Intervention
- Assist provider with removal of blood and debris[9]
- Analgesics
- Antibiotics, if indicated
- Instruct patient to keep ear canal dry
- Follow-up with Otolaryngologist

Evaluation
- Decreased pain
- Ear canal is free of debris, foreign body, and/or blood

Temporomandibular Joint (TMJ) Dislocation

TMJ dislocation can be caused by varied factors. Non-trauma causes such as yawning, chewing, or dental work can cause a TMJ dislocation as well as a mandibular fracture or other blunt trauma. Malocclusion or teeth grinding may be risk factors. Dislocation can be unilateral or bilateral.

Assessment/Analysis
- History of activity prior to observed symptoms and mechanism of injury
- Pain: may be localized to area anterior of the tragus[8]
- Decreased range of motion with mandible
- Inability to close mouth: mucous membranes may become dry
- Malocclusion
- Drooling
- Speaking difficulties
- Palpation at the TMJ elicits increased pain
- X-ray: panoramic view
- MRI for TMJ dislocation from traumatic injury[15]

Interventions
- Establish IV access for crystalloids and medications as needed
- Analgesics
- Assist with manual reduction of mandible
- Assist with procedural sedation, as indicated
- Post-reduction x-ray

- Patient education
  - Diet may include soft foods to allow for joint rest[15]
  - Precipitating factors (if applicable): jaw relaxation, avoiding wide yawning, and/or teeth clenching

Evaluation
- Airway patency
- Effective breathing
- Decreased pain with returned range of motion
- Post reduction films demonstrating normal alignment of TMJ

Trauma

Like any trauma or injury, the approach to facial trauma requires airway, breathing and circulation as top priorities. Since these priorities are for all injuries, they will not be relisted below for the facial injuries but rather implied that this will be the first assessment and management. Assisting to establish an airway may be an immediate intervention. Inspect the mouth for loose teeth and other debris. Displaced teeth can be inadvertently pushed further into the bronchi during intubation and may lead to impaired ventilation.

Zygomatic Fractures

These fractures are often a result of blunt trauma involving a forceful blow. Sometimes referred to as the "cheek bone" the zygoma forms the lateral and inferior orbital wall. Zygomatic fractures often occur concomitantly with an orbital floor fracture, also called a blowout fracture.

Assessment/Analysis
- Mechanism of injury
- Pain
- Facial edema/deformity
- Facial wounds/bleeding
- Periorbital edema and ecchymosis
- Visual impairment (diplopia, blurred vision)
- Bleeding
- Paresthesia on affected side
- Crepitus
- Malocclusion[15]
- Trismus

- Facial X-rays
- Face and head CT scans[15]

Intervention
- Cardiac and pulse oximetry monitoring
- If no suspicion of cervical trauma and hemodynamic stability, head of bed elevated
- Establish IV access for crystalloids, blood products, medications and as needed
- Antibiotics
- Analgesics
- Tetanus immunization, as indicated
- Hospital admission for definitive treatment: possible surgical repair and open reduction
- Suspected eye involvement and/or visual impairment should have urgent ophthalmic consultation[16]

Evaluation
- Airway patency
- Effective breathing
- Hemodynamic stability
- Decreased pain

LeFort Fractures

LeFort fractures are a subset of maxillary fracture patterns. They result from a forceful impact and are often associated with other serious injuries. They can be either unilateral or bilateral sides of the face but all of the fracture patterns involve the pterygoid plates, the wing-shaped region of the sphenoid bone.[17]

- ❖ **LeFort I** is a transverse fracture that separates the lower maxilla from the nasal septum and pterygoid (see Figure 10-4). The patient's maxilla is freely movable similar to loose fitting upper dentures. Facial edema, including periorbital edema and ecchymosis, are usually present along with possible maloccluded teeth
- ❖ **LeFort II** is a pyramidal shaped fracture extending up through the maxilla and across the medial orbits and nasal bones. Similar presentation of symptoms occurs as in the LeFort 1 fracture with the additional findings of crepitus around the orbital perimeters, and possible cerebrospinal fluid (CSF) leaking

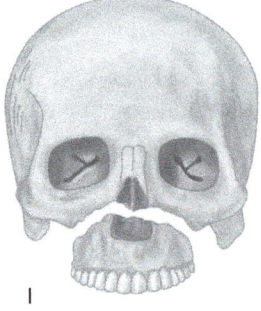
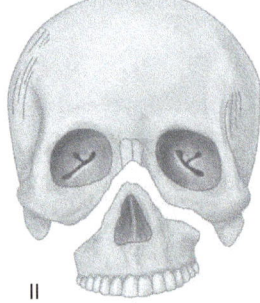
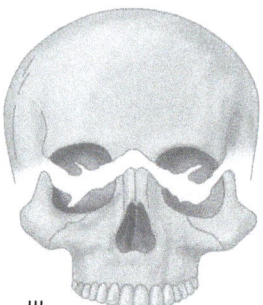

FIGURE 10-4 LeFort fractures levels I, II, and III pictured from left to right

Reproduced with permission from Butterworth J, Mackey DC, Wasnick J: Morgan and Mikhail's Clinical Anesthesiology, 5th ed. New York: McGraw-Hill Education; 2013.

❖ **LeFort III** is a craniofacial disjunction (separation) with fracture pattern extending across the zygoma, orbits, nasal and facial bones. Patients with a LeFort II and LeFort III fracture may have (CSF) leaking

Assessment/Analysis
- Mechanism of injury
- Edema, bleeding, or ecchymosis
- Facial deformity and asymmetry of face
- Malocclusion
- Facial paresthesias
- Periorbital edema and deformity
- Visual impairments
- Crepitus
- Otorrhea (CSF from ears)
- Rhinorrhea (CSF from nose)
- Epistaxis
- Neurologic exam for concomitant traumatic brain injury
- Water's view X-rays, (specific facial bones)
- CT scan of face and head

Interventions
- Airway management may require intubation or surgical airway
- Supplemental oxygen if indicated
- Cardiac and pulse oximetry monitoring
- If no suspicion of cervical trauma and hemodynamic stability, head of bed elevated
- Establish IV access for crystalloids, blood products, and medications as needed
- Antibiotics
- Analgesics and cold compresses for comfort
- Tetanus immunization as indicated
- Hospital admission
- Management of concomitant brain injury
- Surgical repair and open reduction

Evaluation
- Airway patency
- Effective breathing
- Hemodynamic stability
- Decreased pain
- Visual acuity

Laryngeal Trauma

Laryngeal trauma can be an immediate airway emergency. The injury may result in a fractured larynx and/or injury to the surrounding vasculature. Depending on the mechanism, the injury may be referred to as a "clothesline injury," when the victim strikes a straight inanimate object. This type of trauma may occur when the victim is driving a motorcycle or snowmobile, and the impact has a high velocity. Laryngeal trauma may also occur from strangulation. An immediate surgical airway may be required.

Assessment/Analysis
- Hoarseness[15]
- Dyspnea, stridor
- Dysphagia
- Odynophagia[15]
- Hemoptysis
- Bleeding, hematoma
- Pain-may increase with palpation of the anterior neck
- Possible subcutaneous emphysema
- Fiberoptic laryngoscopy
- Laboratory studies
  - CBC
  - Consider blood bank analysis (Type and Screen/Cross), if bleeding and concomitant injuries
- X-ray of neck, cervical spine and chest
- CT scan of neck

Intervention
- Assist with emergent airway as indicated
- Supplemental oxygen if indicated
- Cardiac and pulse oximetry monitoring
- Establish IV access for crystalloid fluids and medications as needed

Evaluation
- Airway patency
- Effective breathing
- Hemodynamic stability
- Decreased pain

Ocular

Ocular complaints, including illness and injury, led to over 2.4 million ED visits between 2007 and 2010. Injury was the leading cause of eye related visits in the 19 to 64-year-old age group and medical causes lead other age groups.[18]

Awareness of the structures of the eye, as pictured in Figure 10-5, guides assessment and intervention aimed at preventing vision loss.

Ocular Assessment

Observation and Comparison to Patient Typical Presentation
- Color of the eye (white sclera, colored iris, or dark pupil)
- Shape of the eye (globe and pupil)
- Drainage (including purulence, blood, or tears)
- Pain (localized or referred)
- PERRLA
  - Pupils equal round and reactive to light and accommodation
  - Includes pupil measurement

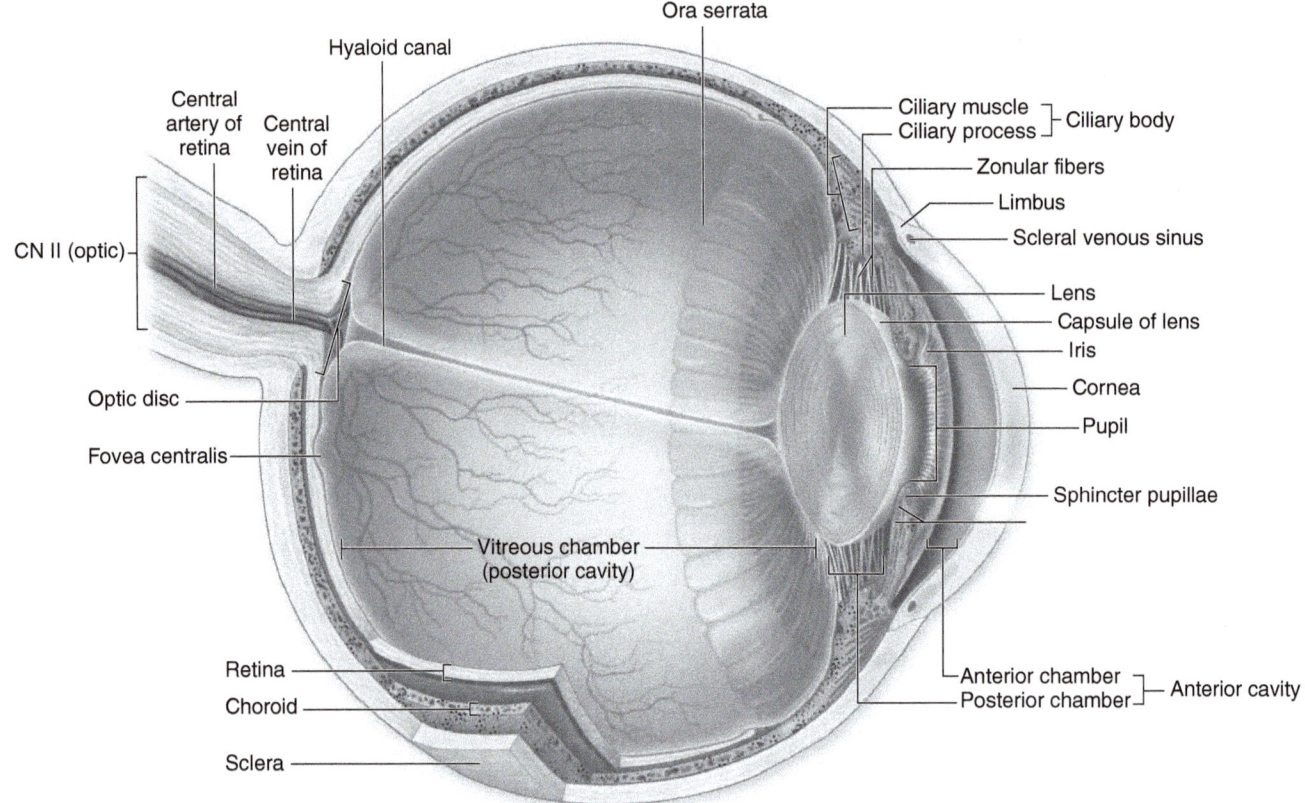

FIGURE 10-5 **Internal anatomy of the eye: Sagittal section**
Reproduced with permission from Mescher A: Junqueira's Basic Histology, 14th ed. New York: McGraw-Hill Education; 2015.

- Extra Ocular Movements (EOM) as pictured in Figure 10-6
  - Intact, limited, or causes pain[19]
  - EOM controlled by Cranial Nerves III, IV, and VI
    - See the Neurological Emergencies chapter (chapter 4) for more on cranial nerves

History of Illness or Injury
- If trauma, assess for concurrent injury
- Assess for vision correction (glasses or contacts)
- Assess for past eye surgeries (cataract, laser, or enucleation)

Vision Characteristics
- Blurred
- Double
- Clouded
- Objects in visual field (e.g. floaters, a curtain, etc.)

Visual Field
- Loss of a visual field
- Visual cuts in the field
- Spots or lines

Visual Acuity
- Considered the vital sign of the eye
- When possible, assess at baseline with vision correction[19]
  - Each eye is tested individually, then together
  - If vision correction is not available, consider "pinhole" visual acuity
    - Example shown in Figure 10-7

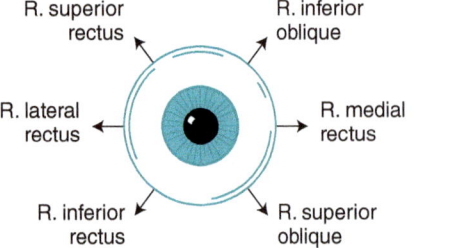 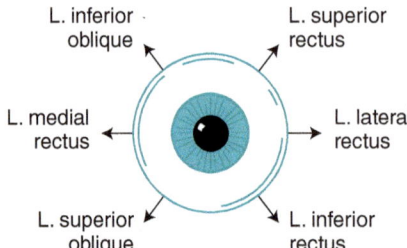

FIGURE 10-6 **Extraocular eye movements. Arrows indicate the directive action each muscle has upon the eye**
Reproduced with permission from Tintinalli J, Stapcyzynski J, Ma OJ, et al: Tintinalli's Emergency Medicine: A Comprehensive Study Guide, 8th ed. New York: McGraw-Hill Education; 2015.

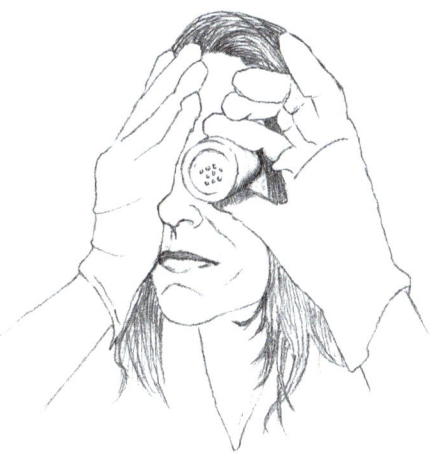

FIGURE 10-7 Pinhole device improvised from paper cup
Reproduced with permission from Iserson KV: Improvised Medicine: Providing Care in Extreme Environments, 2nd ed. New York: McGraw-Hill Education; 2016.

Vision Chart
- Snellen, Tumbling E, or Picture (sailboat)
  - Tested at 6 meters (20 feet)
- Rosenbaum
  - Handheld card tested at 14 inches for nonambulatory patients

Ocular Diagnostics and Interventions

Preventing Elevated Ocular Pressures
- Elevate head of bed and avoid coughing, vomiting, or other Valsalva-like actions
- Prepare for tonometry (measurement of intraocular pressure)
  - Normal intraocular pressure is lower than 20 mm Hg[19,20]

Eye Patch
- Slight pressure on the globe to keep the lid closed
- Patch UNaffected eye if penetrating or foreign object[20,21]
- Stabilize protruding foreign bodies

Eye Shield
- Avoids pressure on the globe[20]
- Shield eye affected by penetrating or foreign object[20]

Slit Lamp Examination
- Magnified view of ocular structures

Medications
- Administer eye drops one at a time into conjunctival sac
- Never administer eye medications with contact lenses in place
- Specific to pupillary response
  - Mydriadic agents dilate pupils
  - Miotic agents constrict pupils
  - Cytoplegic agents dilate by paralyzing ciliary muscle controlling accommodation[20]
- Fluorescein staining: stain demonstrates wounds to cornea or vitreous humor leakage[19,20]

Ocular Evaluation and Patient Education

Use of Safety or Protective Eyewear
- Was eyewear worn when injury occurred
- Can prevent about 90% of sports-related eye injuries[22]
- Patient education to wear protective eyewear appropriately

Contact Lens Care
- Poor care of contacts associated with high risk for Pseudomonas infection
- Swelling, infection, and abrasions are common complications noted during assessment[20]
- Disposable contact lenses reduce complications[23]
- Dry eyes due to overnight wear requires rehydration
- Symptoms related to wear can be reduced by temporary use of glasses instead of contact lenses[23]
- Change contact lens according to manufacturer's directions

Medication Instillation
- Hand hygiene prior to applying gentle retraction of lower lid
- Medication into conjunctival sac (space between lower eyelid and globe of eye)
- Do not touch tip of bottle to eye

Ocular Medical Conditions

Conjunctivitis

Conjunctivitis is an inflammation of the lining of the eyelid where the eyelid is in contact with the sclera. Conjunctivitis can be caused by bacterial, fungal, or viral infections. Contact lens wearers are at particular risk, as are children or those who have poor hand hygiene habits.

Assessment/Analysis
- Inflamed membrane lining eyelid
- Gritty "foreign body" sensation
- Fluorescein staining
  - "Normal" if bacterial
  - Abnormal if viral herpes simplex

Intervention
- Medications
  - Antibiotics for bacterial infection
  - Fluoroquinolones for contact lens wearers[23]
- Patient Education
  - Teach patient hand hygiene and warm compress application
  - Avoid eye make-up
  - Avoid wearing contact lenses until symptoms subside

Evaluation
- Decreased pain
- Infection risk reduction

Uveitis/Iritis

Uveitis is an inflammation of an area of the uveal tract, which includes the iris, ciliary body, and choroid. Anterior uveitis most often involves the iris of the eye. Posterior uveitis most often involved the choroid and is related to a concomitant chronic diagnosis. Without treatment, glaucoma, cataracts, and macular dysfunction are risks for the patient.

- **Anterior Uveitis**
  - Inflammation of iris
    - Pain in affected eye with light in opposite eye related to accommodation
    - Inflammation of cells in anterior chamber noted with slit lamp
    - Caution due to later risk for glaucoma[20]
- **Posterior Uveitis**
  - Rare except for cytomegalovirus related to AIDS[20]
  - Inflammation of the retina or choroid
    - Tearing
    - Red eye
    - Photophobia: often intense
    - Intraocular pressure: low to slightly elevated

Intervention
- Possible steroids or cycloplegic agents
- Dark environment or dark glasses
- Warm compress to eyes
- Eye rest from visual stimulation

Evaluation
- Maintained visual acuity
- Decreased pain

Keratitis

Keratitis is an inflammation of the cornea from bacterial, fungal, amoebic, viral, and photoexposure (ultraviolet) causes. As with conjunctivitis, contact lens wearers are at risk of keratitis.

Assessment/Analysis
- Burns to eyes
- Infections such as mumps, rubella, or infectious mononucleosis
- Microbial keratitis often associated with poor contact lens hygiene[24]
- Extreme pain onset after exposure: 10 to 48 hours later
  - Welding without eye protection
  - Sun exposure from snow or water sports

Intervention
- Medications
  - Antibiotics if bacterial
  - Cycoplegic agents
    - Atropine, scopolamine
- Eye patch for eye rest
- Patient Education: preventative measures based on cause

Evaluation
- Decreased pain
- Infection prevention measures

Glaucoma

Glaucoma is caused by increased pressure in the eye. Increased ocular pressure due to outflow obstruction occurs when the angle in the junction between the iris and cornea is narrowed or completely obstructed. Optic nerve and retinal damage can result from the increased pressure.

Assessment/Analysis
- Pain: sudden, unilateral, or severe
- Headache or photophobia
- Blurred vision or halos around eyes
  - Assess visual acuity
- Abdominal pain: generalized[19]
- Pupil changes: affected side decreased reactivity or fixed
- Intraocular pressure elevated to 40 to 80 mm Hg[19]
  - Recheck hourly

Intervention
- Medications
  - Beta Adrenergic Antagonist (Beta-Blocker) ophthalmic drops, such as timolol
    - Sympathetic nerve blockade reducing aqueous humor production
  - Miotic (parasympathomimetic) ophthalmic drops such as pilocarpine
    - Contracts ciliary muscle enhancing outflow of aqueous humor from the eye
  - Analgesia such as tetracaine or proparacaine

Evaluation
- Regularly recheck intraocular pressures
  - May be needed as often as hourly
- Decreased pain
- Maintain or improve visual acuity

Central Retinal Artery Occlusion

Central retinal artery occlusion is an emergent condition causing sudden unilateral painless vision loss and is usually caused by thrombus or embolus. Central retinal occlusion must be treated immediately because preservation of vision decreases with time to treatment and delays in treatment longer than 1 to 2 hours from onset associated with increased vision complications.

Assessment/Analysis
- Sudden, unilateral, or painless vision loss
- Anxiety
- Visual acuity: light perception or counting fingers
- Ophthalmic exam reveals pale retina[20]

Intervention
- Reduce intraocular pressure
    - Beta blockade
        - Optic drops or oral/IV medication
    - Head of bed elevated 30 degrees
    - Antiemetics as needed
    - Assist with anterior chamber paracentesis
- Focus on reperfusion within 6 hours of onset[25]

Evaluation
- Patient at risk for STEMI or CVA
- Maintain or improve visual acuity

Ocular Trauma

Corneal Abrasion/Laceration

Corneal abrasions or lacerations are caused by an injury to the cornea. Fortunately for the patient, the cornea is very vascular and heals quickly. Corneal abrasion is the most common eye injury causing patients to seek emergency care.

Assessment/Analysis
- Can be very uncomfortable
- Positive fluorescein stain to abrasion/laceration
- Observe for extrusion/dehiscence of globe contents
    - Consider globe rupture if extrusion present or penetrating mechanism of injury

Intervention
- Eye patching does not decrease pain or improve healing[21]
- Consider ophthalmic topical antibiotic therapy
- Topical anesthetic drops should not be given to the patient for long-term use, oral analgesics may be prescribed

Evaluation
- Decreased pain
- Infection prevention measures

Globe Rupture

Globe rupture is a true ophthalmic emergency. Globe rupture is often seen with concurrent injuries and commonly leads to blindness. Since not all globe ruptures are visually obvious, detailed history taking and assessment are required to protect the patient's vision.

Assessment/Analysis
- Change in shape of globe and shape of pupil
- Extruded globe contents
- Vision changes
- Pain
- Photophobia

Intervention
- Elevate the head of the bed
- Do not place pressure to globe
    - Shield the globe and patch/shield unaffected eye
- Do not measure intraocular pressure[19]
- Secure any penetrating objects
- No eye drops
- Antiemetics to reduce vomiting which increases intraocular pressure

Evaluation
- Decreased pain
- Ophthalmology consult for globe repair

Hyphema

A hyphema is a collection of blood in the anterior chamber of the eye, as pictured in Figure 10-8. Hyphema may be caused by blunt trauma or the administration of fibrinolytic therapy. Secondary bleeding within 5 days of the initial hyphema occurs in 30% of hyphema cases and reduces the chance of return to baseline visual acuity.[26]

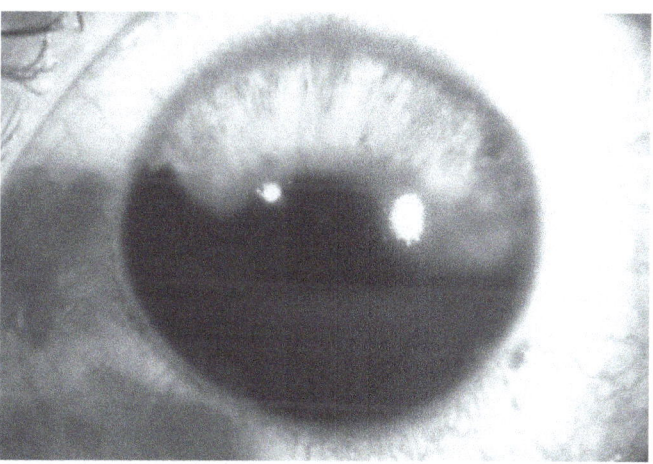

FIGURE 10-8 Hyphema of the eye. Note the subconjunctival hemorrhage also visible in the photograph

Reproduced with permission from Riordan-Eva P, Cunningham E: Vaughan & Asbury's General Ophthalmology, 18th ed. New York: McGraw-Hill Education; 2011.

Assessment/Analysis
- Pain
- Blood visualized in anterior chamber
- Photophobia
- Blurred, clouded, or reddened vision
- Increased Intraocular pressure

Intervention
- Avoid increasing intraocular pressure
    - Antiemetics as needed
    - Head of bed elevated 30 degrees if no c-spine concerns

- Shield affected eye
- Tranexamic acid reduces risk of rebleeding[26]
  - Analgesics
  - Avoid NSAIDs or aspirin: to avoid increased risk of bleeding

Evaluation
- Ophthalmology consult
- Decreased pain
- Maintain or improve visual acuity

Detached Retina

A detached retina can lead to permanent loss of vision. Retinal detachment is usually painless and unilateral occurring when retinal layers separate from the choroid layer. Refer to Figure 10-5 regarding optic anatomy. Blood and vitreous fluid accumulate between the separated layers decreasing supply of oxygen and other nutrients to the retinas leading to blindness.[15] Direct head or eye trauma can be a cause; however, degenerative changes, such as those seen in the elderly, are the most common cause of retinal detachment.[15]

Assessment/Analysis
- Baseline visual acuity
- Visual field deficits
- Mechanism of injury, if applicable
- Cloudy vision, visual cobwebs, or visual veil
- Visual "floaters"[15]
- History of chronic diseases
  - Diabetes
  - Sickle cell disease
  - Hypertension
- History of optic surgeries
- Slit: lamp exam
- Tonometry for intraocular pressure measurement
- May be sudden or gradual[15]
- Normal pupillary reaction

Interventions
- Shield bilateral eyes
- Decrease overall patient movement
- Plan for ophthalmologic consult
- Position as per physician orders
- Plan for hospital admission and surgical repair

Evaluation
- Visual acuity
- Patient anxiety related to change in vision

Chemical Burns

Chemical burns to the eye are another true emergency and delayed treatment may result in permanent loss of vision. Exposure to an alkali causes tissue liquefaction resulting in deep burns to the eye tissue whereas exposure to an acid results in surface damage, which creates a barrier to protect from deeper damage.[19]

Assessment/Analysis
- Painful
- Vision changes with possible corneal clouding
- Redness and swelling of sclera and eyelids

Intervention
- Only life-saving interventions should precede irrigation
  - Defer visual acuity until irrigation is complete
- Eye pH baseline
- Copious irrigation until eye pH is 7.0 to 7.3[19]
  - Ringer's Lactate is closest in pH to tears[27]
  - Saline or sterile water may also be used[20,27]
  - Irrigate from inner canthus towards outer canthus
- Analgesic drops in emergency department only[28]
  - Repeated drops can be toxic to corneal epithelium

Evaluation
- Return to "normal" eye pH
- Decreased pain
- Maintain or improve visual acuity

REFERENCES

1. Cirilli AR. Emergency evaluation and management of the sore throat. *Emerg Med Clin North Am.* 2013;31:501–515.
2. Kahn JH. Retropharyngeal abscess. *Medscape.* http://emedicine.medscape.com/article/764421-overview. Published February 6, 2015. Accessed March 21, 2015.
3. Beaudreau RW. Oral and dental emergencies. In: Tintinalli JE, Stapczynski J, Ma O, et al, eds. *Tintinalli's Emergency Medicine: A Comprehensive Study Guide.* 8th ed. New York, NY: McGraw-Hill; 2016.
4. Hodgdon A. Dental and related infections. *Emerg Med Clin North Am.* 2013;31:465–480.
5. Falcon-Chevere JL, Giraldez L, Rivera-Rivera JO, et al. Critical ENT skills and procedures in the emergency department. *Emerg Med Clin North Am.* 2013;31:29–59.
6. Kasperek ZA, Pollock GF. Epistaxis: an overview. *Emerg Med Clin North Am.* 2013;31:443–454.
7. McGinnis HD. Nose and sinuses. In: Tintinalli JE, Stapczynski J, Ma O, et al, eds. *Tintinalli's Emergency Medicine: A Comprehensive Study Guide.* 8th ed. New York, NY: McGraw-Hill; 2016.
8. Lareau SA, Heitz CR. Face and jaw emergencies. In: Tintinalli JE, Stapczynski J, Ma O, et al, eds. *Tintinalli's Emergency Medicine: A Comprehensive Study Guide.* 8th ed. New York, NY: McGraw-Hill; 2016.
9. Smith D. Dental, ear, nose and throat emergencies. In: Hoyt KS, Selfridge-Thomas J, eds. *Emergency nursing core curriculum.* 6th ed. St. Louis, MO; Elsevier/Saunders: 2007:249–289.
10. Usatine RP, Smith MA, Chumley HS, et al, eds. Ear: foreign body. *The Color Atlas of Family Medicine.* 2nd ed. New York, NY: McGraw-Hill; 2013.
11. Woods CR. Epiglottitis. *UpToDate.* http://www.uptodate.com/contents/search?search=epiglottitis. Published October 2, 2013. Accessed March 21, 2015.
12. Hosmer K. Ear disorders. In: Tintinalli JE, Stapczynski J, Ma O, et al, eds. *Tintinalli's Emergency Medicine: A Comprehensive Study Guide.* 8th ed. New York, NY: McGraw-Hill; 2016.

13. Hwang PH, Patel ZM. Acute sinusitis and rhinosinusitis in adults: treatment. *Up To Date*. http://www.uptodate.com/contents/search?search=acute+sinusitis. Published February 26, 2014. Accessed March 29, 2015.
14. Goldman B. Vertigo. In: Tintinalli JE, Stapczynski J, Ma O, et al, eds. *Tintinalli's Emergency Medicine: A Comprehensive Study Guide*. 8th ed. New York, NY: McGraw-Hill; 2016.
15. Shea SS. Ocular and maxillofacial trauma. In: Hoyt KS, Selfridge-Thomas J, eds. *Emergency Nursing Core Curriculum*. 6th ed. St. Louis, MO: Elsevier/Saunders; 2007:848–878.
16. Ramponi D, White T. Zygomatic arch fracture in a 40-year-old woman. *Adv Emerg Nurs J*. 2014;36(4):299–306.
17. Boswell K. Management of facial fractures. *Emerg Med Clin N Am*. 2013; 31:539–551.
18. Egging D. Ocular trauma. In: Gurney D, ed. *Trauma Nursing Core Course Provider Manual*. 7th ed. Des Plaines, IL: Emergency Nurses Association; 2014:123–136.
19. Centers for Disease Control and Prevention (CDC). *Morbidity and Mortality Weekly*. 2013;62(18):374. http://www.cdc.gov/mmwr/preview/mmwrhtml/mm6218a9.htm. Accessed May 28, 2016.
20. Jayasekara R. Ophthalmic emergencies: Clinician Information. Joanna Briggs Institute JBI141. 2014.
21. Flynn CA, D'Amico F, Smith G. Should we patch corneal abrasions: a meta-analysis. *J Fam Pract*. 1998;47(4):264–70.
22. Weissman BA, Barr JT, Harris MG, Kame RT, McMahon TT, Rah M, Secor GB, Sonsino, J. *Optometric clinical practice guideline care of the contact lens patient, 2e*. St. Louis: American Optometric Association; 2006.
23. Cass SP. Ocular injuries in sports. *Curr Sports Med Rep*. 2012;11(1):11–15.
24. Collier SA, Gronostaj MP, MacGurn AK, et al. Estimated burden of keratitis-United States, 2010. *Morbidity and Mortality Weekly Report (MMWR)*. 2014;63(45):1027–1030.
25. Cugati S, Varma DD, Chen CS, et al. Treatment options for central retinal artery occlusion. *Curr Treat Options Neurol*. 2013;15(1):63–77.
26. Gharaibeh A, Savage HI, Scherer RW, et al. Medical interventions for traumatic hyphema. *Cochrane Database Syst Rev*. 2013;12.
27. Chau J, Lee D, Lo S. Eye irrigation for patients with ocular chemical burns: A systematic review. *The JBI Database of Systematic Reviews and Implementation Reports* 2010;8(12):470–519.
28. Duffy B. Managing chemical eye injuries. *Emerg Nurse*. 2008;16:25–29.

Practice Questions

Question	Rationale
1. The emergency nurse suspects central retinal artery occlusion due to what assessment finding? a. Sudden painless vision loss b. Visual field curtain c. Sudden onset of extreme unilateral eye pain d. Intraocular pressures of 25 mm Hg	*Answer: a* A unique characteristic of central retinal artery occlusion is sudden painless vision loss. Visual field curtain is common in retinal detachment. Sudden extreme unilateral eye pain is most likely to be related to glaucoma. Intraocular pressures of 25 mm Hg is a slightly elevated result and may be related to one of several causes, including uveitis, early glaucoma, or eye trauma.
2. When assessing a patient's history to analyze risk factors for epistaxis, the nurse would want to inquire about a. Recent travel b. Family history of heart disease c. Herbal Supplements d. Diet restrictions	*Answer: c* Specific herbal supplements such as ginseng contain anticoagulation properties that can increase the risk for epistaxis. Although the nurse may collect history about the patient's recent travel locations, dietary restrictions, and family history of heart disease, these are not associated risk factors for epistaxis.
3. The most common site for anterior epistaxis is the a. Sphenopalatine arteries b. Submental region c. Sphenoid sinus region d. Kiesselbach's plexus	*Answer: d* The sphenopalatine artery is often the source for a posterior bleed with epistaxis. Posterior epistaxis is less common, about 10 to 15% of all incidences but has a greater risk for bleeding and/or airway complications. The submental area is the area below the chin and is commonly an area where Ludwig's angina can extend. The sphenoid sinus is located at the base of the skull and the top of the pharynx.
4. A patient complaining of dry, itchy eyes and difficulty removing contact lenses placed 2 days ago is best treated by a. Gentle suction using a manufactured contact lens removal device b. Antibiotic drops to treat corneal abrasions c. Measurement of intraocular pressures d. Gentle flushing of the eyes	*Answer: d* Gentle flushing of an eye dry from extended contact wear is intended to rehydrate tissue and the contact lens. The purpose is not to remove the lens by forceful flushing, but rather to hydrate the tissue and lens to the point that typical removal is possible. A commercial device may cause damage to the eye needing hydration. Antibiotics and ocular pressures are not indicated.
5. How does a periapical abscess differ from a periodontal abscess? a. The periapical abscess involves a minimum of two or more dental caries b. The periapical abscess extends beyond the bone c. The periapical abscess may occur around a healthy tooth d. The periapical abscess can occur in the absence of a dental caries	*Answer: b* A periapical abscess involves the dentin, and can extend down into the pulp and nerve roots. Typically, the periapical abscess arises from untreated dental caries. A periodontal abscess occurs when a pocket can form around the tooth creating a reservoir for bacteria and/or other pathogens. The tooth may remain healthy, but the gum tissue around it is inflamed and becomes infected causing a periodontal abscess.

Question	Rationale
6. Following discharge instructions for a patient with Uveitis, the emergency nurse knows instructions are understood when the patient says a. "I'll just go home and read a book" b. "I'll rest and catch up on my favorite TV show" c. "I'll just go relax on the beach" d. "It's going to be hard to stay away from my computer"	*Answer: d* Treatment for uveitis includes eye rest in dark environments. Eye rest includes time away from television and other "screens" and reading so verbalization of the need to reduce computer usage indicates understanding. Reading and watching TV creates stress on the eye and time at the beach increases exposure to bright lights.
7. Eye drops are administered into the a. Lacrimal sac b. Conjunctival sac c. Cornea d. Canal of Schlemm	*Answer: b* Eye drops are administered into the conjunctival sac by using the index finger to place gentle traction under the eye OR using the index finger and thumb to gently pinch the tissue under the eye to create a pocket between the lower eyelid and the sclera of the globe. Lacrimal sac, cornea, and canal of Schlemm are other anatomical structures of the eye.
8. A patient presents with a sore throat that has recently worsened. His voice is muffled, and he complains of a two day history of fever. He has not eaten or drank because of the pain. Upon inspection, the nurse notes his tonsils appear enlarged and purulent. His painful swallowing is a. Odynophagia b. Trismus c. Halitosis d. Otalgia	*Answer: a* Trismus is the inability to open the mouth. Halitosis is foul breath. Otalgia is ear pain and Odynophagia is pain upon swallowing. All of these are signs and symptoms of a peritonsillar abscess.
9. A 51-year-old patient has come to the emergency department with fever, sore throat and hoarseness for the past 4 days. Today, he felt like he was "choking" in his airway. He has been diagnosed with Ludwig's angina. The nurse's first priority is assuring the following is available a. Cardiac monitoring b. IV antibiotics c. IV hydration d. Cricothyrotomy tray	*Answer: d* A patient with Ludwig's angina has a great risk for airway obstruction due to the edema within the submandibular space, an area that does not provide needed expansion to accommodate swelling without minimizing or occluding the airway. Often these patients are taking directly to the OR with plans for intubation with preparation for a tracheostomy, if needed. Cardiac and pulse oximetry monitoring are indicated as well as IV antibiotics and fluids; however, with the first priority of "airway," an emergency surgical airway kit within reach will prevent a delay if an emergency airway is needed.
10. For a patient with a chemical burn to the eye, the emergency nurse knows that the priority intervention is to a. Baseline visual acuity b. Ophthalmology consult c. Warm compress to the eye d. Irrigation with copious amounts of Ringer's Lactate	*Answer: d* Chemical burns to the eye are an emergency with urgent treatment needed to prevent further vision loss. Irrigation with Ringer's lactate, saline, or sterile water should be done until the pH of the eye reaches about 7.1, or the level of typical tears. Alkali exposure generally requires larger amounts of fluid irrigation. Baseline visual acuity delays treatment. Ophthalmology consult may be needed but is not an initial priority. Warm compress to the eye may provide comfort, but is not a priority treatment.

Question	Rationale
11. The highest priority with approaching the patient who has a dental emergency is a. Level of consciousness b. Airway c. Bleeding d. Infection	*Answer: b* All of these considerations are priorities when managing dental emergencies. As with other emergencies, airway patency is the first priority. Infection could lead to edema that can occlude the airway. Blood loss and decreased level of consciousness can also affect airway patency.
12. Miotic agents act on the eye by a. Constricting the pupil b. Dilating the pupil c. Paralyzing the ciliary muscle d. Paralyzing the suspensory muscle	*Answer: a* Miotic agents constrict the pupil. Examples of miotic agents include opioids, organophosphates, cholinergics, and parasympathomimetics, such as pilocarpine. Dilation is caused by mydriadic agents, such as cocaine, amphetamines, phenylephrine, and anticholinergics, such as atropine and scopalomine. Ciliary muscles are paralyzed by a class of mydriadic agents called cytoplegics, which not only dilates the pupil but also reduces accommodation of the eye. Paralysis of the suspensory muscles occurs with general paralytic medications.
13. For a patient with a penetrating eye injury, a strategy to reduce further injury is to a. Instill cycoplegic agents b. Measure intraocular pressure c. Shield both eyes/stabilize object d. Remove the penetrating object	*Answer: c* Shielding both eyes or shielding the affected eye and patching the unaffected eye. Covering both eyes reduces bilateral eye movement and helps to prevent further injury. Removal of the penetrating object, instillation of any medication, and measuring ocular pressures could cause additional injury.
14. An 18-year-old female visits the emergency department with complaints of ear pain and decreased hearing for the past 2 to 3 days. She reports an increased pain around her ear as she put her pierced earrings on. She has been visiting a friend and swimming in the lake. The nurse anticipates that an otoscopy exam would reveal her tympanic membrane to be a. Edematous and bulging b. Shiny and yellowish in color c. Translucent and pearl gray in color d. Limited in movement	*Answer: c* Typically, the tympanic membrane remains normal with external otitis. She presents with risk factors (hot weather, swimming) and symptoms (pain and tenderness on external ear and decreased hearing). The tympanic membrane is not usually affected with external otitis. With acute otitis media, the TM usually becomes edematous and inflamed from the pressure build up of fluid within the middle ear. The TM may have limited movement on pneumatic otoscopy exam (air insufflation using an otoscope). The TM may be reddened or yellow, which can be signs of a possible bacterial otitis media.
15. An eye patch or eye shield is *not* recommended for which condition? a. Hyphema b. Corneal abrasion c. Globe rupture d. Keratitis	*Answer: b* An eye patch has not been shown to benefit healing or comfort for the patient with a corneal abrasion. An eye patch assists with eye rest for patients with keratitis, but an eye shield is not indicated. An eye shield protects the eye from further damage after globe rupture or hyphema, but a patch is not recommended.

Question	Rationale
16. Zygomatic fractures are often associated with what other type of fractures? a. Tripod fractures b. LeFort I pattern of the maxillary fracture c. LeFort II pattern of the maxillary fracture d. Orbital floor fractures	*Answer: a* A tripod fracture is a zygomatic fracture involving the zygomatic suture lines and is usually caused by a high-velocity blunt force trauma. A LeFort I is a transverse fracture that separates the lower maxilla from the nasal septum and pterygoid. A LeFort II is a pyramidal shaped fracture extending up through the maxilla and across the medial orbits and nasal bones. The zygoma forms the lateral and inferior orbital wall, and because of the close proximity and often-forceful trauma, zygomatic fractures frequently occur concomitantly with fractures of the orbital floor. Orbital floor fractures may be referred to as "blow-out" fractures.
17. Bell's palsy involves which cranial nerve? a. First cranial nerve b. Fifth cranial nerve c. Seventh cranial nerve d. Eighth cranial nerve	*Answer: c* Bell's Palsy involves the seventh cranial nerve, the facial nerve. The facial nerve controls most facial expressions, secretions of tears and saliva as well as taste making it a sensory and motor functioning cranial nerve. Bells palsy involves a paralysis of the seventh cranial nerve that is usually temporary. Trigeminal neuralgia, painful paroxysms involves the fifth cranial nerve. The fifth cranial nerve is the trigeminal nerve and innervates for chewing, and for sensation of touching and pain to the face and mouth. The eighth cranial nerve, the vestibulocochlear nerve is responsible for hearing and equilibrium balance. An acoustic neuroma is a benign tumor on the vestibulocochlear nerve, and if not detected could potentially extend into the cranium. The second cranial nerve is the optic nerve and is responsible for vision. Anosmia, the inability to smell can be caused by damage to the first cranial nerve, the olfactory nerve.
18. A 21-year-old college student comes to the emergency department with complaints of difficulty swallowing, sore throat, right-sided earache, fever and difficulty opening his mouth. Inspection reveals enlarged tonsils with purulence, and the right tonsil is expanded and displacing the uvula. After IV fluid, analgesics and antibiotics are administered, the nurse anticipates the next intervention is to a. Assist with needle aspiration of abscess b. Assist with transfer to the operating room for intubation c. Assist with preparation for hospital admission d. X-ray the neck	*Answer: a* This patient has signs of a peritonsillar abscess. Needle aspiration of the purulent drainage frequently reduces the enlarged abscess and brings relief of symptoms. The aspirate may be collected for a culture and gram stain. A retropharyngeal abscess exists posterior in the pharynx in the deeper space of the neck. A retropharyngeal abscess can be caused by both aerobic and anaerobic pathogens and may pose a greater threat to the airway. CT imaging is often indicated to determine the location and extent of the abscess, but an x-ray will not provide this type of imaging. Because of the precarious location, a retropharyngeal abscess may require intubation and possibly a surgical airway (cricothyrotomy).

Question	Rationale
19. A 77-year-old female presents to the emergency department with her husband. The husband reports that she had a "choking spell" 2 days before, while eating chicken. Since the episode, her oral intake has decreased, and her voice has changed. She has a history of dementia, and he is her primary care giver. Respirations are 24 per minute and slightly labored, and SpO_2 is 90% on room air. The nurse auscultates wheezes on the right side of her chest. The emergency nurse explains the next step for the patient that includes diagnostic testing that has been ordered. Which non-invasive diagnostic test has the greatest sensitivity for detecting a chicken bone foreign body? a. Chest X-ray b. Flexible endoscopy c. CT scan d. Rigid bronchoscopy	*Answer: c* Although radiography films may be done initially and can detect radiopaque objects (coins, pencils, etc.), they do not detect radiolucent foreign bodies such as chicken bones. If the X-rays (i.e. soft tissue radiograph of neck and/or chest x-ray) raise suspicion of a foreign body, laryngoscopy may be implemented; though, this is more invasive than radiography. The CT scan offers detailed diagnostic information about the foreign body such as size and location. These details prove helpful when the history surrounding the aspiration may be incomplete or unknown. Flexible endoscopy and rigid bronchoscopy are tools used in procedures for foreign body removal and may require procedural sedation for patient comfort and cooperation.
20. After reviewing discharge instructions with the patient, for acute rhinosinusitis (sinusitis), all of the following statements indicate the patient's understanding *except* a. "Warm packs to my face may provide relief" b. "Saline irrigation will help my symptoms" c. "These symptoms may last for months and I just have to live with it" d. "Taking pseudoephedrine, as prescribed, will help"	*Answer: c* With symptoms lasting longer than 2 weeks, a bacterial infection may be present and antibiotics may be indicated. Warm packs and saline irrigations may provide relief for acute rhinosinusitis as well as over the counter pseudoephedrine. With prolonged rhinosinusitis, the infection may extend outside of the paranasal sinuses. Complications such as meningitis, intracranial abscess, and cavernous sinus thrombosis and orbital blindness may occur. Thus, prolonged symptoms should not be ignored, and the patient should seek follow-up.
21. A patient with a known history of HIV presents with severe eye pain. Intraocular pressure is measured at 23 mm Hg. What is the most probable cause of the pain? a. Central Retinal Occlusion b. Glaucoma c. Globe rupture d. Posterior Uveitis	*Answer: d* Posterior uveitis is a rare inflammation of the retina or choroid often caused by the cytomegalovirus in patients with HIV/ AIDS. Central retinal occlusion is painless. Glaucoma usually presents with intraocular pressures between 40 and 80 mm Hg. Patients with globe rupture should not have intraocular pressures performed, but if a pressure was recorded, it would be extremely low or possibly zero.
22. How should visual acuity for the nonambulatory patient be tested? a. Finger to nose touch test b. Rosenbaum vision chart c. Snellen vision chart d. Tumbling "E" vision chart	*Answer: b* The Rosenbaum vision chart is a card held in good light at 14 inches from the nonambulatory patient. The patient uses the Snellen vision chart by standing 20 feet (6 meters) away. The tumbling "E" vision chart is also measured from a 20 foot distance and is used for children or patients who do not use the Latin "ABC" alphabet. The finger-to-nose touch test is part of a neurologic test evaluating coordination.

Question	Rationale
23. A 34-year-old male patient involved in a head-on collision at high speed, arrives with suspected cervical spine trauma, closed head injury and a maxillary fracture. The nurse observes clear fluid leaking from his nose and suspects a cerebrospinal fluid (CSF) leak. What LeFort type of maxillary fracture would one anticipate CSF rhinorrhea to be present? a. LeFort II b. LeFort III c. LeFort I and II d. LeFort II and III	*Answer: d* A LeFort I is a transverse fracture that separates the lower maxilla from the nasal septum and pterygoid. The patient's maxilla is freely movable similar to loose fitting upper dentures. A LeFort II is a pyramidal shaped fracture extending up through the maxilla and across the medial orbits and nasal bones. A LeFort III is a craniofacial disjunction (separation) with fracture pattern extending across the zygoma, orbits, nasal and facial bones. CSF from ears and/or nose can occur with LeFort II and LeFort III.
24. Prevention of increased intraocular pressure is *not* accomplished by which of the following? a. Administer antiemetics b. Administration of a miotic agent, such as pilocarpine c. Apply an eye patch d. Elevate head of bed 30 degrees	*Answer: c* An eye patch places pressure on the globe of the eye. Elevating the head of the bed and administration of antiemetics or miotic agents all assist to reduce intraocular pressure.
25. A patient is diagnosed with Bell's palsy in the emergency department. The nurse anticipates the administration of a. Antiemetic b. Artificial tears c. Carbamazepine d. Diuretics	*Answer: b* Bell's palsy involves a dysfunction of the eighth cranial nerve resulting in paralysis with one side of the face. Decreased tearing can occur, and lubricating topical eye drops (artificial tears) are administered to help prevent inflammation to the cornea (keratitis). The patient may have excessive drooling. Diuretics and antiemetics would not relieve symptoms of Bell's palsy. Carbamazepine is the drug of choice for pain relief with trigeminal neuralgia.
26. The nurse teaches the patient about oral rinses of chlorhexidine (0.12%) mouthwash or half-strength hydrogen peroxide twice daily for what following illness? a. Alveolar osteitis (dry socket) following a tooth extraction b. Epiglottitis c. Parotitis d. Vincent Disease	*Answer: d* Necrotizing Ulcerative Gingivitis (NUG), also referred to as Vincent disease or trench mouth, is an aggressive oral infection often associated with malnutrition, poor hygiene or human immunodeficiency virus (HIV). Symptoms include pain, ulceration and bleeding. Along with antibiotics to treat the infection, good oral hygiene is important to review, including an oral rinse, to reduction oral bacteria. The treatment of choice for alveolar osteitis is aimed at controlling bleeding and pain. Treatment for parotitis is rehydration and treatment of the infection of the parotid gland. Epiglottitis treatment often includes antibiotics and can be deemed an airway emergency.

Question	Rationale
27. What is the priority goal of irrigation for a chemical burn to eye? a. Decreased pain b. Eye pH of 7.1 c. Intraocular pressure of 18 mm Hg d. Improving vision	*Answer: b* Following a chemical burn to the eye, rapid return of eye pH to normal pH (7 to 7.3) is the goal of irrigation. While 18 mm Hg is a normal intraocular pressure, it is not the goal of treatment and has nothing to do with irrigation. While improved vision and decreased pain are outcomes of related treatment reaching the goal, they are not the primary goals of irrigation.
28. In a patient suspected of Ludwig's angina, the priority intervention for the nurse is a. Pain management b. Cardiac monitoring c. Positioning of patient d. Egophonic assessment	*Answer: c* Patients experiencing Ludwig's angina are at risk for airway obstruction so initial interventions focused on optimizing airway positioning and airway management. While pain management and cardiac monitoring are included in the care, they are not priority. Egophonic assessment, increased resonance with pulmonary auscultation is associated with lung consolidation or fibrous lung tissue and not with Ludwig's angina. Egophonia involves hearing an "ah" sound upon auscultation when the patient is making an "ee" sound.

Orthopedic and Wound Emergencies

11

Jenna Hannity, MSN, RN, CEN

Orthopedic injuries are common in emergency departments resulting in significant pain, long-term disability, and possible disfigurement. Orthopedic injuries can be life threatening and are often also distracting injuries. The nursing assessment should be completed in the appropriate order, with life threatening injuries managed first. Interventions common to many orthopedic and some wound injuries includes RICE treatment (rest, ice, compression, elevation) and prescribed or OTC medications to manage discomfort. Reassessment is important as missed injuries are a concern and the full extent of injury may take time to manifest. Referral to specialists may be necessary.

Orthopedic

Amputation

Amputation is the removal of part of the body by either accidental or intentional causes and can originate from human or mechanical error. Replantation of the amputated art may or may not be successful. Children tend to have better success with replantation than adults.[1]

There are two common types of amputation, which occur with equal frequency[2]

- ❖ Complete amputation occurs when the appendage is completely severed from the body; examples are a guillotine-type injury or a ragged edge as seen with bombing victims
- ❖ Incomplete amputation occurs when an attachment of the appendage to the body is still present. This often results from crush or tearing injuries. There may be extensive surrounding tissue damage due to a mechanism causing distortion or disruption of the nearby tissues

Assessment/Analysis
- Inspect for bleeding
- Determine the mechanism of injury, time of injury, and extent and location of the injury
- Pain may be present depending on the extent of nerve involvement and damage[2]
- Capillary refill and pulses distal to the injury (partial amputation)
- Stump for condition and amount and type of contamination

Interventions
- Control bleeding using pressure and elevation
  - Do not use a tourniquet unless bleeding cannot be controlled by other means[1]
  - If a tourniquet must be used, place it as close to the amputation site as possible to limit ischemia and nerve compression of extremity[3]
- Establish IV access for crystalloid fluids, blood products, and medications as needed
  - Analgesics
  - Antibiotics
- Immobilize the limb in correct anatomical position
- Clean the site using saline solution irrigation only
  - Do not scrub or use cleaning solutions on the stump[1,2]
- Preserve the amputated part for possible replantation by wrapping in saline-moistened gauze and placing it in a sealed and labeled plastic bag. Place the bag on ice, assuring the part does not freeze or touch the ice directly[1,3,4]
- X-ray to evaluate underlying bony structures and the extent of the damage, including determination of the level of injury and suitability for replantation
- Vascular studies to determine the extent of vascular compromise due to the injury
- Laboratory studies for initial management and pre-operative screening
  - CBC with differential
  - Serum chemistries
  - Consider blood bank analysis (Type and Screen/Cross), if blood loss is significant
  - Coagulation studies
  - Urinalysis and urine drug screen, as indicated
- Maintain NPO status and do not allow the patient to smoke
- Administer tetanus prophylaxis as ordered

- Prepare patient for transfer to an appropriate facility or the operating room
- Provide information and psychosocial support for patient and family

Evaluation
- Effective tissue perfusion and hemodynamic status
- Pain management

Compartment Syndrome

Compartment syndrome occurs when increased pressure within a closed-tissue space compromises circulation to the capillaries, muscles, and nerves within that space, leading to ischemia and necrosis.[4] Compartment syndrome is caused by internal and external compression.

- ❖ External sources of compression include casts, tight dressings, splints, skeletal traction, and prolonged entrapment of a limb-crush injury
- ❖ Internal causes include frostbite, snakebite, fractures, contusions, bleeding into a muscle, and IV infiltration/extravasation

Compartment syndrome is considered a true orthopedic emergency. The key to a positive patient outcome is early recognition, diagnosis, and intervention. If left untreated, devastating and debilitating outcomes such as amputation can result.[2]

Assessment/Analysis
- History of injury to area including fracture, compression, crushing force, or recent surgery
- Pain out of proportion to injury (especially on passive movement) that is progressive, intense, and increases with palpation over the compartment
- Pressure (i.e., palpable tenseness or increased tissue pressure measurement)
- Paresthesia
- Pallor
- Paralysis (or weakness)
- Pulses diminished (late sign)
- Delayed capillary refill

Intervention
- Establish IV access for crystalloid fluids, blood products, and medications as needed
- Administer analgesia as ordered
- Remove all forms of external compression
- Do not apply ice as it promotes further vasoconstriction[1,2]
- Maintain limb at the level of the heart, not above it[3,4]
- Assist with measurement of intracompartmental pressures (see Figure 11-1)
  - When intracompartmental pressures are over 40 mm Hg, surgical decompression by fasciotomy is required[2]
- Frequent reassessment with monitoring of compartment pressures are essential to management

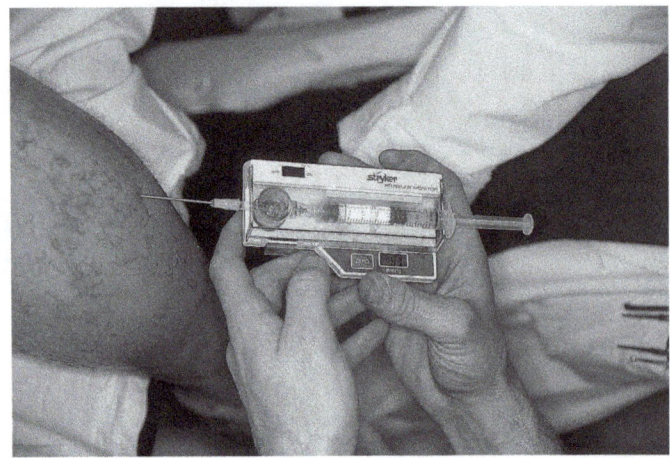

FIGURE 11-1 Measuring intracompartmental pressures. Intracompartmental pressure monitoring can be accomplished with commercially available devices. Normal tissue pressures should be less than 10 mm Hg; orthopaedic consultation is recommended when pressures exceed 30 mm Hg

Reproduced with permission from Knoop KJ, Stack LB, Storrow AB, et al: The Atlas of Emergency Medicine, 4th ed. New York: McGraw-Hill Education; 2016: Photo contributor: Selim Suner, MD MS.

- Anticipate hospital admission with emergent surgery for elevated intracompartmental pressures

Evaluation
- Effective tissue perfusion and hemodynamic status
- Pain management
- Normal neurovascular status

Contusions

A contusion is a closed wound in which a ruptured blood vessel has hemorrhaged into the surrounding tissues. A hematoma is formed when the blood leaks under the skin surface and forms a palpable mass under the skin.[5] Contusions can result from blunt external forces or exertional stresses. At-risk populations include those involved in physical activities, contact sports, or abusive relationships, and patients taking anticoagulant therapy or who have a history of clotting disorders.[1] A contusion differs from ecchymosis in that contusions are caused by trauma whereas ecchymosis results from slow, hemorrhagic leakage of blood into the skin related to aging, medications, or underlying medical condition.[5]

Assessment/Analysis
- Mechanism of injury, time of injury, and past medical history
  - Be alert when obtaining patient history for any red flags indicating maltreatment
- Skin discoloration, size, location, and/or edema at the injured area
- Tenderness with palpation
- Lab studies to rule out thrombocytopenia and/or coagulopathy
  - CBC with differential
  - Coagulation studies

Interventions
- Supportive and based on symptoms
- Rest and elevate affected extremity
- Apply cold packs to decrease swelling and stimulate vasoconstriction
- Administer medications such as mild analgesia as prescribed
- Patient/family education should include trauma prevention and early signs and symptoms of compartment syndrome

Evaluation
- Pain management

Costochondritis

Costochondritis is an acute, self-limiting inflammation of the costal cartilage found at the ribs and sternal junctions and may involve one or several junctions.[6] The inflammation can result from physical exertion or repetitive movements. Costochondritis is most commonly seen in people over 20 years old. Other causes of chest pain (like myocardial infarction) should be ruled out before making this diagnosis.

Assessment/Analysis
- Patient description of the pain including onset, duration, and characteristics
- Past medical history including recent injury and/or surgery
- Palpate for reproducible pain with palpation of the chest wall and pain with movement
- Inspect for swelling, bruising, and/or deformity
- Diagnostic procedures will help rule out other causes of the pain

Interventions
- Analgesia
- Patient education about the importance of rest, deep breathing to prevent respiratory complications, and follow up care

Evaluation
- Pain management

Foreign Bodies

Foreign bodies are any items embedded in various parts of the body, including wood, metal, glass, clothing, gravel, or thorns. Some items, like glass and metal, can be difficult to visually locate, and may require X-ray, but are not likely to cause a tissue reaction if left in place.[7] Foreign bodies which are organic matter are highly reactive in human tissue, lead to infection, and should be removed as quickly as possible. However, they are more difficult to visualize on plain radiographs and may require the use of other radiographic modalities.[7]

Assessment/Analysis
- Description of the injury, its mechanism, time since injury, potential type of foreign body, and location of injury
- Pain assessment
- Inspect the wound and determine if the foreign object is embedded or protruding
- Palpate pulses and assess motor and sensory function distal to the injury

Interventions
- Prepare patient for X-ray as necessary
- Administer medications such as analgesia, antibiotics, and tetanus booster as ordered
- Thoroughly clean the area around the wound
  - Do not soak the affected body part containing organic material such as a wooden splinter: when the foreign body absorbs the liquid, it swells and becomes more prone to disintegrating during removal[7]
- Assist with removal of the object
- Apply appropriate dressings
- Educate the patient about wound care, signs of infection, and follow up care

Evaluation
- Effective tissue perfusion
- Normal neurovascular status
- Pain management

Dislocations

A dislocation is an injury occurring at the articulation of two or more bones causing those bones to move out of the anatomically correct position. Joint subluxation occurs when part of the articular surface contact remains but is not complete.[1,4] Dislocations can be caused by direct or indirect trauma. The extent and severity of dislocation depends on the frequency of the injury-causing act, as well as extrinsic factors, such as amount, direction, and duration of force.[1,2] Dislocations may also include associated soft tissue and vascular or nerve injury. Reduction of dislocation should be completed as soon as possible to prevent permanent dysfunction resulting from compromised vasculature and nerve function.[1]

Assessment/Analysis
- Mechanism of injury, time of injury, and associated injuries
- Pain assessment
- Inspect for blood loss, swelling, ecchymosis, capillary refill, integrity of the skin, deformity/angulation, and compare to opposite extremity
- Palpate affected area for crepitus, abnormal mobility at or between joints, tenderness, temperature of extremity, and pulses distal to the injury
- Determine range of motion: may be reduced range of motion and/or normal function depending on the injury[2]
- Determine sensation surrounding and distal to the injury

Interventions
- Elevate the extremity and apply ice to decrease swelling
- Remove jewelry from the affected area or distal to this area, because it can act as a tourniquet if left in place
- Splint the extremity to provide decreased pain by providing support and position of comfort

- Prepare patient for X-ray before and after reduction
- Establish IV access for crystalloid fluids and medications as needed
- Administer medications such as analgesia and/or procedural sedation medications as ordered
- Assist with reduction as needed
- Prepare the patient for admission, surgery, transfer, and/or discharge
- Patient education about splint care, use of assistive devices, and follow up care

Evaluation
- Normal neurovascular status
- Pain management
- Effective tissue perfusion

Fractures

A fracture is a break in the continuity of a bone. Fractures are painful and temporarily debilitating. Complications of fracture can lead to permanent disability and even death, if not recognized and treated. Fractures are classified by five general divisions with common types pictured in Figure 11-2.

- ❖ Anatomic location: proximal, distal, middle, head, shaft, or base
- ❖ Direction of fracture lines: transverse, oblique, spiral, comminuted, and impacted
- ❖ Relationship of fragments to each other: alignment and apposition
- ❖ Stability: describes the tendency of a fracture to displace after reduction
- ❖ Associated soft tissue injury: simple, compound, or complicated

Fractures can be caused by direct or indirect trauma. A fracture's extent and severity depends on extrinsic factors; amount, direction, and duration of force as well as the frequency of the injury-causing act.[1,2]

Assessment/Analysis
- Mechanism of injury, time of injury, and associated injuries
- Pain assessment
- Inspect for blood loss, swelling, contusion, capillary refill, skin integrity, and deformity/angulation
  - Compare the appearance to opposite extremity if it is not also injured
- For open fractures, assess the size of the wound, for presence of contaminants, and any drainage from the wound
- Palpate affected area for crepitus, abnormal mobility at or between joints, tenderness, temperature of extremity, and pulses distal to the injury. Assess range of motion
  - May be reduced or normal depending on the injury[2]
- Assess sensation surrounding and distal to the injury

Interventions
- Elevate the extremity and apply ice to decrease swelling
- Remove jewelry from the affected area or distal to this area, because it can act as a tourniquet if left in place
- Splint the extremity to provide support and position of comfort, decrease pain, reduce the risk for fat emboli, and to prevent soft tissue injury from fracture fragments[1,2]
- If open fracture is present, cover wound with sterile saline dressings[1,3]
- Establish IV access for crystalloid fluids, blood products, and medications as needed
- Administer medications such as analgesia, procedural sedation medications, antibiotics, and/or tetanus booster as ordered
- Prepare patient for X-ray (pre and post reduction)
- Assist with closed reduction as needed
- Surgery may be required if there is associated vessel damage, to stabilize a bone, when closed reduction has failed or for displaced intra-articular fractures[2]
- Prepare the patient for admission, surgery, transfer, and/or discharge
- Patient education about splint care, use of assistive devices, signs and symptoms of neurovascular compromise, and follow up care

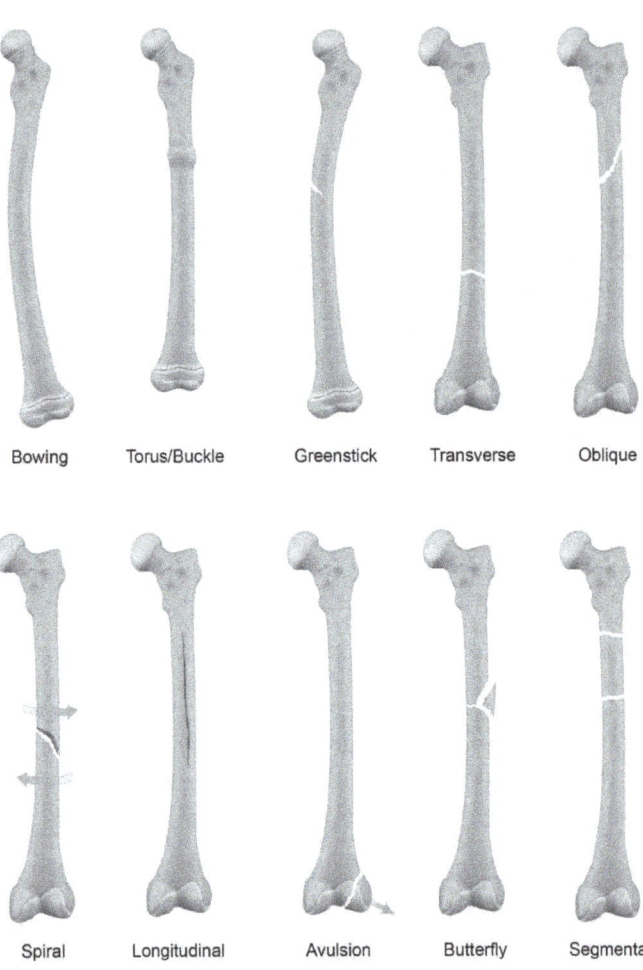

FIGURE 11-2 Type of fracture can provide clues as to mechanism of injury, if unknown or when patient report of mechanism is questioned
Reproduced with permission from Elsayes KM, Oldham SAA: Introduction to Diagnostic Radiology. New York: McGraw-Hill Education; 2014.

Evaluation
- Pain management
- Normal neurovascular status
- Effective tissue perfusion and hemodynamic status

Gout/Pseudogout

Gout and pseudogout are caused by the formation of crystals within the joint space leading to pain and joint inflammation. Gout is inflammation caused by monosodium urate monohydrate crystals,[8] which occurs due to overproduction or reduced secretion of uric acid. Pseudogout is inflammation caused by calcium pyrophosphate crystals.[8] Pseudogout is often idiopathic and clinically indistinguishable from gout.

Gout occurs more often in males than females.[8,9] The first bout of gouty arthritis usually occurs at the first metatarsophalangeal joint and manifests as a red, hot, and swollen joint with intense pain.[9] Thiazide diuretics and foods that are rich in purines can increase the frequency of gout attacks. Treatment in the acute phase is the same for both illnesses, however, no specific therapeutic regimen exists to treat the underlying cause of pseudogout.[8]

Assessment/Analysis
- Presence of fever
- Pain assessment
- History of similar episodes in the past
- Medication history: thiazide diuretics
- Joint edema, erythema, and tenderness on palpation

Interventions
- Establish IV access for crystalloid fluids and medications as needed
- Administer medications as ordered, such as analgesia, corticosteroids, and colchicine
- Collect uric acid lab studies (blood and urine)
- Prepare patient for X-rays as requested
  - Chronic gout may show lesions, whereas new onset gout usually shows no signs on X-ray[8]
- Assist with arthrocentesis if performed to determine presence of crystals
- Patient education about disease process, weight reduction, how to avoid precipitating factors (e.g., low-purine diet), and appropriate follow up

Evaluation
- Pain management

Bursitis

Bursitis is inflammation of the bursa from trauma or infection. Bursa is a small, fluid-filled sac covering the bony prominence among bones, muscles, and tendons. The most common sites of bursitis are the shoulder, elbow, hip, knee, and heel of the foot.[6]

Assessment/Analysis
- History of present complaint including recent surgery, infection, trauma, and/or repetitive use of area, joint involved, and associated symptoms like pain, fever, chills, etc
- Inspect the joint for swelling and redness
- Palpate the joint noting tenderness, warmth, and/or limited range of motion

Interventions
- Ice, rest, and elevate the area
- Immobilize the affected joint with splint
- Administer analgesic or antibiotic medications as ordered
- Assist with orthopedic consultation for possible bursal injection or aspiration

Evaluation
- Pain management

Joint Effusion

Joint effusions involve the collection of fluid in a joint as a result of an inflammatory process, previous surgery, or trauma. The most common effusion site is the knee joint.[6]

Assessment/Analysis
- History of present complaint including recent surgery, infection, and/or trauma, joint involved, and associated symptoms like pain, fever, chills, etc
- Ability to bear weight
- Personal history of substance abuse (risk of septic arthritis)
- Inspect the joint for swelling, redness, and any skin changes
- Palpate the joint noting tenderness and/or limited range of motion

Interventions
- Immobilize the affected joint
- Assist with arthrocentesis
- Laboratory studies for initial management
  - CBC with differential
  - Erythrocyte sedimentation rate (ESR)
  - C-Reactive protein
  - Urinalysis
- Prepare patient for X-ray
- Administer medications such as analgesia, steroids, and/or antibiotics as ordered
- Educate the patient on self-care at home and signs and symptoms needing medical reevaluation

Evaluation
- Pain management

Low Back Pain

Low back pain is usually a benign problem and affects 60% to 80% of patients at some time.[6] Causes include intervertebral disk disease or disk herniation and could lead to spinal cord compromise, such as Cauda equina syndrome (see Chapter 4: Neurologic Emergencies). Low back pain can occur in otherwise healthy people between the ages of 30 and 40 years old.[6] The pain may be localized or radiate to the buttock or lower extremities. Symptoms will vary depending on the involved structures. Risk factors include obesity, poor body mechanics, lifting or moving heavy objects, prolonged sitting, poor office furniture design, and hard floor surfaces.

Assessment/Analysis

- History of present complaint including pain, recent trauma, onset, and associated symptoms like paresthesia, radiation of pain, impaired function of bowel and/or bladder, and/or impaired sexual function
- Inspect the back for abnormal spinal curvature such as lordosis, kyphosis, or scoliosis
- Palpate for point tenderness versus general tenderness, swelling, and/or muscle spasm
- Assess range of motion, deep tendon reflexes, motor function, and sensory testing as needed
- Assess lower lumber/sacral function and sensation
    - Rectal tone
    - Great toe flexion
    - Ability to squeeze buttocks together[10]

Interventions

- Assist patient into position of comfort: pelvic tilt can reduce pain
- Administer analgesia as ordered
- Prepare patient for X-ray
- Intractable pain may require hospital admission
- Patient education about proper body mechanics, home safety such as installing railings and removing loose floor mats, and use of any assistive devices like a walker or cane

Evaluation

- Pain management
- Normal neurological function

Osteomyelitis

Osteomyelitis is an infection of the bone. After an injury, an invasion of organisms may spread to the bone in a variety of ways. It can be a direct invasion to the bone from the outside, such as with a penetrating injury or fracture, or the organisms can invade from another primary source, such as a skin abscess, pneumonia, urinary tract infection, etc. The most common organism causing osteomyelitis is *S. aureus*.[1]

Assessment/Analysis

- Assess for symptoms such as pain, fever, malaise, weakness, irritability, and generalized signs of sepsis
- Obtain thorough patient history including at risk circumstances such as recent fractures, puncture wounds, and IV substance abuse
- Inspect for swelling, redness, and/or warmth over the involved area
- Palpate for tenderness, deformity of the bone, and diminished range of motion
- Lab studies for initial management and pre-operative screening
    - CBC with differential
    - Erythrocyte sedimentation rate (ESR)
    - C-Reactive protein
    - Blood cultures, if indicated

Interventions

- Establish IV access for crystalloid fluids and medications as needed
- Administer analgesia and antibiotic medications
    - Antibiotics may be required for a 6 week period[1]
    - For patients with subsequent ED visits, determine medication adherence
- Immobilize the affected extremity
- Prepare patient for possible admission or transfer for surgical debridement of the infected abscess or bone and antibiotic therapy

Evaluation

- Pain management
- Normal hemodynamic status

Strains/Sprains

A sprain is the stretching, separation, or tear of a supporting ligament. A strain is the separation or tear of muscle fibers from bone. Both can result from direct or indirect trauma. The most common causes are sports-related trauma.[2] Sprains and strains are rare in young children before the closure of the epiphyseal growth plates.[2]

Both strains and sprains are classified by the amount of damage[2,4]

- ❖ First degree: minor tear in the fibers; minimal swelling, minor discomfort, absent or minor ecchymosis
- ❖ Second degree: partial tear, joint intact, more severe swelling, visible ecchymosis
- ❖ Third degree: complete disruption of ligament, joint may be open, minimal to severe swelling, resultant separation of muscle from muscle, muscle from tendon, or tendon from bone

Assessment/Analysis

- Mechanism of injury (especially sudden stretching, twisting, or excessive force to joint), time of injury, and associated injuries
- Pain assessment
- Inspect for swelling, deformity, capillary refill, and ecchymosis
- Palpate for distal pulses and tenderness over affected area
- Assess motor function
- Assess sensation surrounding and distal to the injury

Interventions

- Analgesia
- Ice
- Elevation
- Immobilization

- Patient teaching about any assistive devices, home treatment, signs, and symptoms requiring re-evaluation, and follow up with outside resources

Evaluation
- Pain management
- Normal neurovascular status
- Effective tissue perfusion

Achilles Tendon Rupture

An Achilles tendon rupture can occur in start-and-stop sports, jumping, pushing off, and direct trauma.[4] The patient may report hearing a loud crack or snap or the sensation of something striking the posterior ankle.

Assessment/Analysis
- Mechanism and time of injury
- Pain assessment
- Determine loss of motor function of foot on affected side
  - Thompson test:[11] patient lies supine on exam table with feet hanging over the edge, squeeze each calf bilaterally and observe for plantar flexion
    - If a complete rupture has occurred, there is minimal to no foot movement (positive Thompson's sign), see Figure 11-3
- Patient's ability to stand on ball of foot, plantar flex the foot
- Observe gait: patient may walk flat-footed
- Inspect for swelling, deformity, and ecchymosis
- Palpate for tenderness over affected area

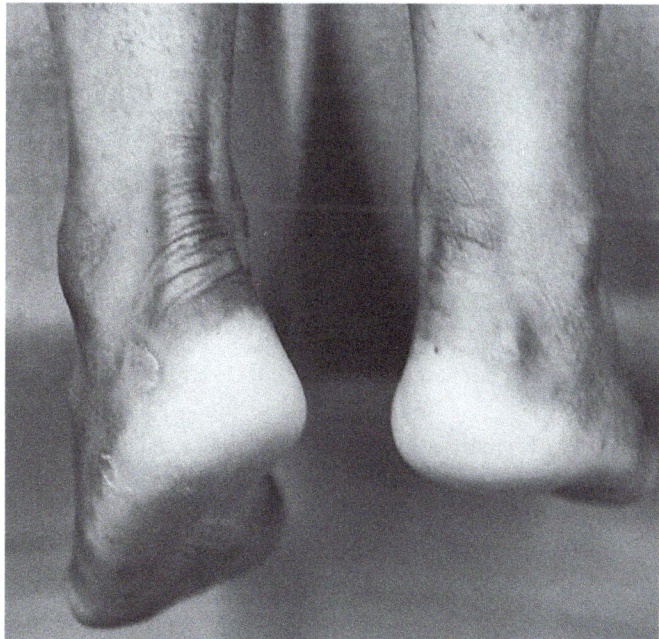

FIGURE 11-3 Achilles Tendon Rupture. Note the loss of the normal resting plantarflexion due to right Achilles tendon rupture. Swelling is also apparent over the injury site
Reproduced with permission from Knoop KJ, Stack LB, Storrow AB, et al: The Atlas of Emergency Medicine, 4th ed. New York: McGraw-Hill Education; 2016: Photo contributor: Kevin J. Knoop, MD, MS.

Interventions
- Ice, elevation
- Administer analgesia as ordered
- Splint the foot in plantar flexion[11]
- Prepare patient for admission, surgery, transfer, and/or discharge

Evaluation
- Pain management

Wound Emergencies

Abrasions

An abrasion is a partial or full thickness wound with denuded skin.[7] It can be mild or severe and may vary in surface area and depth depending on the mechanism of injury. If the abrasion also has embedded foreign bodies, such as gravel, dirt, and/or asphalt, it can cause tattooing of the skin,[12] which may be permanent. Abrasions require vigorous wound cleaning and debridement to remove the foreign bodies, avoid skin discoloration or tattooing, and reduce the risk of infection.

Assessment/Analysis
- Location of wound
- Depth, length, and size of the wound
- Extent of denuded tissue and underlying structures involved
- Tissue swelling, deformity, and/or presence of foreign bodies
- Evidence of wound contamination or presence of exudate
- Pain
- Co-morbidities increasing risk for infection (diabetes, corticosteroid use, etc.)

Interventions
- Superficial wounds may be cleaned with normal saline or tap water[13]
- Dirty or deep wounds may require more extensive preparation. Follow facility protocols
- Anesthesia may be required when removing gravel and other foreign materials from the wound
- If hair removal around the wound is necessary, clip and do not shave to reduce potential for infection[5,14]
- Patient teaching regarding signs and symptoms of infection and wound care at home

Evaluation
- Pain management
- Clean wound

Avulsions

Avulsions are characterized by full-thickness tissue loss preventing wound edge approximation. Avulsions are commonly seen in fingertip and tip of the nose injuries. Small avulsions heal by secondary intention. Larger avulsed areas may require grafting. A "degloving" injury is a severe avulsion, in which the full thickness of skin is peeled away from the hand, foot, or scalp resulting in devascularization of the skin and potential damage to underlying tissue.[12] Flap replacement and grafting are frequently required.

On fingers, rings may be the cause of the degloving (see Figure 11-4).

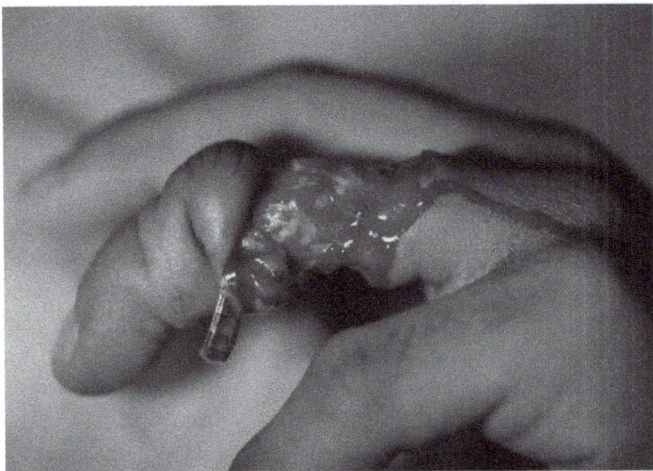

FIGURE 11-4 Finger Degloving Avulsion. Rings being caught and forced proximally are a common cause of finger degloving
Reproduced with permission from Knoop KJ, Stack LB, Storrow AB, et al: The Atlas of Emergency Medicine, 4th ed. New York: McGraw-Hill Education; 2016: Photo contributor: Selim Suner, MD.

Assessment/Analysis
- History of injury including mechanism, time since the injury, location of injury, and any efforts made to preserve avulsed tissue
- Pain assessment
- Inspect for amount of bleeding, extent of injury, and involved structures
- Palpate pulses distal to the injury and areas of tenderness
- Determine sensation surrounding and distal to the injury and range of motion if joint involvement
- CBC with differential if concerned about acute blood loss or infection in an older wound
- Radiographs if associated with possible fracture or foreign body

Interventions
- Elevate affected part
- Apply direct, steady pressure to decrease bleeding
- Establish IV access for crystalloid fluids and medications as needed
- Administer medications such as analgesia, antibiotics, and tetanus booster, as ordered
- Apply a non-adhering dressing[7]
- If degloving injury
  - Realign soft tissue to prevent further damage
  - Cover with sterile dressing
- Prepare patient for hospital admission, transfer, surgery and/or discharge
- Educate patient care of wound and dressing, signs and symptoms of infection, and follow up care

Evaluation
- Hemostasis
- Normal hemodynamic status
- Pain management

Bites

Bites can be caused by animals or humans and can involve contusions, avulsions, lacerations, and puncture wounds. Dog bites make up 80 to 90% of all bites.[15,16] Large dogs can cause serious wounds due to the compressive force of their jaws resulting in crushing-type wounds.[17] Cat bites make up 5 to 15% of all bites and are at high risk for infection.[15] Human bites, 2 to 5% of all bites, are often the result of aggressive acts such as sexual assault and battery.[15] A minor percentage of bites are attributed to smaller animals (rats, ferrets, rabbits), monkeys, reptiles, and farm animals. Regardless of the source, bite wounds are considered contaminated and place the patient at risk of infection.[16,17]

Assessment/Analysis
- Size and location of the wound
- Time elapsed since injury
- Type of animal and its status including health, vaccination history, behavior, current location, and ownership
- Circumstances surrounding the bite (provoked, unprovoked, defensive)
- Inspect for bleeding, crush injury, deep penetrating injury, lacerations, and devitalized tissue
- Assess neurovascular status distal to the wound
- Any signs of infection including redness, drainage, swelling, and pain

Interventions
- Bleeding control using pressure, elevation, and tourniquet if necessary
- Wound irrigation, debridement, and closure assistance as needed
- Administer medications such as antibiotics, analgesia, post-exposure rabies prophylaxis, and/or tetanus booster as ordered
- Prepare for potential healing by secondary intention
  - Bite wounds which cannot be thoroughly cleansed, like cat bites, are usually left open to avoid trapping bacteria in the wound[15]
- Report animal bites as required by hospital policy or municipal laws
- Instruct the patient in wound care and signs of infection indicating that follow up care is required

Evaluation
- Hemostasis
- Pain management
- Clean wound

Snake Bites and Insect Stings

See Chapter 12: Environment and Toxicology Emergencies.

Abscess

An abscess is caused by localized collection of purulent material (pus). Although the pus may eventually erupt on its own, the recommended treatment is to drain and clean the abscess.[16] The wound may then be packed with gauze or have a drain placed. Then it should be covered with a loose, absorbent dressing.

Assessment/Analysis
- Size and location
- Signs of infection including fever, redness, drainage, swelling, and pain

Interventions
- Assist with wound cleaning, incision and drainage, and packing as needed
- Administer medications such as antibiotics and/or analgesia as ordered
  - Antibiotics are generally indicated only if there is fever or recurrence of the abscess[16,18]
- Instruct the patient in wound care and signs of infection indicating required follow up care

Evaluation
- Pain management

Lacerations

Lacerations are open wounds resulting from blunt trauma, which causes tearing or crushing of tissue or wounds from sharp or penetrating mechanisms. The wound may be superficial, only involving the epidermis, or the laceration may extend into fascia and muscle. Healing can be delayed if the laceration occurs over an area of flexion and extension.[7]

Assessment/Analysis
- Mechanism of injury, time of injury, location of injury, and patient history
- Inspect wound depth, length, location, presence of foreign bodies/contaminants, and bleeding
- Palpate pulses distal to injury and areas of tenderness
- Assess motor and sensory function surrounding and distal to the injury and flexion/extension against resistance if there is joint involvement

Interventions
- Control bleeding with local pressure, elevation, and/or tourniquet
- Establish IV access for crystalloid fluids and medications as needed
- Administer medications such as analgesia, sedation for procedures, antibiotics and/or tetanus prophylaxis as ordered
- Cleanse and irrigate the wound and surrounding skin thoroughly
- Assist with wound closure (sutures, staples, skin glue, etc.)
- Apply appropriate dressing
- Prepare patient for admission, transfer, surgery and/or discharge
- Patient education on wound care and signs/symptoms of infection indicating follow up care is required

Evaluation
- Hemostasis
- Normal hemodynamic status
- Pain management

Missile/Penetrating Injuries

Missile injuries are characterized as high-pressure, penetrating wounds and include those caused by gunshot, shrapnel, arrows, and nail guns. Penetrating injuries may also be caused by knives, machetes, paint guns, etc. Puncture wounds caused by paint or grease guns require emergent debridement and extensive irrigation under anesthesia because serious tissue destruction can result from the injected material tracking along fascial planes, neuromuscular bundles, and tendon sheaths.[7] Missile injuries can cause bony, neurovascular, and soft tissue injuries. Some penetrating injuries may also require forensic interventions such as police reporting and preservation of evidence (clothing, bullets, weapons, etc.) for law enforcement.

Assessment/Analysis
- Inspect for active bleeding, depth/length of wound, structures involved, obvious wound contamination
- Patient history including mechanism of injury, time since injury, location of injury, and type of material involved
- Palpate pulses distal to the injury and areas of tenderness
- Assess sensory and motor function surrounding and distal to the injury
- Radiographs of the affected area can help determine foreign body location and/or underlying bony injury

Interventions
- Control local bleeding with pressure, elevation, and/or tourniquet
- Stabilize penetrating objects
- Establish IV access for crystalloids, blood products, and medications as needed
- Administer medications such as analgesia, antibiotics, and tetanus prophylaxis, as ordered
- Clean and irrigate skin around the wound
- Assist with wound care procedures
- Notify law enforcement agencies according to local reporting requirements

- Collect and maintain physical and forensic evidence and chain of custody, as indicated
- Apply appropriate dressings and splints
- Prepare the patient for admission, surgery, transfer, and/or discharge
- Educate the patient about wound care, signs and symptoms of infection, and follow up care

Evaluation
- Hemostasis
- Normal hemodynamic status
- Pain management
- Normal neurovascular status

Pressure Injuries

Pressure injuries, also called pressure ulcers, are local damage to the skin and underlying tissue caused by compression between bony prominence and an external surface.[12] They are classified on a four-grade scale described as follows and illustrated in Figure 11-5.

- Grade 1: non-blanchable erythema of intact skin
- Grade 2: partial-thickness skin loss, involving epidermis, dermis, or both. Superficial and may present as an abrasion or blister
- Grade 3: full-thickness skin loss involving damage to or necrosis of subcutaneous tissue that may extend down to, but not through, underlying fascia
- Grade 4: extensive destruction, tissue necrosis, or damage to muscle, bone or supporting structures, with or without full-thickness skin loss

Contributing factors include[12]

- Those with sensory deficits who cannot detect pressure and therefore do not reposition themselves
- Debility/paralysis making independent repositioning impossible
- Medications or systemic hypoperfusion which reduces blood flow to the tissue
- Use of rigid devices (backboard, cervical collar, splints, etc) which cause pressure on bony prominences
- Malnutrition can increase extent and severity

Assessment/Analysis
- Patient risk factors
- Wound size, location, time, and involved structures
- Presence of infection, drainage, and contaminants
- Pain

Interventions
- Consult with wound care experts for management of existing pressure ulcers
- Administer medications such as analgesia and antibiotics as prescribed
- Prepare patient for possible admission for infected, worsening, or new ulcers
- Patient teaching including repositioning guidelines, wound care, signs and symptoms of infection, and follow up care
- Prevention techniques
  - Patient repositioning and turning at regular intervals
  - Prompt removal from long spine board
  - Padding bony prominences
    - See Figure 11-6 for common areas of pressure
  - Ensuring clean, dry, flat linen behind/under patients
  - Placing long stay patients in a hospital bed/specialty mattress

Evaluation
- Pain management
- Maintenance of skin integrity

Puncture Wounds

A puncture wound is a piercing of the skin by a foreign object, causing a hole in the skin and underlying tissues. Puncture wounds are caused by direct trauma and can be superficial, only involving the skin or can extend through tissue and into the bone, depending on the mechanism of injury. Mechanisms are varied but may include bites, nails, needles, pins, knives, and broken glass. Puncture wounds tend to bleed minimally before sealing themselves off, creating a high risk for infection.[7] Special attention should be given to plantar puncture wounds as they often penetrate to the bone and introduce foreign matter, increasing the risk for osteomyelitis.[12]

Assessment/Analysis
- Mechanism of injury, time since injury, type of injuring object, size and location of the wound, and patient history
- Pain
- Presence of foreign bodies, contaminants, bleeding, or discharge
- Pulses distal to injury and areas of tenderness
- Assess sensory and motor function surrounding and distal to the injury

Interventions
- Perform or assist with wound care
- Apply appropriate dressings or immobilization devices
- Radiographic studies should be completed if the puncture wound is near a joint or bone to rule out underlying fracture and presence of some types of foreign bodies
- Administer medications such as analgesia, antibiotics, and/or tetanus prophylaxis as ordered
  - Routine use of prophylactic antibiotics is not recommended for uncomplicated puncture wounds in healthy individuals as unnecessary antibiotics can predispose patients to superbugs[2,12,18]
- Educate patient about wound care, signs and symptoms of infection, and follow up care

Evaluation
- Pain management
- Normal neurovascular status

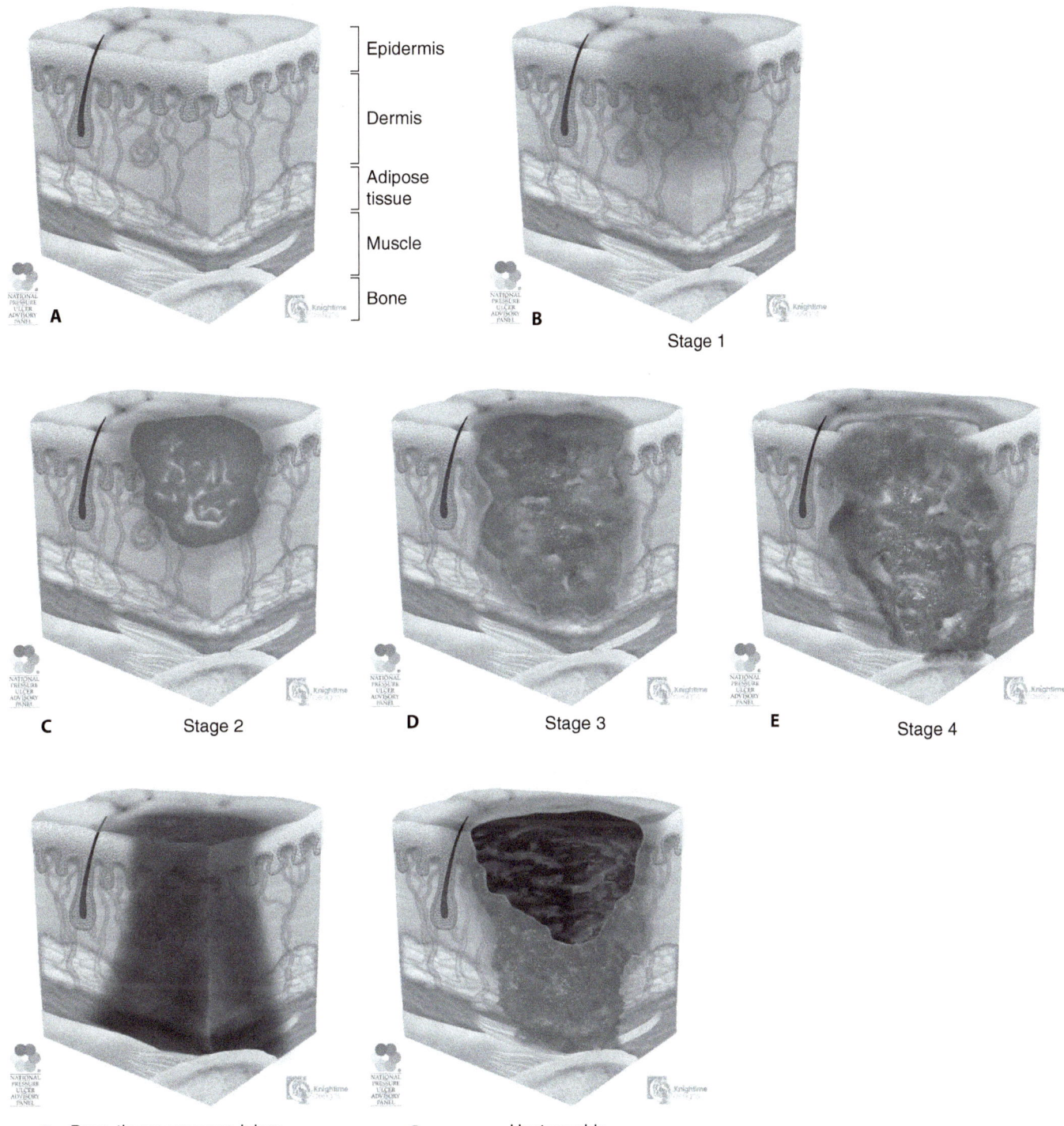

FIGURE 11-5 **National pressure ulcer staging system. (A) Normal Skin (B) Stage 1 Pressure Ulcer (C) Stage 2 Pressure Ulcer (D) Stage 3 Pressure Ulcer (E) Stage 4 Pressure Ulcer (F) Deep Tissue Pressure Injury (G) Unstageable Pressure Ulcer**
Reproduced with permission from the National Pressure Ulcer Advisory Panel, 2016.

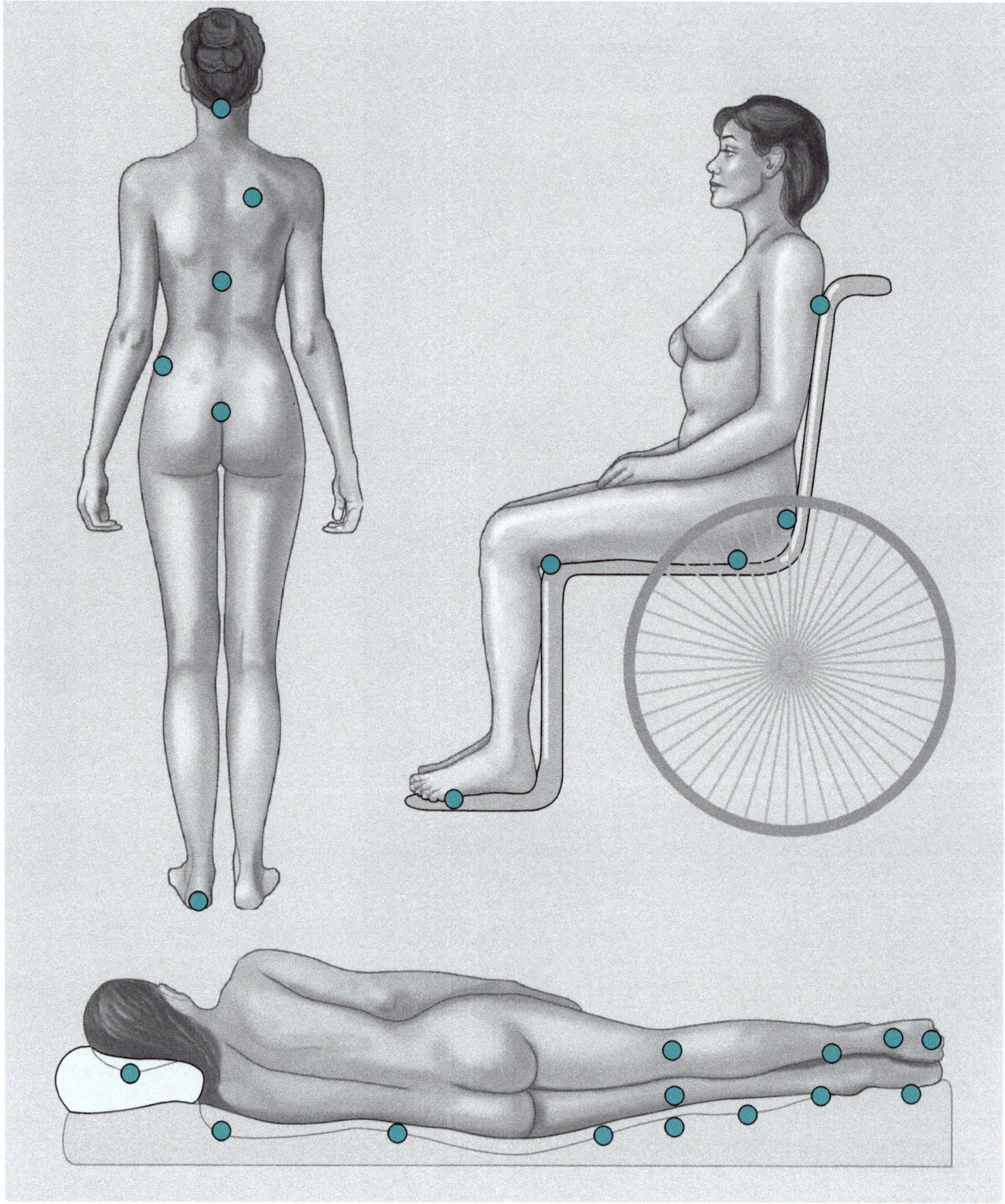

FIGURE 11-6 **Common sites of pressure ulcer development**
Reproduced with permission from Preventing Pressure Ulcers: A Patient's Guide. Washington, DC, US Department of Health and Human Services, USGPO 617-025/68298, 1992.

Blast Injuries

Explosions cause a variety of injuries depending on the size of the explosion and the proximity of the victim to the blast forces. Blast or explosive injuries are classified as primary, secondary, and tertiary. Orthopedic and wound injuries are most likely secondary, such as from flying debris, or tertiary injuries caused by sudden deceleration after being thrown by the blast.[19] Victims of blast explosions can have extensive external injuries which may distract from the search for more serious internal injuries.

Assessment/Analysis
- Consider need for decontamination
- Consider need to activate disaster triage/protocols
- Conduct a thorough trauma head to toe assessment to identify all injuries

Interventions
- Specific to identified injuries

Evaluation
- Pain management

REFERENCES

1. Ramponi DR, Cerepani MJ. Orthopedic trauma. In: Hoyt KS, Selfridge-Thomas J, eds. *Emergency Nursing Core Curriculum*. 6th ed., pp. 891–928. St. Louis, MO: Elsevier/Saunders; 2007.
2. Matamoros, L. Musculoskeletal emergencies and wound management. In: Tscheschlog BA, Jauch A, eds. *Emergency Nursing Made Incredibly Easy!* 2nd ed., pp. 304–347. Philadelphia, PA: Wolters Kluwer Health; 2015.
3. Bratcher CM. Musculoskeletal trauma. In: Gurney D, ed. *Trauma Nursing Core Course Provider Manual*. 7th ed., pp. 193–204. Des Plaines, IL: Emergency Nurses Association; 2014.
4. Halpern JS. Musculoskeletal trauma. In: Hammond BB, Zimmermann PG, eds. *Sheehy's Manual of Emergency Care*. 7th ed., pp. 427–438. St. Louis, MO: Elsevier/Mosby; 2013.
5. Provins-Churbock C. Surface and burn trauma. In: Gurney D, ed. *Trauma Nursing Core Course Provider Manual*. 7th ed. pp. 205–224. Des Plaines, IL: Emergency Nurses Association; 2014.
6. Cerepani MJ, Ramponi DR. Orthopedic emergencies. In: Hoyt KS, Selfridge-Thomas J, eds. *Emergency Nursing Core Curriculum*. 6th ed., pp. 585–603. St. Louis, MO: Elsevier/Saunders; 2007.
7. Ramirez EG. Wounds and wound management. In: Hoyt KS, Selfridge-Thomas J, eds. *Emergency Nursing Core Curriculum*. 6th ed. pp. 738–759. St. Louis, MO: Elsevier/Saunders; 2007.
8. Lazear SE, Roberts A. Medical emergencies. In: Hoyt KS, Selfridge-Thomas J, eds. *Emergency Nursing Core Curriculum*. 6th ed., pp. 483–509. St. Louis, MO: Elsevier/Saunders; 2007.
9. Gout. *Centers for Disease Control and Prevention*. Available at http://www.cdc.gov/arthritis/basics/gout.html. Published on 2015. Accessed March 27, 2016.
10. Crowley, M. Spinal cord and vertebral column trauma. In: Gurney D, ed. *Trauma Nursing Core Course Provider Manual*. 7th ed. pp. 173–192. Des Plaines, IL: Emergency Nurses Association; 2014.
11. Cerepani MJ. Orthopedic and neurovascular trauma. In: Howard PK, Steinmann RS, eds. *Sheehy's Emergency Nursing Principles and Practice*. 6th ed. pp. 313–339. St. Louis, MO: Elsevier/Mosby; 2010.
12. Herr RD. Wound management. In: Hammond BB, Zimmermann PG, eds. *Sheehy's Manual of Emergency Care*. 6th ed. pp. 147–160. St. Louis, MO: Elsevier/Mosby; 2013.
13. Clinical Practice Guideline: Wound Preparation. *Emergency Nurses Association*. Available at https://www.ena.org/practice-research/research/CPG/Documents/WoundPreparationCPG.pdf. Published on 2011.
14. Wafer M. Shock and multisystem trauma emergencies. In: Tscheschlog BA, Jauch A. eds. *Emergency Nursing Made Incredibly Easy!* 2nd ed., pp. 472–509. Philadelphia, PA: Wolters Kluwer Health; 2015.
15. Briggs J. Environmental emergencies. In: Tscheschlog BA, Jauch A, eds. *Emergency Nursing Made Incredibly Easy!* 2nd ed., pp. 437–471. Philadelphia, PA: Wolters Kluwer Health; 2015.
16. Denke NJ. Wound management. In: Howard PK, Steinmann RA, eds. *Sheehy's Emergency Nursing Principles and Practice*. 6th ed., pp. 111–126. St. Louis, MO: Elsevier/Mosby; 2010.
17. Flarity K. Environmental emergencies. In: Howard PK, Steinmann RA, eds. *Sheehy's Emergency Nursing Principles and Practice*. 6th ed. pp. 535–553. St. Louis, MO: Elsevier/Mosby; 2010.
18. Antibiotic "Stewardship" Starts in the ED. *American College of Emergency Physicians*. Available at http://www.acep.org/Content.aspx?id=70630. Published on 2010. Accessed March 13, 2016.
19. Madigan K. Mechanism of injury. In: Gurney D, ed. *Trauma Nursing Core Course Provider Manual*. 7th ed. pp. 761–765. Des Plaines, IL: Emergency Nurses Association; 2014.

Practice Questions

Question	Rationale
1. A patient arrives to the emergency department with a foreign object in the hand received while cutting firewood. The object is not visible in the wound. The emergency nurse knows which intervention is contraindicated? a. Apply a cold pack b. Soak/submerge the wound for cleaning c. Splint the injury d. Determine range of motion	*Answer: b* Soaking or submerging a suspected wooden foreign body could make the object more difficult to remove. Application of a cold pack may reduce swelling making removal easier. There is no indication for splinting or range of motion assessments, but they would not be contraindicated.
2. A patient arrives with a cast to her forearm. She complains of pain that is unrelieved by narcotic pain medication. Her fingers are pale and she complains of tingling. The emergency nurse should anticipate a. Replacing the cast with a splint b. Applying ice to the extremity c. Elevating the extremity above the heart d. Bi-valving or removing the cast	*Answer: d* Patient is displaying signs of compartment syndrome. All external sources of compression should be removed. Once removed, a splint should not replace the cast until the cause of the patient's symptoms is confirmed and treated. Ice and elevating above the heart are contraindicated in suspected compartment syndrome as these actions can decrease blood flow to an already compromised extremity.
3. The following diagnostic test would be used to confirm a shoulder dislocation a. Computed tomography (CT) scan of the shoulder b. Magnetic resonance imaging (MRI) c. Anterior/posterior/lateral X-ray films of the affected joint d. Arthrogram of the affected joint	*Answer: c* Plain films are usually all that are required to confirm dislocations. Arthrogram could be useful if neuromuscular injury is suspected, but is not routine. CT is not needed emergently as plain films will determine if the shoulder is dislocated. MRI is not usually done emergently, but can be done once the joint is relocated, if needed to assess for ligamentous stability and injury.
4. Which of the following foreign bodies is most likely to cause a tissue reaction leading to infection? a. Wooden splinters b. Metal needles c. Glass shards d. Bullets	*Answer: a* Vegetative foreign bodies (such as wood) are highly reactive, often lead to infection, and should be removed as soon as possible. Bullets, glass shards, and metal needles may be left in place if they do not pose a threat to nearby structures and they are not likely to cause a tissue reaction.
5. Amputated parts should be wrapped in saline moistened gauze and placed a. In a bowl of ice b. In a bowl of disinfectant c. In a sealed plastic bag and then into a bowl of ice d. In a biohazard bag	*Answer: c* Amputated parts should not be placed directly on ice or in disinfectant. Sealing in a plastic bag keeps the part from direct contact with ice. This prevents the tissue from freezing and protects the part from tissue changes associated with immersion in melted ice water.

Question	Rationale

6. Wound debridement is
   a. Not necessary for wound healing
   b. Used in place of antibiotics
   c. Used to removed debris so wound healing is enhanced
   d. Best accomplished without analgesia
	Answer: c
	Debridement facilitates removal of waste products, devitalized tissue, and foreign matter found in the wound and therefore enhances wound healing. Many wounds need debridement to heal. Patient comfort should be considered before any painful procedure. Wound debridement facilitates wound healing but does not replace the possible need for antibiotics.

7. Patients with costochondritis often have
   a. Reproducible pain
   b. Elevated troponin levels
   c. Abnormal chest x-rays
   d. Shortness of breath
	Answer: a
	Costochondritis causes reproducible pain with point tenderness upon palpation of the chest wall. Costochondritis does not cause elevated troponin levels, abnormal chest X-rays, or shortness of breath.

8. Which of the following wounds is most at risk for infection?
   a. Puncture wound from a tack into a finger
   b. Plantar puncture wound from a nail through a shoe
   c. Puncture wound from a nail gun to the thigh
   d. Puncture wound from a screwdriver to the hand
	Answer: b
	Plantar puncture wounds are at increased risk of infection, including osteomyelitis, due to increased risk of transmitting and trapping foreign matter including bacteria deep in the tissue. Puncture wounds from nail guns are considered missile injuries. While they have a high-risk mechanism, the primary complication is not infection. Puncture wounds from a tack and a screwdriver may be deep, but the risk of infection is less than from a nail through a shoe.

9. The emergency nurse knows this type of amputation has the best chance of replantation?
   a. Incomplete
   b. Crushing-style
   c. Guillotine-style
   d. Tearing-style
	Answer: c
	Tissue damage is generally minor in a guillotine-style amputation due to the precise cut between the body and the affected part. Crushing and tearing mechanisms cause both more tissue damage because of the distortion and destruction of the involved and surrounding structures, especially the vasculature.

10. When cleaning the stump of an amputation, the emergency nurse knows to
   a. Scrub vigorously to remove debris
   b. Clean the site using normal saline solution irrigation
   c. Clean the site using cleaning solutions (like iodine)
   d. Soak the stump in room temperature water to help remove debris
	Answer: b
	Saline is the only solution indicated for stump care. Vigorous scrubbing can damage the stump. Abrasive cleaning solutions and water can damage the stump. Iodine should not be the potential for effects on tissue damage.

11. An elderly patient arrives after a fall. She has a shortened, externally rotated leg and complains of hip pain. The emergency nurse suspects a
   a. Pelvic fracture
   b. Knee effusion
   c. A knee sprain
   d. Hip contusions
	Answer: a
	Fractures can cause shortening and rotation of the leg on the affected side. An effusion and sprain would cause swelling of the knee, but not shortening compared to the unaffected side. A hip contusion may be a secondary diagnosis for this patient, but would not explain her shortened, externally rotated leg.

Question	Rationale
12. A deadly complication of a long bone fracture is a. Muscle atrophy b. Pressure ulcers c. Fat embolism d. Weight gain	*Answer: c* Fat embolism is a deadly complication of long bone fractures. Muscle atrophy, pressure ulcers, and weight gain are possible side effects of immobility but are generally not deadly.
13. A patient arrives with right knee pain and swelling following a slip during a basketball game. The patient is able to limp and there is visible swelling, but no bony instability. The patient has nearly full range of motion despite the pain. The most likely cause of the patient's discomfort is due to a a. Sprain b. Patellar dislocation c. Fracture d. Abscess	*Answer: a* Sprains are often the result of sports injuries. Fracture of the knee may involve bony instability and the inability to bear weight. Dislocation would affect range of motion. An abscess does not occur acutely due to sports injury, but may occur later due to an infection in an open wound.
14. A patient arrives to the ED following a cat bite to the hand. The cat belongs to her neighbor and is up to date on recommended immunizations. The hand is swollen, red, and painful. The emergency nurse anticipates treatment will include a. Closure with wound glue b. Administration of antibiotics due to the high risk of infection c. Closure with sutures d. Administration of rabies prophylaxis	*Answer: b* Cat bites are high risk for infection. Most bites are not sutured or otherwise closed to prevent the risk of trapping bacteria in the wound. Rabies prophylaxis is not indicated in a vaccinated, asymptomatic animal.
15. A patient arrives to the emergency department reporting a lump on his right arm for several days. He denies trauma. The area is red, swollen, and tender to touch. Circulation, sensation, and movement are intact. The patient has a low-grade fever. The emergency nurse anticipates a. Compartment pressure measurements b. Radiographs to confirm fracture c. Incision and drainage d. Splinting of the affected extremity	*Answer: c* The patient is displaying signs of an abscess. Appropriate treatment includes incision and drainage followed by antibiotic administration. Compartment pressure measurement, radiographs, and splinting are not generally indicated in the presence of an abscess.
16. The emergency nurse is reviewing abscess treatment discharge instructions with a patient. The nurse knows the teaching is effective when the patient states a. I will soak the wound every night so the packing stays moist b. I will take my antibiotics until the swelling goes down c. I will return to my doctor tomorrow to have the wound closed with sutures d. Increased swelling and redness are a signs of infection, which I should have re-evaluated	*Answer: d* Patients should understand signs and symptoms of increasing infection and when to return for re-evaluation. Soaking an abscess is not recommended. Patients should take the full course of antibiotics as prescribed and not stop before the end of the course of antibiotics. After incision and drainage, an abscess should be left open to heal.

Question	Rationale
17. A patient arrives to the emergency department complaining of left shoulder pain. The shoulder is swollen with obvious deformity. The patient is unable to raise the left arm or bring it across the chest. The emergency nurse suspects a(n) a. Radial fracture b. Rotator cuff injury c. Shoulder dislocation d. Arthritic shoulder	*Answer: c* Dislocations present with deformity and limited range of motion. Arthritis is a chronic condition, not an acute process. Rotator cuff injuries result in pain with movement but no significant restriction on range of motion or swelling. Radial fracture should not affect a patient's ability to perform shoulder range of motion.
18. The emergency nurse is reviewing discharge instructions with a patient who received sutures to her face. The nurse knows her teaching is effective when the patient states, "If there are no signs or symptoms of infection, I will have my sutures removed in a. 3 to 5 days" b. 5 to 7 days" c. 7 to 10 days" d. 10 to 14 days"	*Answer: a* Sutures to the face, lips, and eyelids should be removed in 3 to 5 days. Sutures to the eyebrow should be removed in 5 to 7 days. Sutures to the back, chest, arms, hands, and thighs should be removed in 7 to 10 days. Sutures to the lower legs and feet should be removed in 10 to 14 days.
19. The ED nurse knows to anticipate transfer to the OR for the following patient injury a. Puncture wound to the hand b. Paint gun injection to the hand c. Ligament tear in the knee d. Stage 1 pressure ulcer	*Answer: b* High-pressure injuries such as paint gun injections are serious, and immediate surgical intervention is required to drain the paint or oil and to preserve tissue. A simple laceration generally requires nonsurgical wound closure. A ligament tear in the knee may ultimately require surgery but would not require emergency surgery. Stage 1 pressure ulcers require monitoring but not surgical treatment.
20. A patient reports that while playing racquetball he felt a pop followed by severe pain radiating from his heel to the back of his leg and an inability to walk. The emergency nurse should further assess for signs of a. Ankle sprain b. Calcaneus fracture c. Achilles tendon rupture d. Deep vein thrombosis	*Answer: c* Achilles tendon rupture is common in stop-start sports like racquetball and can cause pain from the heel into the leg and an inability to ambulate. Calcaneus fracture and ankle sprains do not include. Pain radiating into the back of the leg with a "pop." Deep vein thrombosis does not have an acute onset (pop) with pain radiating from the heel to the leg and does not significantly affect a patient's ability to walk.
21. The emergency nurse knows discharge teaching was effective when a patient with gout reports a. "Alcohol doesn't affect my risk for gout attacks" b. "Weight reduction will increase my gout attacks" c. "I should drink plenty of water to reduce my risk of gout attacks" d. "I should eat more purine-rich foods to prevent uric acid build up"	*Answer: c* Drinking plenty of water is linked to fewer gout attacks. Alcohol metabolism is thought to increase uric acid production and contributes to dehydrating thus increasing your risk of a gout attack. Weight loss helps reduce the risk of frequent gout attacks. Patients with gout should avoid meats such as liver, kidney and sweetbreads, which have high purine levels and contribute to high blood levels of uric acid.

Question	Rationale
22. A 45-year-old male patient presents to triage complaining of sudden onset of big toe pain. On inspection, the triage nurse notes a red, hot, and swollen great toe. Patient denies trauma. The triage nurse suspects the patient has a. Gout b. Bursitis c. Foot fracture d. Achilles tendon rupture	*Answer: a* Gout. An initial episode of gout is often characterized by spontaneous, intense pain with edema at the metatarsophalangeal joint. Bursitis is often the result of overuse or infection and the common sites are shoulder, elbow, hip, knee, and heel of the foot. Foot fracture is improbable without trauma. Achilles tendon rupture is characterized by heel pain radiating up the back of the leg with difficulty or inability to move the foot.
23. A patient arrives with a splint to his upper extremity. He reports 10/10 pain despite analgesia administration and burning sensation to his arm. The most likely cause of his unrelieved pain is a. A torn ligament b. A history of narcotic dependency c. Compartment syndrome d. Blood loss	*Answer: c* Pain out of proportion to the injury which is not relieved by usual measures is a cardinal sign of compartment syndrome. Torn ligaments do not generally cause consistent, unrelieved pain, especially if they have been appropriately immobilized. Blood loss would not necessarily cause an increase in pain. Although the patient may have a history of narcotic dependency, he also has a fracture and all organic causes of his symptoms should be evaluated before this diagnosis is made.

Environment and Toxicology Emergencies

12

Michael J. Chicarelli, DNP, RN, CEN

Environmental Emergencies

Our environment can be an exciting and beautiful place providing hours of enjoyment, particularly for outdoor enthusiasts. Emergencies related to environmental exposure can include a vast number of specific situations ranging from temperature-related exposure to parasitic infestation. Those at risk include individuals who frequent the outdoors for recreational purposes, as well as those exposed to the environment in situations such as homelessness. Regardless of the circumstances surrounding exposure, the emergency nursing assessment process is approached in a similar way. This chapter discusses common environmental conditions such as temperature-related illness, exposure to noxious substances or organisms, and submersion injury.

Burns

Burns account for an estimated 500,000 emergency department visits each year.[1] In recent years, the management of burn victims has dramatically improved, increasing survival rates.[2] Burns cause varying levels of destruction of tissue, which can lead to long-term concerns including infection and disfigurement. Many burn victims have associated traumatic injuries that increase morbidity and mortality in the prehospital as well as the hospital setting. It is important to remember that burns may be caused by a variety of sources, the most common being thermal. Burns may also be caused by sources of electricity, chemicals, and radiation.[3] Smoke inhalation represents an additional challenge in the setting of burns, increasing complications and patient mortality. Toxic gases, such as carbon monoxide and cyanide, are often released from burning objects commonly found in homes or occupied structures.[4]

Assessment/Analysis
- Airway patency: determine airway involvement
  - Evidence of burns
  - Non-burn findings such as voice changes and carbonaceous sputum
  - At-risk findings, such as singed facial hair
- Breathing: burns to the chest or neck can impair breathing
- Circulation: assess for hypovolemia
- Depth of burn pictured in Figure 12-1
- Body surface area calculation, "rule of nines" as pictured in Figure 12-2

Interventions
- Support airway, breathing, and circulation (ABCs)
- Establish IV access for crystalloid fluids and medications as needed
  - In burns over 10% total body surface area (TBSA), fluid replacement is critical
  - Crystalloid fluids for resuscitation
    - Lactated Ringers recommended by American Burn Association[3]
  - Total amount to be given over 24 hours with half in first 8 hours post-burn
    - Adults: 2–4 mL × %TBSA burned × kg of body weight[3]
    - Pediatrics: 3–4 mL × %TBSA burned × kg of body weight[3]
  - Antibiotics, as ordered
- Warming methods to prevent hypothermia
- Pain management
- Strict aseptic technique to minimize infection
  - *Dry* sterile dressings
    - Moist dressings may increase risk of hypothermia through evaporation
- Consider topical treatments
  - Silver sulfadiazine (Silvadene™) cream
    - Do not use for patients with sulfa allergy

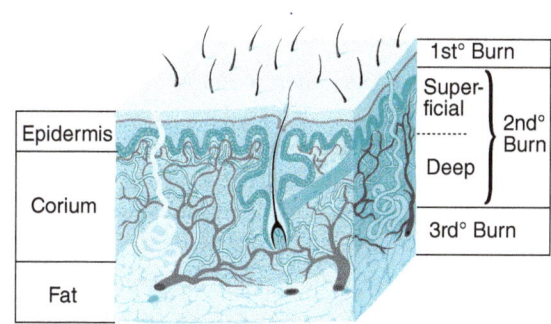

FIGURE 12-1 Layers of the skin showing depth of first-degree, second-degree, and third-degree burns

Reproduced with permission from Doherty G: CURRENT Diagnosis & Treatment: Surgery, 14th ed. New York: McGraw-Hill Education; 2015.

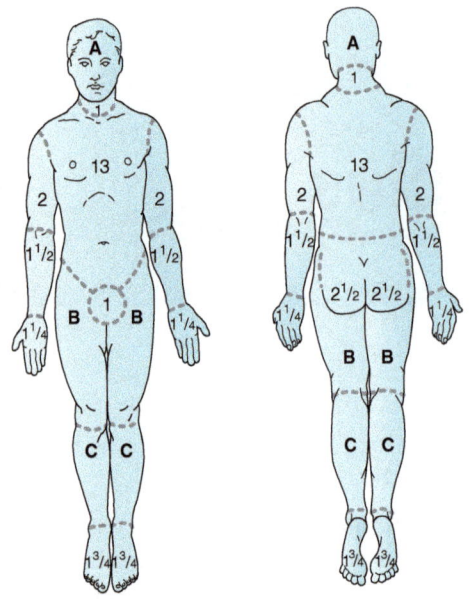
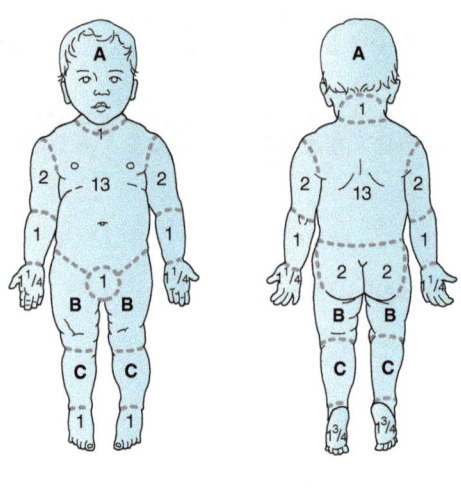

FIGURE 12-2 Table for estimating extent of burns. In adults, a reasonable system for calculating the percentage of body surface burned is the "rule of nines": Each arm equals 9%, the head equals 9%, the anterior and posterior trunk each equal 18%, and each leg equals 18%; the sum of these percentages is 99%

Reproduced with permission from Doherty G: CURRENT Diagnosis & Treatment: Surgery, 14th ed. New York: McGraw-Hill Education; 2015.

- If transferring patient, consult receiving facility before application
- Receiving facility may need to remove (causing patient discomfort) to assess burn
- Urinary catheter placement if strict input and output (I&O) monitoring required due to fluid resuscitation
- Administer tetanus prophylaxis as ordered

Evaluation
- Airway and ventilation status
- Hemodynamic status
- Pain control

Electrical Injuries

Electrical injuries occur when a source of electricity passes through tissue, resulting in damaged nerve pathways and burning of tissue, including skin and organ tissue damage. There are a number of factors influencing the results of contact with an electrical source. The information listed includes a basic description of how current flows and terms to describe electricity.[5]

- Amperes (amps) is the measure of current flow
- Volts is the actual amount of electricity generated by a given source
- Alternating current (AC) is the current found in most commercial and home buildings. This type of current is considered dangerous to cardiac tissue and can lead to ventricular fibrillation. Given a high voltage and amps, alternating current can cause significant internal tissue damage and skin burns. Alternating current can cause muscle tetany, making it difficult for the victim to withdraw from the current
- Direct current (DC) is the type of current found in batteries, low-voltage home appliances, solar panels, and lightning strikes

Electrical burns are the result of electric current rapidly heating the fluid within tissue, causing a thermal burn. The risk associated with electricity contact increases with increased voltage and amperage. Treatment of electrical burns is consistent with the treatment of non-electrical thermal burns. The emergency nurse must be mindful of the potential for cardiac dysrhythmias as well as organ damage/failure among those presenting with exposure to electricity.

Envenomation Emergencies

Envenomation is defined as the injection of a poisonous or toxic substance into tissue via a bite, sting, spine, or fang. This section explores the complexity of the envenomation process as it relates to care in the emergency setting. This section also reviews the various mechanisms by which toxins enter human tissue. Bites and stings can cause a number of serious injuries including infection, lacerations, envenomation, and transmission of infectious disease such as rabies.[1] The most concerning and potentially lethal consequence of this type of injury is anaphylaxis. The emergency nurse must carry a high suspicion for anaphylaxis when assessing an individual with a bite or sting. It is imperative to determine if a patient has a history of allergic reaction to a given insect or animal.[2]

In the United States, the following are common sources of bite and sting injuries

- Hymenoptera
  - Bees
  - Wasps
  - Fire ants
- Snakes
- Mammals such as humans, dogs, rodents, raccoons, skunks, and cats
- Reptiles
- Spiders
- Scorpions

Snakes

Snakebites can be particularly dangerous, depending on the type. The Centers for Disease Control and Prevention (CDC) estimated that between 7000 and 8000 people are bitten each year by venomous snakes in the United States, and about 5 of those bitten die.[6] Mortality rates are likely to be much higher in those not seeking medical treatment.[7] In about 20% of snakebites, the snake does not actually release venom. This is known as a "dry bite" and can be distinguished from an envenomation bite by the absence of edema, marked erythema, and moderate to severe pain.[1] Envenomation edema is pictured in Figure 12-3. In the United States, the most common snake-related bites are from the pit viper family, including rattlesnakes, copperheads, and water moccasins (cottonmouths) and the Elapidae (coral snake) family.[8] Signs and symptoms of snakebites can vary based on the particular snake and the type of venom the snake produces. The venom from a pit viper is hemotoxic, whereas the venom from a coral snake is neurotoxic.[2]

Signs and Symptoms of Envenomation Based on Type of Snake

- **Pit vipers**[9]
  - Assessment
    - Presence of one or two fang marks
    - Local edema with a burning sensation or pain locally
    - Local petechiae and ecchymosis
    - Paralysis
    - Paresthesia
    - Loss of function in effected limb
    - Nausea and vomiting
    - Diaphoresis
    - Visual disturbances
    - Gastrointestinal (GI) bleed/epistaxis
- **Coral snakes**[1]
  - Assessment
    - Mydriasis
    - Seizure
    - Paresthesia
    - Renal failure
    - Hypovolemic shock
    - Respiratory distress/arrest

Assessment/Analysis for all Snakebites

- Airway patency
- Breathing rate and rhythm
- Cardiac rate and rhythm
- Description of snake
  - Presence of one or two fang marks
  - Shape of head
  - Markings or banding on body of snake
- Location of the bite and presence of localized reaction
- Approximate time of bite
- Presence of signs and symptoms as described above based on the type of snake
- Laboratory studies
  - Coagulation studies
  - Complete blood count (CBC) with differential
  - Serum chemistries
  - Urinalysis

Interventions

- Maintain ABCs
- Supplemental oxygen support
- Elevate the affected extremity to the level of the heart, if applicable

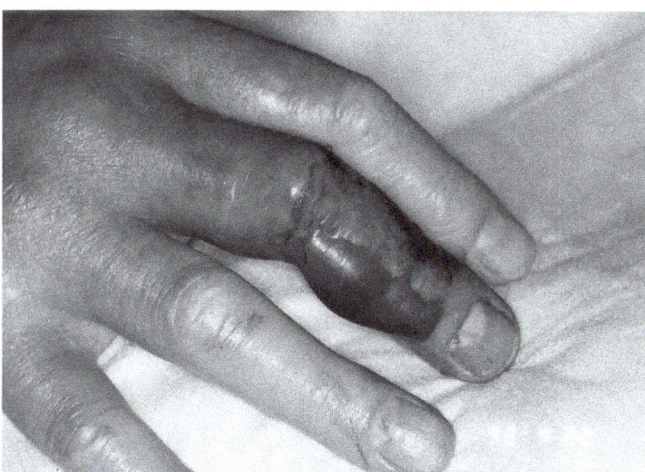

FIGURE 12-3 **Swelling and edema with a hemorrhagic bleb about 6 hours after a rattlesnake bite**
Reproduced with permission from Knoop KJ, Stack LB, Storrow AB, et al: The Atlas of Emergency Medicine, 4th ed. New York: McGraw-Hill Education; 2016: Photo contributor: Sean P. Bush, MD.

- Establish intravenous (IV) access for crystalloid fluids/blood products/medications as needed
  - Prepare to administer antivenin if ordered
  - Antivenin is most effective if administered within 4 to 6 hours of the bite, depending on specific antivenin
  - Effectiveness of antivenin is limited after 12 hours
- Obtain weight for medication calculation
- Analgesics if ordered and safe to administer based on vital signs
- Administer tetanus prophylaxis as ordered

Evaluation
- Airway patency
- Mental status
- Hemodynamic status
- Circulation and neurovascular status in effected extremity
  - Assess for compartment syndrome
- Evaluate and document edema progression at effected site
- Presence of hemorrhage (pit viper bites)
- Pain reassessment

Human and Animal Bites

See Orthopedic and Wound Emergencies chapter (chapter 11).

Bee, Hornet, and Wasp Stings

Bee and wasp stings are very common in the United States. This type of envenomation generally causes a local reaction including burning, stinging, erythema, and edema. Only in rare circumstances do stings cause severe and potentially deadly complications, such as anaphylaxis.[8] Treatment involves the removal of the stinger, if one was left behind. The venom sac at the end of a released stinger will continue to release toxin into the skin tissue; expedited removal is desired. Caution must be taken while removing the stinger so additional toxin is not introduced into the tissue by squeezing the venom sac attached to the stinger. Following stinger removal, ice packs may be applied to the site to reduce inflammation and pain. Antihistamine medications may be administered to treat local discomforts as well as minor allergic reaction. In the case of anaphylaxis, the maintenance of an adequate airway is priority. Medications such as epinephrine and histamine-blocking agents may be required in order to reverse the effects of anaphylaxis.[5]

Assessment/Analysis
- Airway patency
- History, particularly allergy or anaphylaxis due to insect stings
- Local area of sting to determine presence of stinger and venom sac
- Pain

Interventions
- Maintain ABCs
- Supplemental oxygen support
- Establish IV access for crystalloid fluids and medications as needed
  - Especially important when anaphylaxis occurs
- Remove stinger and venom sac if applicable
- Apply cold packs to the sting areas to minimize inflammation
- Administer epinephrine intramuscularly in cases of anaphylaxis
- Administer antihistamine medications, as ordered
- Administer analgesic medications, as ordered
- Administer tetanus prophylaxis, as ordered

Evaluation
- Airway patency
- Hemodynamic status
- Pain reassessment
- Evaluate and document edema/erythema progression at affected site

Aquatic Organisms

Aquatic organism stings such as jellyfish and the Portuguese man-of-war are among the most common found in the marine environment. In most cases, human encounters with aquatic organisms are incidental, and stings usually occur only after the organism has been disturbed. In most cases, a sting from an aquatic organism causes a local skin reaction, as pictured in Figure 12-4, as well as acute pain that usually subsides within

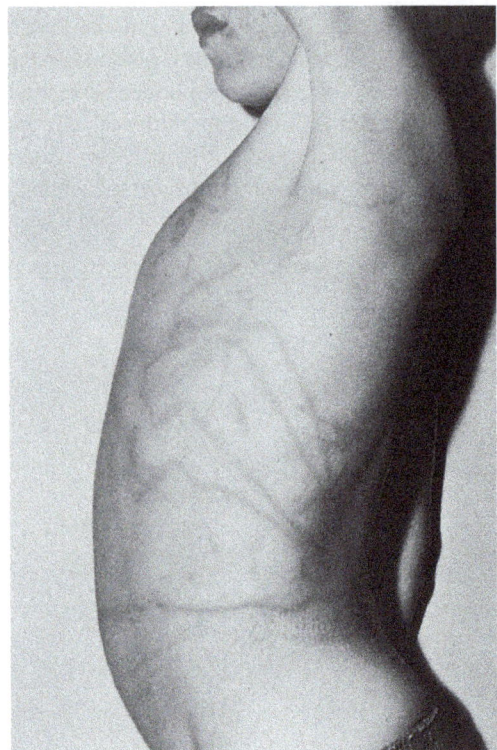

FIGURE 12-4 Localized skin reaction from a jellyfish "sting" envenomation

Reproduced with permission from Halstead BH: Venomous Marine Animals of the World. Washington, DC: US Government Printing Office; 1965.

an hour of the sting. Anaphylaxis is a concern for those who have a known allergy to aquatic organisms or who have been stung for the first time. A jellyfish sting produces a wavy, whip-type erythema pattern as pictured in Figure 12-4.[10] In addition to erythema and pain, a jellyfish sting will produce raised welts 2–3 mm wide.[11]

Treatment is centered on the local affected area as well as monitoring for signs of anaphylaxis. Wound treatment consists of washing the area with salt or seawater to prevent further injection of toxin from remaining nematocysts. Care should be taken not to rub the affected area, and the nurse should wear gloves during the course of wound treatment, particularly upon the removal of remaining tentacles. A solution of 5% acetic acid (vinegar) applied to the area will inactivate any remaining toxin.[2] Topical or systemic antihistamines and/or corticosteroids are sometimes needed. Careful monitoring of airway patency and breathing status can alert the nurse to the progression of anaphylaxis.

Organophosphates and Insecticides

Organophosphates are commonly found in household and commercial insecticides. Nerve agents such as Sarin, Soman, and VX are also organophosphates. When a person is exposed, this chemical disrupts the reuptake of acetylcholine by inhibiting acetylcholinesterase, leading to accumulation of acetylcholine and overstimulation of the central and autonomic nervous system.[1] As with any cholinergic toxidrome, a decrease in blood pressure and heart rate is possible. Classic symptoms of organophosphate exposure may best be remembered using the **SLUDGE** acronym

- **S**—salivation
- **L**—lacrimation
- **U**—urination
- **D**—defecation
- **G**—gastrointestinal distress
- **E**—emesis/expectoration

Organophosphates are readily absorbed dermally, so removal of clothing and washing of the skin reduces exposure. Body fluids and water runoff from decontamination procedures must be handled carefully, as these fluids can lead to further patient and healthcare team exposure. Treatment includes supportive care and the use of IV atropine and IV pralidoxime (2-pyridine aldoxime methyl chloride or 2-PAM) for binding of the organophosphate within the nerve synapse.[12]

Assessment/Analysis
- Airway patency; suction as needed
- Signs of respiratory distress which could lead to failure
- Type of chemical involved
- Type of exposure and exposure time
- Vital signs with focused attention to blood pressure and pulse rate
  - Bradycardia
  - Hypotension
- Mental status
- Miosis
- Vomiting, diarrhea
- Excess salivation
- Polyuria
- Diaphoresis
- General discomfort or agitation
- Paralysis
- Possible seizures
- Laboratory studies
  - CBC with differential
  - Serum chemistries
  - Liver function tests
  - Urinalysis
  - Pregnancy testing, if applicable

Interventions
- Decontamination procedures
  - Environmental safety—decontamination area adjacent/outside of emergency department (ED)—avoid exposure
  - Cautious handling of clothing and body fluids
- Appropriate personal protective equipment (PPE) for healthcare providers
- Supplemental oxygen as needed, airway support; elevated the head of the bed
- Establish IV access for crystalloid fluids and medications as needed
- Prepare to administer atropine and/or pralidoxime (2-PAM)
- Benzodiazepines for seizures
- Administer tetanus prophylaxis, as ordered

Evaluation
- Airway and ventilation status
- Mental status
- Hemodynamic status

Parasite Infestations

Despite significant medical advances, parasite infections remain very common worldwide. Most parasites flourish in warm and moist environments and are common among those with poor diets and of low economic status. In addition, children and immunocompromised patients are at an increased risk for parasitic infections. Parasites enter the human body in a number of ways; however, ingestion of the parasite and inoculation from a bite (mosquito) are the most common. By definition, parasites are living organisms using the body as a host and sustaining themselves at the expense of the host. Clinical features vary based on the type of parasite and the length of time one has been infected. Parasitic disease can go undetected for many years. Common symptoms of parasitic disease include headache, general malaise, intestinal obstruction, fever, and cough. This section discusses a number of common parasitic diseases, including infestation with helminths (parasitic worms), and their characteristics and treatment.[1]

Giardiasis (*Giardia* Infection)

Giardiasis is a gastrointestinal disease caused by the parasite *Giardia* and is the most common parasitic disease in the United States. Giardia can live external to a host for weeks and are introduced to a host via ingestion. Giardia inhabits the GI tract and causes severe diarrhea, fatigue, weight loss, and fever. Diagnosis is made by examining stool samples to identify giardia. People at risk for giardiasis are day care workers, children, and those with poor dietary habits. Treatment includes supportive care and the use of pharmacologic therapies, including the antiprotozoal medication metronidazole, and correction of fluid or electrolyte imbalance.[5]

Taeniasis (Infestation with Flatworms or "Tapeworms")

Taeniasis is an infection of the GI tract caused by the *Taenia* worm. These worms are commonly referred to as "tapeworms" and are ingested by eating undercooked pork or beef. Many individuals with taeniasis have very mild or no symptoms. The most common symptom is the passing of tapeworms upon defecation. Other symptoms may include weight loss, anorexia, and abdominal pain. As with other parasites, diagnosis is made by examining stool specimens. Treatment is pharmacologic and may include the medications praziquantel or niclosamide.[5]

Taenia Solium (Cysticercosis) Infection

The parasite *Taenia solium* causes cysticercosis, a disease in which the parasite larval cysts travel throughout the body and deposit in muscle and brain tissue. Although very rare, this disease has a high rate of morbidity and mortality and can manifest as a first-time seizure due to the destruction of brain tissue by the parasite. A computed tomography (CT) scan will reveal parasitic cysts within the brain.[5]

Malaria

Malaria is a parasitic disease caused from the bite of infected mosquitos. In 2013, the CDC estimated that nearly 200 million cases of malaria occurred worldwide with nearly 500,000 deaths (mostly children). Although very rare in the United States, nearly 1,500 malaria cases are diagnosed each year, with most individuals diagnosed returning from travel to areas where malaria is prevalent.[13] Malaria is caused by a number of parasites introduced via a mosquito bite. The most common parasite in human infections is *Plasmodium falciparum*, which causes widespread destruction of erythrocytes through hemolysis. Symptoms begin with a "flulike" prodrome including fever, chills, malaise, and headache. Late symptoms include splenic enlargement or rupture and encephalopathy leading to seizures, coma, and death.[5]

Toxic Plant Exposure

Determination of a specific plant toxin can present an interesting challenge for emergency providers. Often, individuals presenting with symptoms of toxic plant exposure are unaware of the name of the contacted or ingested plant. A wide variety of potentially toxic plants, including those used for decorative purposes, are found in homes or in landscapes.[2] Plant intoxication may be the result of either an intentional or accidental ingestion. Children and adolescents make up the largest demographic presenting for emergency care.[1] Toxins found in most plants can be categorized into three types: calcium oxalate, cardiac glycosides, and anticholinergics. The goal of therapy in the emergency setting should include the support of ABCs and the reduction of effects related to the associated toxin.[2]

Examples of Toxic Plants

- Anticholinergic[5]
  - Jimson weed
  - Mandrake
  - Henbane
- Glycosides[5]
  - Foxglove
  - Milkweed
  - Oleander
  - Apricot and cherry pits
  - Elderberry
  - Holly
  - Lily of the valley
- Carboxylic acid[5]
  - Rhubarb leaves
  - Caladium
  - Elephant's ear

Assessment/Analysis

- Type and section of plant (e.g. leaf, stem, flower, bulb, etc.) ingested/exposed
- Symptoms related to the class of the plant exposure
  - Calcium oxalate–producing plants—manifest as GI distress, including oral mucosa pain, nausea, vomiting, and diarrhea
  - Glycosides—can present with nausea and vomiting and bradycardia
  - Anticholinergic plants—produce hallucinations, confusion, and agitation
- Contact dermatitis: localized reaction with edema, pain, and itching
- Current medication and allergy list (medications and substances)

Interventions

- Supplemental oxygen support as needed
- Establish IV access for crystalloid fluids/blood products/medications as needed
- Consult a poison control center
- Treat symptoms

Evaluation

- Airway patency
- Hemodynamic monitoring
- Cardiac rate and rhythm

- Core temperature
- Mental status
- Evaluate effectiveness of pharmacologic therapy

Radiation and Hazardous Material Exposure

Radiation is found in many natural sources within our environment, although the word itself invokes fear among the general public. Background radiation describes the low levels of radiation exposure humans are subjected to constantly from natural sources. From a health perspective, radiation exposure becomes concerning when one is exposed to a powerful source in a short period of time. Tissue damage from radiation exposure is highly dependent on the type and dose of radiation absorbed as well as the overall time exposed to the source. Radiation can be divided into two distinct categories, ionizing and non-ionizing. Ionizing radiation has the ability to destroy human tissue by causing alterations in DNA that lead to abnormal cell growth, which ultimately can cause tumors and cancer-related disease. The higher the ionizing value of a particle, the higher the likelihood that tissue damage will occur. Types of ionizing radiation particles can be divided further into subcategories.[14]

Alpha Radiation—This type of particle is highly ionizing, causing extensive damage to tissue. Although this particle can cause serious damage to human tissue, it has very low penetration potential. The alpha particle is the least penetrating type of ionizing radiation and will not penetrate clothing or skin. The greatest health concern with this type of radiation is related to internal consumption. Once inhaled or ingested, the highly ionizing alpha particle is brought close to internal tissues, leading to cell destruction.[1]

Beta Radiation—This type of ionizing radiation particle is much smaller than the alpha particle, which allows more penetration of tissue, although it is less ionizing than the alpha particle. Beta particles will only penetrate intact skin to a depth of a few millimeters and can be shielded easily by wood, heavy clothing, plastics, or glass. Like the alpha particle, ingestion or inhalation of beta particles can cause significant tissue damage over time.[1]

Gamma Radiation—The type of radiation most emergency nurses are familiar with, gamma radiation, is used in medical diagnostic imaging equipment, such as x-ray machines. Gamma radiation is highly energetic, penetrates tissue very well, and is difficult to shield against. In most cases, lead is required to properly shield against this type of radiation.[1]

Radiation Exposure Protection: Time, Distance, and Shielding

Basic protection methods can be used to minimize exposure radiation and its harmful effects.

- ❖ **Time**—It is important to minimize the time spent near the source. In a patient care setting, real-time dosimetry can serve as an indicator for exposure time. Dosimeters measure the amount of radiation received. Healthcare workers should consider wearing a dosimeter that can be read in real time during the decontamination and care process in order to monitor the maximum allowable dose received[1]
- ❖ **Distance**—Given the opportunity, distancing from the radiation source can provide protection. As mentioned in the section on types of ionizing radiation, alpha and beta particles can be easily blocked and do not have the ability to travel great distances in the air[1]
- ❖ **Shielding**—Proper shielding can provide a great deal of protection. Knowing the type of radiation particle involved is important to the shielding strategy. Alpha and beta particles require minimal physical shielding; however, since inhalation and ingestion are very damaging, the use of proper face/respiratory protection is imperative. For gamma radiation, lead shielding offers the best protection[1]

Acute Radiation Syndrome

Acute radiation syndrome (ARS) refers to the effects on the human body when it is exposed to ionizing radiation. The onset of ARS can occur shortly after exposure, and it can last for weeks. Treatment is highly dependent on the type of exposure and is mostly supportive.[5]

Assessment/Analysis
- Signs and Symptoms of ARS
  - GI symptoms including nausea, vomiting, and diarrhea
    - In severe cases, sloughing of the GI tissue can occur, leading to hemorrhage
  - Immunodeficiency
  - Thrombocytopenia
  - Internal bleeding
  - General malaise
  - Altered mental status

Types of Radiation Exposure

- **Exposure**—Exposure occurs when an individual comes into contact with an ionizing radiation–emitting source but does not have the source making direct contact. Imagine ionizing radiation exposure as a beam of light; the light can make contact with skin but does not actually make physical contact, and exposure is discontinued when the light source is removed[1]
- **Contamination**—Contamination of ionizing radiation occurs when the source of the radiation is physically in contact with the body or clothing[1]
- **Incorporation**—Incorporation is the process of the body incorporating and distributing the source of ionizing radiation to various organ systems. This type of exposure is common with ingestion or inhalation of isotopes. A common example of incorporation is an ingested iodine isotope that is incorporated by the thyroid[1]

- Bleeding and skin burns
- Type of exposure and time exposed

Interventions
- Ensure protection for self and others
- Determine if field decontamination has occurred
- Support ABCs
- Decontamination process if required, and only by those experienced in decontamination
- Provide supplemental oxygen if required
- Establish IV access for crystalloid fluids/blood products/medications as needed
  - Prepare to provide medications such as chelation agents (for incorporation), antidiarrheal, antiemetics, blood and blood products upon order[5]
- Provide analgesics if ordered
- Avoid nonsteroidal anti-inflammatory agents[5]

Evaluation
- Airway patency
- Hemodynamic monitoring
- Cardiac rate and rhythm
- Pain management
- Mental status
- Intake and output

Submersion Injury

Submersion injury is simply the inability to effectively ventilate due to being submerged in a substance where oxygen is not readily available. Submersion can lead to significant hypoxia followed by death if the individual is not removed from the substance and hypoxia is not corrected. Water is commonly the primary culprit in submersion injuries; however, submersion in any substance, wet or dry, can lead to a submersion injury. Some of the less common substances include mud, liquid and dry chemicals, earth, grain, and salt. Children are at most risk for submersion injuries.[1] Once an individual is submersed, panic often sets in, and drowning can occur very quickly.

Assessment/Analysis
- Airway and breathing stabilization
- Auscultate lung sounds
- Monitor pulse oximetry. Consider capnography
- Injury mechanisms and concurrent trauma
- Type of substance involved in submersion, consider hazardous material
- Length of time submersed
- Knowing the temperature of the substance could be helpful in the setting of hypo/hyperthermia

Interventions
- Maintain ABCs
- Consider cervical spine precautions
- Prepare for potential rapid sequence intubation (RSI)
- Establish IV access for crystalloid fluids and medications as needed
  - Infuse warmed fluids
- Maintain or support normal body temperature

Evaluation
- Airway patency, including clearing obstructions and foreign material
- Respiratory effort
- Effectiveness of oxygenation
- Hemodynamic stability
- Core temperature

Temperature-related Emergencies

Heat-related Emergencies

Heat-related emergencies occur when an individual is exposed to extreme high temperatures for a period of time and the body fails to regulate its temperature using the usual physiologic processes.[15] Once the body exceeds the normal temperature of 98.6°F (37°C), a series of heat-related symptoms can occur, ranging from minor symptoms such as muscle cramps, to major symptoms such as cardiovascular failure and death. Older adults, infants, athletes, and outdoor enthusiasts are at higher risk for heat-related emergencies. The key intervention for all types of heat-related illness is removal from the high-temperature environment and active cooling techniques. The progression of heat-related illness can be described in three stages known as heat cramps, heat exhaustion, and heat stroke.[1]

Heat Cramps—The cramping of large skeletal muscles due to physical exertion in a warm or hot environment. The muscle cramping is related to hyponatremia from heavy perspiration and excessive oral fluid intake.[1]

Assessment/Analysis
- Muscle cramps
- Fatigue
- Core temperature may be within normal limits
- Mild tachycardia
- Profuse perspiration
- Headache
- Dizziness
- Nausea and vomiting
- Serum chemistries

Interventions
- Remove patient from heat and place in a cool environment (shade, indoors, temperature controlled environment) if possible
- Begin oral fluid replacement if vomiting does not prohibit
- Give oral electrolyte solutions

- Establish IV access for crystalloid fluids/medications as needed
  - Especially if not tolerating oral intake
- Monitor intake and output
- Pain management

Evaluation
- Effectiveness of oral or IV replacement therapy
- Monitor vital signs, including temperature
- Decreased pain

Heat Exhaustion—The consequence of progressing heat cramps. Characterized by moderate to severe dehydration and weakness. If left untreated, heat exhaustion can progress to heat stroke.[1]

Assessment/Analysis
- Muscle cramps
- Fatigue and weakness
- Skin warm to the touch
- Altered mental status
- Core temperature may be elevated as high as 104° F (39°C).
- Tachycardia/dysrhythmias
- Profuse perspiration
- Headache
- Dizziness
- Pale skin due to vasoconstriction
- Laboratory studies
  - Serum chemistries, especially potassium and creatine kinase (CK)

Interventions
- Remove patient from heat and place in a cool environment (shade, indoors, temperature-controlled environment) if possible
- Active cooling with fans, water-soaked towels, ice pack to posterior neck and axillae (not directly on skin)
- Establish IV access for crystalloid fluids/medications as needed
- Pain management

Evaluation
- Effectiveness of IV replacement therapy
- Mental status reevaluation
- Monitor vital signs
- Cardiac monitoring
- Intake and output

Heat Stroke—The most concerning stage of heat-related illness; a medical emergency. Heat stoke is defined as a core temperature greater than 102.5°F (39.2°C)[5] and can reach temperatures exceeding 106°F (41°C).[16] At this stage of heat illness, the body has lost thermoregulation abilities. Cardiovascular failure and central nervous system damage is a key concern. Treatment of heat stroke is focused on maintaining ABCs while aggressive cooling takes place.[1]

Assessment/Analysis
- Assess ABCs and stabilize
- Severe muscle cramps
- Altered level of consciousness including coma
- Hot skin
- Dry skin due to inability to perspire
- Core temperature: may exceed 106°F (41°C)
- Tachycardia/dysrhythmias
- Rhabdomyolysis
- Disseminated intravascular coagulation (DIC)
- Laboratory studies
  - Serum chemistries with liver function tests
  - CBC with differential
  - Coagulation studies
  - Serum creatine kinase

Interventions
- Remove patient from heat and place in a cool environment (shade, indoors, temperature-controlled environment) if possible
- Active cooling with ice packs or ice bath
- Establish IV access for crystalloid fluids and medications as needed
  - Infuse-room temperature (72°F/22.2°C) fluids
- Electrolyte replacement

Evaluation
- Patent airway, effective breathing
- Mental status reevaluation
- Hemodynamic stability
- Intake and output
- Core temperature—goal is to reduce to 102°F (38.9°C) and slow/stop efforts to avoid overcooling[2]

Cold-related Emergencies

Cold exposure claims the lives of nearly 700 people in the United States each year.[1] Many deaths occur in urban areas due to poorly heated dwellings or homelessness. The use of drugs and alcohol intoxication are risk factors contributing to the morbidity and mortality of cold-related injuries.[1] This section reviews the two most common cold-related emergencies: hypothermia and frostbite.

Hypothermia—A medical emergency defined as a core temperature less than 95°F (35°C). Hypothermia can occur in a number of ways, including exposure to a very cold environment, submersion in cool liquids, and through some disease processes such as hypoglycemia (in infants).[17] Those at risk for hypothermia include the very young and very old, as well as those experiencing acute drug or alcohol intoxication. Hypothermia can lead to cardiovascular and central nervous system (CNS) collapse. Altered mental status and cardiac dysrhythmias (ventricular fibrillation) are common with hypothermia and are the main contributors to mortality. The treatment goal for hypothermia is elevating core temperature and prevention of cardiovascular collapse.[5]

Assessment/Analysis
- Airway patency and breathing effectiveness
- Core temperature of less than 95°F (35°C)
- Determine length and type of exposure
- Altered level of consciousness including coma
- ECG changes[18]
  - Bradycardia
  - Prolonged PR and QT intervals
  - Atrial fibrillation
  - Ventricular fibrillation
  - J wave (also called Osborn wave) on ECG[18] as pictured in Figure 12-5

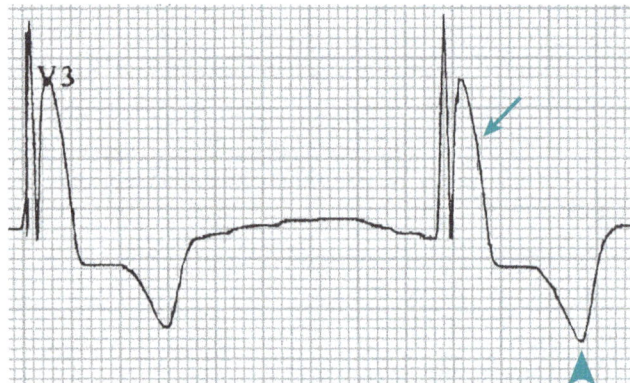

FIGURE 12-5 A large Osborn wave (J wave) (*arrow*) follows the QRS and is distinct from the T wave (*arrowhead*), common in hypothermia
Reproduced with permission from Knoop KJ, Stack LB, Storrow AB, et al: The Atlas of Emergency Medicine, 4th ed. New York: McGraw-Hill Education; 2016.

Interventions
- Support airway and breathing
- Supplemental oxygen
- Cardiac monitoring
- Remove wet clothing
- Obtain core temperature
- Establish IV access for crystalloid fluids and medications as needed
  - Infuse warmed IV fluids
- External rewarming
  - Elevated ED room temperature
  - Heat lamps
  - Blankets, including heated or forced air
  - Heat packs
- Internal rewarming
  - Diagnostic peritoneal lavage (DPL)
  - Gastric lavage
  - Bladder irrigation
  - In extreme cases, continuous arterial venous rewarming (CAVR) through dialysis or ECMO/ECLS (extracorporeal membrane oxygenation/extracorporeal life support)
- If in cardiac arrest, continue resuscitation until 86°F (30°C)
  - At this temperature, defibrillation and medications may begin to be more effective[5]

Evaluation
- Patent airway and effective breathing
- Hemodynamic stability
- Mental status reevaluation
- Core temperature—goal is to avoid overwarming, stop core rewarming efforts at 93°F[2] (33.8°C)
- Monitor vital signs
- Cardiac monitoring—important to continuously monitor during rewarming because of the potential for rewarming cardiac arrhythmias
- Strict intake and output monitoring

Frostbite—The destruction of tissue due to the formation of ice crystals within the tissue. Crystals formed in the freezing process cause individual cells to rupture and ultimately die. Once frostbite occurs, the damage to cells is irreversible. Although frostbite most frequently occurs in the hands and feet, it can involve any limb or skin surface. Treatment is centered on rewarming of the tissue to prevent damage to unaffected tissue. It is imperative to ensure that once rewarming has begun, it can be sustained, as refreezing of the tissue will cause further damage.[2,19]

Assessment/Analysis
- Determine length and type of exposure
- Assess mental status and signs of concurrent hypothermia
- Pale, yellow or black skin
- Edema
- Blisters (to be left intact) as pictured in Figure 12-6
- Eschar
- Circulation and motor status of affected limb

Interventions
- Treatment for hypothermia as listed in hypothermia section
- Gentle and slow rewarming of tissue
- Do not rub or massage affected tissue
- Analgesics as ordered

Evaluation
- Patent airway and effective breathing
- Mental status reevaluation
- Pain control
- Core temperature
- Vital signs
- Distal circulation/movement/sensation of affected extremity
  - Assess for compartment syndrome

Initial symptoms seen 2 to 4 days post-exposure mimic those found in a viral syndrome and include arthralgias/myalgia, fever, nausea/vomiting, abdominal pain, and headache. The red or purple flat petechial rash giving RMSF part of its name appears 2 to 5 days after the fever, although some patients do not develop a rash. Later signs and symptoms include CNS depression, renal failure, respiratory failure, and myocarditis. Treatment is based on supportive care and the use of the antibiotic doxycycline.[5]

Assessment/Analysis

- Obtain history of tick bite or activity that may have led to a tick bite (camping, hiking, etc)
- Identify the anatomic location of the tick bite and assess for existing embedded ticks
- Assess for rash, GI symptoms, and headache or CNS depression
- Laboratory studies
    - Antigen antibodies: Immunoglobulin G or M
    - Serum chemistries
    - CBC with differential

Interventions

- Maintain patent airway and effective breathing, particularly if CNS depressed
- Remove tick
    - Avoid crushing or squeezing
    - Remove gently, attempting to remove intact
    - If parts remain, use splinter removing techniques
    - Save tick for identification
- Establish IV access for crystalloid fluids and medications as needed
- Analgesics for pain
- Doxycycline administration as ordered
- Administer tetanus prophylaxis as ordered

Evaluation

- Monitor airway and breathing
- Hemodynamic stability
- Monitor sensorium
- Education on the use of DEET-containing sprays to avoid future tick bites
- Education on inspection of skin after high-risk outdoor activities

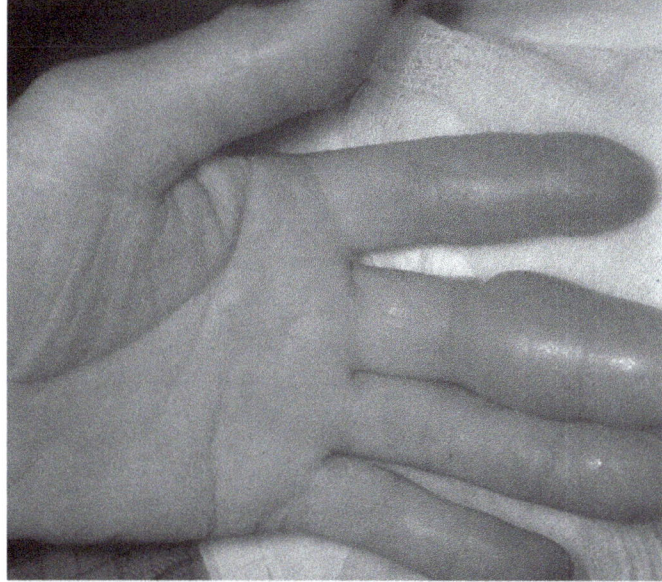
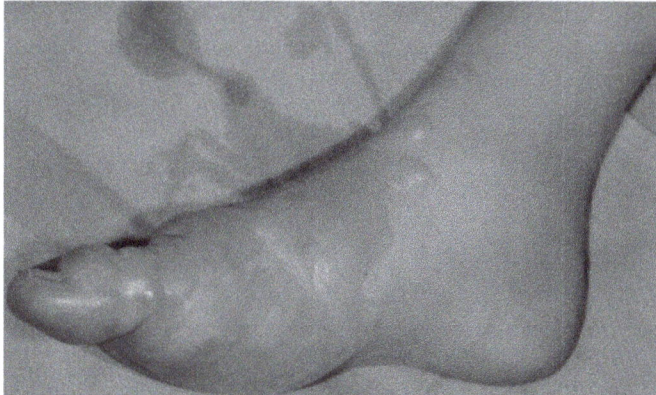

FIGURE 12-6 Intact frostbite blisters on the hand and the foot
Reproduced with permission from Kasper DL, Fauci AS, Hauser S, et al: Harrison's Principles of Internal Medicine, 19th ed. New York: McGraw-Hill Education; 2015.

Vector-borne Illnesses

Tick-borne Illness

Like mosquitoes, ticks are insects that feed on the blood of animals and in the process can serve as a vector in the transmission of disease. Common diseases transmitted by ticks include Lyme disease, Rocky Mountain spotted fever, and tularemia. In the United States, Rocky Mountain spotted fever is the most severe of the tick-borne illness, whereas Lyme disease is the most common.[5] Those at risk for tick bite include children and outdoor enthusiasts including campers and hikers. In most cases, tick bites go unnoticed initially, because of the small size of the tick. Ticks also tend to settle in anatomy covered with hair, adding to the difficulty finding the tick.[2] Once the tick becomes engorged with blood, it is much larger and easily seen. Some patients with a tick-borne illness may have no memory of a tick bite.

Rocky Mountain Spotted Fever (RMSF)

In the United States, Rocky Mountain spotted fever is reported nationally, although over 60% of cases are reported in states of Oklahoma, Missouri, Arkansas, Tennessee, and North Carolina.

Lyme Disease

In the United States, more than 30,000 cases of Lyme disease are reported each year, although it is estimated that the actual number of cases may be as high as 200,000 to 300,000 per year.[5] The rate of Lyme disease transmission is directly related to the amount of time a tick feeds on the victim. If ticks are removed within 36 hours of attachment, the risk for acquiring Lyme disease is very low.[5] Signs and symptoms of Lyme disease are very similar to RMSF in the early stages, and treatment is the same. Lyme disease progression is characterized in three stages.[2]

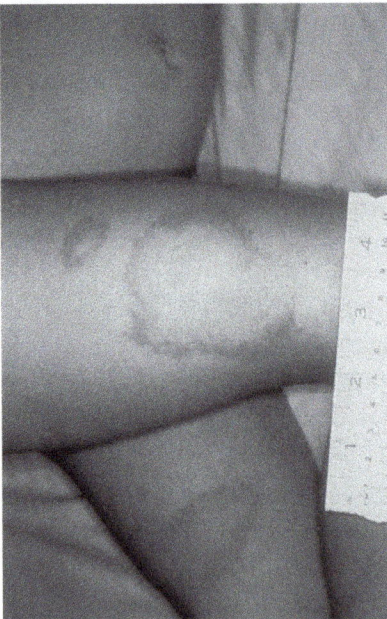

FIGURE 12-7 Erythema migrans. The typical rash of Lyme disease is shown evolving in concentric rings around the site of the tick bite
Reproduced with permission from Willey JM, Sherwood L, Woolverton C: Prescott, Harley & Klein's Microbiology, 7th ed. New York: McGraw-Hill Education; 2007.

- ❖ First stage (day 0 to 4 weeks): local erythematous "bull's eye" rash as pictured in Figure 12-7; flulike signs and symptoms including fever, chills, headache, fatigue, joint and muscle aches. Symptoms typically subside after a few weeks and may go unnoticed
- ❖ Second stage (4 weeks to several months): symptoms include facial palsy, headache, CNS depression, neck stiffness, ataxia, cardiac atrioventricular (AV) block arrhythmias, joint and muscle pain, and encephalitis
- ❖ Third stage (many weeks to years): chronic arthritis, myocarditis, and neuropathy

Assessment/Analysis
- History of tick exposure
- Identify anatomic location of the tick bite and assess for existing embedded ticks
- Assess for rash, GI symptoms, and headache or CNS depression
- Laboratory studies
  - Organism-specific immunoassay testing
  - Serum chemistries
  - CBC with differential

Interventions
- Airway support, particularly if CNS depressed
- Remove any discovered ticks
- Establish IV access for crystalloid fluids and medications as needed
- Analgesics for pain
- Doxycycline administration, as ordered
- Administer tetanus prophylaxis, as ordered

Evaluation
- Monitor airway and breathing
- Hemodynamic stability
- Education on the use of DEET-containing sprays to avoid future tick bites
- Education on inspection of skin after high-risk outdoor activities

Rabies

A neurotropic virus causes rabies, and rabies has a very high mortality rate because treatment options and effectiveness are the morbidity and mortality rates are high. The virus is spread to humans via saliva from a bite of an infected wild or domestic animal. The virus finds its way to the central nervous system via peripheral nerves, where it causes encephalopathy and eventually death. The incubation period for the rabies virus is typically 1 to 3 months, making early treatment following an animal bite imperative. Rabies in the prodromal period presents as generalized viral symptoms such as fever, chills, weakness, headache, nausea, and vomiting. Later symptoms include CNS depression and ultimately coma.[5]

Assessment/Analysis
- Presence of viral syndrome symptoms or mental status changes
- Obtain information regarding the history of an animal bite or bat exposure
- Examine for the presence of a healing or healed animal bite (possible fang marks)
- History related to an unprovoked animal bite is valuable
- Quantity of animal saliva exposure

Interventions
- Supplemental oxygen support
- Support airway, breathing, and circulation
- Establish IV access for crystalloid fluids and medications as needed
- If domesticated animal, obtain history of animal vaccinations, if possible
- Report animal bites as required by hospital policy/municipal laws
- Post-exposure vaccination[17]
  - For those not previously vaccinated
  - Given in combination with human rabies immune globulin (HRIG)
  - Appropriate for bite and non-bite exposures
  - Vaccination should occur at regular intervals starting at day zero and following on days, 3, 7, and 14[17]
- Administer tetanus prophylaxis, as ordered

Evaluation
- Patent airway and effective breathing
- Hemodynamic stability
- Education on post-rabies vaccination schedule

Toxicology

Acids and Alkalis

Acids and alkalis are in a category of chemicals referred to as corrosives, which can cause substantial injury to tissues including mucous membranes, skin, and eyes. Acids are defined as solutions or substances with a low pH (a pH of less than 7). Common acids include hydrochloric, sulfuric, and nitric acids. Acids cause coagulation necrosis.

Alkalis have a pH of greater than 7. Drain cleaners and fertilizers are examples of alkaline substances. Chemical names of alkalis include potassium hydroxide and ammonium hydroxide. Alkalis cause tissue liquefaction necrosis soon after contact with the skin.

As with many substances, intentional ingestion or exposure of caustics is possible.[2] On receiving a patient with acid or alkali exposure, the emergency nurse should assess for suicidal ideation.

Hydrofluoric acid is abundant in the manufacturing industry, which happens to be where most exposures occur. Hydrofluoric acid is a weak acid that has the ability to penetrate deep into tissues. The fluoride ion causes demineralization of bone and can lead to hypocalcemia. Calcium gluconate in the form of a paste or gel is applied to the affected areas in order to bind the fluoride ions and spare the calcium found in the bone tissue. In some cases, other forms of calcium, such as calcium chloride or calcium carbonate, are used for the same reasons.[5]

Assessment/Analysis

- Obtain past medical, medication, and allergy history
- Obtain history of exposure
  - Determine concentration and agent involved in exposure
  - Length of time exposed
  - Route of exposure
- Assess airway and respiratory effort if ingested orally or inhaled. Airway compromise typically results from increasing edema
- Abnormal respiratory patterns such as stridor
- If inhaled or ingested orally, drooling/failure to clear airway secretions may be a symptom of airway edema and should be acted on immediately
- Examine affected site(s), including oral mucosa for chemical burns or blisters
- Examine eyes for injury
  - Pale or white milky-appearing conjunctiva indicates corneal injury

Interventions

- Support airway, breathing, and circulation
- Establish IV access for crystalloid fluids and medications as needed
- Administer calcium if ordered
- Analgesics for pain if ordered
- Eye irrigation until a pH of 7.2 to 7.4 is obtained, if ordered
- Brush off dry chemicals, then irrigate
- Irrigation with water or saline for skin burns
- Laboratory studies: serum electrolytes, especially calcium
- Cardiac monitoring (due to risk of hypocalcemia with hydrofluoric acid)

Evaluation

- Airway patency and hemodynamic monitoring
- Pain management
- Mental status reevaluation
- Intake and output

Carbon Monoxide

Carbon monoxide (CO) is an odorless and colorless gas produced as a byproduct of the combustion of fossil fuels. According to the CDC, carbon monoxide poisoning is the leading cause of death related to unintentional poisoning.[20] Estimates suggest that CO contributes to nearly 15,000 emergency department visits with more than 500 attributed deaths despite emergency care.[1] In the United States, nearly 4000 individuals die from carbon monoxide inhalation, and a large percentage die prior to emergency care.[5] Although most inhalation occurrences are accidental, some are intentional in the setting of suicidal ideation.[21] Carbon monoxide inhalation is particularly harmful, as it binds to the hemoglobin found in red blood cells. The binding competes with oxygen binding, leading to tissue hypoxia and falsely high pulse oximetry readings. In addition, carbon monoxide can cause direct tissue damage at the cellular level via a number of inflammatory mechanisms.[22]

Assessment/Analysis

- History of exposure
  - Length of time exposed
  - Source of exposure (with house fires, consider cyanide inhalation)
  - Space in which inhalation occurred
- Headache, lethargy
- If female of childbearing age, determine pregnancy status
- Mental status
- Skin inspection
  - Bright red skin and mucous membranes
  - A classic, though rare, sign found in moderate to severe carbon monoxide inhalation
- Cardiac dysrhythmias
- Hypotension
- Suicidal ideation—assess if inhalation was intentional
- Laboratory studies
  - Arterial blood gases
  - CBC with differential
  - Carboxyhemoglobin level
  - Cardiac biomarkers (enzymes)
- Oxygen saturation is often falsely elevated because of competition and binding of carbon monoxide to hemoglobin

Interventions
- Supplemental oxygen support; attempt to achieve 100% delivery, regardless of oxygen saturation readings
- Maintain airway and breathing
- Prepare for possible rapid sequence intubation by provider
- Establish IV access for crystalloid fluids and medications as needed

Evaluation
- Airway patency and effective breathing
- Hemodynamic stability
- Level of consciousness
- If discharged from emergency department, ensure safe environment

Cyanide

Cyanide commonly refers to any substance containing a cyano group attached to a positively charged ion (such as potassium cyanide). Cyanide is naturally occurring and can be found in the pits of many fruits such as apricots, peaches, and cherries.[2] It is also used in manufacturing and production plants and by jewelers. Cyanide works by disrupting cellular processes, leading to the dysfunction of cellular respiration and causing tissues to become hypoxic and ultimately die. The ingestion or inhalation of cyanide can lead to death very quickly, potentially within minutes if inhaled. More commonly, exposure to cyanide occurs as a byproduct of the combustion of household items in house fires, particularly furniture or carpeting.[4,23]

The effects of cyanide poisoning can be reversed by the use of medications such as hydroxocobalamin, amyl nitrite, and sodium thiosulfate, which are often kept in a kit for emergency use.[5] These medications act either by directly binding to the cyanide or by increasing the efficiency of natural excretion. From an emergency nursing perspective, treatment is centered on supportive care.

Assessment/Analysis
- Early signs
  - Anxiety
  - Nausea
  - Tachycardia
  - Hypertension
  - Headache and dizziness
  - Bitter almond smell on breath
- Advanced signs
  - Bradycardia
  - Cardiovascular collapse
  - Hypotension
  - Decrease in mental status
  - Progressive metabolic acidosis
  - Seizures
  - Bright red blood (upon phlebotomy)
- Circumstances surrounding ingestion or inhalation, including total time of exposure
- Concurrent injury, particularly related to burns in the setting of house fire
- Vital signs including continuous pulse oximetry
- Laboratory studies
  - Arterial blood gas
  - Cyanide level

Interventions
- Maintain airway and breathing.
  - Prepare for early intubation
  - High flow oxygen
- Establish IV access for crystalloid fluids and medications as needed
- Prepare to administer reversal medications if ordered
- Seek assistance from a poison control center

Evaluation
- Airway patency and effective breathing
- Hemodynamic status
- Cardiac rate and rhythm

Drug Interactions

With the increase in the number of therapeutic pharmaceutical medications, the possibility of drug interactions must be taken into account. Any person using medications is at risk for a drug interaction. Obviously, when two or more medications are taken, the risk for a drug–drug interaction exists. As more medications are added, the risk increases substantially. Medication interactions with food or herbal supplements can also pose a threat. Drug interactions can have a number of effects based on the drug and the type of interaction. There are three main categories of drug interaction[24]

- Intensification of one drug by the other drug
  - Example: Warfarin™ and St. John's wort (herbal medication)
- Reduction of one drug by the other drug
  - Example: Diazepam™ is inhibited by amiodarone
- Creation of adverse effects when the drugs are combined
  - Example: Disulfiram (Antabuse™) or metronidazole (Flagyl™) combined with alcohol

The emergency nurse must obtain a full medication history, including over-the-counter medications and herbal medications, in the emergency department. Careful analysis and medication reconciliation are two ways to prevent drug interactions. Consultation of pharmacy resources or poison centers can also provide the emergency nurse with a wealth of information regarding potential drug interactions.

Overdose and Intentional Ingestions

Accidental and intentional medication overdose are common presentations in emergency departments. The CDC estimates that 44 people in the United States die each day from prescribed analgesics alone.[25] Medication overdose can be attributed to a number of factors, including misunderstanding of medication dosing times, forgetfulness, and the misconception that "more is better." Regardless of the cause, certain medication overdoses can lead to significant morbidity and death. This section discusses general treatment concepts related to common medications involved with intentional or accidental overdose.

General Treatment Interventions: Reducing Absorption of the Medication

Reducing medication absorption is implemented through different methods. It is imperative the emergency nurse obtain information about any medications potentially contributing to the overdose, as some absorption-reducing treatments may cause further harm.[1] Given the multiple and variable existing medications, the following are general concepts to apply to most medication overdoses.

- Therapies for reducing medication in stomach or GI system
  - Induction of vomiting (syrup of ipecac)[1]
    - Generally not recommended; clinical evidence is not clear on effectiveness
    - Can cause electrolyte and acid–base balance disturbances
    - Frequent and violent vomiting can cause Mallory-Weiss tears
    - Aspiration pneumonia
  - Gastric lavage[25]
    - Gastric lavage has not been clinically shown to improve recovery even when implemented within 60 minutes of ingestion
    - Associated with high risk of aspiration, esophageal perforation, and electrolyte imbalance
    - Do not perform lavage on overdoses of medications that may alter mental status unexpectedly, such as tricyclic antidepressants and analgesics (airway concern)
    - Not recommended for acid or alkali overdose due to re-irritation of the esophagus
    - Lavage, through gastric tube, with slightly warm tap water; 200 to 300 mL at a time until clear
  - Binding agents[1]
    - Activated charcoal works by binding substances within the stomach through its multiple pores and trapping it for elimination
    - Charcoal can be given orally or by nasogastric/orogastric (NG/OG) tube following lavage (if performed)
    - Activated charcoal does not bind to metals such as lead, iron, or lithium
    - Most effective if administered within 1 hour of ingestion
    - Do not administer activated charcoal to patients who may require GI endoscopy as it will obstruct the view from the scope

Improving Elimination

Following decontamination of the gastric contents, improving the speed at which the medication is eliminated from the body can prove to be beneficial. Elimination can be enhanced in a variety of ways

- Administration of a cathartic agent[1]
  - Cathartic agents such as magnesium citrate, sorbitol, or polyethylene glycol will improve GI elimination
  - Stimulates gastric motility
  - Use with caution in children
  - Repeat doses should not be given
  - Can be given with activated charcoal to improve elimination of the charcoal itself, which has bound the toxic substances
- Hemodialysis[1]
  - Hemodialysis is used primarily to remove toxins from the blood and correct acid–base imbalances
  - Substances such as toxic alcohols, salicylates, and acetaminophen can successfully be removed from the blood using hemodialysis
  - Requires central vascular access

Medication-Specific Overdose Considerations

- Acetaminophen overdose[1]
  - Initial symptoms mild or absent
  - At high levels, very hepatotoxic
  - Significant liver damage has occurred when signs and symptoms do become present
  - Serial acetaminophen blood level and liver function tests (every 4 hours) should be monitored
  - Activated charcoal is effective if given within 2 hours of ingestion
  - Medication therapy with N-acetylcysteine (also known as NAC, Mucomyst™, or Acetadote™) is effective in preventing liver damage, particularly when given within 8 to 10 hours of ingestion
- Nonsteroidal anti-inflammatory drug (NSAID) overdose[1]
  - Gastric irritation is common; may use antacids or proton pump inhibitor medications to treat
  - Ibuprofen
    - Can cause GI symptoms, acidosis, bradycardia, liver and renal failure
    - Treat with activated charcoal
  - Aspirin
    - Metabolic acidosis due to metabolism forming ketoacids
    - Respiratory alkalosis due to tachypnea
    - Assess for tinnitus or ringing in the ears
    - Treat with activated charcoal
    - Treat with IV sodium bicarbonate or, if severe, dialysis
- Tricyclic antidepressant overdose[1]
  - Used in the management of depression
  - Overdose can lead to anticholinergic effects, neurotoxicity, and cardiotoxicity

- Cardiac monitoring for prolonged QRS, PR, or QT intervals
- Do not induce vomiting because of potential CNS depression
- Treatment includes systemic alkalization by administering IV sodium bicarbonate to minimize acidosis or activated charcoal for absorption
• Calcium channel and beta blocker overdose[26]
- Cardiotoxic
- Results in bradycardia, arrhythmias, and reduction of contractility
  • Atropine may be required for bradycardia
- May develop hypotension requiring fluid resuscitation
- Strict cardiac monitoring is imperative
- Activated charcoal, glucagon, or lipid emulsions may be considered
- High-dose insulin for calcium channel overdose continues to be studied and acts by treating cardiac suppression causes by calcium channel blockers. Insulin has a positive inotropic effect on the cardiac tissue as well as improving calcium uptake[5]

General Overdose Assessment, Intervention, and Evaluation Considerations

Assessment/Analysis
- History regarding the overdose
  - Intentional versus unintentional
  - Name of medication or medications
  - Amount of medication taken and dose
  - Approximate time of ingestion
  - Route of ingestion
  - Witness to the ingestion
  - Emesis prior to arrival
- Laboratory studies
  - Toxicity screening
  - Serum lactate
  - Serum chemistries and liver function tests
  - Arterial or venous blood gas
  - Coagulation studies

Interventions
- Maintain airway, support effective breathing
- Vital sign monitoring including cardiac monitoring
- Establish IV access for crystalloid fluids and medications as needed
- Consult a poison control center
- Assist with gastric lavage, if indicated
- Administer activated charcoal and a cathartic as ordered
- Prepare to administer antidotes (if one exists) for known medication ingestions

Evaluation
- Maintain airway patency and effective breathing
- Hemodynamic stability
- Vital signs and cardiac monitoring
- Monitor for possible evolving deterioration
- Evaluation of effectiveness of antidotes, activated charcoal, or reversal agents
- Need for suicidal precautions or other protective measures

Substance Abuse

Substance abuse contributes to a significant number of ED visits every year. The problem appears to be growing, as well as the number of substances being abused. Many emerging substances such as "bath salts" have gained attention. This section discusses commonly abused substances, as well as typical nursing interventions associated with each.[27]

Alcohol Use and Abuse

Alcohol is one of the most widely abused substances in the United States. It is estimated that approximately 70% of overdose ED visits involve alcohol abuse.[1] There is no specific demographic associated with alcohol abuse, although males tend to have a higher rate than females. Chronic use of alcohol not only causes destruction of the liver and other GI organs but also increases the risk of trauma-related injury. People with chronic alcohol use are also at risk for developing life-threating delirium tremens upon the discontinuation of use. This condition constitutes a medical emergency.[2]

Assessment/Analysis
- Airway patency due to risk for aspiration
- Mental status and ability to self-maintain an open airway
- Potential head injury
- Tremors
- Nystagmus
- Ataxia
- Jaundice
- Hepatomegaly
- Approximate amount of alcohol ingested
- Approximate time of last drink
- History of alcohol use
  - Chronic versus binge
  - Use of substitutes such as mouthwash or hand sanitizer
- Sign of withdrawal: assess/score symptoms applying withdrawal assessment scale such as Clinical Institute Withdrawal Assessment for Alcohol (CIWA)
- Laboratory studies
  - Blood or breath alcohol level
  - Serum chemistries
  - Liver function tests
  - Possibly coagulation studies
  - Possibly toxicology screen
  - Point-of-care blood glucose

- Preexisting conditions such as GI bleed, seizures, and liver disease

Interventions
- Acute intoxication
  - Patent airway—Assist with airway intervention, as needed
  - Effective breathing
  - Aspiration precautions (protect airway)
  - Supplemental oxygen support if indicated
- Establish IV access for crystalloid fluids and medications as needed
  - IV fluids and electrolyte replacement upon order
- Administer medications as ordered for withdrawal, agitation, or delirium
  - Benzodiazepines

Evaluation
- Maintain airway patency
- Continuous evaluation for agitation, withdrawal, or seizure activity

Opiate Abuse

Opiates are commonly prescribed for moderate to severe pain. The euphoric effects produced by opiates can lead to addiction and abuse. In the United States, prescription drug abuse has increased dramatically in recent years. Street versions of opium, such as heroin, have also become a popular abuse drug. In many cases, opiate abuse begins with high-cost, prescription-grade medications. Once addiction occurs, many abusers turn to lower-cost options, such as heroin. Opium causes CNS depression leading to respiratory failure usually due to apnea. Fortunately, an antidote exists and is effective if given prior to prolonged apnea. Naloxone (Narcan) is the antidote for opium, and it works by competing with CNS opiate receptor sites. Naloxone can be given IV, intramuscularly (IM), intranasally, or subcutaneously.[1]

Assessment/Analysis
- Airway and breathing status
- Time and type of last opiate use
- Previous administered doses of naloxone in the prehospital period
- Mental status
- Constricted pupils (pinpoint pupils)
- Constipation
- Hypotension
- Laboratory studies
  - Toxicology screen
  - Glucose level
  - Pregnancy testing
  - Arterial blood gas (ABG)
- Chest x-ray

Interventions
- Assist with RSI, airway support
- Establish IV access for crystalloid fluids and medications as needed
- Cardiac monitor, vital signs including pulse oximetry, consider capnography
- Administer naloxone, which may be administered IV, IM, intranasally, or subcutaneously
  - Typical dose, for adults, is 0.4 to 2 mg initially, repeated every 3 minutes until respiratory depression is reversed, not to exceed 10 mg
  - Prepare for possible agitation upon administration from abrupt withdrawal

Evaluation
- Patent airway, effective breathing
- Hemodynamic stability
- Relapse of CNS and respiratory depression

Cocaine Abuse

Cocaine is a powerful vasoconstrictor, producing euphoric effects by stimulating the CNS, which makes it a very popular drug of abuse. Cocaine causes the release of catecholamines and discontinues the reuptake of norepinephrine and dopamine. Vasoconstriction caused by using the drug can produce cardiac symptoms such as angina and myocardial infarction. Cocaine can be abused by a number of administration routes. The most common method for cocaine abuse is intranasal use, although it can also be smoked or injected.[2]

Assessment/Analysis
- Airway and breathing status
- Time, type, and route of last use
- Polysubstance use or abuse
- Mental status
- Dilated pupils
- Cardiac symptoms including angina and palpitations
- Hypertension
- Hyperthermia
- Tachycardia
- Anxiety
- Hallucinations
- Seizures
- Coma
- Vital sign and cardiac monitoring
- Laboratory studies
  - Cardiac enzymes
  - Toxicology screen
  - Serum chemistries
  - CBC with differential

Interventions
- Support ventilations
- Protect airway
- Assist with RSI
- Cardiac monitor, frequent vital signs, and pulse oximetry
- Electrocardiogram (ECG)
- Establish IV access for crystalloid fluids and medications as needed
- Benzodiazepines for agitation and hypertension[5]
- Ensure patient and staff safety

Evaluation
- Maintain airway patency and effective breathing
- Hemodynamic stability
- Continuous cardiac and vital sign monitoring, including temp

Amphetamine Abuse

Amphetamine is a synthetic drug stimulating the CNS, leading to an increase in energy, insomnia, and a feeling of euphoria. This drug is also used prescriptively to treat attention deficit disorder (ADD) and as a means of weight reduction. Crystal methamphetamine or "crystal meth" is a form of amphetamine that can be snorted, injected, body packed, or smoked. Crystal meth abuse is increasing in the United States.[2]

Assessment/Analysis
- Airway and breathing status
- Mental status
- Information surrounding abuse history
  - Time, type, and route of last use
  - Purpose of drug use (abuse, ADD, weight loss, etc)
  - Polysubstance use or abuse
- Dilated pupils
- Cardiac symptoms including angina and palpitations
- Hypertension
- Tachycardia
- Hyperthermia
- Anxiety, appears "jumpy" or unable to remain focused
- Seizures
- Skin lesions
- Hallucinations
- Toxicology screen

Interventions
- Maintain airway and support breathing
- Supplemental oxygen if indicated
- ECG and continuous cardiac monitoring
- Establish IV access for crystalloid fluids and medications as needed
- Cooling measures if hyperthermia is present
- Provide medications upon order for anxiety
  - Benzodiazepines for hyperactivity, hypertension, and seizures
  - Haloperidol for psychotic symptoms
- Protect from potential seizure activity

Evaluation
- Airway and ventilation status
- Continuous cardiac and vital sign monitoring
- Reevaluate and monitor core temperature
- Patient and staff safety

Synthetic Cathinones—"Bath Salts"

Synthetic cathinones, also known as "bath salts", have recently become a popular drug of abuse. This class of drug was recognized in 2010 when emergency departments were reporting adverse medical effects. Reports of abuse increased from 300 in 2010 to more than 6000 in 2011.[28] Cathinone is a psychoactive chemical similar in structure to amphetamine and found in the leaves of the khat plant. The effect of cathinone ingestion is also similar to amphetamine use in that it produces inhibition of dopamine, serotonin, and norepinephrine reuptake as an indirect sympathomimetic. The clinical effects are also similar. The various routes of administration for synthetic cathinones include oral ingestion, inhalation, or intravenous injection.[28]

Assessment/Analysis[1,23]
- Airway and breathing status
- Information surrounding abuse history
  - Time, type, and route of last use
  - Purpose of drug use (abuse, weight loss, treatment for ADD, etc)
  - Polysubstance use or abuse
- Vital sign and cardiac monitoring
- ECG
- Core temperature
- Mental status
- Hypertension
- Increased mental awareness
- Nausea and vomiting
- Anorexia
- Tachycardia
- Severe hyperthermia
- Anxiety, appears "jumpy" or unable to remain focused
- Seizures
- Agitation
- Tremors
- Hallucinations
- Laboratory studies
  - Serum chemistries and urinalysis
    - Concern for rhabdomyolysis

Interventions

- Support airway and breathing
- Supplemental oxygen support if indicated
- Protect airway
- Establish IV access for crystalloid fluids and medications as needed
- Cooling measures if hyperthermia is present
- Provide medications upon order for anxiety
  - Benzodiazepines for hyperactivity, hypertension, and seizures
- Protect from potential seizure activity

Evaluation

- Airway patency and effective breathing
- Hemodynamic stability
- Continuous cardiac and vital sign monitoring
- Reevaluate and monitor core temperature
- Communicable Diseases: please refer to chapter 9, beginning on page 193

REFERENCES

1. ENA. *Sheehy's Emergency Nursing Principles and Practice*. 6th ed. St. Louis, MO: Mosby; 2010.
2. Hoyt KS, Selfridge-Thomas J, eds. *Emergency Nursing Core Curriculum*. 6th ed. Philadelphia, PA: Elsevier Saunders; 2007.
3. American Burn Association. *Advanced Burn Life Support Providers Manual*. Chicago, IL; Author: 2007.
4. MacLennan L, Moiemen N. Management of cyanide toxicity in patients with burns. *Burns*. 2015;41:18–24.
5. Tintinalli JE, Stapczynski S, Ma OJ, et al. *Tintinalli's Emergency Medicine: A Comprehensive Study Guide*. 8th ed. New York, NY: McGraw-Hill; 2016.
6. Venomous snakes. *Centers for Disease Control and Prevention Web site*. http://www.cdc.gov/niosh/topics/snakes/default.html. Accessed November 6, 2015.
7. McGhee S, Finnegan A, Clochesy JM, et al. Effects of snake envenomation: a guide for emergency nurses. *Emerg Nurse*. 2015;22:24–29.
8. Quan D. North American poisonous bites and stings. *Crit Care Clin Toxicol*. 2012;28:633–659.
9. Smith S, Sammons SS, Carr J, et al. Bedside management considerations in the treatment of pit viper envenomation. *J Emerg Nurs*. 2014;40:537–545.
10. Goldsmith LA, Katz SI, Gilchrest BA, et al. *Fitzpatrick's Dermatology in General Medicine*. 8th ed. New York, NY: McGraw-Hill Education; 2012.
11. Daly JS, Scharf MJ. Bites and stings of terrestrial and aquatic life. In: *Fitzpatrick's Dermatology in General Medicine*. 8th ed. New York, NY: McGraw-Hill Education; 2012.
12. King AM, Aaron CK. Organophosphate and carbamate poisoning. *Emerg Med Clin North Am*. 2015;33:133–151.
13. Malaria. *Centers for Disease Control and Prevention Web site*. http://www.cdc.gov/Malaria. Accessed November 6, 2015.
14. Kazzi Z, Buzzell J, Bertelli L, et al. Emergency department management of patients internally contaminated with radioactive material. *Emerg Med Clin North Am*. 2015;33:179–196.
15. Raukar N, Lemieux R, Finn G, et al. Heat illness—A practical primer. *R I Med J*. 2015;98:28–31.
16. Gaudio FG, Grissom CK. Cooling methods in heat stroke. *J Emerg Med*. 2016;50:607–616.
17. Rabies. *Centers for Disease Control and Prevention Web site*. http://www.cdc.gov/rabies/medical_care. Accessed March 16, 2016.
18. Bayés-de-Luna A, Goldwasser D, Fiol M, et al. Surface electrocardiography. In: Fuster V, Walsh RA, Harrington RA, eds. *Hurst's The Heart*. 13 ed. New York, NY: McGraw-Hill; 2011.
19. McIntosh SE, Opacic M, Freer L, et al. Wilderness medical society practice guidelines for the prevention and treatment of frostbite: 2014 update. *Wilderness Environ Med*. 2014;25 Suppl:S43–S54.
20. Carbon monoxide poisoning. *Centers for Disease Control and Prevention Web site*. http://www.cdc.gov/co/default.htm. Accessed November 6, 2015.
21. Hampson NB, Piantadosi CA, Thom S, et al. Practice recommendations in the diagnosis, management, and prevention of carbon monoxide poisoning. *Am J Respir Crit Care Med*. 2012;11:1095–1101.
22. Rose JJ, Xu Q, Wang L, et al. Shining a light on carbon monoxide poisoning. *Am J Respir Crit Care Med*. 2015;192:1145–1147.
23. Borron SW, Bebarta VS. Asphyxiants. *Emerg Med Clin North Am*. 2015;33: 89–115.
24. Lehne RA. *Pharmacology for Nursing Care*. 8th ed. St. Louis, MO: Elsevier Saunders; 2013.
25. Benson BE, Hoppu K, Troutman WG, et al. Position paper update: gastric lavage for gastrointestinal decontamination. *Clin Toxicol*. 2013;51: 140–146.
26. Graudins A, Lee HM, Druda D. Calcium channel antagonist and beta-blocker overdose: antidotes and adjunct therapies. *Br J Clin Pharmacol*. 2016;81:453–461.
27. Injury prevention & control: Prescription drug overdose. *Centers for Disease Control and Prevention Web site*. http://www.cdc.gov/drugoverdose/index.html. Accessed November 6, 2015.
28. Mello NK, Mendelson JH. Cocaine and other commonly abused drugs. In: Kasper D, Fauci A, Hauser S, et al, eds. *Harrison's Principles of Internal Medicine*. 19th ed. New York, NY: McGraw-Hill; 2015.

Practice Questions

Question	Rationale
1. A 41-year-old male patient presents to the emergency department after an exposure to an organophosphate insecticide. After decontamination, he is experiencing profuse salivation and is urinating and defecating frequently. The emergency nurse anticipates which medication will be ordered? a. An antiemetic and antidiarrheal medication b. IV atropine c. IV atropine and IV pralidoxime (2-PAM) d. Epinephrine and diphenhydramine	*Answer: c* Atropine and pralidoxime (2-PAM) are the agents used to treat an organophosphate exposure. Atropine works by reducing symptoms (SLUDGE) while pralidoxime (2-PAM) works by binding the organophosphate, which is considered curative. IV atropine alone will not eliminate the organophosphate from the nerve synapse; it will only reduce the symptoms of SLUDGE. Epinephrine and diphenhydramine are not indicated, and antiemetics and antidiarrheals are not priority for this patient.
2. The emergency nurse encounters a patient who has a hydrofluoric acid exposure to the right hand and fingers. The emergency nurse recognizes hydrofluoric acid as an acid leading to what type of emergency? a. Full-thickness chemical burn blistering b. Bradycardia c. Anaphylaxis d. Bone damage and severe pain	*Answer: d* Hydrofluoric acid easily passes through the skin and exchanges its fluoride ion with calcium. This causes bone destruction and severe pain as a result. Generally, hydrofluoric acid does not cause a significant skin burn, although it might create erythema in the area. The application of calcium (i.e., calcium gluconate gel) to the skin acts to withdraw the hydrofluoric acid from the tissue, which spares bone destruction. Blistering is not typically seen with hydrofluoric acid exposure. Anaphylaxis and bradycardia are not common with hydrofluoric acid exposure.
3. An adult patient involved in a car fire enters the emergency department. Once stabilized, the emergency nurse determines that the patient has burns to the anterior chest, left anterior arm, and right posterior leg. Using the rule of nines, the emergency nurse estimates the total surface burn area as a. 18% b. 27% c. 32% d. 36%	*Answer: c* Using the rule of nines, the anterior chest scores at 18%, the anterior and posterior arms are each 4.5%, and the anterior and posterior legs count for 9% each. The total surface area for the patient described above is 31.5% and has been rounded to 32%.

Question	Rationale
4. The emergency nurse is assessing a person bitten on the left hand by a rattlesnake. The nurse identifies two fang marks on the hand with some minor edema and bleeding. The patient complains of minor pain, and vital signs are within normal limits. Upon reassessment an hour later, the emergency nurse finds no change in the patient's assessment. This can best be explained by which phenomenon? a. This patient is immune to snake venom b. A "dry bite" that did not involve envenomation c. Not enough time has passed for the snake venom to cause symptoms d. The patient was not bitten by a snake	*Answer: b* Dry bites occur in approximately 20% of pit viper snakebites. Dry bites are characterized by the presence of fang marks without symptoms of envenomation such as pain, edema, or systemic changes such as vital sign abnormalities. It is possible that this patient was not bitten by a snake. The emergency nurse must take a careful history to determine the accuracy of the patient's description of the snake and if in fact it is poisonous.
5. The acronym SLUDGE as seen in insecticide and organophosphate exposures stands for a. Salivation, Lacrimation, Urination, Defecation, Gastrointestinal distress, and Emesis b. Salivation, Lacrimation, Urination, Gastrointestinal distress, and Elimination c. Salivation, Liquidation, Urination, Defecation, Gastrointestinal distress, and Emesis d. Salivation, Lacrimation, Urination, Defecation, Gastritis, and Erection	*Answer: a* The acronym SLUDGE references the words Salivation, Lacrimation, Urination, Defecation, Gastrointestinal distress, and Emesis. These are common symptoms of an exposure to an organophosphate insecticide.
6. A female patient presents to the emergency department with severe diarrhea, fatigue, and weight loss. The emergency nurse performs a history and assessment. Which historical finding suggests the patient may have giardiasis? a. Patient works in a meat processing plant b. Patient traveled to New Mexico recently c. Patient works in a day care center d. Patient is a vegan	*Answer: c* Giardiasis is a parasitic disease causing severe diarrhea, fatigue, fever, and weight loss. Those traveling outside the United States, day care workers, children, and individuals with poor dietary habits are most at risk for ingesting the giardiasis parasite.
7. The emergency nurse is caring for a patient contaminated with gamma radiation particles. The emergency nurse understands what principle for ensuring healthcare team safety by minimizing exposure? a. Gamma radiation has little or no risk with exposure b. Decontamination will keep the nurse and staff safe c. Distance and shielding from the patient d. Time, distance, and shielding	*Answer: d* The principle of time, distance, and shielding is the preferred method to minimize exposure to ionizing radiation. By minimizing time near the source of radiation, the amount of ionizing radiation absorbed is reduced. Distance from a source of ionizing radiation also minimizes exposure. The use of shielding such as lead aprons and thyroid shields can provide the most benefit. Respiratory protection is also warranted in order to prevent inhalation of a radioactive substance.

Question	Rationale
8. A patient presents to the emergency department following a near drowning in a nearby lake. The patient is receiving high-flow oxygen and is maintaining his airway. The nurse notes coarse lung sounds throughout all lung fields. What is the emergency nurse most concerned about with initial treatment in a near drowning? a. Sepsis due to inhalation of dirty water b. Aspiration pneumonia and hypothermia c. Physical trauma due to the violent nature of near drowning d. Hyperthermia	*Answer: b* Aspiration pneumonia and hypothermia are both likely in near drowning episodes, and each should be considered in any submersion event. Bacterial pneumonia is a concern as well, although much later. Near-drowning patients are at risk for hypothermia. Sepsis is not a threat in this present scenario. A near drowning is not typically associated with traumatic injuries, although more information may be collected after initial treatment.
9. A patient presents to the emergency department following collapse at a distance running event. The emergency nurse immediately suspects a heat-related emergency. What signs and symptoms would the nurse expect to see with heat stroke as opposed to heat exhaustion? a. Core temperature 102.5°F (39.2°C), warm skin, profuse perspiration, and altered mental status b. Core temperature 104.5 (40.2°C), hot skin, lack of perspiration, and altered level of consciousness c. Headache, pale skin, and profuse perspiration d. Muscle cramps, mild tachycardia, headache, and lack of perspiration	*Answer: b* Heat stroke is a medical emergency and is differentiated from heat exhaustion by a core temperature of greater than 104.0°F (40°C) and the lack of perspiration.
10. A 34-year-old male patient presents to the emergency department after exposure to very cold temperatures during a hunting trip. The nurse assesses both of his feet and notes edema with cold, pale skin. He has circumferential blisters to both feet. Given his history and assessment findings, the nurse suspects frostbite. Which of the following interventions would be *contraindicated* for this condition? a. Slow rewarming of his feet using warm water b. Obtaining a core temperature c. Rubbing or massaging both of his feet to stimulate circulation d. Providing ordered analgesics for pain	*Answer: c* Frostbite is the freezing of tissue. At the cellular level, ice crystals form within the tissue, causing cellular damage. Rubbing or massaging the affected areas can cause further damage to the tissue. The other listed interventions are appropriate for the treatment of frostbite.
11. A patient is diagnosed with carbon monoxide poisoning. The patient is awake and alert but is evasive when a history on the circumstances surrounding the inhalation exposure is obtained. The emergency nurse should be concerned with a. Decreased perfusion to the patient brain causing confusion b. Intentional inhalation of carbon monoxide and possible suicidal ideation c. Possible illegal activity prior to the inhalation d. A safe ride home for the patient	*Answer: b* It is important to consider suicidal ideation for unexplained carbon monoxide inhalation. Although carbon monoxide inhalation can be caused by faulty heating appliances within the home, it is also a common means of suicide attempt/completion.

Question	Rationale

12. What substance does activated charcoal not absorb?
  a. Acetaminophen
  b. Amitriptyline (tricyclic antidepressant)
  c. Ibuprofen
  d. Lithium
	Answer: d
	Activated charcoal is very effective at absorbing a variety of substances. It does not effectively absorb heavy metals such as iron and lead and medications such as lithium. Activated charcoal does effectively bind to ibuprofen, acetaminophen, and most tricyclic antidepressants if taken within 2 hours of the ingestion (the closer to time of ingestion, the greater the chance of effectiveness).

13. A 22-year-old male patient presents to the emergency department following a party at which his friends state he used "bath salts." The emergency nurse knows "bath salts" are similar to amphetamines and can have which of the following effects?
  a. Constricted pupils
  b. Hallucinations, hypotension, and bradycardia
  c. Sedation, CNS depression, and airway compromise
  d. Severe hyperthermia, anxiety, agitation, and tremors
	Answer: d
	Cathinone, or "bath salts," is very similar to amphetamines and inhibits dopamine, serotonin, and norepinephrine reuptake. Common symptoms include hyperthermia, anxiety, agitation, and tremors due to the increased levels of these neurotransmitters.

14. As an emergency nurse caring for a patient who used cocaine, what related condition must be considered and evaluated?
  a. Pneumonia due to ineffective airway clearance
  b. Slow gastric motility leading to constipation
  c. Myocardial infarction
  d. Exsanguination from a nosebleed
	Answer: c
	Cocaine is a potent vasoconstrictor, causing constriction of the coronary arteries. This vasoconstriction can exacerbate angina or can lead to a myocardial infarction. A complete cardiac evaluation may be performed in the emergency setting. Pneumonia, slow gastric motility and exsanguination are not typically seen shortly after cocaine use.

15. A 42-year-old male patient has overdosed on a tricyclic antidepressant. The emergency nurse anticipates the following treatments *except*
  a. Induced vomiting to remove pill fragments from the stomach
  b. Activated charcoal
  c. Systemic alkalization
  d. Cardiac monitoring
	Answer: a
	The induction of vomiting is contraindicated in the care of a tricyclic antidepressant (TCA) overdose. A TCA overdose can cause CNS depression leading to an unprotected airway. Vomiting increases the risk for aspiration pneumonia and airway occlusion. Activated charcoal may bind with TCA, preventing further absorption, and cardiac monitoring is indicated because TCA can cause arrhythmias.

16. A 31-year-old female patient arrives at the emergency department via EMS, with severe hypothermia after being found sleeping outside in freezing temperatures. What ECG abnormality would be anticipated given this history?
  a. Elevated Q wave
  b. J waves
  c. Tented T waves
  d. Sine wave
	Answer: b
	Severe hypothermia can lead to arrhythmias including ventricular fibrillation. On ECG, one common finding is J waves, most commonly seen in the precordial leads. J waves are typically seen when the body core temperature falls below 89.6°F (32°C). Elevated Q waves could indicate myocardial injury; tented T waves and cardiac sine waves indicate hyperkalemia.

Question	Rationale
17. A patient has experienced an acute exposure to a radioactive material while working in a laboratory. The patient states the substance he was working with was an alpha radiation emitter. He was not using personal protective equipment and believes he might have inhaled some of the substance. With knowledge about alpha radiation, the emergency nurse knows that a. Alpha radiation is low ionizing and will not cause tissue destruction b. Alpha radiation is highly ionizing and is very destructive to tissue c. Alpha radiation is moderately ionizing and is very destructive to tissue d. Alpha radiation is highly ionizing and is low penetrating, so tissue destruction is not a concern	*Answer: b* Alpha radiation is highly ionizing and is known to cause extensive damage to tissue. It also happens to have very low penetration compared to other types of radiation. When an alpha emitter is inhaled, it has the potential to cause injury to lung tissue. Even though the penetration is low, with inhalation it is very close to the lung tissue and can penetrate it. Destruction of lung tissue can occur, leading to deterioration of the tissue and ineffective blood oxygenation.
18. A 22-year-old male patient presents to the emergency department following a first-time seizure. The nurse learns from his family that the patient had recently traveled outside of the United States. A CT scan shows multiple foreign bodies in the brain tissue. What disease does the emergency nurse suspect the patient has? a. Cysticercosis b. Taeniasis c. Malaria d. Giardiasis	*Answer: a* Cysticercosis is a disease in which parasite larval cysts travel throughout the body and deposit in muscle and brain tissue. In many cases, a first-time seizure is the primary indicator of the parasite infection. Taeniasis is usually from eating undercooked pork or beef and has associated symptoms of weight loss and abdominal pain. Early symptoms of malaria are flu-like with fever and chills. Giardiasis leads to GI symptoms such as diarrhea.
19. An emergency nurse is caring for a patient who was burned over 30% of the body surface area following a natural gas explosion at home. After stabilizing the patient's airway and breathing, what would be the next highest nursing intervention priority? a. IV pain and sedation medication b. Urinary catheter placement c. Application of warming devices to maintain body temperature d. Ensure adequate IV access	*Answer: d* Fluid replacement in burn patients is critical. Following stabilization of the ABCs, IV fluid replacement must begin as soon as possible. Ensuring that the patient has good IV access to begin fluid replacement is paramount. Although maintaining the patient's body temperature is important, it can be done simultaneously starting with warm IV fluid.
20. When removing embedded jellyfish stingers or tentacles from a victim who has been stung, the emergency nurse recognizes a. The remnants left behind from a jellyfish sting are harmless b. Gloves must be worn in order to prevent secondary toxin exposure c. Rinsing the sting area with hydrogen peroxide will neutralize jellyfish toxin d. Jellyfish tentacles do not contain stingers that could release toxin	*Answer: b* The remnants of jellyfish stingers or tentacles contain unreleased toxin. The nurse must don gloves in order to prevent becoming a victim of a sting as well. To neutralize jellyfish toxin, an acetic acid solution such as vinegar should be used. Isopropyl alcohol is a secondary substitute, although it is not as effective in neutralizing the toxin.

Question	Rationale
21. Following atropine and 2-PAM treatment of a patient with organophosphate exposure, the nurse knows the patient is improving when a. Heart rate decreases b. Respiratory rate decreases c. Blood pressure decreases d. Urination decreases	*Answer: d* Organophosphate exposure results in SLUDGE symptoms: Salivation, Lacrimation, Urination, Defecation, GI upset, and Emesis. Treatment should reverse SLUDGE symptoms—in this case, it should decrease urination. Hypotension and bradycardia are also signs of organophosphate exposure, so increasing hypotension or bradycardia would not indicate effective treatment. Respiratory rate may not be affected in organophosphate exposure.
22. Following a prolonged extrication from a burning house, a patient arrives without obvious burns and no signs of inhalation injury. Vital signs are Pulse—58; Respirations—20; BP—102/58 mm Hg. The patient responds to verbal stimuli. Upon drawing the patient's blood for testing, the nurse notices bright red blood. The nurse suspects that the patient was exposed to what toxin? a. Carbon monoxide b. Carboxylic acid c. Cyanide d. Glycosides	*Answer: c* Cyanide exposure, most likely from chemical fumes released by burning carpet or furniture, results in hypotension, bradycardia, and bright red blood. Carbon monoxide exposure may result in cherry-red skin color, not a change in blood color. Carboxylic acid and glycosides are toxins found in plant material and exposure is commonly through ingestion or topical contact.

Professional Issues in Emergency Nursing

13

Dino Johnson, MHA, BSN, RN

Emergency department (ED) nursing encompasses more than just taking care of patients at the bedside. Professional issues arise on a regular and frequent basis, and the ED nurse must be able to navigate through complex situations and understand how the nursing role relates to the department, the hospital, the system/community, and the healthcare industry. This chapter examines several professional ED issues through the perspective of the nurse, the patient, the system, and triage.

Nurse

Critical Incident Stress Management

The ED nurse will face a multitude of incidents and situations possibly leading to personal stress, depersonalization of patients, emotional exhaustion, and ultimately burnout. A method to lessen these effects is having a Critical Incident Stress Management (CISM) system in place. It is up to the team, in partnership with leadership, to establish criteria to activate such a system. Any number of incidents may result in activation of the CISM system, including unexpected deaths, a pediatric death, a negative event regarding a teammate, or a violent incident involving a staff member. Staff may choose to participate after an event, but they should not be forced to participate or share their thoughts or feelings about the event.[1]

Assessment/Analysis
- Consider debriefing
  - Staff crying or visible signs of distress from team members
  - Withdrawal or uncharacteristic mood change following an event
  - Perseveration of discussion regarding an incident
  - An unexpected outcome
  - An error is made during the care of a patient leading to a bad outcome
  - A staff member is assaulted

Implementation[1]/Interventions
- Debrief the event with the involved parties, including
  - Disclosure of facts regarding the incident
  - Disclosure of emotional reactions to the event
  - Normalization of responses
  - "Normal responses to abnormal events"
  - Discussion of what can be improved
  - Planning for the future
  - Having a reassuring and supportive environment as facilitated by a peer or leader
- Offer 1:1 sessions with trained professionals
- Chaplain, Social Work, or Employee Assistance services

Evaluation
- Staff turnover rates
  - Considering the reasons for turnover
- Staff satisfaction
- Morale indicators or evaluation tools
- Reduction in negative outcomes

Ethical Dilemmas

The ED nurse may encounter several ethical dilemmas throughout his or her nursing career. As a result, two factors to consider when selecting an organization for employment are the mission and the values. Inevitably, because of the complexity of the ED setting, an ethical dilemma will present, causing the employee and organizational relationship to strengthen or to become strained. Ethical dilemmas might include requests to perform duties that may be against the RN's personal beliefs, such as administering emergency contraception or resuscitating a patient who has a very low quality of life. Excessive ED boarding or low staffing levels that threaten patient safety are other system issues ED nurses may encounter.[2] The RN is often left balancing organizational needs, personal needs, patient needs, and the needs of colleagues. Ultimately, it is important to have a framework from which to work. Several ethical dilemma decision-making tools are available.[2] The FOUR TOPICS CHART, pictured in Appendix 13, is one example of a framework for ethical decision making.

Assessment/Analysis
- Is there an applicable policy, protocol, guideline, or procedure in place at your organization?
- What is the stance of the professional organization on the dilemma (i.e., Emergency Nurses Association)?
- What is the stance of regulatory agencies such as The Joint Commission or your state department of health?

- What is your understanding of the role of the organization in the decision? (That is, does your organization have an ethics committee or something similar?)

Implementation
- Define the dilemma[3]
- Define the values, ethical principles, and laws involved[3]
- Consider all alternatives[3]
- Involve all stakeholders in the discussion
- Escalate up the chain of command as appropriate

Evaluation
- Was the desired outcome reached from the perspective of the clinical team and from the perspective of the patient?
- Were there any negative outcomes?
- What can be applied to future similar scenarios?
- Does a policy or protocol need to be written or modified?
- Are there any regulatory, risk, or legal implications?

Evidence-Based Practice

Evidence-based practice (EBP) is the intentional use of current best evidence to make decisions about the care of the patients. It means combining individual expertise with the most recent clinical evidence from research.[4] See Figure 13-1 for elements included in decision making related to using evidence. The emergency department is constantly changing to meet the needs of patients and improve outcomes. Emerging research will shift indicated treatments and diagnostics based on the patient condition, and the ED nurse must evolve to continually meet new treatment expectations based on evidence and experience.

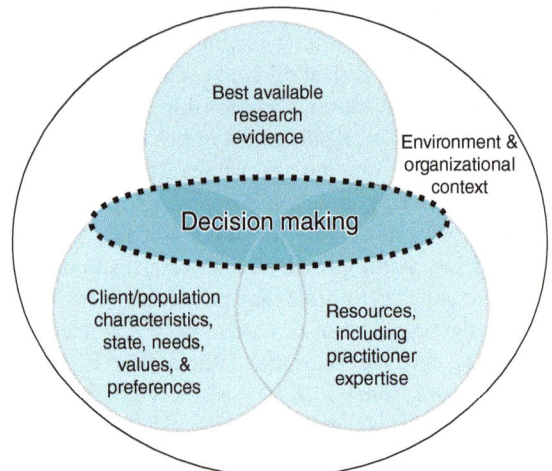

FIGURE 13-1 Elements included in decision-making related to using evidence
Reproduced with permission from Weiner IB, Craighead WE: Corsini's Encyclopedia of Psychology, 4th ed. Hoboken: Wiley; 2009.

Assessment/Analysis
- Order sets (i.e., diagnostic imaging, labs, medications)
- Policies, procedures, and protocols
- Practice patterns by self and department
- Information from governing bodies such as The Joint Commission (TJC), state department of health (DOH), and Centers for Medicare & Medicaid Services (CMS)
- Current information and new research from practice-related journals and articles
- Updates from organizations that seek to improve outcomes, such as the American Heart Association, Emergency Nurses Association, American Academy of Emergency Physicians, or the Institute of Healthcare Improvement

Implementation/Interventions
- Standardize treatments based on best practices
  - Protocols and pathways
  - Antibiotics and other medications
  - Imaging and other diagnostic tests
- Standardize nursing care based on best practices
- Structured review of emerging practices and research

Evaluation
- Outcome metrics
  - Patient return rates
  - Hospital readmission rates
  - Mortality rates
  - Left without being seen rates
- Throughput metrics
  - Door to percutaneous coronary intervention (PCI) or transfer time in the ST-segment elevation myocardial infarction (STEMI) population
  - Door to tissue plasminogen activator (tPA) for the stroke population
  - Door to provider times
  - ED length of stay for admitted and discharged patients
- Patient satisfaction scores, Hospital Consumer Assessment of Healthcare Providers and Systems (HCAHPS)
- Feedback from nursing staff regarding functional nursing care processes and barriers to providing optimal care

Lifelong Learning

Practice in the emergency department is continually evolving to meet patient demand and ongoing quality improvement measures. The emergency nurse must find ways to stay current with evidence-based practices and a constantly changing environment. The emergency nurse can never stop attempting to improve personal practice. Many states require continuing education credits for RN licensure renewal.

Assessment/Analysis
- State licensing requirements for ongoing education requirements
- Resources for ongoing education such as journals, Internet resources, nursing educators, organizational support
- Opportunities for attending formal education from colleges and universities

- Transparency in hospital-based quality and process improvement committees

Implementation
- Read current professional journals
- Attend conferences
- Attend available classes
- Become involved in local, state, or national committee work pertinent to nursing practice
- Implement and share new learning
- Attain professional nursing certification

Evaluation
- Continuing education credits acquired
- Evaluate effectiveness of practice changes through process and outcome measures

Research

Clinical research is when the clinician applies interventions or observes human participants, patients, or volunteers. It is conducted in ways designed to produce generalized scientific knowledge.[5] Nursing research drives ED nursing practice forward and is a key component in establishing evidence-based care. Publicized research is generally structured with an introduction, method, background, discussion, and a conclusion. For an emergency nurse, staying current with evidence-based practice may involve reviewing individual research studies or a set of synthesized studies in the form of systematic reviews or a meta-analysis.[6]

Assessment/Analysis[7]
- The study's validity
- The study's importance
- The study's level of evidence
  - An example Level of Evidence table is shown in Figure 13-2
  - An example Evidence Hierarchy is shown in Figure 13-3
- The study's relevance to your patients

Implementation
- Identify best practices from research
- Using the principles of EBP described previously, apply the learning

	CLASS I Benefit >>> Risk Procedure/treatment SHOULD be performed/administered	**CLASS IIa** Benefit >> Risk Additional studies with focused objectives needed IT IS REASONABLE to perform procedure/administer treatment	**CLASS IIb** Benefit ≥ Risk Additional studies with broad objectives needed; additional registry data would be helpful Procedure/treatment MAY BE CONSIDERED	**CLASS III** Risk ≥ Benefit Procedure/treatment should NOT be performed/administered SINCE IT IS NOT HELPFUL AND MAY BE HARMFUL
LEVEL A Multiple populations evaluated[a] Data derived from multiple randomized clinical trials or meta-analyses	■ Recommendation that procedure or treatment is useful/effective ■ Sufficient evidence from multiple randomized trials or meta-analyses	■ Recommendation in favor of treatment or procedure being useful/effective ■ Some conflicting evidence from multiple randomized trials or meta-analyses	■ Recommendation's usefulness/efficacy less well established ■ Greater conflicting evidence from multiple randomized trials or meta-analyses	■ Recommendation that procedure or treatment is not useful/effective and may be harmful ■ Sufficient evidence from multiple randomized trials or meta-analyses
LEVEL B Limited populations evaluated[a] Data derived from a single randomized trail or nonrandomized studies	■ Recommendation that procedure or treatment is useful/effective ■ Evidence from single randomized trial or nonrandomized studies	■ Recommendation in favor of treatment or procedure being useful/effective ■ Some conflicting evidence from single randomized trial or nonrandomized studies	■ Recommendation's usefulness/efficacy less well established ■ Greater conflicting evidence from single randomized trial or nonrandomized studies	■ Recommendation that procedure or treatment is not useful/effective and may be harmful ■ Evidence from single randomized trial or nonrandomized studies
LEVEL C Very limited population evaluated[a] Only consensus opinion of experts, case studies, or standard of care	■ Recommendation that procedure or treatment is useful/effective ■ Only expert opinion, case studies, or standard of care	■ Recommendation in favor of treatment or procedure being useful/effective ■ Only diverging expert opinion, case studies, or standard of care	■ Recommendation's usefulness/efficacy less well established ■ Only diverging expert opinion, case studies, or standard of care	■ Recommendation that procedure or treatment is not useful/effective and may be harmful ■ Only expert opinion, case studies, or standard of care
Suggested phrases for writing recommendations[b]	should is recommended is indicated is useful/effective/beneficial	is reasonable can be useful/effective/beneficial is probably recommended or indicated	may/might be considered may/might be reasonable usefulness/effectiveness is unknown/unclear/uncertain or not well established	is not recommended is not indicated should not is not useful/effective/beneficial may be harmful

Axes: SIZE OF TREATMENT EFFECT (horizontal); ESTIMATE OF CERTAINTY (PRECISION) OF TREATMENT EFFECT (vertical)

FIGURE 13-2 An example of a Levels of Evidence table
Reproduced with permission from Krumholz HM, Anderson JL, Bachelder BL, et al: ACC/AHA 2008 performance measures for adults with ST-elevation and non-ST-elevation myocardial infarction: a report of the American College of Cardiology/American Heart Association Task Force on Performance Measures (Writing Committee to Develop Performance Measures for ST-Elevation and Non-ST-Elevation Myocardial Infarction) Developed in Collaboration With the American Academy of Family Physicians and American College of Emergency Physicians Endorsed by the American Association of Cardiovascular and Pulmonary Rehabilitation, Society for Cardiovascular Angiography and Interventions, and Society of Hospital Medicine, *J Am Coll Cardiol*. 2008;52(24):2046–2099.

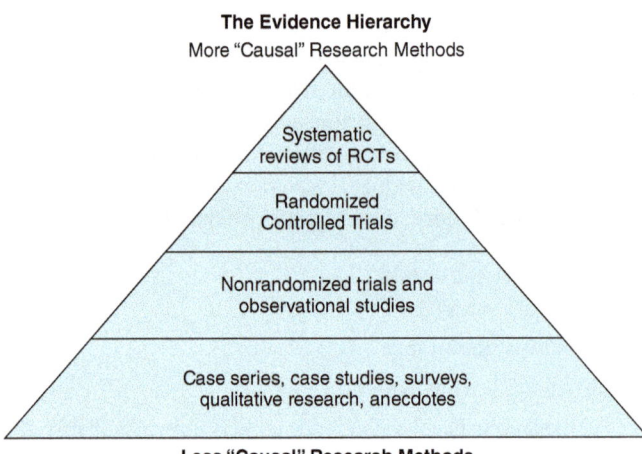

FIGURE 13-3 An example Evidence Hierarchy diagram
Reproduced with permission from South-Paul J, Matheny S, Lewis E: CURRENT Diagnosis & Treatment: Family Medicine, 4th ed. New York: McGraw-Hill Education; 2015.

Evaluation
- Outcomes
- Experiences with the research application

Patient

Discharge Planning

Discharge planning in the emergency department is increasingly important as performance expectations rise. Several factors influence the discharge plan, such as the diagnosis, the patient's social structure and cognitive abilities, required treatments, and the patient's ability to access future healthcare. Each unique diagnosis requires specific instructions and patient teaching. The patient's understanding of the discharge instructions is linked to readmission rates and patient satisfaction.[7] A personalized discharge instruction sheet, including the discharge diagnosis and follow-up instructions, should be given to every patient. The patient or legal guardian should sign these instructions.[8] Discharge planning involves both patient education and a plan for follow-up care.

Assessment/Analysis
- Medical screening exam
- Patient's cognitive abilities
- Appropriate diagnosis
- Discharge vital signs
  - Documented reason for discharge with abnormal vital signs
- Patient's discharge requests
- Timeliness of follow-up
- Patient's ability to receive follow-up care due to factors such as mobility, ability to pay, and other life demands

Implementation
- Patient teaching on diagnosis and medications
- Clear policies and standards of discharge planning[9]
  - Includes special populations such as substance abuse patients, behavioral health patients, or patients who have received narcotics or sedation during their ED visits[8]
- Work with all members of the care team to develop a framework for safe patient discharge[8]

Evaluation
- Patient understanding using teach-back methods[8]
- Patient satisfaction scores
- Outcome metrics such as 72-hour return rate
- Safety events related to the discharge process

End-of-Life Issues

Organ and tissue donation. Notification of death to an organ procurement organization (OPO) is a Joint Commission requirement in the ED setting.[10] More than 123,000 patients are on the national transplant list.[11] All 50 states have some form of consent and/or registry laws through their Department of Motor Vehicles, which increases the likelihood of family consent following death.[11] In the event of a "care versus organ donation" conflict, a trained organ procurement specialist should be consulted, as they are skilled in conflict resolution and are familiar with the governing laws.[11] Both organs and tissues can be donated, and the OPO will determine appropriate harvest following consent.

Assessment/Analysis
- Criteria for potential donors
- Accessing and notifying the local OPO
- Readiness of the patient's family

Implementation
- Policies and procedures regarding notification after death
- A standard referral process to an OPO
- Facilitate communication between the family and the OPO

Evaluation
- Appropriate referral rates
- Timeliness of referrals

Advance Directive. An advance directive is a document discussing the patient's wishes in various situations, should the patient be unable to make independent decisions.[11] A power of attorney specifies who is legally allowed to make decisions when the patient is not able.[12] Patients often come to the emergency department without advance directives, and the team may not know the identity of the person with durable power of attorney. Often times, the emergency department is not the ideal place for end-of-life discussions or experiences due to factors such as shorter length of stay (LOS), poor design without room for families, and patients presenting with complex medical conditions.[12]

Assessment/Analysis
- Patient prognosis and end-of-life care needs
- Documentation regarding patient wishes during end-of-life care
- Institutional policies regarding end-of-life care and the use of advance directives in the emergency department setting

Implementation
- Collaborate with other members of the team to determine the appropriate course of action

- Attempt to reach the patient's durable power of attorney based on the available information
- Education regarding advance directives and end of life[13]

Evaluation
- Staff satisfaction and feedback
- Family feedback
- Structure within the community regarding end-of-life discussions in the primary care setting

Family Presence. Family presence during resuscitation may increase understanding, help with grieving, and alleviate guilt or disappointment.[12] When family is present, it is recommended a liaison be with them to assist in communication, education, and support.[12] The majority of family members report they would like to be present during resuscitative efforts.[13] Additional benefits of family presence include seeing the amount of resources committed to saving their family member and seeing the teamwork and professionalism of the care team.[14] The family can also provide critical information to the patient care team about the patient.[15] Reasons that oppose family presence, such as code team disruption or psychological trauma to the family, are not supported in the literature.[14]

Assessment/Analysis
- Family and patient wishes
- Team readiness
- Safety of the environment

Implementation
- Ensure available liaison
- Coordinate with multidisciplinary teams such as social services, pastoral care, and medical staff
- Establish family presence guidelines or policies
- Educate team on family presence benefits

Evaluation
- Discuss family's perception and understanding
- Debrief with involved team members

Withholding, withdrawing, and palliative care. Emergency nurses play a key role during end-of-life care, including withholding care, withdrawing care, or initiating palliative care. The International Council of Nurses declares it is the RN's responsibility to provide patients with a peaceful ending of life.[15] Providing palliative care in the ED setting is often difficult because of time constraints, lack of information about the patient, and societal expectations of emergency care.[16] Treatment in palliative care focuses on patient comfort and may include treating pain, dyspnea, nausea/vomiting, constipation, and agitation.[16]

Assessment/Analysis
- Identify patients who may benefit from palliative care[16]
- Availability of documentation indicating patient's wishes, such as an advance directive, if unable to respond
- Durable power of attorney's wishes
- Patient's wishes if able to respond

Implementation
- Collaborate with providers and other care team members supporting palliative philosophies of care[16]
- Collaborate with specialized palliative care providers[16]
- Provide staff education on topics concerning palliative care and end-of-life care[16]

Evaluation
- Patient and family feedback
- Patient satisfaction
- Policies and procedures regarding end-of-life care

Forensic Evidence Collection

Emergency nurses need to have the ability to recognize patterns of injury, document observations, and preserve evidence in a manner consistent with legal standards.[17] Emergency nurses preserve evidence collected in the emergency department, document and photograph care, and testify in legal proceedings.[18] Visible wounds should be documented and photographed prior to medical treatment if possible, and should include a form of patient identification in the photo, such as a patient label/sticker.[19] Examples of injuries requiring evidence collection are gunshot wounds, stab wounds, and injuries from assaults or sexual assaults.

Assessment/Analysis
- Wounds requiring evidence collection
- Local and state laws regarding evidence collection
- Patient history and events leading up to injury

Implementation
- Document patient and witness statements verbatim[18]
- Photograph injuries
- Follow protocols and procedures regarding evidence collection
- Collaborate with local law enforcement agencies to develop chain-of-custody protocols[18]

Evaluation
- Law enforcement feedback
- Legal team feedback
- Patient feedback

Pain Management and Procedural Sedation

Pain is the most common reason for seeking emergency care, but only 60% of patients reporting pain receive medication, and 74% of patients presenting with pain are discharged in moderate to severe pain.[17] The Joint Commission requires pain assessments in the emergency setting, as well as reassessments after intervention and treatment.[20] It is important that the treatment and management of pain be guided by the patient's perception of pain, not the clinician's interpretation of the patient's pain experience.[21] Treatment of pain includes both pharmacological and nonpharmacological interventions. Painful interventions may require procedural sedation. Procedural sedation is the administration of sedatives or dissociative agents, with or without analgesics, allowing the patient to tolerate unpleasant procedures while maintaining cardiorespiratory function. It is intended to result in a depressed level of consciousness, but allows the patient to maintain independent oxygenation and airway control.[21] Nurses who assist with procedural sedation should have ongoing training on medications used for sedation, assessment of patients undergoing sedation, and recognition of the signs and symptoms of a distressed, sedated patient. Nurses should be audited by nurse experts and have proper licensing and education.[22] After sedation, a patient should remain in the clinical area with the same level of monitoring as during the procedure until the level of consciousness and vital signs return to their pre-procedural baseline.[23]

Assessment/Analysis
- Patient's reported pain level
  - Scale for the appropriate age/cognitive level
  - Scale for nonverbal or sleeping/comatose patients
- Vital signs
- Nonpharmacological interventions (ice, elevation, heat, or distraction)
- Patient's condition/diagnosis
- Informed consent for procedural sedation
- Oxygenation
- Equipment such as airway adjuncts, suction, and monitoring equipment[23]
- Respiratory rate
- Definitive airway supplies
- Capnography[23]
- Heart rhythm
- Discharge plan

Implementation
- Pain assessment/reassessment policies
- Procedural sedation policies
- Reversal agents for sedation medications

Evaluation
- Pain level before and after intervention
- Patient's return to baseline vital signs and cognition after procedural sedation
- Patient satisfaction
- Outcomes related to pain management and sedation

Patient Safety

One of the core principles for healthcare workers is to "do no harm." However, after the release by the Institute of Medicine of the landmark paper "To Err Is Human" proclaiming that as many as 98,000 people were killed each year by medical errors, patient safety came to light as a major issue in American healthcare. Modern medical error beliefs are focused on systems thinking.[23] When an error occurs, it is often attributed to a series of breakdowns across a system rather than to individual failures. This line of thinking acknowledges that humans will make mistakes and, through highly reliable systems, errors can be reduced or prevented.[24] Tasks that are highly repetitive are at particular risk for error when people go on "autopilot."[24] Culture is a large part of safety, and it is important to have a culture that embraces reporting by responding respectfully and in a nonpunitive manner.[24]

Assessment/Analysis
- Team dynamics
- Error report structure
- Current guidelines supporting safe practice[25]
- Ability to coach and challenge team members and leaders when safe practices are breached or threatened[25]

Implementation
- Standardization[24]
- Simplification[24]
- A culture that does not focus on placing blame
- Built-in redundancies[24]
- Improved teamwork and communication[24]
- Platform to learn from mistakes[24]
- Error reporting system[25]

Evaluation
- Error prevention techniques
  - Example: reducing possible error by interrupting the flow or pattern of an error, as illustrated in the "Swiss Cheese Model" pictured in Figure 13-4

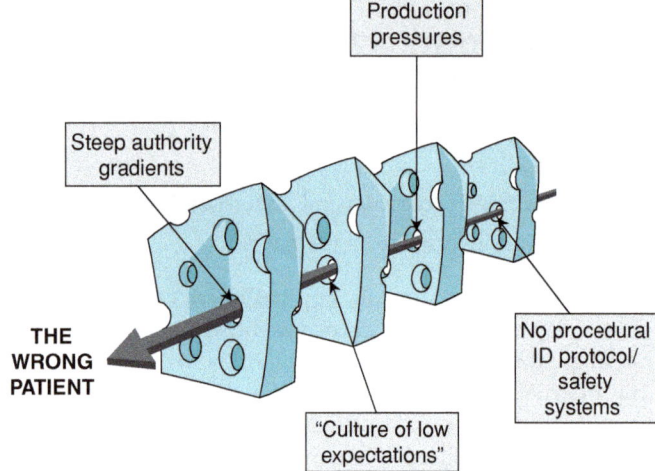

FIGURE 13-4 Swiss Cheese model of error occurrence
Reproduced with permission from Reason J: Human error: models and management, *BMJ*. 2000;320(7237):768–770.

- Platform for sharing learning[24,25]
- Patient outcomes related to errors
- Events after an error is made[24]

Patient Satisfaction

Satisfaction is measured and publicly reported for emergency departments. These reports serve as a measure of the patient's perception of the care received. Several practices have been shown to improve the patient's experience in the emergency department, such as frequent rounding, patient callbacks, updating patients on the plan of care and expected timelines, bedside report, and using the "manage up" technique during handoffs.[25] The healthcare provider (HCP) must be mindful of the patient's expectations and understand how expectations influence care decisions. For example, research indicates that antibiotics may be overprescribed if the HCP perceives the patient expects them.[26] Evidence further suggests that patients want acknowledgement of their pain level and clear explanations of what to expect during the ED stay. Tools such as AIDET (Acknowledge, Introduce, Duration, Explanation, and Thank You) are designed to help the HCP remember to highlight areas patients report improve their experience.[26] Complaints are more commonly related to service than to quality of care.[27]

Assessment/Analysis
- Current patient satisfaction scores
- Current practices and initiatives to promote patient satisfaction

Implementation
- Processes to promote regular patient rounding
- Scripting to promote explanations including timelines and expectation management
- Callbacks for discharged patients
- Bedside report during handoff of care

Evaluation
- Effectiveness of current practices
- Patient satisfaction scores

Transfer and Stabilization

Safe stabilization and transfer is a concept that has legal and practice implications in the emergency department.[28] Within the context of transferring a patient, the Emergency Medical Treatment and Labor Act (EMTALA) was established in 1986 and mandates that hospitals participating in Medicare provide a medical screening exam and stabilizing treatment, and that they have an explicit accepting hospital prior to transferring a patient.[29] Having agreements with other facilities and EMS agencies can enhance a smooth transfer process.[29] Before transferring a patient, the emergency department must provide stabilization care within the capabilities of the department or facility.

Assessment/Analysis
- Patient appropriateness for transfer
- Services offered at each facility to identify where transfer agreements may benefit
- Medical records and how they will be communicated to accepting facility[29]

Implementation
- Develop transfer agreements with facilities and EMS agencies

- Review and evaluate patient transfers
- Document standards for transfers, including patient consent and understanding

Evaluation
- Review cases of transferred patients to ensure EMTALA standards are met
- Review cases for documentation elements and identify gaps
- Feedback from receiving facilities

Transitions of Care

External, Internal, and Shift Handoffs. Handoffs of care are continuous in the emergency department as patients flow in and out of the department and shifts change. Patient handoffs are one of the greatest sources of potential errors and risk when compared to anything else the emergency RN does.[29]

> There are two main categories of handoffs to consider: (1) when a patient remains stationary and the nurse or other healthcare provider performs a handoff, such as a shift handoff, or conversely, (2) when a patient moves from place to place, such as from the emergency department to an inpatient floor during admission.[30]

All types of handoffs have the potential for missing information or misinformation, but also offer the chance for a new clinician to see and evaluate the patient. The new clinician also provides a new set of eyes to assess the patient, which can be of benefit.[30] One study suggests that transferring care between providers was a greater predictor of hospital complications and errors than the patient's severity of illness.[30]

Because of the number of errors related to patient handoff, the Joint Commission (TJC) implemented a patient safety goal mandating that facilities implement a standardized approach to patient handoffs, including the opportunity to ask and respond to questions. Although this is no longer an active national patient safety goal, it is still relevant and should be followed.[30] Key elements included from the TJC regarding handoffs include interactive communication, up-to-date and accurate information, limited interruptions, a process for verification, and an opportunity to review any relevant historical data.[30] See Table 13-1 for an example of a model used to improve safe handoffs.

The discharged patient is also at risk when handing care back to a receiving facility, such as a skilled nursing facility or adult family home. Checklists incorporating key elements have been shown to decrease errors for the external handoff.[30] An example Discharge Checklist can be viewed in Table 13-2. Further, communication is a key element for safe handoff, so creating and maintaining a linkage between the electronic medical records (EMRs) of facilities sharing patients, such as between hospitals and skilled nursing facilities, can improve handoff safety.[30]

TABLE 13-1 Elements of Safe Handoff using the Anticipate Mnemonic

Administrative	Accurate information, such as name and location
New information	A clinical update, including brief history and diagnosis, updated medication and problem list, current baseline status, and recent procedures and significant events
Tasks	The "to do" list, best expressed in "if/then" statements
Illness	The primary provider's assessment of the patient's severity of illness
Contingency plans	Statements that assist in cross-coverage, including things that have and have not worked in the past

Reproduced with permission from Vidyarthi AR: Triple handoff. AHRQ WebM&M (serial online); Septmeber 2006. Available at http://webmm.ahrq.gov/case.aspx?caseID=134

TABLE 13-2 An Example of a Discharge Checklist

Discharge medications
Review with the patient
Highlight changes from hospital
Specifically inform patient about side effects

Discharge summaries
Dictate in a timely fashion
Include discharge medications (highlight changes from admission)
List outstanding tests and reports that need follow-up
Give copies to all providers involved in the patient's care

Communication with patient/family
Provide patient with medication instructions, follow-up details, and clear instructions on warning signs and what to do if things are not going well
Confirm that patient comprehends your instructions
Include a family member in these discussions if possible

Communication with the primary physician
Make telephone contact with primary care physician prior to discharge

Follow-up plans
Discharge clinic
Follow-up phone calls
Appointments or access to primary providers

Reproduced with permission from Forster A. Discharge fumbles. AHRQ WebM&M (serial online); December 2004. Available at http://webmm.ahrq.gov/case.aspx?caseID=84

Assessment/Analysis
- Method for exchanging information between HCPs
- Current practices around handoffs
- Patient's condition during handoff
- Identified key elements that require communication between HCPs

Implementation
- Use phonetic alphabet for clarity
  - Alpha, Bravo, Charlie instead of A, B, C
- Read-back
- Formulate pre-transfer of care coordination process for admitted and discharged patients[30]
- Perform bedside handoffs
- Standardize handoff content and structure between HCPs
- Develop checklists or "ticket to ride" for transports between nursing and ancillary services such as diagnostic imaging[30]

Evaluation
- Patient satisfaction
- Adverse events related to handoffs
- Effectiveness of implemented standards related to handoffs
- Feedback from external sites receiving and sending patients
- Feedback from departments that receive ED patients

Patient Boarding

Patients who have an accepting admitting provider, but are unable to leave the emergency department because of inpatient space constraints or bed availability, are considered "boarded" in the emergency department. ED boarding is fraught with patient safety risks both for the boarded patient and for subsequent patients arriving for emergency care, who must wait, sometimes for long periods of time, for ED care because of maximized ED capacity. Studies show that boarding leads to adverse patient outcomes and limits access to care for other patients.[30] Patients with medical admissions tend to board more than patients with other types of admissions, such as surgical or critical care patients.[31] Studies suggest that ED boarding contributes to a longer length of stay for the patient and increased complications, such as skin breakdown, infection, and pulmonary or cardiac complications.[32] Other studies suggest that patients prefer to board in inpatient areas as opposed to emergency departments.[32] The Institute for Healthcare Improvement (IHI) states that holding inpatients in alternative locations is a result of ineffective hospital flow processes.[31]

Assessment/Analysis
- ED flow and bottlenecks
- Boarding hours data
- Inpatient and ED length of stay
- Use of alternative treatment areas
  - Hallway spaces
  - Facility-specific temporary bed locations
- Capacity constraints
- Arrival rates and admission rates by hour of day and day of week

Implementation
Process improvement strategies focus on throughput (moving patients to their intended dispositions). Suggested strategies
- Move boarders to inpatient halls[33]

- Level surgical and procedural schedules across the full 7-day week[34]
- Schedule early cardiac catheterization procedures[34]
- Develop a bed management system with a person overseeing and placing patients[34]
- Implement discharge lounges[34]
- Expedite inpatient discharges[34]
- Monitor bed turnaround times[34]
- Simplify admission protocols[34]
- Discharge inpatients who have pending tests that they can receive as outpatients[34]

Evaluation
- Boarding times
- Patient outcomes related to holding
- Process measures that indicate appropriate throughput, such as bed request time to ED depart
- ED and inpatient length-of-stay metrics

Cultural Considerations

Interpretive Services. Federal law prohibits discrimination related to language proficiency.[34] ED staff often use the most readily available resources they have to interpret, which may be another staff member or family member. However, this informal process creates multiple potential issues such as misinformation, inaccuracy, and incompleteness. Relying on family to interpret may limit true comprehension by the patient and create privacy concerns.[35] Approximately 20% of staff members who try to interpret have insufficient language skills to perform interpreter functions.[36] In the absence of an interpreter, pictures may be used to help close the language barrier.[36] Patients with lower English proficiency report decreased satisfaction with their HCPs.[36] "Title VI of the Civil Rights Act of 1964 requires providers who participate in Medicaid, Medicare, or other federally funded programs to provide language assistance."[37]

Assessment/Analysis
- Patient's language skills and the need for an interpreter upon arrival
- Effect of interpreter use on the patient's length of stay[37]
- Institutional policies and procedures regarding the use of interpreters and available resources

Implementation
- Use certified and trained interpreters whenever possible[37]
- Ask for exact translation[37]
- Place interpreter out of the line of sight of the patient so the patient is speaking directly to the provider[37]
- Speak directly to the patient and watch the patient when the interpreter speaks
- Write down key points and instructions and ask the interpreter to transcribe for the patient[37]
- Check for comprehension by asking the patient to summarize[37]
- Use phone or video interpreters if a person is not available

Evaluation
- Patient satisfaction
- Feedback from staff/providers regarding interpreter availability

HIPAA, Privacy, and Mandatory Reporting. The Health Insurance Portability and Accountability Act (HIPAA) is one of the most widely known and important laws protecting patients' health information. HIPAA establishes standards around the disclosure of an individuals' protected health information (PHI).[37] Practically speaking, in the ED setting, healthcare information is anything about the patient's health or treatment in written, oral, or recorded form, including any identifiable information such as name, social security number, or date of birth.[38] Protecting a patient's privacy is a core duty in emergency nursing. However, factors such as crowding, visitors, department physical layout, and process designs make patient privacy a challenge.[38] ED staff should ask the patient for permission to discuss personal information in front of visitors.[38] Patients presenting with law enforcement officers provide a unique challenge, and where not required by law, the patient should provide consent before speaking in front of law enforcement officers regarding healthcare concerns.[38] Filming and photographing of wounds should also involve patient consent, when not required by law.[38] As devices such as smartphones become more and more prevalent, the ED staff must remain vigilant regarding patient privacy and ensure that photos and videos are not taken that compromise the privacy of other patients in the emergency department.

Some circumstances do require the reporting of protected health information (PHI), but only the minimum necessary information should be disclosed. There are 12 national priorities in which healthcare institutions are allowed to report without consent of the patient, as listed in Table 13-3. Minors

TABLE 13-3 The 12 National Priorities for Which Protected Health Information May Be Disclosed or Used without Written Authorization

1. As required by law (statute, regulation, or court order)
2. For public health reporting (e.g., vital statistics, disease, adverse event reporting)
3. For reporting abuse, neglect, or domestic violence
4. For health oversight activities (e.g., inspections, audits)
5. For judicial and administrative proceedings
6. For law enforcement purposes (e.g., criminal investigations) under certain circumstances
7. For disclosures about deceased persons to medical examiners, coroners, and funeral directors
8. For organ, eye, and tissue donation purposes
9. For some types of research (e.g., in cases where an institutional review board has waived the authorization requirement)
10. To avert a serious threat to the health or safety of the public
11. For specialized government functions, such as military missions or correctional activities
12. For workers' compensation claims

Reproduced with permission from Tintinalli J, Stapczynski J, Ma OJ, et al: Tintinalli's Emergency Medicine: A Comprehensive Study Guide, 8th ed. New York: McGraw-Hill Education; 2015.

may have special considerations. Under EMTALA obligations, all people presenting for care must receive a medical screening exam, so minors may not require parental consent in emergency situations.[38] However, in non-emergent situations, every attempt to contact the minor's guardian(s) should be made and documented.[38] Exceptions to the notification of guardians vary by state, but generally speaking, minors can seek testing and care for sexually transmitted diseases; prenatal and pregnancy-related care; alcohol, substance abuse, and mental health services; or sexual and physical abuse evaluation and treatment without parental consent.[38] Each state will have laws defining the ages for any exceptions.

Assessment/Analysis
- Institutional policy and procedures regarding privacy
- Physical layout of the emergency department and nontraditional bed spaces such as hallways

Implementation
- Develop policies on visitors and access to patients
- Develop policies on what information will be disclosed to outside agencies such as law enforcement and public health
- Design physical layout to avoid accidental overhearing of private health information

Evaluation
- Patient feedback and satisfaction
- Patient and/or staff complaints regarding privacy concerns or breaches

Decision Making and Informed Consent. Shared decision making can improve the patient's perception of care and satisfaction and can also help decrease the reporting of pain after the ED visit.[38] Patients need information about their care to make a reasoned and informed decision.[38] The ED RN will work with the provider to provide such information to patients and answer questions as appropriate. The informed consent process is one of the most frequently occurring examples of decision making in the ED environment. Key elements of informed consent include the diagnosis, nature, and purpose of treatment; risks and consequences to treatment; alternatives with risks and benefits; and prognosis if treatment is or is not accepted.[38] Generally speaking, it is always better to give the patient more, not less, information during the course of treatment.[38] It is also important to allow the patient the opportunity to ask questions and to never attempt to coerce a patient into treatment.[38] If a patient appears uninterested, has no questions, or agrees too easily, reassess the patient for learning or language barriers.[38] Once verbal consent is obtained, it is preferred, for proper record keeping, to have a written consent covering the topics discussed.[38] Some circumstances may not require informed consent, such as during an emergency or with a public health matter.[38] During situations where consent is needed but the patient is unable to provide it, and no emergency exists, ED staff must find a surrogate decision maker such as a spouse, adult child, or relative.[38] Documentation such as an advance directive may determine who the surrogate decision maker is for a patient.[38]

Assessment/Analysis
- Patient's capacity to make decision
- Patient's acuity or condition
- The need for surrogate decision maker
- Patient's understanding of the situation
- Documentation of consent
- Patient's willingness to participate in care

Implementation
- Develop a policy to clearly define informed consent process
- Encourage staff to use principles that involve patients in decisions when applicable or appropriate

Evaluation
- Patient satisfaction
- Audit consent documentation

System

Delegation of Tasks to Assistive Personnel

Delegation of tasks to assistive personnel is one way to maximize nursing resources in a safe and efficient manner. The RN can delegate tasks in order to focus on more complex patient care needs.[39] Each ED RN must be familiar with individual state laws regarding delegation, as well as the organization's policies and procedures. A core principle of delegation is that the RN delegating must provide an assessment of the patient before and after the delegated task to identify what aspects of a task can be delegated and to evaluate the outcome of the delegated task. The RN must be clear in what he or she is delegating and must provide an opportunity for questions to the assistive personnel.

Assessment/Analysis
- Tasks that may be delegated
- Competence and scope of practice of assistive personnel
- Review the stance on delegation for the individual state's board of nursing

Implementation
- Provide clear direction to assistive personnel
- Develop policies to help guide what can and cannot be delegated

Evaluation
- Evaluate delegated task for desired outcome
- Ongoing feedback from nursing and assistive personnel on delegation challenges and barriers

Disaster Management (Preparedness, Mitigation, Response, Recovery)

Disasters follow a cycle of various durations that includes response, recovery, mitigation of risk, prevention, and preparedness. This has come to be known as the disaster life cycle.[40] See Figure 13-5.

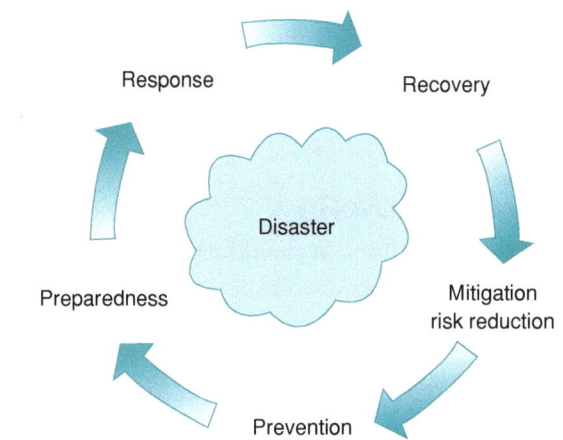

FIGURE 13-5 **The disaster life cycle**
Reproduced with permission from Stone CK, Humphries R: CURRENT Diagnosis & Treatment Emergency Medicine, 7th ed. New York: McGraw-Hill Education; 2011.

Disasters come in many forms, including natural disasters, mass casualty incidents, or internal disasters caused by critical staffing levels or a large water leak in the department's ceiling.[41] Most hospitals do not have disasters; therefore, hospital personnel must plan and drill to learn the hospital's disaster management response plan.[41] TJC requires hospitals have an emergency management plan activated twice a year by drill or actual response, with community involvement required in at least one of the activations.[41]

When a disaster occurs, there are typically two waves of patients seeking care.[41] The first wave is composed of those who self-refer to the ED, or self-extricate from the scene, which typically occurs within 30 to 90 minutes from the disaster event.[41] The second wave of patients is transported by EMS and generally includes higher acuity patients requiring more resources. The second wave typically arrives 60 minutes after the disaster event.[41]

The National Response Framework (NRF), created by the Stafford Act, establishes a structure and process to implement a systematic and coordinated effort of federal assistance during a disaster.[41] The Stafford Act also establishes that the Federal Emergency Management Agency (FEMA) serves as the primary coordinating agency during a disaster and during the recovery phase.[41]

While FEMA coordinates at the federal level, the National Incident Management System (NIMS) establishes and defines how to systematically approach disasters from the local level up to the federal level.[41] Components of NIMS include preparedness, communication and information management, and resource management. The Hospital Incident Command System (HICS) works in conjunction with NIMS to provide standardized approaches to disaster response, including common terminology, modular organization, management by objectives, incident action planning, manageable span of control, incident facilities and locations, comprehensive resource management, establishment and transfer of command, chain and unity of command, accountability, dispatch/deployment, and information and intelligence management.[41] An important factor in mitigating disaster risk is the early detection of symptom clusters. Emergency departments may well be the front door for detection of potential disease outbreaks, bioterrorist events, or mass exposure to harmful elements. Early detection of exposures could greatly reduce morbidity and mortality in the event of a disaster.[41] There are several approaches to surveillance, including case-based identification and environmental or laboratory-based surveillance.[42]

Assessment/Analysis
- Disaster response plan
- The department, hospital, or community hazard vulnerability analysis (HVA)[42]
- Triage protocols during disaster response[43]

Implementation
- Develop a personal and family disaster plan[43]
- Train in the use of personal protective equipment (PPE)[43]
- Train on decontamination techniques[43]
- Develop a disaster drill schedule
- Complete disaster training for ED staff
- Store critical supplies—water, lights, charts

Evaluation
- Review lessons learned from events at other locations
- Debrief disaster drills

Federal Regulations

Emergency Medical Treatment and Active Labor Act (EMTALA). EMTALA is a federal law imposed on hospitals operating emergency departments and birthing units. There are several aspects to EMTALA, but the primary intent of the law is to ensure that any person presenting to the emergency department seeking care has a medical screening exam (MSE) completed by a qualified individual, receives stabilizing treatment, and is transferred appropriately if the facility is unable to meet the needs of the patient.[38] The standards of medical screening, stabilization, and transfer must be completed, regardless of the ability to pay. There are several nuances to the concept of a person presenting to the emergency department. The law further clarifies that EMTALA applies to anyone presenting to the hospital property requesting an evaluation or treatment of a medical condition. Hospital property is further defined as "the physical area immediately adjacent to the provider's main building, other areas and structures not strictly contiguous to main building but are located within 250 yards of the main building."[38] If an ambulance presents to the hospital grounds, EMTALA law also applies. When an ambulance service must wait for extended periods of time to hand off to a busy emergency department, the continuum of care is delayed, posing a potential EMTALA risk.[38]

The hospital must maintain a list of providers on call. On-call specialty providers are obligated to respond to emergent medical conditions and accept transfers from hospitals without the ability to care for a patient in compliance with EMTALA.[38] EMTALA obligations end once a patient is admitted to the hospital, although it does apply for observation-status patients.[38]

Assessment/Analysis
- Patients or potential patients presenting to the hospital property for treatment
- Incidence of diversion of ambulances
- Ambulance intake process for timeliness
- Triage intake practices

Implementation
- Educate staff who may have first contact with patients presenting to the hospital for care
- Develop policies that clearly define the geographical boundaries for the hospital in compliance with EMTALA obligations
- Develop a policy defining who can perform a MSE
- Develop a transfer process with clear documentation of accepting provider and facility

Evaluation
- Audit transfer documents
- Feedback from receiving facilities
- Triage process
- Training and education effectiveness

Performance Improvement

Healthcare delivery is continuously evolving and changing. As such, process improvement (PI) models are used to quickly adapt to ever-changing needs. There are several PI methods available, but some of the more common methods include PDSA (Plan, Do, Study, Act), Lean, and Six Sigma. Regardless of method, the point is to continuously improve to meet the demands of customers, payers, and staff while providing the highest quality care possible. Not all change equates to improvement. For example, if an electronic medical record is introduced, but is not modified to meet the needs of the emergency department, the improvement is insignificant. If an order set is developed applying best practices, but it is not consistently implemented, process improvement is marginalized.[43] However, change, combined with front-line staff input and the use of a proven PI methodology, can result in the improvement of the delivery of care in the emergency department.[44]

Assessment/Analysis
- PI method used across organization
- Educational opportunities to acquire the skills for performance improvement

Implementation
- Adopt a single methodology
- Ensure that all are using the same method and approach[44]

Evaluation
- Results to original plan or hypothesis[44]
- Outcomes reviewed periodically

Emergency Triage

Triage is the practice of sorting patients by acuity upon arrival to the emergency department. A reliable and validated five-level triage system should be used.[44] Emergency nurses complete a specific triage educational program, including a didactic component and an orientation with a nurse experienced in triage.[45] Further, the triage RN should have verified training in BLS, ACLS, ENPC, TNCC, and GENE. Certification in emergency nursing is also recommended.[46] Many other qualities and skills can ensure the success of the ED RN performing triage: the ability to work under extreme stress, to appropriately delegate tasks, and to make rapid and accurate decisions. Strong communication skills, a diverse knowledge base, and strong interpersonal skills will also ensure success.[46]

Assessment/Analysis
- Patient to identify objective and anecdotal findings of primary chief complaint
- RN skill set, training, and experience level

Implementation
- Develop a triage educational program
- Implement a peer review process[46]
- Provide continuing education[46]

Evaluation
- Accuracy of triage acuity designation
- Patient satisfaction
- Review case studies for learning opportunities

Appendix 13

The FOUR TOPICS CHART is one example of an ethical-decision making framework.

The Four Topics Chart

Medical Indications	Preferences of Patients
The Principles of Beneficence and Nonmaleficence 1. What is the patient's medical problem? Is the problem acute? chronic? critical? reversible? emergent? terminal? 2. What are the goals of treatment? 3. In what circumstances are medical treatments not are the probabilities of success of various treatment options? 4. In sum, how can this patient be benefited by medical and nursing care, and how can harm be avoided?	The Principle of Respect for Autonomy 1. Has the patient been informed of benefits and risks of diagnostic and treatment recommendations, understood this information, and given consent? 2. Is the patient mentally capable and legally competent, or is there evidence of incapacity? 3. If mentally capable, what preferences about treatment is the patient stating? 4. If incapacitated, has the patient expressed prior preferences? 5. Who is the appropriate surrogate to make decisions for an incapacitated patient? What standards should govern the surrogate's decisions? 6. Is the patient unwilling or unable to cooperate with medical treatment? If so, why?
Quality of Life	**Contextual Features**
The Principles of Beneficence and Nonmaleficence and Respect for Autonomy 1. What are the prospects, with or without treatment, for a return to normal life and what physical, mental, and social deficits might the patient experience even if treatment succeeds? 2. On what grounds can anyone judge that some quality of life would be undesirable for a patient who cannot make or express such a judgment? 3. Are there biases that might prejudice the provider's evaluation of the patient's quality of life? 4. What ethical issues arise concerning improving or enhancing a patient's quality of life? 5. Do quality-of-life assessments raise any questions that might contribute to a change of treatment plan, such as forgoing life-sustaining treatment? 6. Are there plans to provide pain relief and provide comfort after a decision has been made to forgo life-sustaining interventions? 7. Is medically assisted dying ethically or legally permissible? 8. What is the legal and ethical status of suicide?	The Principles of Justice and Fairness 1. Are there professional, interprofessional, or business interests that might create conflicts of interest in the clinical treatment of patients? 2. Are there parties other than clinician and patient, such as family members, who have a legitimate interest in clinical decisions? 3. What are the limits imposed on patient confidentiality by the legitimate interests of third parties? 4. Are there financial factors that create conflicts of interest in clinical decisions? 5. Are there problems of allocation of resources that affect clinical decisions? 6. Are there religious factors that might influence clinical decisions? 7. What are the legal issues that might affect clinical decisions? 8. Are there considerations of clinical research and medical education that affect clinical decisions? 9. Are there considerations of public health and safety that influence clinical decisions? 10. Does institutional affiliation create conflicts of interest that might influence clinical decisions?

Reproduced with permission from Jonsen AR, Siegler M, Winslade WJ: *Clinical Ethics: A Practical Approach to Ethical Decisions in Clinical Medicine*, 8th edition. New York: McGraw-Hill; 2015.

REFERENCES

1. Pack M. Critical incident stress management: a review of the literature with implications for social work. *Int Social Work* [serial online]. 2013;56(5):608–627.
2. Jonsen AR, Siegler M, Winslade WJ. Introduction. In: Jonsen AR, Siegler M, Winslade W, eds. *Clinical Ethics: A Practical Approach to Ethical Decisions in Clinical Medicine*. 8th ed. New York, NY: McGraw-Hill; 2015.
3. Toren O, Wagner N. Applying an ethical decision-making tool to a nurse management dilemma. *Nurs Ethics* [serial online]. 2010;17(3):393–402.
4. What is Evidence-Based Practice (EBP)? *Duke University Medical Center Library & Archives*. http://guides.mclibrary.duke.edu/c.php?g=158201&p=1036021. Published December 2014. Updated December 8, 2015. Accessed December 12, 2015.
5. Jonsen AR, Siegler M, Winslade WJ. Contextual features. In: Jonsen AR, Siegler M, Winslade WJ, eds. *Clinical Ethics: A Practical Approach to Ethical Decisions in Clinical Medicine*. 8th ed. New York, NY: McGraw-Hill; 2015.
6. Spring B, Persell SD. Evidence-based behavioral practice. In: Feldman MD, Christensen JF, Satterfield JM, eds. *Behavioral Medicine: A Guide for Clinical Practice*. 4th ed. New York, NY: McGraw-Hill; 2014.

7. Aron DC. Chapter 3. Evidence-Based Endocrinology and Clinical Epidemiology. In: Gardner DG, Shoback D, eds. *Greenspan's Basic & Clinical Endocrinology*. 9th ed. New York, NY: McGraw-Hill; 2011.
8. Bush K. Position Statement Review Committee. Safe discharges from the emergency setting position statement. *Emergency Nurses Association Website*. https://www.ena.org/practice-research/Practice/Position/Pages/SafeDischarge.aspx. Published June 2013. Accessed December 12, 2015.
9. Eckerline CA, Brantley JC. Legal aspects of emergency care. In: Stone C, Humphries RL, eds. *CURRENT Diagnosis & Treatment Emergency Medicine*. 7th ed. New York, NY: McGraw-Hill; 2011.
10. Han C, Barnard A, Chapman H. Emergency department nurses' understanding and experiences of implementing discharge planning. *J Adv Nurs* [serial online]. 2009;65(6):1283–1292.
11. Weaver L, Hobgood C. Death notification and advance directives. In: Tintinalli JE, Stapczynski J, Ma O, Yealy DM, Meckler GD, Cline DM, eds. *Tintinalli's Emergency Medicine: A Comprehensive Study Guide*. 8th ed. New York, NY: McGraw-Hill; 2016.
12. Marco CA. Ethical Issues of Resuscitation. In: Tintinalli JE, Stapczynski J, Ma O, Cline DM, Cydulka RK, Meckler GD, eds. *Tintinalli's Emergency Medicine: A Comprehensive Study Guide*. 7th ed. New York, NY: McGraw-Hill; 2011.
13. Clarke R. Improving end-of-life care in emergency departments. *Emerg Nurse* [serial online]. 2008;16(7):34–37.
14. Goshorn EC, Kan JA, Vicario SJ. Basic & advanced cardiac life support. In: Stone C, Humphries RL, eds. *CURRENT Diagnosis & Treatment Emergency Medicine*. 7th ed. New York, NY: McGraw-Hill; 2011.
15. Leske J, McAndrew N, Brasel K. Experiences of families when present during resuscitation in the emergency department after trauma. *J Trauma Nurs* [serial online]. 2013;20(2):77–85.
16. Gurney D. Position Statement Review Committee. Palliative and end-of-life care in the emergency setting position statement. *Emergency Nurses Association Website*. https://www.ena.org/practice-research/Practice/Position/Pages/PalliativeEndOfLifeCare.aspx. Published 2002. Updated September 2013. Accessed December 13, 2015.
17. Zalenski RJ, Zimny E. Palliative care. In: Tintinalli JE, Stapczynski J, Ma O, Yealy DM, Meckler GD, Cline DM, eds. *Tintinalli's Emergency Medicine: A Comprehensive Study Guide*. 8th ed. New York, NY: McGraw-Hill; 2016.
18. Fowler DR. Chapter e263.2. Forensics. In: Tintinalli JE, Stapczynski J, Ma O, Cline DM, Cydulka RK, Meckler GD, eds. *Tintinalli's Emergency Medicine: A Comprehensive Study Guide*. 7th ed. New York, NY: McGraw-Hill; 2011.
19. Forensic evidence collection position statement. *Emergency Nurses Association Website*. https://www.ena.org/practice-research/Practice/Position/Pages/ForensicEvidence.aspx. Published 1998. Revised July 2010. Accessed December 13, 2015.
20. Masteller M, Prahlow A, Walsh M, Thomas S, Wolfenbarger R, Prahlow J. Proper handling of bullet evidence in trauma patients. *Trauma* [serial online]. 2014;16(3):189–194.
21. Ducharme J. Acute pain management in adults. In: Tintinalli JE, Stapczynski J, Ma O, Cline DM, Cydulka RK, Meckler GD, eds. *Tintinalli's Emergency Medicine: A Comprehensive Study Guide*. 7th ed. New York, NY: McGraw-Hill; 2011.
22. Colvin C. Procedural sedation and analgesia. In: Stone C, Humphries RL, eds. *CURRENT Diagnosis & Treatment Emergency Medicine*. 7th ed. New York, NY: McGraw-Hill; 2011.
23. Jacques K, Dewar A, Gray A, Kerslake D, Leal A, Open M. Procedural sedation and analgesia in the emergency department. *Trauma* [serial online]. 2015;17(3):166–174.
24. Wachter RM. Basic principles of patient safety. In: Wachter RM, ed. *Understanding Patient Safety*. 2nd ed. New York, NY: McGraw-Hill; 2012.
25. Patient safety in emergency health care archived position statement. *Emergency Nurses Association Website*. https://www.ena.org/SiteCollectionDocuments/Position%20Statements/Archived/PatientSafety.pdf. Published 2005. Revised December 2010. Archived July 2015. Accessed December 15, 2015.
26. Baker S. *Excellence in the Emergency Department: How to Get Results*. Gulf Breeze, FL: Fire Starter Publishing; 2009.
27. Smith CD, Weinberger SE. Barriers to providing high-value care. In: Moriates C, Arora V, Shah N, eds. *Understanding Value-Based Healthcare*. New York, NY: McGraw-Hill; 2015.
28. Bongale S, Young I. Why people complain after attending emergency departments. *Emerg Nurse* [serial online]. 2013;21(6):26–30.
29. Mechem C. Emergency medical services. In: Tintinalli JE, Stapczynski J, Ma O, Yealy DM, Meckler GD, Cline DM, eds. *Tintinalli's Emergency Medicine: A Comprehensive Study Guide*. 8th ed. New York, NY: McGraw-Hill; 2016.
30. Wachter RM. Transition and handoff errors. In: Wachter RM, ed. *Understanding Patient Safety*. 2nd ed. New York, NY: McGraw-Hill; 2012.
31. Beaulieu P, Position Statement Review Committee. Holding, crowding, and patient flow position statement. *Emergency Nurses Association Website*. https://www.ena.org/practice-research/Practice/Position/Pages/Holding.aspx. Published May 2014. Updated July 2014. Accessed December 21, 2015.
32. Hodgins M, Moore N, Legere L. Full house: the incidence and impact of boarding admitted patients in the emergency department. *NENA Outlook* [serial online]. 2010;33(1):13–15.
33. Viccellio P, Zito J, Singer A, et al. Patients overwhelmingly prefer inpatient boarding to emergency department boarding. *J Emerg Med* [serial online]. 2013;45(6):942–946.
34. Rabin E, Kocher K, Weber E, et al. Solutions to emergency department "boarding" and crowding are underused and may need to be legislated. *Health Affairs* [serial online]. 2012;31(8):1757–1766.
35. Lie D, Liao SS. Cultural sensitivity training. In: McKean SC, Ross JJ, Dressler DD, Brotman DJ, Ginsberg JS, eds. *Principles and Practice of Hospital Medicine*. New York, NY: McGraw-Hill; 2012.
36. Iserson KV. Communications. In: Iserson KV, ed. *Improvised Medicine: Providing Care in Extreme Environments*. New York, NY: McGraw-Hill; 2012.
37. Fortin AH VI, Dwamena FC, Frankel RM, Smith RC. Adapting the interview to different situations and other practical issues. In: Fortin AH VI, Dwamena FC, Frankel RM, Smith RC, eds. *Smith's Patient-Centered Interviewing: An Evidence-Based Method*. 3rd ed. New York, NY: McGraw-Hill; 2012.
38. Siff JE. Legal issues in emergency medicine. In: Tintinalli JE, Stapczynski J, Ma O, Yealy DM, Meckler GD, Cline DM, eds. *Tintinalli's Emergency Medicine: A Comprehensive Study Guide*. 8th ed. New York, NY: McGraw-Hill; 2016.
39. Isaacs C, Kistler C, Platts-Mills T, et al. Shared decision-making in the selection of outpatient analgesics for older individuals in the emergency department. *J Am Geriatr Soc* [serial online]. 2013;61(5):793–798.
40. Delegation. ANA and National Council of State Boards of Nursing Joint Position Statement. *American Nurses Association Website*. http://www.nursingworld.org/MainMenuCategories/Policy-Advocacy/Positions-and-Resolutions/ANAPositionStatements/Position-Statements-Alphabetically/Joint-Statement-on-Delegation-American-Nurses-Association-ANA-and-National-Council-of-State-Boards.html. Published 2005. Accessed December 22, 2015.
41. Starr GA, Allen TW, Stewart CE. Disaster medicine. In: Stone C, Humphries RL, eds. *CURRENT Diagnosis & Treatment Emergency Medicine*. 7th ed. New York, NY: McGraw-Hill; 2011.
42. Grey MR, Spaeth KR. Surveillance systems and bioterrorism. In: Grey MR, Spaeth KR, eds. *The Bioterrorism Sourcebook*. New York, NY: McGraw-Hill; 2006.
43. Emergency management and preparedness for all-hazards position statement. *Emergency Nurses Association Website*. https://www.ena.org/practice-research/Practice/Position/Pages/AllHazards.aspx. Published June 2008. Updated February 2012. Accessed December 23, 2015.
44. King ES, Myers JS. Principles and models of quality improvement: plan-do-study-act. In: McKean SC, Ross JJ, Dressler DD, Brotman DJ, Ginsberg JS, eds. *Principles and Practice of Hospital Medicine*. New York, NY: McGraw-Hill; 2012.
45. Standardized ED triage scale and acuity categorization: joint ENA/ACEP position statement. *Emergency Nurses Association Website*. https://www.ena.org/SiteCollectionDocuments/Position%20Statements/Joint/StandardizedEDTriageScaleandAcuityCategorization.pdf. Accessed December 27, 2015.
46. Triage qualifications position statement. *Emergency Nurses Association Website*. https://www.ena.org/practice-research/Practice/Position/Pages/TriageQualifications.aspx. Published 2010. Updated February 2011. Accessed December 27, 2015.

Practice Questions

Question	Rationale
1. While debriefing a pediatric code, you notice the primary RN is not contributing to the conversation. When asked if she'd like to let the group know how she feels about the case, she declines. The most appropriate response is to let her know 　a. This is a safe place to share 　b. Everyone is required to share during a debrief 　c. You are available if she'd like to talk later 　d. The group would like to hear her perspective	*Answer: c* No one should be forced to share during a debriefing after a stressful event. Telling the staff member the debrief is a safe place, stating it is required to share, or telling her the group would like to hear her perspective can all be viewed as pressuring someone to share who is not ready to do so yet.
2. There are several tools available for ethical decision making. One option is 　a. The Four Topics Chart 　b. Google it 　c. Maslow's Hierarchy 　d. Stakeholder Analysis	*Answer: a* The Four Topics chart is a tool known to help individuals or teams make difficult ethical decisions. Using a common search engine such as Google does not often provide evidence-based answers. All stakeholders should be involved in the decision, but a stakeholder analysis does not provide answers to ethical dilemmas. Maslow's Hierarchy is not a relevant decision-making tool for ethical dilemmas.
3. Which of the following elements are *not* part of evidence-based practice (EBP)? 　a. Personal experience 　b. Research studies 　c. Patient perception 　d. The experience of a colleague in a similar situation	*Answer: c* Patient perception. Enhancing patient perception or experience may be a reason to use evidence-based practice, but it is not an element of EBP. Personal experience, the experience of those around you, and research studies are all a part of EBP.
4. To advance the emergency nurse's learning, all are good sources of information *except* 　a. Social media 　b. *Journal of Emergency Nursing* (JEN) 　c. Emergency Nursing Association Website 　d. The nurse educator for your department	*Answer: a* Social media is not a valid source of information and often contains misinformation or invalid studies. The JEN, ENA website, and the nurse educator are all trusted sources of information.
5. Research is often broken down into which of the following structures? 　a. Introduction, Method, Background, Discussion, and Conclusion 　b. Introduction, Background, Interpretation, and Conclusion 　c. Abstract, Background, Discussion, Interpretation, and Conclusion 　d. Introduction, Abstract, Goals, Background, and Conclusion	*Answer: a* Research studies are broken down into the Introduction to describe what the study is about, the Method to describe how the study was conducted, the Background to describe the population of the study, the Discussion to analyze the results, and the Conclusion to discuss the findings.

Question	Rationale
6. A provider prints discharge instructions. Which element *must* be completed prior to discharging the patient? a. Vital signs b. Medical screening exam (MSE) c. Co-pay is collected d. A review of the patient's labs	*Answer: b* The medical screening exam is required to discharge a patient to meet EMTALA obligations. Vital signs, the collection of a co-pay, and the review of the patient's labs are all elements of the discharge process, but not mandated or required to discharge a patient.
7. A 94-year-old man with terminal lung cancer and advanced dementia presents to the emergency department via ambulance. He requires emergent rapid sequence intubation. During the handoff, the EMT states that he believes the patient is a DNR patient. The team should a. Provide comfort measures to the patient b. Intubate the patient c. Start attempting to call the patient's power of attorney (POA) to clarify code status d. Ask the patient if he'd like to be intubated	*Answer: b* If a patient requires lifesaving intervention and the code status is unclear, the team should proceed with the measure until clarification can be made. The emergency nurse should not use information the EMT "believes" until information can be verified.
8. During a resuscitation code, the spouse of the patient is standing in the corner of the room crying. You should a. Ask the spouse to leave to not cause further psychological trauma b. Assign a team member to stand with her to explain what's going on c. Continue with the code as if the spouse isn't present d. Ask the spouse to leave, so she doesn't disrupt the team members involved in the code	*Answer: b* Evidence supports that family presence has been shown to be helpful to the family during a resuscitation. Opposing views such as psychological trauma or team member disruption are not shown to be valid concerns. Of course, each situation must be assessed, but generally speaking, family presence is encouraged. Assigning a liaison to help the family understand what's going on has been shown to improve the family experience.
9. A patient arrives after sustaining a gunshot wound. What should the RN do with the clothing the patient was wearing? a. Place them in a patient belongings bag and put them in a safe place b. Throw them away because they're soiled with excessive amounts of blood c. Place them in the approved collection bag/ device for evidence d. Leave them in place for the police to decide what to do	*Answer: c* Evidence collection is an important part of ED nursing. Placing the clothing in a bag, if it is not an approved bag or device, can affect the chain of custody and the evidence on the clothing. Throwing them away may result in the loss of evidence, and leaving them on is not a likely option while treating the patient.

Question	Rationale
10. What is the most common reason for seeking care in the emergency department? a. Sutures b. Behavioral health complaints c. Rash d. Pain	*Answer: d* Pain is the most common reason for ED visits. Although suture placement, behavioral health, and rash are all common reasons for an ED visit, they are not the most common.
11. During the course of a procedural sedation, a patient's respiratory rate drops to 10 breaths/minute. The nurse should a. Stop the procedure b. Assess the patient's vital signs and capnography values c. Do nothing. A decreased respiratory rate is normal during sedation d. Reposition the patient's airway to ensure patency	*Answer: b* A decreased respiratory rate requires an assessment of the patient and his ventilation status. The procedure should not be stopped if the patient is tolerating a respiratory rate of 10. A respiratory rate of 10 is slightly below normal and should not be ignored. If an obstructed airway is suspected, repositioning the patient's airway is not likely to help increase the respiratory rate.
12. You had labs drawn last week for a routine physical. You work in the same system where you had the labs drawn. While at work, you decide to obtain your results a. It is OK to look in the electronic medical record (EMR) for the results because they're your labs, therefore not a HIPAA concern b. You should go to medical records and sign a release of information to obtain your labs c. You should ask a co-worker to print them for you, which is OK because you gave her verbal consent d. You should get permission from your manager to look up your labs	*Answer: b* Any time you are accessing medical records without a clinical reason to do so, you are at risk for violating HIPAA laws. You should not go into your own records without proper authority to do so. Asking a co-worker to do it is only placing her at risk, and your verbal consent is not valid. Your manager's permission does not release information in the appropriate manner required for accessing medical records.
13. The disaster life cycle is a. Response, Recovery, Mitigation of Risk, Prevention, and Preparedness b. React, Recover, Evaluate, and Prepare c. React, Triage, Coordinate, Treat, and Recover d. Response, Triage, Prevent, and Prepare	*Answer: a* The disaster life cycle is Response, Recovery, Mitigation of Risk, Prevention, and Preparedness.
14. A patient collapses in the ED parking lot and appears to be in acute distress. The parking lot is located 75 yards from the ED entrance. The triage RN should a. Call 911 to pick up the patient b. Bring the patient in for stabilization treatment c. Do nothing since the patient is outside d. Call security to determine what is going on out there	*Answer: b* The patient is on hospital property and within 250 yards of the entrance; therefore EMTALA law applies to this patient. There is no need to call 911, as the patient is close enough for staff to respond. Although you may request security to come with you, they are not the appropriate personnel to respond to a clinical situation.

Question	Rationale
15. The primary purpose of triage is to a. Ensure the patient is properly registered with his legal name b. Get patients to a physician immediately c. Prioritize patients needing immediate treatment over those who can wait d. Assess the patient to determine resources needed when he is placed in a room	*Answer: c* The primary purpose of triage is to sort the patients to determine who will see the provider first. Registration, the assigning of an acuity level, and assessing the patient are all elements of triage, but the primary purpose is to appropriately sort the patients.
16. Generally, documentation requirements for a patient being discharged from the emergency department to return to home at a skilled nursing facility include a. Discharge instructions including results from medical screening exam b. Discharge instructions and EMTALA transfer process c. Discharge instructions and updating the medical power of attorney d. Discharge instructions and EMS transport documentation	*Answer: a* The hospital should provide documentation validating the results of the patient's medical screening exam, a requirement of the EMTALA law. Discharge instructions meet this requirement. Emergency departments or hospitals may have agreements in place to use an EMTALA transfer process returning the patient to a skilled nursing facility similar to an interhospital transfer, though those agreements are local or state specific in nature. While updating the medical POA and providing transport documentation may be appropriate for some patients, they would generally not be required, unless part of a broader local agreement.
17. An adult patient who is the suspected victim of domestic abuse is being treated in your emergency department. You know you are required to a. Make a mandatory report to your state agency b. Call the local law enforcement agency for patient protection c. Allow the patient to determine reporting plan d. Flag the patient's chart for care management follow-up	*Answer: c* An adult patient who does not also qualify as a "vulnerable" patient, such as frail elderly or developmentally disabled, may chose to report abuse and may also choose *not* to report abuse. An emergency nurse reporting the situation to law enforcement or other state agency could be violating the patient's privacy rights, as protected by HIPAA laws. Care management may not be needed for this patient.
18. A patient is being treated in the emergency department for a Jimson weed exposure. Upon arrival, ED staff called the poison control center help line. Three hours later, the poison control center calls for an update. To comply with HIPAA laws, the nurse a. Cannot release any information b. Can share information about the overdose c. Should ask the charge nurse what to do d. Should have the provider speak with the poison control center	*Answer: b* When initially called about the patient's case, the poison control center became a consultant on the case and is thereby part of the patient's treatment team. Therefore, HIPAA laws provide for sharing relevant information with the poison control center. Statements regarding HIPAA and consultants, such as poison control centers, can be found in 45 CFR (Code of Federal Regulations) 164.501 under the heading of Treatment. For more information, conduct an Internet search using the search terms "*45 CFR 164.501.*" The other answer options are not correct.

Answer Page for 150 Question CEN Prep Quiz

1.	2.	3.	4.	5.
6.	7.	8.	9.	10.
11.	12.	13.	14.	15.
16.	17.	18.	19.	20.
21.	22.	23.	24.	25.
26.	27.	28.	29.	30.
31.	32.	33.	34.	35.
36.	37.	38.	39.	40.
41.	42.	43.	44.	45.
46.	47.	48.	49.	50.
51.	52.	53.	54.	55.
56.	57.	58.	59.	60.
61.	62.	63.	64.	65.
66.	67.	68.	69.	70.
71.	72.	73.	74.	75.
76.	77.	78.	79.	80.
81.	82.	83.	84.	85.
86.	87.	88.	89.	90.
91.	92.	93.	94.	95.
96.	97.	98.	99.	100.
101.	102.	103.	104.	105.
106.	107.	108.	109.	110.
111.	112.	113.	114.	115.
116.	117.	118.	119.	120.
121.	122.	123.	124.	125.
126.	127.	128.	129.	130.
131.	132.	133.	134.	135.
136.	137.	138.	139.	140.
141.	142.	143.	144.	145.
146.	147.	148.	149.	150.

Randomized 150 Question CEN Prep Quiz

Question	Rationale
1. A patient enters the emergency department complaining of a racing heart, palpitations, and shortness of breath with an onset 30 minutes prior to arrival. The nurse places the patient on the cardiac monitor and notes that the heart rate is 190 bpm. What cardiac rhythm would the nurse expect to see? a. Normal sinus rhythm b. Sinus tachycardia c. Supraventricular tachycardia d. Ventricular fibrillation	*Answer: c* Supraventricular tachycardia is defined as a heart rate greater than 150, narrow complex, and regular rhythm. The signs and symptoms correlate with supraventricular tachycardia. Sinus tachycardia is a heart rate between 100 to 150. Normal sinus rhythm is a heart rate between 60 to 100. Ventricular fibrillation has no heart rate and the patient would be unresponsive.
2. A 34-year-old male being treated for an acute asthma exacerbation is showing improvement after treatment. However, he is tachycardic and complaining of dry mouth. His pupils appear dilated. This is likely a side effect of a. Albuterol b. Prednisone c. Magnesium sulfate d. Atropine sulfate	*Answer: d* Atropine sulfate is an anticholinergic, a parasympatholytic causing dilated pupils, decreased salivation, and tachycardia. Anticholinergics also dilate the bronchi and stimulate the release of epinephrine and norepinpherine, which is why medications such as atropine may beneficial in reactive airway diseases. Albuterol is a β_2 adrenergic agonist, a sympathomimetic that causes skeletal muscle tremors, anxiety, tachycardia, headache, palpitations, and hypertension. Prednisone can cause hyperglycemia, and magnesium sulfate can cause irregular heartbeat, hypotension, or muscle weakness.
3. A patient presents to the emergency department with a primary concern of suicidal ideation. He has attempted suicide four times before, overdosing on medications each time. Which of the following statements is *not* true? a. It is important to realize someone who has overdosed four times in the past is at decreased risk for suicide b. Suicidal "contracts" made with patients have not been shown to decrease suicide c. Firearms are used in the United States more than any other means to die by suicide d. Mental illness is a risk factor which is important to consider	*Answer: a* A past history of suicide attempts is a strong indicator of future suicidal risk. Although suicide contracts are still sometimes used, there is a lack of evidence to support the efficacy of contracts and contracts are not considered legally binding documents. Always consider the individual in front of you and their risk factors. Firearms should always be considered when assessing an individual for suicide. Access to lethal means has been shown to be an important factor which is modifiable. Firearms should be removed and access should be restricted if an individual expresses suicidal ideation. Any mental illness diagnosis should be considered a risk factor for suicide. Both bipolar disorder and depression are two of the most common mental illnesses increasing suicide risk.

Question	Rationale
4. A patient complains of chest pain unrelieved with rest. The ECG shows T wave inversion, but no elevation in his Troponin level. Based on the signs and symptoms, the patient is most likely experiencing? a. Stable angina b. Unstable angina c. Non-STEMI d. STEMI	*Answer: b* Unstable angina is defined as continued chest pain remaining after cessation of activity or chest pain relieved by nitroglycerin and without elevation in cardiac enzymes. Stable angina is characterized by chest pain relieved with cessation of the activity. Non-STEMI is defined as chest pain often with T wave inversion and/or ST segment depression and elevation in the cardiac enzymes. STEMI is characterized by chest pain with ST elevation and elevation in the cardiac enzymes.
5. A patient arrives with a splint to his upper extremity. He reports 10/10 pain despite analgesia administration and burning sensation to his arm. The most likely cause of his unrelieved pain is a. A torn ligament b. A history of narcotic dependency c. Compartment syndrome d. Blood loss	*Answer: c* Pain out of proportion to the injury which is not relieved by usual measures is a cardinal sign of compartment syndrome. Torn ligaments do not generally cause consistent, unrelieved pain, especially if they have been appropriately immobilized. Blood loss would not necessarily cause an increase in pain. Although the patient may have a history of narcotic dependency, he also has a fracture and all organic causes of his symptoms should be evaluated before this diagnosis is made.
6. A 28-year-old male patient is being discharged from the emergency department following a diagnosis of epididymitis. The ED nurse knows the patient understands his discharge instructions when he makes the following statement a. I may not ever be able to have kids b. I need to wear support, like a jock strap, when I am up walking c. I can keep running in preparation for the marathon I'm in next month d. My antibiotic is only needed if the pain doesn't get better	*Answer: b* Epididymitis can be from a sexually transmitted infection. Other causes can be from urological procedures such as a cystoscopy. Pain is a hallmark of the illness, and elevating and supporting the penis especially during physical activity decreases the pain. Often, the patient may be advised not to resume vigorous physical activity until they have followed up with their primary care physician or urologist. Infertility typically is not related to epididymitis. Antibiotics may be prescribed if a STD is suspected, and the patient should complete the entire course of antibiotics.
7. A patient experiences point tenderness at McBurney's point during an abdominal assessment. What other findings may coincide with this symptom? a. History of chronic intermittent pain b. Hematochezia c. Elevated WBC d. Pain radiates to the right shoulder	*Answer: c* McBurney's point is located midway between the umbilicus and the anterior superior iliac crest in the RLQ. If point tenderness is localized at this point, it may be an indication of an acute appendicitis. An elevated WBC, in the presence of other suspecting symptoms, has a greater diagnostic value for appendicitis. Acute pain is associated with appendicitis. The risk of perforation increases if symptoms are present more than 48 hours. Hematochezia is bright red or maroon rectal bleeding and is suggestive of a lower GI bleeding or a massive upper GI bleed. Pain radiating to the right shoulder can be symptomatic for acute cholecystitis

Question	Rationale

8. The emergency nurse knows the patient understands discharge homecare instructions for treatment and monitoring of a small (<10%) pneumothorax when the patient states
   a. "I'm glad I can go home; I am flying to Hawaii in two days"
   b. "I'm glad I can keep practicing my snorkeling in the local pool"
   c. "I need to come back in two days to have a tube placed in the side of my chest"
   d. "If I cut back on my smoking, this will never happen again"
	Answer: b
	Patients discharged with a small pneumothorax should be counseled not to fly or dive but surface snorkeling will be safe as long as the patient is warned not to free dive while snorkeling. The patient would only require chest tube if the pneumothorax increases in size and the patient starts having symptoms of shortness of breath. Smoking will increase risk but reduction will not eliminate risk of recurrence.

9. A patient with respiratory distress is placed on capnography. The following wave forms would be anticipated with COPD?
   a. Flat and extended
   b. Tall and narrow
   c. "Shark fin" shaped
   d. Curved
	Answer: c
	Patients with COPD and asthma exacerbations will have a wave form that appear like a "shark fin" as the CO_2 is slow to escape during exhalation due to alveolar trapping. This waveform usually correlates with a higher CO_2 level. ABG assessment is a good correlation tool with capnography. A flat and wider waveform may indicate little ventilation and perfusion occurring (lower CO_2 level). Other abnormal waveforms require assessing the patient's breathing pattern, rate, and depth of respirations. If the patient is mechanically ventilated or receiving supplemental oxygen, assuring that the tubing and circuitry are connected and working properly.

10. You are working the evening shift and are concerned several of the patients in the emergency department currently are at risk for violence. You know the patient with the highest risk for violence is
   a. An 88-year-old male who is confused and is using a loud voice to get his point across
   b. A 40-year-old woman coming in on the ambulance who has been violent in the ambulance
   c. A 24-year-old male who is intoxicated and has a laceration to his foot
   d. A 23-year-old patient with a diagnosis of schizophrenia who has hallucinations
	Answer: b
	Although each of these patients present with risk factors, the best predictor of violent behavior is a history of violent behavior. The woman who is violent in the ambulance has demonstrated recent violence and is at the highest risk. The 88-year-old male demonstrates risks of being male, confusion, and using a loud voice, which may indicate an escalation of behaviors. An intoxicated male in his twenties demonstrates a risk for violence related to the intoxication and being male. A patient with schizophrenia who has hallucinations may be at risk if the hallucinations are causing paranoia. In this case, we do not know the content of the hallucinations.

Question	Rationale

11. A patient is being treated in the emergency department for a Jimson weed exposure. Upon arrival, ED staff called the poison control center help line. Three hours later, the poison control center calls for an update. To comply with HIPAA laws, the nurse
  a. Cannot release any information
  b. Can share information about the overdose
  c. Should ask the charge nurse what to do
  d. Should have the provider speak with the poison control center
	Answer: b
	When initially called about the patient's case, the poison control center became a consultant on the case and is thereby part of the patient's treatment team. Therefore, HIPAA laws provide for sharing relevant information with the poison control center. Statements regarding HIPAA and consultants, such as poison control centers, can be found in 45 CFR (Code of Federal Regulations) 164.501 under the heading of Treatment. For more information, conduct an Internet search using the search terms "*45 CFR 164.501*." The other answer options are not correct.

12. Afterload is increased by
  a. Increased preload
  b. Decreased preload
  c. Increased systemic vascular resistance
  d. Decreased systemic vascular resistance
	Answer: c
	Afterload is the amount of "load" or resistance that the heart must beat against to generate a cardiac output, like trying to open a door against the wind. The resistance to the blood flow within the systemic circulation is referred to as systemic vascular resistance (SVR). SVR is increased in conditions such as vasoconstriction and aortic valve stenosis. SVR is decreased in vasodilation. Many antihypertensives decrease SVR.
	    Preload is the filling pressures of the atria and ventricles at end diastole. Preload is influenced by many variables such as circulating blood volume and myocardial contractility.

13. The most common presentation for a patient with bipolar in a manic state is
  a. Suicidal ideation
  b. Depressed mood and irritability
  c. Elevated mood and psychomotor agitation
  d. Both depressed mood and elevated mood
	Answer: c
	Patients who are experiencing a bipolar manic state often present with an elevated mood frequently accompanied by irritability and psychomotor agitation. Bipolar disorder does convey an increased risk for suicide but the risk is greater during the depressive episodes of bipolar. Episodes of bipolar include mania or hypomania and depression. In the manic state, someone would not have a depressed mood.

14. A patient presents to the emergency department with hypertension, left side weakness, and an inability to speak. The patient appears frustrated and anxious but is able to follow commands. The emergency nurse understands the patient has likely had a stroke in what area of the brain?
  a. Huntington's area: Located in the left Parietal lobe
  b. Cushing's area: Located in the right Limbic lobe
  c. Broca's area: Located in the dominant frontal lobe
  d. Wernicke's area: Located in the right temporal lobe
	Answer: c
	Interruption of blood flow to Broca's area affects the motor component of speech. The patient is able to understand and follow commands so the patient can still processes speech. Inability to understand commands would indicate a receptive aphasia secondary to damage in Wernicke's area. Huntington and Cushing's area do not exist as anatomical features of the brain.

Question	Rationale
15. A 45-year-old man arrives by EMS after being "accidently" stabbed in the chest by his girlfriend an hour earlier. Upon arrival, he is restless and complains of shortness of breath. He is on a non-rebreather mask with high flow oxygen. Vital signs are T-97.4°F (36.3°C); P-116; R-32; BP-82/56; SpO_2-81%. Decreased breath sounds are auscultated on the left side and a stat chest x-ray confirms a tension pneumothorax. What intervention should occur next? a. A needle thoracostomy b. Obtain a type and crossmatch lab c. A chest tube placement d. Prepare for surgery	*Answer: a* Immediate decompression of tension pneumothorax is a top priority with the goal of restoring adequate ventilation and perfusion to the lungs. Chest tube placement is the definitive treatment, after decompression to relieve the trapped air. Depending on the amount of internal blood loss and patient symptoms, blood products may be needed after his airway and breathing are stabilized. Surgical intervention may be required following his trauma resuscitation.
16. An adult patient who is the suspected victim of domestic abuse is being treated in your emergency department. You know you are required to a. Make a mandatory report to your state agency b. Call the local law enforcement agency for patient protection c. Allow the patient to determine reporting plan d. Flag the patient's chart for care management follow-up	*Answer: c* An adult patient who does not also qualify as a "vulnerable" patient, such as frail elderly or developmentally disabled, may chose to report abuse and may also choose *not* to report abuse. An emergency nurse reporting the situation to law enforcement or other state agency could be violating the patient's privacy rights, as protected by HIPAA laws. Care management may not be needed for this patient.
17. A patient is brought into the emergency department by EMS. EMS states the patient's car was hit on the driver's side by another vehicle. The patient's head shattered the side window and there is a laceration on the left side of the skull. EMS states the patient was unconscious at the scene but was alert and talking on the way in. He complained of a severe headache and had weakened grips on the right side. Upon arrival, however, the patient has again lost consciousness and has a left fixed and dilated pupil. The ED nurse suspects the patient has a. A subdural bleed b. An epidural bleed c. A diffuse axonal injury d. A concussion	*Answer: b* Epidural bleeds are associated with trauma and often have a lucid period prior to rapid deterioration. Because the bleeding is arterial, usually from the middle meningeal artery, with a hematoma developing between the skull and tough covering of the brain. Injury side pupil dilation and opposite side motor weakness is consistent with this type of injury.

Question	Rationale
18. A 41-year-old male patient presents to the emergency department after an exposure to an organophosphate insecticide. After decontamination, he is experiencing profuse salivation and is urinating and defecating frequently. The emergency nurse anticipates which medication will be ordered? a. An antiemetic and antidiarrheal medication b. IV atropine c. IV atropine and IV pralidoxime (2-PAM) d. Epinephrine and diphenhydramine	*Answer: c* Atropine and pralidoxime (2-PAM) are the agents used to treat an organophosphate exposure. Atropine works by reducing symptoms (SLUDGE) while pralidoxime (2-PAM) works by binding the organophosphate, which is considered curative. IV atropine alone will not eliminate the organophosphate from the nerve synapse; it will only reduce the symptoms of SLUDGE. Epinephrine and diphenhydramine are not indicated, and antiemetics and antidiarrheals are not priority for this patient.
19. A patient arrives to the emergency department with complaints of chest pain. On assessment, a pericardial friction rub and diffuse ST elevations are noted. The patient is most likely experiencing what condition? a. Pericarditis b. Non-STEMI c. STEMI d. Pericardial tamponade	*Answer: a* Pericarditis is an inflammation of the pericardial lining. Classic signs and symptoms include pain relieved when leaning forward, pericardial friction rub, and diffuse ST elevations. Non-STEMI signs and symptoms include ST depression or T wave inversions with elevation in cardiac enzymes. STEMI signs and symptoms include ST elevation in two or more leads, without the presence of a pericardial friction rub. Pericardial tamponade is an accumulation of fluid, pus, or blood in the pericardial sac compressing the heart preventing full myocardial expansion. The patient will have muffled heart sounds instead of a pericardial friction rub.
20. Which of the following would not be an indicator of potential abuse? a. Elderly dementia patient with patterned bruising b. Toddler who has bruising in various stages of healing c. Husband refuses to let the nurse interview his wife alone d. Stories of a child's injuries change	*Answer: b* Patients who have patterned bruising, especially in the shape of objects, should be investigated for abuse. Care providers who refuse to allow the patient to be interviewed alone may raise suspicion of abuse. When stories are inconsistent or if the descriptions of the events do not match the injury, the nurse should discuss these findings with his or her team and report as local laws mandate. It is not unusual for toddlers at the cruising age to have bruising from falls.
21. One key characteristic of panic attacks which is often most difficult for patients is a. Embarrassment over the attacks b. Fear of recurrent attacks c. Associated nausea d. That they are not taken seriously	*Answer: b* Panic attacks are associated with a fear of reoccurrence. This fear may be debilitating to patients. The panic attacks may be associated with a wide range of physiological systems and sometimes social impact such as embarrassment. Panic attacks are often taken seriously due to the associated physical symptomology.

Question	Rationale
22. The emergency nurse encounters a patient who has a hydrofluoric acid exposure to the right hand and fingers. The emergency nurse recognizes hydrofluoric acid as an acid leading to what type of emergency? a. Full-thickness chemical burn blistering b. Bradycardia c. Anaphylaxis d. Bone damage and severe pain	*Answer: d* Hydrofluoric acid easily passes through the skin and exchanges its fluoride ion with calcium. This causes bone destruction and severe pain as a result. Generally, hydrofluoric acid does not cause a significant skin burn, although it might create erythema in the area. The application of calcium (i.e., calcium gluconate gel) to the skin acts to withdraw the hydrofluoric acid from the tissue, which spares bone destruction. Blistering is not typically seen with hydrofluoric acid exposure. Anaphylaxis and bradycardia are not common with hydrofluoric acid exposure.
23. A 38-year-old male presents to the emergency department complaining of weakness and numbness of the lower extremities. He had a fever with "the flu" a few weeks ago, but no other medical history. He states the numbness started in his feet but has now progressed to the level of his hips and he is so weak he can barely stand. Exam shows depressed deep tendon reflexes and symmetrical weakness of the lower extremities. The ED nurse anticipates this patient will need a. Admission to the ICU on an insulin infusion b. Ultrasound cardiovascular exam of bilateral lower extremities for arterial occlusion c. Lumbar puncture to rule out meningitis d. Admission to the ICU and mechanical ventilation	*Answer: d* Ascending symmetrical weakness and numbness with loss of deep tendon reflexes indicates Guillain-Barré Syndrome. One quarter of all patients with Guillain-Barre require mechanical ventilation due to respiratory failure as the syndrome progresses to breathing muscles. The patient's history does not suggest he has hyperglycemia and would need an insulin infusion. He is not exhibiting signs of arterial occlusion in the lower extremities or signs associated with meningitis.
24. An adult patient involved in a car fire enters the emergency department. Once stabilized, the emergency nurse determines that the patient has burns to the anterior chest, left anterior arm, and right posterior leg. Using the rule of nines, the emergency nurse estimates the total surface burn area as a. 18% b. 27% c. 32% d. 36%	*Answer: c* Using the rule of nines, the anterior chest scores at 18%, the anterior and posterior arms are each 4.5%, and the anterior and posterior legs count for 9% each. The total surface area for the patient described above is 31.5% and has been rounded to 32%.
25. Upon entering a room with a patient complaining of a headache, the patient is found to be pacing the room and refusing to lie on the bed. The patient complains of sharp pain behind the right eye. The right eye is swollen and drooping with tear production noted. What medication is considered to be most effective for this type of headache? a. Hydromorphone IV with a Normal Saline bolus b. Proparacaine drops to the affected eye c. High flow oxygen through a non-rebreather mask d. Compazine™/Benadryl™/Toradol™ combination	*Answer: c* The unilateral pain behind the right eye, inability to sit still, and agitation are indicative of a cluster headache. High flow oxygen is the preferred treatment for cluster headaches. Compazine™/Benadryl™/Toradol™ combination is the treatment for a migraine headache, which involve bilateral pain, nausea, and photophobia. Opioids are not usually the first line treatment for suspected cluster headaches, and proparacaine eye drops would not be indicated.

Question	Rationale
26. A 45-year-old female patient enters into the emergency department with complaints of intermittent chest pain that has happened at rest, during sleep, and with exercise. The patient was diagnosed with Prinzmetal's angina. What question should the nurse ask the patient? a. Do you smoke cigarettes? b. How long have you been exercising? c. Do you have any respiratory conditions? d. Does cold exposure relieve the chest pain?	*Answer: a* Cigarette smoking causes vasoconstriction which can cause vasospasm of the coronary arteries. The length of time exercising and any respiratory conditions does not directly address the causes of Prinzmetal's angina. Cold exposure causes vasoconstriction and would worsen rather than relieve the chest pain.
27. The emergency nurse suspects central retinal artery occlusion due to what assessment finding? a. Sudden painless vision loss b. Visual field curtain c. Sudden onset of extreme unilateral eye pain d. Intraocular pressures of 25 mm Hg	*Answer: a* A unique characteristic of central retinal artery occlusion is sudden painless vision loss. Visual field curtain is common in retinal detachment. Sudden extreme unilateral eye pain is most likely to be related to glaucoma. Intraocular pressures of 25 mm Hg is a slightly elevated result and may be related to one of several causes, including uveitis, early glaucoma, or eye trauma.
28. While palpating the abdomen of a patient, the emergency nurse observes rebound tenderness. Rebound tenderness raises the possibility for all of the conditions *except* a. Appendicitis b. A perforated colon c. Constipation d. Cholecystitis	*Answer: c* Although rebound tenderness does not have 100% sensitivity for appendicitis, peritonitis (a perforated colon) or cystitis, patients presenting with any of these conditions may have rebound tenderness noted during physical assessment. Some of the common symptoms associated with constipation are abdominal discomfort, bloating, and straining during bowel evacuation.
29. A 17-year-old male patient is being discharged from the emergency department. He had presented with abdominal pain in his right and left lower quadrants. Besides mild nausea and some tenderness with palpation in his lower abdomen, he has no other symptoms. His CBC, ultrasound, and CT scan results were negative for any findings. The ED nurse's discharge instructions should include a. Avoid greasy foods and consider an over-the-counter proton pump inhibitor, such as Omeprazole b. Increase your fiber intake and drink 6 to 8 glasses of water per day to relieve your constipation c. If symptoms continue or new ones develop, rest and follow-up with your primary care provider in 3 days d. If pain persists and/or worsens or a fever or vomiting appear, return to the emergency department	*Answer: d* This patient did not appear acutely ill; however, his symptoms could be in the early stage for appendicitis or small bowel obstruction. Given his age, there is a greater likelihood for an early appendicitis that could progress. Discharge instructions, both written and verbal, should emphasize returning for medical care should an acute infectious process, such as appendicitis, evolve. Avoiding greasy foods is encouraged if cholelithiasis is suspected. The patient does not report a history of colicky RUQ abdominal pain suggesting gallstones. Proton pump inhibitors are typically prescribed when a patient has a history of gastroesophageal reflux disease (GERD) or ulcer. Although increasing fiber and water intake is healthy, his symptoms and imaging results do not suggest constipation. The risk of a perforated appendix is likely with symptoms lasting more than 2 days. Waiting 3 days to follow-up with one's primary care provider, for new or continued symptoms, is too long of a wait with possible appendicitis.

Question	Rationale
30. A seven-month old girl is brought into the emergency department by her mother. The mother states the little girl was fine at daycare today, but tonight she found the toddler "jerking her arms and legs with her eyes rolled back in her head." The child is warm to the touch with a rectal temp of 100.9°F (38.3°C), rhinorrhea, and tachycardia. Otherwise the child has clear lung sounds and appears well hydrated. The ED nurse reassures the patient's mother by telling her a. There was nothing the mother could do to prevent the illness b. Two-thirds of patients will never experience a second episode c. Anti-seizure medications are very effective these days d. A CT scan is non-invasive and will reveal any brain damage	*Answer: b* The patient is presenting with a febrile seizure. CT scans and anti-seizure medications are not appropriate for this patient since febrile seizures rarely cause permanent damage to the brain, and often do not recur.
31. A 45-year-old male patient presents to triage complaining of sudden onset of big toe pain. On inspection, the triage nurse notes a red, hot, and swollen great toe. Patient denies trauma. The triage nurse suspects the patient has a. Gout b. Bursitis c. Foot fracture d. Achilles tendon rupture	*Answer: a* Gout. An initial episode of gout is often characterized by spontaneous, intense pain with edema at the metatarsophalangeal joint. Bursitis is often the result of overuse or infection and the common sites are shoulder, elbow, hip, knee, and heel of the foot. Foot fracture is improbable without trauma. Achilles tendon rupture is characterized by heel pain radiating up the back of the leg with difficulty or inability to move the foot.
32. The emergency nurse is assessing a person bitten on the left hand by a rattlesnake. The nurse identifies two fang marks on the hand with some minor edema and bleeding. The patient complains of minor pain, and vital signs are within normal limits. Upon reassessment an hour later, the emergency nurse finds no change in the patient's assessment. This can best be explained by which phenomenon? a. This patient is immune to snake venom b. A "dry bite" that did not involve envenomation c. Not enough time has passed for the snake venom to cause symptoms d. The patient was not bitten by a snake	*Answer: b* Dry bites occur in approximately 20% of pit viper snakebites. Dry bites are characterized by the presence of fang marks without symptoms of envenomation such as pain, edema, or systemic changes such as vital sign abnormalities. It is possible that this patient was not bitten by a snake. The emergency nurse must take a careful history to determine the accuracy of the patient's description of the snake and if in fact it is poisonous.

Question	Rationale
33. A patient presents with a maculopapular rash on his trunk, fever, fatigue, and diarrhea. He states, he is an IV drug user sex worker. What is the likely cause of his symptoms? a. Measles b. MRSA c. HIV d. Herpes Zoster virus	*Answer: c* Given his history and symptoms, he likely has primary HIV infection. MRSA and measles have similar rashes however, the history is highly suspicious for HIV. Herpes Zoster rash has vesicles. This patient should be tested and provided counseling on follow up community resources. He should also be counseled and provided with measures for safe sex practices as well as needle exchange information.
34. When assessing a patient's history to analyze risk factors for epistaxis, the nurse would want to inquire about a. Recent travel b. Family history of heart disease c. Herbal Supplements d. Diet restrictions	*Answer: c* Specific herbal supplements such as ginseng contain anticoagulation properties that can increase the risk for epistaxis. Although the nurse may collect history about the patient's recent travel locations, dietary restrictions, and family history of heart disease, these are not associated risk factors for epistaxis.
35. Patient teaching for patients with COPD should include all of the following *except* a. Encourage adequate fluid intake b. Limit the use of antihistamines, antitussives, and decongestants c. Avoid exercise as it may exacerbate symptoms d. Encourage small, frequent meals	*Answer: c* It is important to encourage exercise as it helps to increase energy and decrease shortness of breath. COPD patients should drink plenty of fluids to help thin secretions; limit the use of medications that have a dehydrating effect; and eat small meals frequently to minimize abdominal distension that can reduce lung capacity.
36. A young professional woman has delayed pregnancy until timing is more appropriate with her lifestyle. She had a positive pregnancy test at 9 weeks gestation and has seen the nurse practitioner in her obstetrician's office for her first prenatal visit at 11 weeks gestation. She is currently 12 4/7 weeks gestation and is having spotting of bright red bleeding. Terrified that something is going wrong with the pregnancy, she comes to your ED. She has no pain with the bleeding but did have some menstrual like cramping earlier that has gone away. FHT are 135 bpm. After checking her cervix, it is closed. There is a small amount of darker blood in her vagina but no active bleeding is seen. Patient is suspected of having a. Threatened abortion b. Inevitable abortion c. Missed abortion d. Complete abortion	*Answer: a* Threatened abortion: cervix remains closed; inevitable abortion: cervix dilates to 3 cm; missed abortion: no bleeding or cramping are present; complete abortion: some bleeding, mild contractions and product of conception is passed and cervical os is closed. You may confuse the somewhat similar symptoms of threatened abortion and complete abortion but this patient still has FHTs.

Question	Rationale
37. A 68-year-old arrives via EMS with complaints of shortness of breath. Symptoms started about 3 hours prior to arrival. According to the patient's wife, he had flu-like symptoms for the past three days. He has no other significant past medical history. Upon arrival, he is on oxygen at 4 liters via nasal cannula. Vital signs are T-96.2°F (35.7°C); P-98; R-24; BP-110/62; SpO$_2$-93% on room air. According to his presentation, what condition would the nurse suspect? a. Pulmonary embolism (PE) b. Sepsis c. ARDS d. DIC	*Answer: b* This patient has a suspected infection, and sepsis is often diagnosed in the presence of a suspected or actual infection along with some of the following signs and symptoms: some of the diagnostic criteria of fever greater than 38.3°C. (100.9°F.), or hypothermia (core temperature less than 36.0°C or 96.8°F), heart rate greater than 90 per minute, tachypnea, altered mental status, significant edema, hyperglycemia (glucose >140 mg/dL in the absence of diabetes). Although pulmonary embolism could be a possible diagnosis for this patient, none of the known risk factors are listed upon arrival such as recent surgery, history of blood clots, or DVT. Adult respiratory distress syndrome (ARDS) usually follows an acute illness or injury and results in extreme shortness of breath as the lungs become less compliant. Disseminated intravascular coagulation (DIC) is a coagulopathy involving systematic circulation and a rapid consumption of clotting factors.
38. Ventricular tachycardia commonly leads to what rhythm? a. Third degree heart block b. Pulseless electrical activity (PEA) c. Supraventricular tachycardia d. Ventricular fibrillation	*Answer: d* Ventricular tachycardia commonly leads to ventricular fibrillation. Ventricular tachycardia does not commonly lead to third degree heart block, pulseless electrical activity (PEA), and supraventricular tachycardia.
39. The priority in the assessment of a patient with homicidal ideation is a. Ensuring the individual that they are targeting is informed b. Assessing for immediate danger c. Developing a plan to ensure the patient and others are safe d. Calling the police to inform them of the risk	*Answer: b* During the assessment phase, the nurse should ensure immediate safety is ensured. The other answers represent appropriate interventions which do not represent the priority.
40. The emergency nurse is discharging an otherwise healthy 75-year-old male patient diagnosed with cystitis. He is prescribed Bactrim™ and Pyridium™. All of the following statements demonstrate his understanding of his discharge instructions *except* a. "I need to drink at least 8 glass of water a day" b. "I need to take all of my Bactrim as it is prescribed" c. "If my urine turns a rusty orange color I should come back here" d. "I need to follow up with my doctor next week"	*Answer: c* Pyridium™ may be prescribed for dysuria and urinary frequency and can turn the urine orange or a reddish orange color. Patients should be informed of this and not to be alarmed if they observe this. Increasing oral fluid intake and completing the prescribed antibiotic are essential teaching points for the patient to understand. Follow-up with their primary care physician may be prescribed if the infection's etiology may need further study.

Question	Rationale

41. The most common site for anterior epistaxis is the
  a. Sphenopalatine arteries
  b. Submental region
  c. Sphenoid sinus region
  d. Kiesselbach's plexus
	Answer: d
	The sphenopalatine artery is often the source for a posterior bleed with epistaxis. Posterior epistaxis is less common, about 10 to 15% of all incidences but has a greater risk for bleeding and/or airway complications. The submental area is the area below the chin and is commonly an area where Ludwig's angina can extend. The sphenoid sinus is located at the base of the skull and the top of the pharynx.

42. A patient with a history of T6 cord injury presents with a headache, high blood pressure, nasal congestion, and appears flushed and diaphoretic. The first action would be to
  a. Start two large bore IVs and initiate a fluid bolus
  b. Give IV Mannitol 0.9 mg/kg with 10% of the total dose as a bolus followed by an infusion of the rest over the next 60 minutes
  c. Check the patient's indwelling urinary catheter for kinks
  d. Obtain a 12 lead ECG
	Answer: c
	This patient appears to be suffering from autonomic dysreflexia, a dangerous complication of spinal cord injuries that can be triggered by something as simple as a distended bladder. Of the given answers, unkinking the catheter tubing is the only intervention that would remove a stimulus that could trigger autonomic dysreflexia.

43. The emergency nurse knows discharge teaching was effective when a patient with gout reports
  a. "Alcohol doesn't affect my risk for gout attacks"
  b. "Weight reduction will increase my gout attacks"
  c. "I should drink plenty of water to reduce my risk of gout attacks"
  d. "I should eat more purine-rich foods to prevent uric acid build up"
	Answer: c
	Drinking plenty of water is linked to fewer gout attacks. Alcohol metabolism is thought to increase uric acid production and contributes to dehydrating thus increasing your risk of a gout attack. Weight loss helps reduce the risk of frequent gout attacks. Patients with gout should avoid meats such as liver, kidney and sweetbreads, which have high purine levels and contribute to high blood levels of uric acid.

44. A patient with extreme anxiety and hyperventilation has the following ABG values
pH 7.48, CO_2 27, HCO_3 25. These values show
  a. Compensated respiratory acidosis
  b. Uncompensated respiratory acidosis
  c. Compensated respiratory alkalosis
  d. Uncompensated respiratory alkalosis
	Answer: d
	The patient has an elevated pH and a decreased CO_2, which indicates respiratory alkalosis. The HCO_3 is within normal range, so the body is not compensating.

Question	Rationale
45. A 53-year-old patient presents to the emergency department by ambulance with a chief complaint of nausea and dizziness with headache. EMS started an IV and gave a 500 mL normal saline bolus and 4 mg of Zofran™ prior to arrival. Vital signs are P-70; R-20; BP-169/59, SPO$_2$ 99% on room air. The patient states his main complaint is his headache, which has been going on for a few days but is now much worse. He also states he's been "bumping into things, lately and I might need my glasses checked." Eyes are reactive, but the left pupil is 2 mm larger than the right. On exam the ED nurse notes no unilateral deficits. The priority is to a. Obtain labs, ECG, and a full set of vitals b. Notify the emergency provider with anticipating an order for a stat non-contrast head CT c. Obtain a visual acuity exam and collect a detailed medical history d. Apply high flow oxygen via non-rebreather mask	*Answer: b* This patient has symptoms of a posterior stroke, which can often be missed because they do not present with unilateral weakness. Headache with nausea and visual disturbance coupled with the difference in pupil size (anisocoria) should raise the nurse's concern of a cerebrovascular accident. Other options such as obtaining labs and a visual acuity exam are not the priorities for this. High flow oxygen is treatment for cluster headaches.
46. A patient complains of chest pain, dyspnea, and dizziness for two hours prior to arrival. The patient is placed on the cardiac monitor. The patient's heart rate is 30 and the ECG shows asynchronous but regular P-to-P and R-to-R intervals. The patient is experiencing which of the following dysrhythmias? a. Normal sinus rhythm with first degree AV block b. Second degree AV block type 1 c. Second degree AV block type 2 d. Third degree heart block	*Answer: d* The patient symptoms of chest pain, dyspnea, and dizziness combined with the ECG findings indicate a third degree heart block. Normal sinus rhythm with first degree AV block is a prolonged PR interval and the heart rate is 60 to 100. The second degree AV block type 1 has a PR interval that varies with a QRS segment being dropped. The second degree AV block type 2 PR interval is not prolonged, but the QRS segment is dropped.
47. A patient complaining of dry, itchy eyes and difficulty removing contact lenses placed 2 days ago is best treated by a. Gentle suction using a manufactured contact lens removal device b. Antibiotic drops to treat corneal abrasions c. Measurement of intraocular pressures d. Gentle flushing of the eyes	*Answer: d* Gentle flushing of an eye dry from extended contact wear is intended to rehydrate tissue and the contact lens. The purpose is not to remove the lens by forceful flushing, but rather to hydrate the tissue and lens to the point that typical removal is possible. A commercial device may cause damage to the eye needing hydration. Antibiotics and ocular pressures are not indicated.

Question	Rationale
48. Generally, documentation requirements for a patient being discharged from the emergency department to return to home at a skilled nursing facility include a. Discharge instructions including results from medical screening exam b. Discharge instructions and EMTALA transfer process c. Discharge instructions and updating the medical power of attorney d. Discharge instructions and EMS transport documentation	*Answer: a* The hospital should provide documentation validating the results of the patient's medical screening exam, a requirement of the EMTALA law. Discharge instructions meet this requirement. Emergency departments or hospitals may have agreements in place to use an EMTALA transfer process returning the patient to a skilled nursing facility similar to an interhospital transfer, though those agreements are local or state specific in nature. While updating the medical POA and providing transport documentation may be appropriate for some patients, they would generally not be required, unless part of a broader local agreement.
49. A 17-year-old male presents to the emergency department with complaints of weakness. He is tachypneic, tachycardia, and hypotensive. A glucometer check in the waiting room reveals a glucose reading of 406. The triage nurse anticipates which immediate action? a. Transport to ED treatment area b. Assess airway c. Establish IV d. Administer insulin	*Answer: b* This patient is presenting with symptoms of hypovolemic shock, possibly a nonhemorrhagic origin such as DKA. Although he would need all of the above interventions, a patent airway is the top priority.
50. A patient presents to the ER through triage with a headache. She was seen at urgent care 6 days ago for a sinus infection but now reports "I thought I was all better, but suddenly tonight it is much worse." The patient is febrile at 103.6°F (39.8°C) and complains of a stiff neck, which is a very painful to move. The triage nurse prioritizes which interventions for this patient? a. IV access, labs, and blood cultures followed by antibiotics b. Lumbar puncture and head CT scan, followed by antibiotics c. Head CT scan, followed by LP and antibiotics only after CT results d. Lumbar puncture, head CT scan with antibiotics after LP results	*Answer: a* The question asks the nurse to prioritize interventions for a patient with suspected bacterial meningitis. Initiation of antibiotics in these patients should not be delayed while waiting for neuroimaging or LP results. Head CT would be performed prior to lumbar puncture to rule out the risk of herniation secondary to a space-occupying lesion.
51. A patient arrives in the emergency department after being involved in a motor vehicle crash (MVC). The patient struck the steering wheel with her chest. The patient is diagnosed with blunt chest trauma and pericardial effusion and then becomes unresponsive and hypotensive. What is the priority intervention? a. Continue to monitor the patient b. Pericardiocentesis c. Administer Dopamine intravenously d. Needle-chest decompression	*Answer: b* The patient is unstable and needs immediate intervention such as a pericardiocentesis. If the RN simply continues to monitor the patient, the patient will become worse. Administering Dopamine intravenously may be needed, but it is not the priority intervention. The patient is not displaying signs or symptoms related to tension pneumothorax in which needle-chest decompression would be the recommended intervention.

Question	Rationale

52. A patient with angioedema related to smoke inhalation has the following ABG values
pH 7.35, CO_2 53, HCO_3 28. These values show
  a. Compensated respiratory acidosis
  b. Uncompensated respiratory acidosis
  c. Compensated respiratory alkalosis
  d. Uncompensated respiratory alkalosis
	Answer: a
	The patient has a pH on the low end of normal with an elevated CO_2, indicating respiratory acidosis. The elevated HCO_3 indicates the body is compensating, otherwise the pH would be even lower. It is helpful to remember that CO_2 is an acid and HCO_3 is an alkaline. The body uses these to balance the pH. If the CO_2 gets to high or the HCO_3 is too low, the pH drops. If the CO_2 gets too low or the HCO_3 gets too high, the pH increases.

53. A patient has just been in a traumatic MVC in which a passenger is killed. The patient does not appear injured, but is visibly distressed. The emergency nurse enters the room and understands the patient may have all of the following characteristics of a situational crisis *except*
  a. The nurse may need to take control of the situation
  b. Reactions can differ based on individuals
  c. Culture can often play a role in the way someone responds to situational crisis
  d. People with preexisting mental health diagnosis react better to crisis situations
	Answer: d
	Patient with mental illness often present with increased reactions to situational crisis. During a situational crisis, a nurse may need to take control to ensure safety of the individual. Reactions to situational crisis can vary based on past experiences, mental health, culture, and an individual's coping mechanisms.

54. Damage control resuscitation for traumatic hypovolemic shock focuses on preventing all of the following complications *except*
  a. Infection
  b. Blood loss
  c. Coagulopathy
  d. Metabolic acidosis
	Answer: a
	Damage control resuscitation does not prevent infection. Infection control measures include hand hygiene and aseptic technique. Administering combined blood products to replenish clotting factors and blood volume and maintaining adequate perfusion are part of damage control resuscitation interventions.

55. While shopping, Jane notices a dull headache beginning. Jane is 35 weeks pregnancy and has noticed additional swelling and heartburn over the past two weeks. Upon arrival to the emergency department, Jane begins to have a seizure. The nurse knows to expect what treatment to be ordered
  a. Oxytocin
  b. D_{50}
  c. Magnesium sulfate
  d. Phenytoin
	Answer: c
	In a pregnant patient experiencing seizures, preeclampsia should be suspected. Magnesium sulfate reduces seizure activity through an unknown mechanism, but has been shown to be more effective than other seizure medications, such as phenytoin. Oxytocin and D_{50} are not indicated at this time.

Question	Rationale
56. Which of the following findings indicate a patient with an asthma exacerbation is not improving? a. Peak flow levels are 75% of predicted b. Lung sounds are diminished throughout and without wheezing c. There is audible end expiratory wheezing noted d. SpO$_2$ measurements have improved	*Answer: b* Lack of wheezing with diminished breath sounds indicates severe obstruction of air flow and requires immediate intervention. Evaluations that show improvement of symptoms include an improved peak flow greater than 70% of predicted, improvement of SpO$_2$ measurements, and a transition from wheezing on inspiration and expiration to end expiration only.
57. A 65-year-old patient presents to the emergency department with a new onset of psychosis. He has no history of mental illness per his and his wife's report. The nurse begins the assessment. All of the following statements are true *except* a. This is unlikely a new onset of mental illness b. Toxicology screen would be important to assess c. Sudden cessation of alcohol use could be a factor d. Medication such as steroids could be a factor	*Answer: a* It would be unlikely this presentation would be a new onset of mental illness. If the patient has a history of mental illness, this could be causing the psychosis. Toxicology and medication review could reveal a cause for the psychosis. Cessation of alcohol use could lead to alcohol withdrawal which can present with psychosis.
58. The primary purpose of triage is to a. Ensure the patient is properly registered with his legal name b. Get patients to a physician immediately c. Prioritize patients needing immediate treatment over those who can wait d. Assess the patient to determine resources needed when he is placed in a room	*Answer: c* The primary purpose of triage is to sort the patients to determine who will see the provider first. Registration, the assigning of an acuity level, and assessing the patient are all elements of triage, but the primary purpose is to appropriately sort the patients.
59. How does a periapical abscess differ from a periodontal abscess? a. The periapical abscess involves a minimum of two or more dental caries b. The periapical abscess extends beyond the bone c. The periapical abscess may occur around a healthy tooth d. The periapical abscess can occur in the absence of a dental caries	*Answer: b* A periapical abscess involves the dentin, and can extend down into the pulp and nerve roots. Typically, the periapical abscess arises from untreated dental caries. A periodontal abscess occurs when a pocket can form around the tooth creating a reservoir for bacteria and/or other pathogens. The tooth may remain healthy, but the gum tissue around it is inflamed and becomes infected causing a periodontal abscess.
60. A patient reports that while playing racquetball he felt a pop followed by severe pain radiating from his heel to the back of his leg and an inability to walk. The emergency nurse should further assess for signs of a. Ankle sprain b. Calcaneus fracture c. Achilles tendon rupture d. Deep vein thrombosis	*Answer: c* Achilles tendon rupture is common in stop-start sports like racquetball and can cause pain from the heel into the leg and an inability to ambulate. Calcaneus fracture and ankle sprains do not include. Pain radiating into the back of the leg with a "pop." Deep vein thrombosis does not have an acute onset (pop) with pain radiating from the heel to the leg and does not significantly affect a patient's ability to walk.

Question	Rationale
61. A critically injured trauma patient arrives in the emergency department following ejection from the car that he was driving. He was unresponsive, hypotensive, and intubated at the scene. During transport via medical helicopter, he received 2 units of crystalloids, 2 units of packed red blood cells, 1 unit of fresh frozen plasma, and Tranexamic Acid (TXA) IV. Current vital signs are T-97.8°F (36.6°C); P-128; R-16 (assisted); BP-80/48. The emergency nurse anticipates the one of the following lab tests is needed for guiding blood product administration a. Hematocrit and hemoglobin b. INR c. Thromboelastography d. Platelet count	*Answer: c* Thromboelastography (TEG) provides a visual graphic about the clotting process. The graphic provides information about specific clotting factors that are deficient and can guide administration of blood components. The other lab tests do not provide complete information about any coagulopathy.
62. A patient has a history of hypertension and hyperlipidemia and states that he developed sudden onset of upper back pain with dyspnea. The patient's blood pressure was 160/80 upon arrival with a heart rate of 104. A contrast CT scan was completed and an ascending aortic aneurysm was noted. What is the first priority to be completed for this patient? a. Administer intravenous fluids b. Administer an antihypertensive c. Administer a beta-blocker d. Administer analgesics	*Answer: b* To prevent aortic dissection, it is important to decrease the blood pressure keeping the systolic between 100 to 120 mm Hg. Adding intravenous fluids would further increase the vascular volume and increase the blood pressure. Administering a beta-blocker to reduce myocardial contractility and analgesics for the pain are necessary, but they are not the first priority.
63. Environmental factors contributing to reducing the risk for violence include all of the following *except* a. Use of metal detectors b. Training for staff in de-escalation techniques c. Rooms free of potential weapons d. Limiting access for non-patients	*Answer: b* The training of staff in de-escalation would not be considered an environmental factor reducing the risk for violence. It is important to keep rooms free of items that could be used as weapons and to maintain an easy exit at all times.
64. The ED nurse knows to anticipate transfer to the OR for the following patient injury a. Puncture wound to the hand b. Paint gun injection to the hand c. Ligament tear in the knee d. Stage 1 pressure ulcer	*Answer: b* High-pressure injuries such as paint gun injections are serious, and immediate surgical intervention is required to drain the paint or oil and to preserve tissue. A simple laceration generally requires nonsurgical wound closure. A ligament tear in the knee may ultimately require surgery but would not require emergency surgery. Stage 1 pressure ulcers require monitoring but not surgical treatment.

Question	Rationale
65. A patient recently underwent a pericardiocentesis. What sign or symptom would indicate the procedure was unsuccessful? a. Narrowing pulse pressure b. Increased blood pressure c. Heart rate of 75 d. Increase in urine output	*Answer: a* A narrowed pulse pressure indicates poor heart function such as an unsuccessful pericardiocentesis. Signs and symptoms of cardiac tamponade include hypotension, muffled heart tones, and jugular vein distention. An increase in blood pressure and urine output indicates a successful procedure because there is an increase in blood flow to the heart, kidneys, and the rest of the body. Typically, patients with cardiac tamponade will have a rapid heartbeat greater than 100 bpm to compensate for the hypotension.
66. The acronym SLUDGE as seen in insecticide and organophosphate exposures stands for a. Salivation, Lacrimation, Urination, Defecation, Gastrointestinal distress, and Emesis b. Salivation, Lacrimation, Urination, Gastrointestinal distress, and Elimination c. Salivation, Liquidation, Urination, Defecation, Gastrointestinal distress, and Emesis d. Salivation, Lacrimation, Urination, Defecation, Gastritis, and Erection	*Answer: a* The acronym SLUDGE references the words Salivation, Lacrimation, Urination, Defecation, Gastrointestinal distress, and Emesis. These are common symptoms of an exposure to an organophosphate insecticide.
67. A 41-year-old female patient presents to the emergency department with a suspected infection. The patient develops fever, tachycardia, rigors and hypotension. Her vital signs are T-102.6°F (39.2°C); P-118; R-20; BP-84/52; SpO_2-92% on room air. The following lab test is a sensitive marker for decreased tissue perfusion? a. Procalcitonin b. INR c. Lactate level d. ABG	*Answer: c* When a patient with a suspected or known infection develops sepsis with possible deterioration to septic shock, a serum lactate is a sensitive indicator for tissue hypoxia. The INR or international normalized ratio measures the clotting ability of varied clotting factors. Although procalcitonin is a marker of an inflammatory response, the lack of non-specificity minimizes the useful utility in identifying sepsis and septic shock. An ABG may not be immediately indicated as this patient is not in severe respiratory distress, and the patient has a pulse oximetry of 92% on room air.
68. A patient presents with urticarial rash, angioedema, and hoarse voice after consuming crab cakes. His airway is patent; what is the priority of care? a. Administer 0.01 mL/kg epinephrine (1 mg/mL concentration) IM to max dose of 0.5 mg b. Administer H1/H2 blockers c. Administer corticosteroid d. Administer oral Diphenhydramine	*Answer: a* The patient is displaying symptoms of anaphylaxis. Once airway patency is established immediate administration of epinephrine is the first priority. Epinephrine in the 1 mg/mL should primarily be given via intramuscular or subcutaneous routes for patient safety. The patient should be instructed to avoid shellfish in the future and to carry an *epinephrine* auto-injector for future reactions. The other options would be the next interventions.

Question	Rationale
69. You enter the room of a 2-year-old child who arrived in cardiac arrest after being hit by a car. Trauma resuscitation efforts are discontinued 90 minutes later and the child is pronounced dead. The grieving parents remain with their child. One of the most important nursing interventions is a. Assist with funeral arrangements b. Remind them the death was not their fault c. Call the Coroner/Medical Examiner and organ donation service d. Support their bereavement and provide a quiet calm area for them	*Answer: d* The ED nurse often encounters situational crises that occur suddenly and are often catastrophic. The nurse's role is to support the individual or family's coping. Allowing open communication and providing a calm atmosphere can encourage their grieving. Funeral arrangements can be made later. Suggesting fault should not be assigned may be perceived that someone is to blame. Notifying other agencies may be required, but can be delegated or prioritized once the family is provided immediate support.
70. Following discharge instructions for a patient with Uveitis, the emergency nurse knows instructions are understood when the patient says a. "I'll just go home and read a book" b. "I'll rest and catch up on my favorite TV show" c. "I'll just go relax on the beach" d. "It's going to be hard to stay away from my computer"	*Answer: d* Treatment for uveitis includes eye rest in dark environments. Eye rest includes time away from television and other "screens" and reading so verbalization of the need to reduce computer usage indicates understanding. Reading and watching TV creates stress on the eye and time at the beach increases exposure to bright lights.
71. A patient collapses in the ED parking lot and appears to be in acute distress. The parking lot is located 75 yards from the ED entrance. The triage RN should a. Call 911 to pick up the patient b. Bring the patient in for stabilization treatment c. Do nothing since the patient is outside d. Call security to determine what is going on out there	*Answer: b* The patient is on hospital property and within 250 yards of the entrance; therefore EMTALA law applies to this patient. There is no need to call 911, as the patient is close enough for staff to respond. Although you may request security to come with you, they are not the appropriate personnel to respond to a clinical situation.
72. What should be done expediently in intubated patients to prevent aspiration? a. Obtaining a chest x-ray b. Elevating the head of the bed c. Gastric tube placement d. Providing IV sedation	*Answer: c* Gastric tube placement should be performed immediately following endotracheal intubation to decompress the stomach and reduce the risk of aspiration. A chest X-ray is helpful in confirming tube placement, but will not reduce the risk of aspiration. Elevating the head of the bed is helpful to reduce aspiration and ventilator-associated pneumonia (VAP), but can be performed prior to intubation. Sedating intubated patients helps to reduce the risk of dislodgement and discomfort to the patient.
73. A female patient presents to the emergency department with severe diarrhea, fatigue, and weight loss. The emergency nurse performs a history and assessment. Which historical finding suggests the patient may have giardiasis? a. Patient works in a meat processing plant b. Patient traveled to New Mexico recently c. Patient works in a day care center d. Patient is a vegan	*Answer: c* Giardiasis is a parasitic disease causing severe diarrhea, fatigue, fever, and weight loss. Those traveling outside the United States, day care workers, children, and individuals with poor dietary habits are most at risk for ingesting the giardiasis parasite.

Question	Rationale
74. A patient suffered severe abdominal and chest wall trauma. During the initial assessment, abdominal sounds are auscultated in the lower left chest. The nurse suspects the patient has a. A ruptured diaphragm b. A tension pneumothorax c. A flail chest d. Hyper-resonant abdominal sounds	*Answer: a* A ruptured diaphragm is more likely to occur on the left side of the chest as there are not solid organs (such as the liver) to protect it from blunt or penetrating force. When this occurs, the intestines herniate into the chest cavity, displacing the lungs. Therefore, abdominal sounds may be heard. This phenomenon will not occur with a tension pneumothorax or flail chest.
75. Eye drops are administered into the a. Lacrimal sac b. Conjunctival sac c. Cornea d. Canal of Schlemm	*Answer: b* Eye drops are administered into the conjunctival sac by using the index finger to place gentle traction under the eye OR using the index finger and thumb to gently pinch the tissue under the eye to create a pocket between the lower eyelid and the sclera of the globe. Lacrimal sac, cornea, and canal of Schlemm are other anatomical structures of the eye.
76. A 45-year-old man arrives by EMS after being stabbed in the chest an hour earlier. Upon arrival, he is restless and complains of shortness of breath. He is on a non-rebreather mask with high flow oxygen. Vital signs are T-97.4°F (36.3°C); P-116; R-32; BP-82/56; SpO_2-81%. Diminished breath sounds are auscultated on his left side and tracheal deviation is noted toward his right side. What type of injury and shock are suspected? a. Pericardial tamponade (obstructive shock) b. Pericardial tamponade (distributive shock) c. Tension pneumothorax (obstructive shock) d. Tension pneumothorax (distributive shock)	*Answer: c* Obstructive shock is a classification of shock when blood flow is decreased. The hypoperfusion is caused by a pathological obstruction as seen with a tension pneumothorax, pericardial tamponade and pulmonary embolus.
77. The emergency nurse is caring for a patient contaminated with gamma radiation particles. The emergency nurse understands what principle for ensuring healthcare team safety by minimizing exposure? a. Gamma radiation has little or no risk with exposure b. Decontamination will keep the nurse and staff safe c. Distance and shielding from the patient d. Time, distance, and shielding	*Answer: d* The principle of time, distance, and shielding is the preferred method to minimize exposure to ionizing radiation. By minimizing time near the source of radiation, the amount of ionizing radiation absorbed is reduced. Distance from a source of ionizing radiation also minimizes exposure. The use of shielding such as lead aprons and thyroid shields can provide the most benefit. Respiratory protection is also warranted in order to prevent inhalation of a radioactive substance.

Question	Rationale
78. A patient recently brought to the emergency department is demonstrating a clinical picture of cardiogenic shock following an acute MI. The ED nurse anticipates observing all of the following signs with this patient *except* 　a. Elevated brain natriuretic peptide (BNP) 　b. S3 heart sound 　c. Bradycardia 　d. Hepatomegaly	*Answer: c* With cardiogenic shock, tachycardia usually is part of the clinical picture as the heart attempts to increase cardiac output and tissue perfusion. One of the hallmarks of cardiogenic shock is heart failure and the signs and symptoms that accompany this. An elevated BNP, S3 heart sound and hepatomegaly are all indicative of heart failure.
79. Four patients arrive at the front desk of the emergency department. Which patient should the RN assess first? 　a. 68-year-old male with chest pain, diaphoresis, pale skin, and vomiting 　b. 18-year-old male with chest pain worse upon movement and deep breathing 　c. 45-year-old female with abdominal pain, vomiting, and diarrhea 　d. 53-year-old female with pleuritic chest pain, productive cough, and dyspnea	*Answer: a* The symptoms of the 68-year-old male with chest pain, diaphoresis, and vomiting could indicate he is having an acute myocardial infarction and would be the first patient for the RN assesses. The 53-year-old female with pleuritic chest pain, productive cough, and dyspnea would be important to see, however not as important as the 68-year-old male patient. The 45-year-old with abdominal pain, vomiting, and diarrhea is not as critical as the 68-year-old male patient. The 18-year-old female patient with chest pain worsening with deep breathing and movement can wait to be seen.
80. You had labs drawn last week for a routine physical. You work in the same system where you had the labs drawn. While at work, you decide to obtain your results 　a. It is OK to look in the electronic medical record (EMR) for the results because they're your labs, therefore not a HIPAA concern 　b. You should go to medical records and sign a release of information to obtain your labs 　c. You should ask a co-worker to print them for you, which is OK because you gave her verbal consent 　d. You should get permission from your manager to look up your labs	*Answer: b* Any time you are accessing medical records without a clinical reason to do so, you are at risk for violating HIPAA laws. You should not go into your own records without proper authority to do so. Asking a co-worker to do it is only placing her at risk, and your verbal consent is not valid. Your manager's permission does not release information in the appropriate manner required for accessing medical records.
81. A 31-year-old female arrives to the emergency department after being stung by a bee and she is "deathly" allergic to bee stings. She does not carry her epinephrine autoinjector with her. After stabilization, she responds to treatment. After a period of observation, she is ready for discharge. Part of discharge teaching should include 　a. The importance of calling 911 　b. The instructions about where to obtain a first aid kit 　c. Education about administering a nebulizer treatment 　d. Instructions about availability and use of an epinephrine autoinjector	*Answer: d* Although calling 911 is an important teaching step, it does not stop the rapid immune response seen in anaphylactic shock. Epinephrine is the single most important administered medication to stop or slow the rapid evolving anaphylactic shock, and patient/family education about emergency treatment is essential.

Question	Rationale
82. Which of the following findings would be of concern immediately following endotracheal intubation? a. The color on the exhaled CO_2 indicator is yellow b. Upon auscultation, sounds are heard over the epigastrium c. Bilateral chest rise and fall is noted with ventilation d. Chest x-ray shows the tip of the endotracheal tube just above the right main bronchus	*Answer: b* Auscultation of the epigastrium should be performed immediately following endotracheal intubation. Sounds heard over the epigastrium with the absence of chest rise and fall indicates intubation of the esophagus. The next step should be auscultation of the lungs, with bilateral breath sounds indicating proper placement. Evaluation of the color on the CO_2 indicator should reveal a change from purple to yellow. Finally, a chest x-ray should be performed to confirm placement of the endotracheal tube. Because the right main bronchus is superior to the left, it is more common to enter. This would be indicated by diminished lung sounds on the left. To resolve, gently pull pack on the endotracheal tube so it rests just above the right main bronchus.
83. A patient presents to the emergency department following a near drowning in a nearby lake. The patient is receiving high-flow oxygen and is maintaining his airway. The nurse notes coarse lung sounds throughout all lung fields. What is the emergency nurse most concerned about with initial treatment in a near drowning? a. Sepsis due to inhalation of dirty water b. Aspiration pneumonia and hypothermia c. Physical trauma due to the violent nature of near drowning d. Hyperthermia	*Answer: b* Aspiration pneumonia and hypothermia are both likely in near drowning episodes, and each should be considered in any submersion event. Bacterial pneumonia is a concern as well, although much later. Near-drowning patients are at risk for hypothermia. Sepsis is not a threat in this present scenario. A near drowning is not typically associated with traumatic injuries, although more information may be collected after initial treatment.
84. A patient presents with a sore throat that has recently worsened. His voice is muffled, and he complains of a two day history of fever. He has not eaten or drank because of the pain. Upon inspection, the nurse notes his tonsils appear enlarged and purulent. His painful swallowing is a. Odynophagia b. Trismus c. Halitosis d. Otalgia	*Answer: a* Trismus is the inability to open the mouth. Halitosis is foul breath. Otalgia is ear pain and Odynophagia is pain upon swallowing. All of these are signs and symptoms of a peritonsillar abscess.
85. A woman who is pregnant comes in the emergency department with irregular contractions that began 2 hours ago and are occurring more frequently. She is 31 2/7 weeks gestation. Baby is active and fetal heart tones are ranging 150 to 155 bpm. Her contractions are palpable and occurring every 10 minutes. What symptom will suggest preterm labor? a. Patient feels like she needs to void b. There is evidence of cervical change and dilation c. Regular contractions at 5 minutes apart d. Patient feels better sitting up	*Answer: b* Pre-term labor is defined as: contractions that become regular (begin and end in a rhythmic regular pattern of timed intervals) and cause cervical changes which is considered preterm labor (up to 2 cm change). Regular contractions could be associated to Braxton-Hicks contractions that can present in a regular pattern but do not change cervical dilation. In some cases pre-term labor can be associated to urinary tract infections (UTI), but the need to void is not specific to a UTI; bedrest and positioning do not affect pre-term labor.

Question	Rationale
86. A 51-year-old patient has come to the emergency department with fever, sore throat and hoarseness for the past 4 days. Today, he felt like he was "choking" in his airway. He has been diagnosed with Ludwig's angina. The nurse's first priority is assuring the following is available a. Cardiac monitoring b. IV antibiotics c. IV hydration d. Cricothyrotomy tray	*Answer: d* A patient with Ludwig's angina has a great risk for airway obstruction due to the edema within the submandibular space, an area that does not provide needed expansion to accommodate swelling without minimizing or occluding the airway. Often these patients are taking directly to the OR with plans for intubation with preparation for a tracheostomy, if needed. Cardiac and pulse oximetry monitoring are indicated as well as IV antibiotics and fluids; however, with the first priority of "airway," an emergency surgical airway kit within reach will prevent a delay if an emergency airway is needed.
87. A chest tube is placed in a patient to evaluate blood from a hemothorax following a significant chest trauma. An emergency thoracotomy is indicated when a. There is greater than 750 mL of initial blood return b. There is no blood return, but increasing dyspnea c. Blood return is greater than 200 mL per hour for 4 hours d. A second chest tube needs to be placed	*Answer: c* Emergency thoracotomy would not be required for an initial blood return of 750 mL. It is required if chest tube insertion results in greater than 1500 mL of blood return initially, or greater than 200 mL per hour for 4 consecutive hours. Autotransfusion-returning the shed blood, may be another intervention to consider. If there is no blood return, placement of the chest tube should be questioned, especially with increasing dyspnea, but an emergency thoracotomy would not be warranted. The need for a second chest tube, particularly if it is on the opposite side, does not require immediate thoracotomy unless there is significant blood loss.
88. During the course of a procedural sedation, a patient's respiratory rate drops to 10 breaths/minute. The nurse should a. Stop the procedure b. Assess the patient's vital signs and capnography values c. Do nothing. A decreased respiratory rate is normal during sedation d. Reposition the patient's airway to ensure patency	*Answer: b* A decreased respiratory rate requires an assessment of the patient and his ventilation status. The procedure should not be stopped if the patient is tolerating a respiratory rate of 10. A respiratory rate of 10 is slightly below normal and should not be ignored. If an obstructed airway is suspected, repositioning the patient's airway is not likely to help increase the respiratory rate.
89. A patient diagnosed with a deep vein thrombosis (DVT) suddenly becomes short of breath, tachycardic, tachypneic, and restless. What complication does the nurse suspect? a. Acute myocardial infarction b. Pulmonary embolism c. Pericardial tamponade d. Congestive heart failure	*Answer: b* Patients with DVTs are at high risk for pulmonary embolism. Sudden onset of shortness of breath, tachycardia, tachypnea, and restlessness are manifestations of pulmonary embolism. Acute myocardial infarction, pericardial tamponade, and congestive heart failure are not a complication of DVT.

Question	Rationale
90. A triage nurse would anticipate a diagnosis of shingles with a patient presenting with complaints of a. Painful, bilateral flank pain b. A generalized, urticarial rash; with a history of exposure to chickenpox c. A painful, itchy rash appearing with tiny blisters along a unilateral dermatome of the trunk d. A generalized, pruritic rash that appears to have small blisters	*Answer: c* Herpes Zoster, also known as shingles, is characterized by a maculopapular rash, which is very painful and itchy, and commonly appears on the trunk and follows a unilateral dermatome.
91. The emergency nurse is reviewing discharge instructions with a patient who received sutures to her face. The nurse knows her teaching is effective when the patient states, "If there are no signs or symptoms of infection, I will have my sutures removed in a. 3 to 5 days" b. 5 to 7 days" c. 7 to 10 days" d. 10 to 14 days"	*Answer: a* Sutures to the face, lips, and eyelids should be removed in 3 to 5 days. Sutures to the eyebrow should be removed in 5 to 7 days. Sutures to the back, chest, arms, hands, and thighs should be removed in 7 to 10 days. Sutures to the lower legs and feet should be removed in 10 to 14 days.
92. A patient arrives to the emergency department complaining of left shoulder pain. The shoulder is swollen with obvious deformity. The patient is unable to raise the left arm or bring it across the chest. The emergency nurse suspects a(n) a. Radial fracture b. Rotator cuff injury c. Shoulder dislocation d. Arthritic shoulder	*Answer: c* Dislocations present with deformity and limited range of motion. Arthritis is a chronic condition, not an acute process. Rotator cuff injuries result in pain with movement but no significant restriction on range of motion or swelling. Radial fracture should not affect a patient's ability to perform shoulder range of motion.
93. An ED nurse enters a patient's room to collect a patient history. The patient's chief complaint is "hearing voices" and has a history of psychosis. Currently, he is quiet and calm. To ensure safety, the nurse should a. Turn the television on to provide a distraction for the patient b. Offer a meal to the patient if he answers all of the questions c. Confirm an escape route by positioning between the door and patient d. Place the patient in 4-point restraints	*Answer: c* Delusions, hallucinations and/or a loss of reality may lead to dangerous judgments made by the patient suffering from psychosis. The ED nurse must provide safety. One way to assist with this safety is not to become trapped in a patient's room. The nurse should always have an escape route in case the patient becomes threatening or violent. Turning a TV on would not ensure a low stimulating environment, which is more therapeutic for the patient with psychosis. Bribing the patient is not therapeutic and would not be effective since the patient's rational reasoning skills are not intact. 4-point restraints are not indicated if the patient presents no imminent danger to self or others.

Question	Rationale
94. Three young children in the same family are diagnosed with chicken pox. Discharge instructions noted for this family include all of the information *except* a. Chicken pox is caused by the varicella zoster virus (VZV) and is very contagious b. The rash which develops, is pruritic in nature c. A person may develop a mild fever and is contagious from 1 to 2 days before the outbreak of the chicken pox rash d. There is no risk of exposure to immunocompromised individuals	*Answer: d* An immunocompromised individual diagnosed with chicken pox is at risk for developing complications such as VZV dissemination to the visceral organs, pneumonia, hepatitis, encephalitis, and DIC.
95. A patient presents to the emergency department following collapse at a distance running event. The emergency nurse immediately suspects a heat-related emergency. What signs and symptoms would the nurse expect to see with heat stroke as opposed to heat exhaustion? a. Core temperature 102.5°F (39.2°C), warm skin, profuse perspiration, and altered mental status b. Core temperature 104.5 (40.2°C), hot skin, lack of perspiration, and altered level of consciousness c. Headache, pale skin, and profuse perspiration d. Muscle cramps, mild tachycardia, headache, and lack of perspiration	*Answer: b* Heat stroke is a medical emergency and is differentiated from heat exhaustion by a core temperature of greater than 104.0°F (40°C) and the lack of perspiration.
96. For a patient with a chemical burn to the eye, the emergency nurse knows that the priority intervention is to a. Baseline visual acuity b. Ophthalmology consult c. Warm compress to the eye d. Irrigation with copious amounts of Ringer's Lactate	*Answer: d* Chemical burns to the eye are an emergency with urgent treatment needed to prevent further vision loss. Irrigation with Ringer's lactate, saline, or sterile water should be done until the pH of the eye reaches about 7.1, or the level of typical tears. Alkali exposure generally requires larger amounts of fluid irrigation. Baseline visual acuity delays treatment. Ophthalmology consult may be needed but is not an initial priority. Warm compress to the eye may provide comfort, but is not a priority treatment.

Question	Rationale
97. A mother drives her 6-year-old son, with a peanut allergy, to the emergency department after he developed urticaria. The child weighs 20 kg. The emergency nurse observes edema around his lips and hears inspiratory wheezes when auscultating lung sounds. The next action should be a. Establish an IV and administer a 400 mL 0.9 NS fluid bolus b. Apply a cardiac monitor and continuous pulse oximetry c. Administer 0.15 mL epinephrine IM (1 mg/mL concentration of epinephrine) d. Administer 0.015 mL epinephrine IM (0.1 mg/mL concentration of epinephrine)	*Answer: c* This child's allergic reaction is deteriorating to symptoms of anaphylaxis. He is developing angioedema, and his lung sounds have wheezing. Epinephrine is the most important treatment for suspected anaphylaxis. The correct concentration for epinephrine, when administered IM, is 1 mg/mL (or 1:1,000). The correct concentration is 0.1 mg/mL when epinephrine is administered IV (or 1:10,000). Cardiac monitoring and pulse oximetry are indicated but can immediately follow administration of epinephrine. IV establishment and a fluid bolus (20 mL/kg) may be indicated if the child's symptoms continue and anaphylactic shock is suspected.
98. An ill-appearing 50-year-old male arrives at the emergency department via EMS. His chief complaint is abdominal pain, vomiting, and fever of 101°F (38.3°C) for the past 12 hours. His abdominal pain is diffuse with muscle rigidity upon palpation of his abdomen. Past medical history is noncontributory except for a screening colonoscopy 24 hours earlier. This patient may be experiencing the following condition a. Appendicitis b. Diverticulitis c. Perforated ulcer d. Peritonitis	*Answer: d* A perforation may have occurred from the colonoscopy causing spillage of bowel contents into the peritoneal cavity. If left untreated, sepsis will ensue. His history of having a recent colonoscopy would raise the index of suspicion for a perforated colon. Typically pain from appendicitis becomes localized in the RLQ and pain from diverticulitis becomes localized in the LLQ. Although a ruptured appendix or perforated ulcer can cause diffuse abdominal pain with peritonitis, his history of a recent colonoscopy coincides with the potential cause of his peritonitis.
99. The emergency nurse is reviewing abscess treatment discharge instructions with a patient. The nurse knows the teaching is effective when the patient states a. I will soak the wound every night so the packing stays moist b. I will take my antibiotics until the swelling goes down c. I will return to my doctor tomorrow to have the wound closed with sutures d. Increased swelling and redness are a signs of infection, which I should have re-evaluated	*Answer: d* Patients should understand signs and symptoms of increasing infection and when to return for re-evaluation. Soaking an abscess is not recommended. Patients should take the full course of antibiotics as prescribed and not stop before the end of the course of antibiotics. After incision and drainage, an abscess should be left open to heal.

Question	Rationale
100. The ED nurse is in the hall when they hear screaming from a room down the hall. The nurse responds and finds a patient's wife yelling and screaming. She is standing in the corner, appears red in the face, and is breathing rapidly. Her husband is hiding under the covers. The nurse attempts to de-escalate the situation. The first action of the nurse is to a. Approach the patient with arms extended b. Yell at the patient's wife to calm herself or Security will be called c. Manage personal reactions d. Ask for PRN lorazepam to calm the wife	*Answer: c* The first step to manage a disruptive situation is for the nurse to calm himself or herself. Approaching the patient at this time would not be indicated; first establish safety and maintain a safe distance. Yelling is rarely effective when attempting to calm someone. Calling for Security may be an intervention but threatening is rarely an effective means to de-escalate someone. Family members would only be treated if the family member was also a patient.
101. A mother presents to triage with her 4-year-old son and reports the child may have measles. The only noted symptoms are a cough and runny nose over the past 3 days. The child attends a large daycare. As a triage nurse, what history and symptoms increase suspicion of measles? a. Fever, malaise, and rash noted to the child's face. The child is up to date with immunizations b. Cough, fever, weight loss, and diarrhea c. Nausea, vomiting, and diarrhea with a rash noted to the patient's lower extremities. No history of immunizations d. Fever, malaise, cough, and runny nose. No history of immunizations. A rash noted on a child's face and trunk spreading distally onto the lower extremities	*Answer: d* Fever, malaise, cough, runny nose, and conjunctivitis are symptoms of Measles. Since the child has not received his immunizations, the child is at risk. A maculopapular rash occurs; typically about 14 days post exposure and spreads from the head to the trunk and distally to the lower extremities.
102. What is the most common reason for seeking care in the emergency department? a. Sutures b. Behavioral health complaints c. Rash d. Pain	*Answer: d* Pain is the most common reason for ED visits. Although suture placement, behavioral health, and rash are all common reasons for an ED visit, they are not the most common.
103. A 34-year-old male patient presents to the emergency department after exposure to very cold temperatures during a hunting trip. The nurse assesses both of his feet and notes edema with cold, pale skin. He has circumferential blisters to both feet. Given his history and assessment findings, the nurse suspects frostbite. Which of the following interventions would be *contraindicated* for this condition? a. Slow rewarming of his feet using warm water b. Obtaining a core temperature c. Rubbing or massaging both of his feet to stimulate circulation d. Providing ordered analgesics for pain	*Answer: c* Frostbite is the freezing of tissue. At the cellular level, ice crystals form within the tissue, causing cellular damage. Rubbing or massaging the affected areas can cause further damage to the tissue. The other listed interventions are appropriate for the treatment of frostbite.

Question	Rationale

104. A patient returns from CT with a change in condition. Earlier the patient was confused and restless but now the patient only responds to a sternal rub. The patient's pulse has decreased from 120 bpm to 64 bpm. Blood pressure was 150/70 mm Hg and is now 180/40 mm Hg. Breathing has become increasingly irregular in both rate and depth. The nurse recognizes that
  a. This is Cushing's Triad: increasing pulse pressure with systolic hypertension, bradycardia, and irregular respirations, a sign of increasing pressure inside the skull
  b. This is Honing's Sign: hypertension, tachypnea with a normal pulse rate, and a sign of increasing intracranial pressure
  c. This is Kehr's Sign: indication that there is bleeding inside the peritoneal cavity, possibly a ruptured spleen
  d. This is Homer's Triad: deterioration in mentation with a decrease in heart rate indicates bleeding in the brain
	Answer: a
	Increasing hypertension with a widening pulse pressure, bradycardia, and irregular respiratory patterns is Cushing's Triad. Don't be fooled by the "normal" pulse of 64 bpm. It clearly is trending down from previous tachycardia. Kehr's sign is pain in the left shoulder when the patient is prone. Honing's Sign and Homer's Triad are not actual clinical signs.

105. Virchow's triad is
  a. Jugular venous dissention (JVD), muffled heart sounds, and hypotension
  b. Tachycardia, mental status changes, and decreased urine output
  c. Damaged vascular endothelium, venous stasis, and hypercoagulability of blood
  d. Lower extremity fracture, abdominal or thoracic, and head injuries
	Answer: c
	Virchow's triad is a group of simultaneous factors that increases the risk for thrombosis development. A hypercoagulable state may follow recent surgery. Vascular endothelial injury may occur after catheter insertion or recent trauma, and venous stasis can result from pregnancy, immobility, or obesity. JVD, muffled heart sounds, and hypotension, referred to as Beck's triad, are a cluster of symptoms associated with pericardial tamponade. Tachycardia, mental status changes and decreased urine output can be early signs of shock. Waddel's triad describes an injury pattern that may occur when a pedestrian is struck by a car. A triad of injuries involving lower extremities, the abdomen or thorax, and head are potentially involved is this injury pattern.

106. The highest priority with approaching the patient who has a dental emergency is
  a. Level of consciousness
  b. Airway
  c. Bleeding
  d. Infection
	Answer: b
	All of these considerations are priorities when managing dental emergencies. As with other emergencies, airway patency is the first priority. Infection could lead to edema that can occlude the airway. Blood loss and decreased level of consciousness can also affect airway patency.

Question	Rationale
107. A patient arrives to the emergency department reporting a lump on his right arm for several days. He denies trauma. The area is red, swollen, and tender to touch. Circulation, sensation, and movement are intact. The patient has a low-grade fever. The emergency nurse anticipates a. Compartment pressure measurements b. Radiographs to confirm fracture c. Incision and drainage d. Splinting of the affected extremity	*Answer: c* The patient is displaying signs of an abscess. Appropriate treatment includes incision and drainage followed by antibiotic administration. Compartment pressure measurement, radiographs, and splinting are not generally indicated in the presence of an abscess.
108. A patient is diagnosed with carbon monoxide poisoning. The patient is awake and alert but is evasive when a history on the circumstances surrounding the inhalation exposure is obtained. The emergency nurse should be concerned with a. Decreased perfusion to the patient brain causing confusion b. Intentional inhalation of carbon monoxide and possible suicidal ideation c. Possible illegal activity prior to the inhalation d. A safe ride home for the patient	*Answer: b* It is important to consider suicidal ideation for unexplained carbon monoxide inhalation. Although carbon monoxide inhalation can be caused by faulty heating appliances within the home, it is also a common means of suicide attempt/completion.
109. Miotic agents act on the eye by a. Constricting the pupil b. Dilating the pupil c. Paralyzing the ciliary muscle d. Paralyzing the suspensory muscle	*Answer: a* Miotic agents constrict the pupil. Examples of miotic agents include opioids, organophosphates, cholinergics, and parasympathomimetics, such as pilocarpine. Dilation is caused by mydriadic agents, such as cocaine, amphetamines, phenylephrine, and anticholinergics, such as atropine and scopalomine. Ciliary muscles are paralyzed by a class of mydriadic agents called cytoplegics, which not only dilates the pupil but also reduces accommodation of the eye. Paralysis of the suspensory muscles occurs with general paralytic medications.

Question	Rationale
110. A 22-year-old construction worker arrives via EMS after falling from a second story building. He was intubated prior to arrival. He is currently unresponsive to verbal stimuli and is not moving his extremities. FAST exam is negative. A total of 2 liters of crystalloid IV fluid has infused. His current vital signs are T-98.1°F (36.7°C); P-48; R-14 (assisted); BP-78/40. His skin is warm and dry. What type of shock is suggested by the symptoms? a. Neurogenic shock b. Hypovolemic shock c. Cardiogenic shock d. Obstructive shock	*Answer: a* This patient's mechanism of injury would raise the index of suspicion that he has sustained a spinal cord injury. Neurogenic shock occurs with a loss of sympathetic tone in cervical and upper thoracic complete spinal cord lesions, and the balance between the sympathetic nervous system (fight or flight) and the parasympathetic nervous system (slow and dilate) are not synergistic. Bradycardia and hypotension are the result of increased parasympathetic tone and are often present in neurogenic shock. Hypotension may not improve with fluid challenges, and a vasopressor infusion may be needed to improve perfusion. With hypovolemic shock, typically when the intravascular space is depleted, the heart responds with tachycardia. An exception to a tachycardic response would be if the patient were on a *B*-blocker or other heart slowing medication. Tachycardia and hypotension are two common symptoms for cardiogenic shock. The classification of obstructive shock includes pericardial tamponade, tension pneumothorax and pulmonary embolus. This patient's injury and presentation do not have the common presenting symptoms for obstructive shock.
111. A 25-year-old female patient was involved in a head on collision with significant chest wall trauma. A tracheobronchial injury is suspected when a. There is a contusion noted to the upper chest b. The patient is unable to speak c. The chest tube insertion fails to evacuate subcutaneous emphysema d. The patient has increasing dyspnea	*Answer: c* Tracheobronchial injuries are often the result of rapid deceleration. They should be suspected when chest tube insertion fails to evacuate subcutaneous emphysema. Contusions to the chest wall and increasing dyspnea can be indicative of many injuries and is therefore not specific to tracheobronchial injuries. The inability to speak would be indicative of a laryngeal injury.
112. A wife brings her husband to the emergency department reporting he has not been sleeping and has been up all night every night working on new business plans for over a week. The patient states nothing is wrong. The ED nurse suspects he may be experiencing a manic episode. During the assessment the nurse should a. Offer a PRN of an antidepressant to stabilize his mood b. Assess if he is hearing or seeing things c. Ask the wife to leave the room to determine if her reports are valid d. Tell the patient that in order to complete his project, he will need to provide a urine sample	*Answer: b* Assessing if the patient is hallucinating (hearing or seeing things) is an important question. Due to his lack of sleep, it would not be an unusual finding. Offering a PRN of an antidepressant is not indicated. Antidepressants are not used alone in bipolar disorder and during a manic phase would not be the treatment of choice. Asking the wife to leave may not be necessary; typically in mania, the patient presents with little insight into his/her mental illness or current functioning. Using someone's illness as a means to get him to do something should not be done in practice. In this case, using his "project" as a means to get a urine sample would not be appropriate.

Question	Rationale
113. The ED nurse is in the room alone assessing a patient when he discloses that he wants to kill his neighbor. He appears anxious. He has a detailed plan and explains he is going to kill him after he leaves the emergency department. The nurse's next actions include all of the following actions *except* a. Informing the authorities about the threat to the neighbor b. Walking the patient to the secure room c. Asking the patient if they have a weapon d. Leave the patient alone while the nurse obtains a PRN antianxiety medication for him	*Answer: d* The nurse should consider and consult with other team members about the threats. The nurse may call the police if there is a good faith belief that the disclosure is necessary to prevent or lessen a serious imminent threat to the patient or other. Walking the patient to a secure room is appropriate. The nurse should ask for additional staff to complete the interview. Asking if the patient has a weapon should be done as soon as additional staff is available. A patient should not be left alone if they have stated a credible threat to kill someone.
114. A patient arrives after sustaining a gunshot wound. What should the RN do with the clothing the patient was wearing? a. Place them in a patient belongings bag and put them in a safe place b. Throw them away because they're soiled with excessive amounts of blood c. Place them in the approved collection bag/ device for evidence d. Leave them in place for the police to decide what to do	*Answer: c* Evidence collection is an important part of ED nursing. Placing the clothing in a bag, if it is not an approved bag or device, can affect the chain of custody and the evidence on the clothing. Throwing them away may result in the loss of evidence, and leaving them on is not a likely option while treating the patient.
115. A patient at 26 weeks gestation is brought to the emergency department. She was watching television with her husband and son when she felt something warm and wet. Concerned that she may have ruptured her membranes, she ran to the bathroom and discovered she was bleeding. She saturated a mini pad but the bleeding stopped after the initial gush. She has had no bleeding since but she came in to the ED because she is scared the baby may have been bleeding. The ED nurse suspect a. Ruptured ovarian cyst b. Vasa previa c. Placenta abruptio d. Placenta Previa	*Answer: d* Painless bright bleeding during pregnancy is usually caused by the placenta becoming separated either completely or sometimes partially. It is due to the placenta implantation being close or over the cervical os. Rupture ovarian cyst will not cause painless bleeding; placenta abruptio is related to painful bleeding or board-like abdomen; vasa previa is much more serious and if ruptured the bleeding would not stop.
116. What substance does activated charcoal not absorb? a. Acetaminophen b. Amitriptyline (tricyclic antidepressant) c. Ibuprofen d. Lithium	*Answer: d* Activated charcoal is very effective at absorbing a variety of substances. It does not effectively absorb heavy metals such as iron and lead and medications such as lithium. Activated charcoal does effectively bind to ibuprofen, acetaminophen, and most tricyclic antidepressants if taken within 2 hours of the ingestion (the closer to time of ingestion, the greater the chance of effectiveness).

Question	Rationale
117. For a patient with a penetrating eye injury, a strategy to reduce further injury is to a. Instill cycoplegic agents b. Measure intraocular pressure c. Shield both eyes/stabilize object d. Remove the penetrating object	*Answer: c* Shielding both eyes or shielding the affected eye and patching the unaffected eye. Covering both eyes reduces bilateral eye movement and helps to prevent further injury. Removal of the penetrating object, instillation of any medication, and measuring ocular pressures could cause additional injury.
118. A female patient presents to the emergency department with psychological concerns. During the suicide assessment, she admits that she is considering suicide by firearm. Which of the following risk factors is most important to consider? a. She recently broke up with her boyfriend b. She has a diagnosis of depression c. She has a detailed plan to die by suicide d. She comes into the emergency department alone	*Answer: c* All of these items could be risk factors for suicide. However, the one that is most concerning and increases the risk is a detailed plan to die by suicide. Patients who have a plan and means (such as access to a firearm) to follow through with the plan are at highest risk. Additionally, firearms are used in more suicides than any other means, so access to a firearm is an alarming risk factor. Situational stressors often contribute to suicidal ideation and depression conveys an increased risk for suicide. Presenting to the emergency department alone could be for a variety of reasons. However, social isolation is a risk factor.
119. A focused assessment with sonography in trauma (FAST) exam is the preferred radiological exam in trauma because it a. Requires minimal training to perform b. Can be done quickly at bedside to identify internal trauma c. Is more definitive than other radiological exams d. Is less expensive than other tests	*Answer: b* A FAST exam can be performed at the bedside and requires a skilled provider to perform the test. This ultrasound screening test is helpful in identifying blood (internal bleeding), such as a hemothorax. Although there are other radiological exams that provide clearer pictures, such as CT. The FAST exam is beneficial as it can be done rapidly and does not require moving the patient to another location.
120. A 41-year-old male presents with complaints of increasing dyspnea and chest pain. While collecting a history from a patient, the nurse notices documentation in the patient's health history that raises suspicion of a pulmonary embolism. What risk factor was noted? a. Factor V deficiency b. Von Willebrand's disease c. Factor V Leiden d. Fragile X Syndrome	*Answer: c* The natural clotting process contains intrinsic responses to slow or stop the clotting process to prevent abnormal blood clots. Factor V Leiden, also known as thrombophilia, is a mutated gene. People who have this gene have a greater tendency for developing blood clots. A hypercoagulable condition exists. The clotting system normally applies activated protein C (APC), an anticoagulant, to limit clot formation. With Factor V Leiden, a mutated gene causes resistance to APC. Factor V plays a role in the normal clotting development by converting prothrombin to thrombin. People with a Factor V deficiency have a greater risk for bleeding, especially following surgery or childbirth. Von Willebrand's disease is an inherited condition and is caused by a lack of the Von Willebrand factor, one of the factors involved with clotting. Bleeding episodes can be severe for people who have Von Willebrand. Additional clotting factors may be required, such as fresh frozen plasma, for patients with Factor V deficiency or Von Willebrand's to decrease bleeding. Fragile X syndrome is an inherited condition from an altered gene. It affects both sexes and can cause severe cognitive and behavioral challenges.

Question	Rationale
121. During a resuscitation code, the spouse of the patient is standing in the corner of the room crying. You should a. Ask the spouse to leave to not cause further psychological trauma b. Assign a team member to stand with her to explain what's going on c. Continue with the code as if the spouse isn't present d. Ask the spouse to leave, so she doesn't disrupt the team members involved in the code	*Answer: b* Evidence supports that family presence has been shown to be helpful to the family during a resuscitation. Opposing views such as psychological trauma or team member disruption are not shown to be valid concerns. Of course, each situation must be assessed, but generally speaking, family presence is encouraged. Assigning a liaison to help the family understand what's going on has been shown to improve the family experience.
122. An 18-year-old female visits the emergency department with complaints of ear pain and decreased hearing for the past 2 to 3 days. She reports an increased pain around her ear as she put her pierced earrings on. She has been visiting a friend and swimming in the lake. The nurse anticipates that an otoscopy exam would reveal her tympanic membrane to be a. Edematous and bulging b. Shiny and yellowish in color c. Translucent and pearl gray in color d. Limited in movement	*Answer: c* Typically, the tympanic membrane remains normal with external otitis. She presents with risk factors (hot weather, swimming) and symptoms (pain and tenderness on external ear and decreased hearing). The tympanic membrane is not usually affected with external otitis. With acute otitis media, the TM usually becomes edematous and inflamed from the pressure build up of fluid within the middle ear. The TM may have limited movement on pneumatic otoscopy exam (air insufflation using an otoscope). The TM may be reddened or yellow, which can be signs of a possible bacterial otitis media.
123. A patient arrives to the ED following a cat bite to the hand. The cat belongs to her neighbor and is up to date on recommended immunizations. The hand is swollen, red, and painful. The emergency nurse anticipates treatment will include a. Closure with wound glue b. Administration of antibiotics due to the high risk of infection c. Closure with sutures d. Administration of rabies prophylaxis	*Answer: b* Cat bites are high risk for infection. Most bites are not sutured or otherwise closed to prevent the risk of trapping bacteria in the wound. Rabies prophylaxis is not indicated in a vaccinated, asymptomatic animal.
124. What medications are expected to be ordered for the patient with Cushing's Triad? a. Atropine b. Mannitol c. Octreotide d. Hypotonic solution IV, such as 0.45% NaCl	*Answer: b* Mannitol is an osmotic diuretic that decreases intracranial pressure. A Hypotonic IV solution such as 0.45% NaCl would not have an osmotic diuretic effect. Atropine and octreotide would not be appropriate.

Question	Rationale
125. Hematochezia has the following characteristics a. Black or "tarry" blood from rectum often associated with upper GI bleeds b. Vomiting of blood or "coffee ground" emesis c. Bright red or maroon rectal bleeding and can be associated with upper or lower GI bleeding d. Bleeding from the ligament of Treitz	*Answer: c* Hematochezia is bright red or maroon rectal bleeding and is usually indicative of lower GI bleeding. However, hematochezia can also occur with a very rapid upper GI bleed (>1000 mL). Melena is black or "tarry" stool from rectum. Although melena is often associated with upper GI bleeding, it can also occur with intake of specific substances such as iron, licorice and beets (pseudomelena). Vomiting blood or "coffee ground" emesis is referred to as hematemesis. The ligament of Treitz is a smooth muscle that is connected to the junction of the duodenum and jejunum and is referred as a landmark separating an upper GI and lower GI bleed.
126. An eye patch or eye shield is *not* recommended for which condition? a. Hyphema b. Corneal abrasion c. Globe rupture d. Keratitis	*Answer: b* An eye patch has not been shown to benefit healing or comfort for the patient with a corneal abrasion. An eye patch assists with eye rest for patients with keratitis, but an eye shield is not indicated. An eye shield protects the eye from further damage after globe rupture or hyphema, but a patch is not recommended.
127. A patient arrives in the emergency department complaining of chest pain, palpitations, and shortness of breath. The cardiac monitor displays supraventricular tachycardia (SVT). What common signs and symptoms would the nurse anticipate the patient to have? a. Dizziness and dyspnea b. Hypertension and nausea c. Clear mentation and respiratory rate of 16 d. Heart rate of 130 and respiratory rate of 28	*Answer: a* Dizziness and dyspnea are classic signs and symptoms of SVT. Patients may be hypertensive and nauseous when they are in SVT, but these are common signs and symptoms. Clear mentation and a respiratory rate of 16 are normal findings. Heart rate of 130 and a respiratory rate of 28 indicate tachycardia and tachypnea. However, the heart rate needs to be above 150 to be classified as SVT.
128. A 32-year-old male patient involved in a motorcycle crash presents with multiple injuries. He was wearing a helmet and does not appear to have any head or facial trauma. He is dyspneic, tachycardic, and tachynpneic with road rash and redness to his anterior chest. Close inspection reveals tracheal deviation to the left with diminished lung sounds on the right. The priority intervention is to a. Perform immediate needle decompression to the right 2nd intercostal space b. Prepare for immediate endotracheal intubation c. Perform immediate needle decompression to the left 2nd intercostal space d. Anticipate chest tube insertion	*Answer: a* Tracheal deviation is the hallmark sign of a tension pneumothorax. It is identified by absent or diminished lung sounds on the affected side and tracheal deviation away from the affected side. Immediate needle decompression is the primary intervention. In this case, the assessment indicates the tension pneumothorax is on the right side. Once needle decompression is successful, additional interventions would include preparing for endotracheal intubation and chest tube insertion.

Question	Rationale
129. A patient's wife is concerned that her husband is at risk for suicide. Her husband has a diagnosis of bipolar disorder. When educating her about the diagnosis and suicide risk, the ED nurse should include the following statement a. The risk for suicide is highest for patients in the depressive state of bipolar b. The risk for suicide is highest during the impulsive manic state of bipolar c. The risk for suicide is not significantly higher than the general public d. The risk for suicide is the same in the depressive and manic states	*Answer: a* During the depressive state of bipolar disorder, the patient is at higher risk for suicide. Bipolar disorder, carries an increased risk for suicide. During the manic state, patient may engage in risky and dangerous behaviors. However, the suicide risk is lower during manic states.
130. A 22-year-old male patient presents to the emergency department following a party at which his friends state he used "bath salts." The emergency nurse knows "bath salts" are similar to amphetamines and can have which of the following effects? a. Constricted pupils b. Hallucinations, hypotension, and bradycardia c. Sedation, CNS depression, and airway compromise d. Severe hyperthermia, anxiety, agitation, and tremors	*Answer: d* Cathinone, or "bath salts," is very similar to amphetamines and inhibits dopamine, serotonin, and norepinephrine reuptake. Common symptoms include hyperthermia, anxiety, agitation, and tremors due to the increased levels of these neurotransmitters.
131. A young patient presents to the emergency department with her mother. The patient has a history of hydrocephalus and had a shunt placement 4 months ago. The patient is now complaining of a severe headache whenever she is sitting up and her fontanels are depressed. The concern for this patient is a. Shunt malfunction, which is common in the first 2 years after placement b. Shunt infection, which is caused by the patient's normal flora and can lead to septic shock c. Overdrainage of the shunt, which requires supportive therapy, seizure protocols, and surgery to replace the shunt d. Shunt dislodgement: the distal end of the shunt has moved	*Answer: c* The depressed fontanels and headache when she is sitting up are signs that the shunt is draining too much. If the patient had signs of increasing intracranial pressure (ICP) such as increased irritability and changes in her level of consciousness, a malfunctioning shunt would be a more likely cause for symptoms.

Question	Rationale
132. A 75-year-old male has just arrived to the emergency department, following a MVC when his car, which he was driving, left the road and hit a telephone pole. He was restrained with no airbags to deploy. He is restless, complaining of chest pain and shortness of breath. His lung sounds are clear and equal and skin is cool and pale. His last set of vital signs are P-118; R-28; BP-88/40; SpO$_2$-86% on a non-rebreather mask with high-flow oxygen. While auscultating a manual BP, the nurse notes a significant drop (about 20 mm Hg) when he inhales. Identify the term describing this physical finding a. Muffled heart tones b. Pulsus paradoxus c. Pulsus alternans d. Diminished perfusion	*Answer: b* During normal inspiration, negative intrathoracic pressure increases resulting in increasing blood flow. However, in pericardial tamponade with the pericardial pressure already increased, adding more pressure during end-inspiration further weakens the stroke volume and decreases the blood pressure. Pulsus paradoxus occurs when the BP decreases (>10 mm Hg) during inspiration. Muffled heart tones can be a sign of pericardial tamponade and is one of the components of Beck's triad. However, the sound of muffled heart tones is heard through auscultating heart sounds and not the BP. Pulsus alternans describes a pulse pattern that alternates between strong and weak without a change in the pulse rate. Although this may be observed in a patient with an arterial line, pulsus alternans is not auscultated during a BP assessment. He is exhibiting signs of decreased perfusion such as hypotension, tachycardia, and restlessness. However, the variation is auscultating a BP related to the respiratory cycle does not indicate diminished perfusion.
133. As an emergency nurse caring for a patient who used cocaine, what related condition must be considered and evaluated? a. Pneumonia due to ineffective airway clearance b. Slow gastric motility leading to constipation c. Myocardial infarction d. Exsanguination from a nosebleed	*Answer: c* Cocaine is a potent vasoconstrictor, causing constriction of the coronary arteries. This vasoconstriction can exacerbate angina or can lead to a myocardial infarction. A complete cardiac evaluation may be performed in the emergency setting. Pneumonia, slow gastric motility and exsanguination are not typically seen shortly after cocaine use.
134. A 42-year-old male patient has overdosed on a tricyclic antidepressant. The emergency nurse anticipates the following treatments *except* a. Induced vomiting to remove pill fragments from the stomach b. Activated charcoal c. Systemic alkalization d. Cardiac monitoring	*Answer: a* The induction of vomiting is contraindicated in the care of a tricyclic antidepressant (TCA) overdose. A TCA overdose can cause CNS depression leading to an unprotected airway. Vomiting increases the risk for aspiration pneumonia and airway occlusion. Activated charcoal may bind with TCA, preventing further absorption, and cardiac monitoring is indicated because TCA can cause arrhythmias.
135. A 31-year-old female patient arrives at the emergency department via EMS, with severe hypothermia after being found sleeping outside in freezing temperatures. What ECG abnormality would be anticipated given this history? a. Elevated Q wave b. J waves c. Tented T waves d. Sine wave	*Answer: b* Severe hypothermia can lead to arrhythmias including ventricular fibrillation. On ECG, one common finding is J waves, most commonly seen in the precordial leads. J waves are typically seen when the body core temperature falls below 89.6°F (32°C). Elevated Q waves could indicate myocardial injury; tented T waves and cardiac sine waves indicate hyperkalemia.

Question	Rationale
136. A patient has experienced an acute exposure to a radioactive material while working in a laboratory. The patient states the substance he was working with was an alpha radiation emitter. He was not using personal protective equipment and believes he might have inhaled some of the substance. With knowledge about alpha radiation, the emergency nurse knows that a. Alpha radiation is low ionizing and will not cause tissue destruction b. Alpha radiation is highly ionizing and is very destructive to tissue c. Alpha radiation is moderately ionizing and is very destructive to tissue d. Alpha radiation is highly ionizing and is low penetrating, so tissue destruction is not a concern	*Answer: b* Alpha radiation is highly ionizing and is known to cause extensive damage to tissue. It also happens to have very low penetration compared to other types of radiation. When an alpha emitter is inhaled, it has the potential to cause injury to lung tissue. Even though the penetration is low, with inhalation it is very close to the lung tissue and can penetrate it. Destruction of lung tissue can occur, leading to deterioration of the tissue and ineffective blood oxygenation.
137. A 35-year-old female presents with dyspnea and tachycardia. Her history includes use of birth control pills, cigarette smoking, and a severe iodine allergy. In addition to a D-dimer test, the nurse would anticipate an order for a. A chest x-ray b. An ECG c. A CT scan d. A ventilation/perfusion scan	*Answer: d* This patient has risk factors for a pulmonary embolus (PE), which are difficult to diagnose with a chest x-ray. An ECG may be ordered to rule out other causes for her symptoms, but would not definitively diagnose a PE. A CT scan is the most reliable test, but is contraindicated because of her iodine allergy. In this case, a ventilation/perfusion scan would be the preferred alternative.
138. An elderly female patient arrives via ambulance with complaints of multiple episodes of watery diarrhea and abdominal tenderness. While assessing the patient and placing her in a gown, her clothing is noted to be grossly contaminated with feces. While reviewing records sent from a long-term care facility, additional information stating she has had a recent, lengthy hospitalization and has been taking prescribed antibiotics for the past week is noted. The patient is alert and oriented with stable vital signs. The patient becomes anxious, tearful and is incontinent of stool. What measures are implemented while caring for the patient? a. Assist the patient to the bedside commode, instruct the patient to use the call light when further assistance is needed and use hand sanitizer as you leave the patient room b. Provide support while acknowledging the patient's concern and provide peri-care placing an incontinent brief on the patient c. Instruct the patient to calm down and clean the patient will maintaining standard precautions d. Provide support to the patient while acknowledging her anxiety. Provide peri-care while maintaining contact precautions. Assure all caregivers follow strict hand washing practice while caring for the patient	*Answer: d* This patient is at risk for potential *C. difficile* as noted by her complaint of watery diarrhea, abdominal pain, recent hospitalization, and antibiotic therapy. It is important to provide support, maintain standard and contact precautions, and follow strict hand washing practice. *C. difficile* is shed in feces, spread via caregiver hands who have touched a contaminated surface or item. Use of alcohol gel-based hand sanitizer does not kill the bacteria.

Question	Rationale
139. Proper isolation precautions for the nurse performing phlebotomy for a patient with mumps includes a. Gown and gloves b. Gown, gloves, and mask c. Gown, gloves, N-95 (or equivalent) mask d. Gown, gloves, N-95 (or equivalent) mask, and negative airflow	*Answer: b* Mumps is transmitted via coughing, sneezing, or direct contact with infected saliva. Proper isolation precaution type for mumps is droplet isolation, consisting of gown, gloves, and a standard surgical-type or procedure mask. Goggles or other eye protection should be considered for interventions resulting in exposure to respiratory fluids, such as during intubation or a bronchoscopy. Airborne precautions would require an N-95 level mask, which is not indicated for treatment of a patient with mumps.
140. A 22-year-old male patient presents to the emergency department following a first-time seizure. The nurse learns from his family that the patient had recently traveled outside of the United States. A CT scan shows multiple foreign bodies in the brain tissue. What disease does the emergency nurse suspect the patient has? a. Cysticercosis b. Taeniasis c. Malaria d. Giardiasis	*Answer: a* Cysticercosis is a disease in which parasite larval cysts travel throughout the body and deposit in muscle and brain tissue. In many cases, a first-time seizure is the primary indicator of the parasite infection. Taeniasis is usually from eating undercooked pork or beef and has associated symptoms of weight loss and abdominal pain. Early symptoms of malaria are flu-like with fever and chills. Giardiasis leads to GI symptoms such as diarrhea.
141. Which of the following tests is NOT helpful in distinguishing non-cardiogenic pulmonary edema from congestive heart failure (CHF)? a. ABGs b. Chest x-ray c. CT chest d. BNP	*Answer: a* Presentation of patients with pulmonary edema is similar whether it is cardiogenic or non-cardiogenic in nature. Radiological and laboratory tests help to distinguish the two. Patients with cardiogenic pulmonary edema, such as CHF will show a widened mediastinum on a chest x-ray and a CT chest. In addition, they will show an elevated BNP level. ABGs are not reliable to distinguish as they may be abnormal due to either cause.
142. An emergency nurse is caring for a patient who was burned over 30% of the body surface area following a natural gas explosion at home. After stabilizing the patient's airway and breathing, what would be the next highest nursing intervention priority? a. IV pain and sedation medication b. Urinary catheter placement c. Application of warming devices to maintain body temperature d. Ensure adequate IV access	*Answer: d* Fluid replacement in burn patients is critical. Following stabilization of the ABCs, IV fluid replacement must begin as soon as possible. Ensuring that the patient has good IV access to begin fluid replacement is paramount. Although maintaining the patient's body temperature is important, it can be done simultaneously starting with warm IV fluid.

Question	Rationale
143. A 64-year-old female patient presents with a significantly swollen tongue and lips. She is extremely anxious and is drooling. The emergency nurse positions the patient and opens the airway with a jaw thrust. The priority intervention for this patient is a. Insert an oral airway b. Prepare for cricothyrotomy c. Apply oxygen via non-rebreather mask d. Obtain SpO_2 measurement	*Answer: b* The patient is showing symptoms of airway obstruction associated with angioedema. Insertion of an oral airway is dangerous as it could cause further swelling and completely obstruct the airway. It is important to anticipate immediate intubation and prepare for cricothyrotomy as insertion of an endotracheal tube may not be possible. Patients with an airway obstruction often have extreme anxiety and placement of a non-rebreather mask may worsen it. Although SpO_2 measurement is helpful and may be done simultaneously with other interventions, the priority is airway securement.
144. A 94-year-old man with terminal lung cancer and advanced dementia presents to the emergency department via ambulance. He requires emergent rapid sequence intubation. During the handoff, the EMT states that he believes the patient is a DNR patient. The team should a. Provide comfort measures to the patient b. Intubate the patient c. Start attempting to call the patient's power of attorney (POA) to clarify code status d. Ask the patient if he'd like to be intubated	*Answer: b* If a patient requires lifesaving intervention and the code status is unclear, the team should proceed with the measure until clarification can be made. The emergency nurse should not use information the EMT "believes" until information can be verified.
145. A 46-year-old patient is diagnosed with pertussis and is being discharged. Further teaching is needed when the patient states a. "I will need to make sure my family also takes the prescribed antibiotics" b. "I should get the Tdap vaccination every 10 years" c. "The antibiotics will help me to feel better in a few days" d. "I can expect to have this cough for 2 to 3 months"	*Answer: c* Pertussis is an infection that more often affects adolescents and adults as immunization duration decreases. Antibiotic use does not shorten the course of the illness, which typically lasts 2 to 3 months, but will reduce the spread to others. Those in close contact should also complete a course of antibiotics to reduce the spread of the illness. It is important to teach patients the importance of vaccination every 10 years to ensure immunity.
146. A 56-year-old female patient who has history of lung cancer and metastasis to the bone arrives to the emergency department via EMS, with severe shortness of breath and chest pain. She is pale, and her vital signs are T-98.6°F (37.0°C) oral; P-110; R-34, BP-78/54; SpO_2-82% on room air. She is alert, and has an increased work of breathing. Physical assessment reveals bilateral clear lung sounds on auscultation and heart sounds are muffled. Based on her history and current symptoms, what condition and type of shock do her symptoms suggest? a. Severe sepsis and distributive shock b. Anaphylaxis and distributive shock c. Tension pneumothorax and obstructive shock d. Pericardial tamponade and obstructive shock	*Answer: d* Two common signs of pericardial tamponade are chest pain and dyspnea, and the most common cause is a malignancy. Auscultating heart sounds through the fluid surrounding the heart creates the muffled sounds that are heard. An abnormal temperature and infection usually accompany septic shock whereas muffled heart tones are not part of the clinical presentation for septic shock. Urticaria, angioedema, and respiratory stridor are classic symptoms in anaphylactic shock, and she is not presenting with these. She does not have unilateral decreased breath sounds with auscultation. This sign is classic for a tension pneumothorax.

Question	Rationale
147. Family members bring their elderly mother to the emergency department for decreased mental status and refusal to eat. They mention their mother was discharged from the hospital two weeks prior following treatment for pneumonia. The patient's vital signs are T-95.6°F (35.3°C); P-56; R-12; BP-96/56; SpO₂ 94% on room air. Following airway management, the priority intervention is a. Hypertonic saline b. Active or Passive rewarming c. Thyroid hormone replacement d. Antibiotics	*Answer: c* Frequently preceded by infectious illness, myxedema coma symptoms include bradycardia, hypotension, hypothermia, and decreased respiratory effort. Treatment priority for this life-threatening disease is airway management followed by replacement of thyroid hormone. While passive rewarming is recommended, active rewarming may increase vasodilation causing further hypotension. Hypertonic saline and antibiotics are not indicated from the information in the scenario.
148. A patient is brought in by ambulance with aphasia and right-sided weakness. The stroke protocol was activated in the field. EMS states the patient lives alone, and had been seen working in her garden 2 hours prior to the 911 call. The patient can follow commands but only repeat the words "no, not." Her right-sided hand grasps are significantly weaker than her left, and she has some moderate right-sided arm drift. She cannot hold her right leg up against gravity at all. The doctor is in the room on patient arrival and listens to the EMS report. The doctor asks the paramedic, "Did you check a blood sugar?" Why was this question asked? a. Hypertension and diabetes increase the risk for stroke b. High blood sugar can inhibit the effectiveness of alteplase (tPA) c. Hypoglycemia can mimic stroke symptoms, but is easily reversible d. Hyperglycemia can increase the chances of hemorrhagic stroke	*Answer: c* Low blood sugar should be checked on patients presenting with altered mental status including symptoms associated with stroke. While a history of hypertension and diabetes are risk factors for stroke, reducing potential stroke mimics, such as hypoglycemia is a more immediate priority.
149. A 46-year-old patient comes to the emergency department with complaints of a "stomachache." She said the pain began about 12 hours prior to arrival and she suspects the cause as "some vegetables I ate." Vital signs are within normal limits and she ambulates without difficulty from triage to her room. Shortly after arrival, she has a black tarry stool in the bedside commode. What test does the nurse anticipate for a stool specimen? a. Hemoglobin and Hematocrit b. Orthostatic vital signs c. Fecal occult blood test d. Stool sample of ova and parasites	*Answer: c* A "pseudomelena" can occur as a result of ingesting certain substances such as iron, beets, licorice, bismuth, and charcoal. The stool may look "tarry" and black but testing for occult blood will be negative. Measuring the hemoglobin and hematocrit may be deferred until GI bleeding is confirmed. Orthostatic vital signs may be helpful if she were complaining of dizziness and weakness while ambulating. Stool for ova and parasites should be tested if an infectious process or ingestion of contaminated food or water is suspected.

Question	Rationale
150. A 72-year-old male arrives to the ED via EMS following flu-like symptoms with fever for the past five days. He is talking but confused. His vital signs are T-102°F (38.9°C); P-112, R-20; BP-92/58; SpO_2-91% on room air. His urine is foul smelling. The emergency nurse anticipates the immediate interventions a. Assist with securing an airway with endotracheal intubation b. Obtain a clean catch urine specimen and other ordered labs c. Insert an indwelling Foley catheter and measure an accurate output d. Obtain IV access, labs and administer prescribed antibiotics following collection of blood cultures	*Answer: d* This patient's flu-like symptoms, fever and foul smelling urine suggest a urinary tract infection and possibly pyelonephritis. Pyelonephritis is a serious infection of the urinary tract that involves the kidney and renal structures. IV fluids and antibiotics are indicted. This patient is also exhibiting signs of possible sepsis with a fever, tachycardia and hypotension, warranting a set blood cultures before antibiotic administration. A clean catch urine specimen and other labs such as a CBC with differential and serum chemistries are also indicated; however, antibiotic administration is equally a high priority. Supplemental oxygen for his lower pulse oximetry may be needed; however, he is not exhibiting respiratory failure.

Index

Page references for figures are indicated by *f*, for tables by *t*, and for test boxes by *b*.

A

Abdomen
    acute, 106–107, 123*b*, 124*b*, 127*b*, 130*b*
    pain, 105, 105*f* (*See also* Gastrointestinal emergencies)
    physical assessment sequence, 123*b*
    rebound tenderness, 123*b*, 127*b*
    trauma, 119–121, 120*f*, 130*b*
    trauma, FAST evaluation, 120, 120*f*, 130*b*
Abducens nerve, 64*f*, 64*t*, 86*b*, 87*b*
Abnormal vaginal bleeding (AVB), 136
Abortion
    complete, 163*b*
    inevitable, 163*b*
    missed, 163*b*
    threatened/spontaneous, 143–144, 143*t*, 163*b*
AVPU scale, 63
Abrasions, 241–242, 242*f*
Abruptio placenta, 146–147, 147*f*, 161*b*, 162*b*
Abscess, 243, 250*b*
Abstinence, with STD, 159*b*
Abuse reporting, 287*b*, 288, 296*b*
Acetaminophen overdose, 267
Achilles tendon rupture, 241, 241*f*, 251*b*, 252*b*
Acid exposure, 265, 272*b*
Acidosis, respiratory, 60*b*
Acid reflux, 126*b*
Acoustic neuroma, 231*b*
Acrocyanosis, 159*b*
Activated charcoal, 275*b*
Acute abdomen, 106–107, 124*b*
    appendicitis, 106, 123*b*, 124*b*
    peritonitis, 106–107, 124*b*
    physical assessment, 123*b*
    rebound tenderness, 123*b*, 127*b*
    traumatic, 130*b*
Acute arterial obstruction, 22–23, 33*b*
Acute coronary syndrome (ACS), 5–9
    angina, 5, 26*b*, 31*b* (*See also* Angina)
    aortic aneurysm, 8–9, 27*b*, 29*b*
    aortic dissection, 9, 27*b*, 29*b*
    cardiopulmonary arrest, 9–10, 30*b*
    dysrhythmias, 10–19, 26*b*–28*b*, 30*b*–32*b*
    non-ST-segment elevation, 5, 6–7, 26*b*, 31*b*, 35*b*
    ST-segment elevation, 5, 7–8, 7*t*, 26*b*, 31*b*, 34*b*, 35*b*
Acute kidney injury (AKI), 191–192, 205*b*
Acute myocardial infarction (AMI), 28*b*
Acute otitis externa (AOE), 217
Acute otitis media (AOM), 217–218
    tympanic membrane, 230*b*
Acute radiation syndrome (ARS), 259–260
Acute renal failure (ARF), 191–192, 205*b*
Acute respiratory distress syndrome (ARDS), 47, 48–49, 103*b*
Addison's disease, 186
Adrenal crisis, 186, 204*b*
Adrenal disorders, 186
Adrenal insufficiency, 186
Advance directions, 282–283
Afterload, increased, 91, 99*b*, 104*b*
Aggressive violent behavior, 165–166, 173*b*, 175*b*
AIDS, 191, 191*f*
Airborne precautions, 193
Airway
    obstruction, 45, 45*f*, 58*b*
    upper, 45, 45*f* (*See also* Respiratory emergencies)
Alcoholic cirrhosis, 111–112, 112*f*, 127*b*
Alcohol use and abuse, 268–269
Alkalis, 265
Alkalosis, respiratory, 60*b*
    noncompensated, 54*b*
Allergic reactions, 179–180, 179*f*, 202*b*
Alpha radiation, 259, 276*b*
Alternating current electrical injuries, 254
Alzheimer's disease, 64–65
Ammonium hydroxide, 265
Amperes (amps), 254
Amphetamine abuse, 270
Amputation, 235–236, 248*b*, 249*b*
    guillotine-style, 249*b*
    stump care, 249*b*
Anaphylactic shock (anaphylaxis), 94–95, 95*f*, 99*b*, 179–180, 179*f*, 202*b*, 209*b*
    children, allergic, 101*b*
    epinephrine, 95, 101*b*, 102*b*
Anemia, 180, 202*b*
Aneurysm, aortic, 8–9, 27*b*, 29*b*
Angina
    Prinzmetal, 5, 26*b*
    stable, 26*b*, 31*b*
    unstable, 5, 26*b*, 31*b*
Angioedema, 58*b*, 179–180, 179*f*, 209*b*
    after smoke inhalation, arterial blood gas, 60*b*
    children, allergic, 101*b*
Anisocoria, 82*b*
Anosmia, 231*b*
Antidiuretic hormone (ADH), 183
Anxiety, 166–167
Aortic aneurysm, 8–9, 27*b*, 29*b*
Aortic dissection, 9, 27*b*, 29*b*
APGAR criteria, 152, 152*t*
Aphasia
    Broca's, 71, 80*b*
    Wernicke's, 71, 80*b*

Appendicitis, 106, 124*b*
　McBurney's point, 106, 123*b*
　rebound tenderness, 123*b*
Appendix, perforated, 124*b*
Aquatic organism envenomation, 256–257, 256*f*, 276*b*
Arterial blood gas (ABG), 102*b*
　interpretation, 52*t*, 60*b*
Aspiration, 37–38, 55*b*
　prevention, after endotracheal intubation, 60*b*
Aspiration pneumonia, near-drowning, 274*b*
Aspirin overdose, 267
Asthma, 38–39
　adverse drug effects, 62*b*
　emergencies, 60*b*
　exercise, 55*b*
　severe, 56*b*
　spacer, 55*b*
Asystole, 19, 30*b*, 32*b*
Atrial fibrillation, 13–14, 13*f*, 30*b*, 32*b*
Atrial flutter, 13, 13*f*
Atrioventricular (AV) block, 14–16
　first degree, 14–15, 15*f*, 27*b*
　second degree, type I, 15, 15*f*, 27*b*
　second degree, type II, 15–16, 15*f*, 27*b*, 32*b*
　third degree, 16, 16*f*, 27*b*
Autonomic dysreflexia (hyperreflexia), 77–78, 81*b*
AVPU scale, 63

B

Babinski reflex, 64
Back pain, 239–240
Bacterial endocarditis, 19–20, 20*f*, 31*b*, 35*b*
Bacterial vaginosis (BV), 140*t*–141*t*
Bag-valve mask, 54*b*
Banana bag, 206*b*
Bariatric surgery, postoperative risks, 206*b*
Barrett's esophagus, 110
Basilar skull fracture, 74–75, 74*f*
　Battle sign, 74, 74*f*, 87*b*
　periorbital ecchymosis, 74, 75*f*, 87*b*
Bath salts, 270–271, 275*b*
Battle sign, 74, 74*f*, 87*b*
Becks triad, 100*b*, 101*b*, 125*b*
Bee envenomation, 256
Bell-clapper deformity, 134, 134*f*
Bell's palsy, 55*b*, 214, 231*b*, 233*b*
Benign prostatic hypertrophy (BPH), 136
Beta blocker overdose, 268
Beta radiation, 259
$β_2$-transferrin, CSF, 75, 85*b*
Bigeminy, 17, 17*f*
Bi-pap, 40, 40*f*, 54*b*, 57*b*
Bipolar disorder, 167–168
　depression, 168, 177*b*
　mania, 173*b*, 176*b*
Bites, 242–243, 250*b*
Bladder trauma, 135, 158*b*
Blast injuries, 247
Blood dyscrasias, 180–181, 202*b*
　anemia, 180, 202*b*
　hemophilia, 181, 202*b*
　leukemia, 181
　thrombocytopenia purpura, 180–181, 180*f*
Blunt cardiac trauma, 24–25, 27*b*, 29*b*, 33*b*
Boarding, patient, 286–287
Bowel obstructions, 118–119, 118*t*, 129*b*
Bowel sounds, 123*b*, 129*b*
Bradycardia, sinus, 10, 10*f*, 31*b*, 32*b*
BRAT diet, 129*b*

Broca's aphasia, 71, 80*b*
Bronchitis, 41, 56*b*
Brown-Sequard syndrome, 75, 87*b*
Brudzinski sign, 69
Burns, 253–254, 253*f*, 254*f*, 272*b*
　fluid replacement, 253, 276*b*
　hypovolemic shock, 99*b*
　ocular chemical, 226, 229*b*, 234*b*
　rule of nines, 272*b*
Bursitis, 239, 252*b*

C

Calcaneus fracture, 251*b*
Calcium channel blocker overdose, 268
Calcium hydroxide, 265
Calcium imbalance, 184–185, 204*b*, 207*b*
Calculi, renal, 133–134, 157*b*
Candida albicans, 126*b*
Capnography, 52, 52*f*
　shark fin waves, 52, 61*b*
Carbon monoxide, 265–266, 274*b*
Cardiac tamponade, 21–22, 26*b*, 27*b*
　pericardial, 92, 92*f*, 99*b*, 100*b*
Cardiac trauma, blunt, 24–25, 27*b*, 29*b*, 33*b*
Cardiogenic shock, 61*b*, 91–92, 101*b*, 102*b*
　vasopressors, 91, 99*b*
Cardiopulmonary arrest, 9–10, 30*b*
Cardiopulmonary resuscitation (CPR), 9–10, 32*b*
Cardiovascular emergencies, 5–35
　acute coronary syndrome, 5–9, 26*b*–32*b*, 34*b*–35*b*
　cardiac tamponade, 21–22, 26*b*, 27*b*
　dysrhythmias, 10–19, 26*b*–28*b*, 30*b*–32*b*
　hypertension, 21, 33*b*
　infective endocarditis, 19–20, 20*f*, 31*b*, 35*b*
　pericarditis, 22, 26*b*, 35*b*
　peripheral vascular disease, 22–24, 23*f*, 28*b*, 31*b*, 33*b*
　trauma, blunt cardiac, 24–25, 27*b*, 29*b*, 33*b*
Caries, dental, 213
Cat bites, 242–243, 250*b*
Cathinones, synthetic, 270–271, 275*b*
Cauda equina syndrome, 75, 87*b*
Cavity, dental, 213
Central cord syndrome, 75, 87*b*
CEN prep quiz, 297–337
　answers, 338
Central retinal artery occlusion, 224–225, 228*b*
Cerebral perfusion pressure (CPP), 67
Cerebrospinal fluid (CSF)
　$β_2$-transferrin, 75, 85*b*
　glucose test, 75, 85*b*
　halo sign, 75, 85*b*
Certification, CEN
CEN prep quiz, 297–337
CEN prep quiz, answers, 338
　rationale, 1
　test preparation, 2–3, 4*t*
Chancroid, 140*t*–141*t*
Charcoal, activated, 275*b*
Chemical burns, ocular, 226, 229*b*, 234*b*
Chest compressions, neonatal resuscitation, 153
Chest wall trauma, 50, 50*f*, 59*b*
Chicken pox, 196–197, 197*f*, 209*b*
Childhood diseases, 193–199
　chicken pox, 196–197, 197*f*, 209*b*
　diphtheria, 198–199
　fever, 188–189, 190*t*, 206*b*
　herpes zoster, 197–198, 197*f*, 209*b*
　measles, 193–194, 194*f*, 208*b*
　mumps, 194–195, 194*f*, 207*b*

pertussis, 195–196, 196f
respiratory emergencies, 37
Chlamydia, 140t–141t
Cholangitis, 111
Cholecystitis, 111, 111f
Cholelithiasis, 111, 111f, 124b
pancreatitis, 130b
Chronic kidney disease (CKD), 191–192
Chronic obstructive pulmonary disease (COPD), 39–40, 40f, 56b, 61b
Chronic venous insufficiency (CVI), 23–24, 23f, 33b
Chvostek sign, 184
Cigarette smoking, Prinzmetal angina, 5, 26b
Cincinnati Prehospital Stroke Scale (CPSS), 71, 87b
Cirrhosis, 111–112, 112f, 127b
Clavicle fractures, 50
Clostridium difficile infection (CDI), 193, 208b
Clostridium perfringens, 126b
Clotting
Factor V Leiden, 93, 100b
thromboelastography, 97, 103b
Cluster headaches, 67, 81b
Cocaine abuse, 269–270, 275b
Coffee ground emesis, 124b
Cognitive impairment, vascular, 65
Cold-related emergencies, 261–262, 262f, 263f, 274b, 275b
Colonoscopy, perforated ulcer, 124b
Communicable diseases, 193–200
childhood diseases, 193–199, 194f, 196f, 197f, 207b–209b (See also Childhood diseases)
Clostridium difficile, 193, 208b
isolation precautions, 193
multi-drug resistant organisms, 199–200 (See also Multi-drug resistant organisms (MDROs))
Compartment syndrome, 236, 236f, 248b, 252b
Complete abortion, 163b
Complete cord injuries, 75–76
Complete heart block, 16, 16f, 27b
Concussion, 73
Conjunctivitis, 223–224
Consciousness
level, 63, 86b, 89b
loss of, 89b
Consent, informed, 288
Constipation, 123b
Contact lens
care, 223
dry, itchy eyes, 229b
Contact lens infections
conjunctivitis, 223–224
keratitis, 224, 230b
Contact precautions, 193
Contamination, radiation, 259b
Contralateral, 64
Contusions, 236–237, 249b
Coral snakes, 255–256
Cord syndrome, 75, 87b
Corneal abrasion/laceration, 225
Coronary artery disease (CAD), vomiting, 125b
Costochondritis, 237, 249b
Costovertebral angle (CVA) pain
pyelonephritis, 132
renal trauma, 135, 158b
Cranial nerves, 64, 64f, 64t, 86b, 87b
Cricothyrotomy, 58b
Critical Incident Stress Management (CISM) system, 279
Crohn's disease (CD), 116–117, 117t, 129b
Croup, 40–41, 54b
Crystal methamphetamine (crystal meth), 260
Cullen's sign, 120, 120f

Cultural considerations, 287
Cushing's triad, 68, 83b, 88b
Cyanide, 266, 277b
Cyclopegics, 224, 230b
Cyst, ovarian, 139, 158b
Cysticercosis, 258, 276b
Cystitis, 131–132, 162b
rebound tenderness, 123b

D

Damage control resuscitation, 97, 103b
Debridement, 249b
Debriefing, 293b
Decerebrate posturing, 63, 64
Decision making, 288
Decorticate posturing, 63, 64
Deep tendon reflexes, 63
Deep vein thrombosis (DVT), 24, 28b, 33b, 251b
obstructive shock, 93–94, 102b (See also Obstructive shock)
pulmonary embolus, 47–48, 55b, 58b, 93–94, 100b
Dehydration, 182–183, 203b, 204b
Delegation of tasks to assistive personnel, 288
Delivery, emergent, 148–153
APGAR criteria, 152, 152t
meconium aspiration, 152
placenta accreta, 152, 160b
placenta delivery, 152
umbilical cord prolapse, 152–153
Dementia
Alzheimer's, 64–65
vascular, 65
Dental caries, 213
Dental conditions and abscesses, 212–213, 230b
periapical abscess, 213, 228b
periodontal abscess, 213
post tooth extraction, 212–213
pulpitis, 212
Dental emergencies, 212–213, 230b
periapical abscess, 213, 228b
periodontal abscess, 213
post tooth extraction, 212–213
pulpitis, 212
Depression, 168
bipolar disorder, 168, 177b
Detached retina, 226, 228b
Diabetes insipidus (DI), hypernatremia, 184
Diabetic ketoacidosis (DKA)
hyperglycemia, 186–187, 187t
hypovolemic shock, 103b, 205b
rehydration, 205b
Diaphragm injuries, 50
rupture, 60b
Diffuse axonal injury (DAI), 73–74
Diphtheria, 198–199
Direct current electrical injuries, 254
Disaster management, 288–289, 289f, 295b
Discharge planning, 282, 296b
Dislocation, 237–238
shoulder, 248b, 251b
temporomandibular joint, 219–220
Disseminated intravascular coagulation (DIC), 103b, 182, 203b
abruptio placenta, 146
Distributive shock, 94–96
anaphylactic, 94–95, 95f, 99b, 101b
neurogenic, 77, 87b, 94, 99b, 101b
septic, 95–96, 95f, 157b, 192
Diverticula, 114
Diverticulitis, 114, 124b
Diverticulosis, 114

DNR, 283, 294b
Domestic abuse reporting, 287b, 288, 296b
Donation, organ and tissue, 282
Droplet precautions, 193
Drug interactions, 266
Duodenal ulcers, 109–110, 110f, 124b
Dysfunctional uterine bleeding (DUB), 136
Dysrhythmias, 10–19
   asystole, 19, 30b, 32b
   atrial fibrillation, 13–14, 13f, 30b, 32b
   atrial flutter, 13, 13f
   atrioventricular block, 14–16, 15f, 27b, 32b
     (See also Atrioventricular (AV) block)
   idioventricular rhythm, 16–17, 16f, 32b
   junctional rhythm, 14, 14f, 32b
   premature atrial contractions, 12, 12f
   premature junctional contractions, 14
   premature ventricular contractions, 17, 17f, 30b
   sinus arrhythmia, 11, 11f
   sinus bradycardia, 10, 10f, 31b, 32b
   sinus pause/arrest, 12–13, 12f, 28b
   sinus tachycardia, 10–11, 11f, 26b, 33b
   supraventricular tachycardia, 11–12, 11f, 26b, 28b
   ventricular fibrillation, 18–19, 18f, 26b, 30b
   ventricular tachycardia, 17–18, 17f, 27b

E

Eclampsia, 147–148
Ectopic pregnancies, 144–145, 144f
Effusion, joint, 239
Egophonia, 234b
Egophony, 55b
Eighth cranial nerve, 231b
Electrical injuries, 254
Electrolyte imbalance, 183–186
   calcium, 184–185, 204b, 207b
   potassium, 185–186, 202b, 204b, 206b
   sodium, 183–184
Embolus
   fat, long bone fracture, 250b
   pulmonary, 47–48, 55b, 58b, 93–94, 100b
   venous thromboembolism, 24, 28b, 33b, 93–94
Emergency triage, 290, 296b
Emergent delivery, 148–153
Emesis, coffee ground, 124b
EMTALA, 285, 289–290, 294b, 295b, 296b
Endocarditis, infective, 19–20, 20f, 31b, 35b
Endocrine conditions, 186–188
   adrenal, 186, 204b
   glucose-related, 186–187, 187t, 205b
   thyroid disorders, 187–188, 188f, 205b, 207b
End-of-life issues, 282–283, 294b
Endolymphatic hydrops, 219
Endoscopy, emergent, 115t, 127b
Endotracheal intubation, 54b, 57b, 59b
   complications, 59b
   gastric tube placement, 59b
   neonatal resuscitation, 153
Envenomation, 254–257
   aquatic organisms, 256–257, 256f, 276b
   bee, hornet, and wasp stings, 256
   snakes, 255–256, 255f, 273b
Environmental emergencies, 253–264
   acute radiation syndrome, 259–260
   burns, 253–254, 253f, 254f
   cold-related emergencies, 261–262, 262f, 263f, 274b, 275b
   electrical injuries, 254
   heat-related emergencies, 260–261, 274b
   insecticides, 257
   organophosphates, 257, 272b, 273b, 277b
   parasite infestations, 257–258, 276b
   rabies, 264
   radiation and hazardous material, 259–260, 273b
   submersion injury, 260, 274b
   toxic plant exposure, 258–259
   vector-borne illnesses, 263–264
Eosinophilic esophagitis (EE), 110–111
Epididymitis, 132, 163b
Epidural hemorrhage, 74, 80b
Epiglottitis, 41–42, 42f, 216–217, 216f, 233b
Epinephrine, anaphylactic shock, 95, 101b, 102b
Epistaxis, 213–214, 213f, 228b
Error prevention techniques, 284, 284f
Erythema migrans, Lyme disease, 264, 264f
Esophageal foreign bodies, 115, 115t, 128b, 232b
Esophageal varices, 113–114
Esophagitis, 110–111, 126b
Essential hypertension, 21, 33b
Ethical dilemmas, 279–280, 291b, 293b
Evidence-based practice (EBP), 280, 280f
Evidence Hierarchy, 281, 282f
Exercise
   asthma, 55b
   pulmonary embolus, 55b
Exophthalmos, 188, 188f
Expressive aphasia, 71, 80b
Extracellular fluid (ECF), 182
Extraocular movements, 221f
Eye
   anatomy, internal, 221f, 228b
   assessment, 221–223, 222f, 223f
   diagnostics and interventions, 223
   evaluation, 223
   extraocular movements, 221f
Eye drop administration, 223, 229b
Eye emergencies. See Ocular emergencies
Eye patch, 223
Eye shield, 223

F

Facial nerve disorders, 214–215
   Bell's palsy, 55b, 214, 231b, 233b
   trigeminal neuralgia, 214–215, 231b
Facial nerve palsy, 214
Factor V, 100b
Factor V deficiency, 100b
Factor VIII deficiency, 181
Factor V Leiden, 93, 100b
Factor XI deficiency, 181
Family presence, resuscitation, 283, 294b
FAST evaluation
   abdominal trauma, 120, 120f, 130b
   respiratory emergencies, 59b
   stroke, 72
Fat embolism, long bone fracture, 250b
Febrile seizures, 70–71, 81b, 189
Federal regulations, 289–290
Fever, 188–189, 190t, 206b
Fibrillation
   atrial, 13–14, 13f, 30b, 32b
   ventricular, 18–19, 18f, 26b, 30b
Fifth cranial nerve, trigeminal neuralgia, 214–215, 231b
Fire exposure
   ABG values, 60b
   endotracheal intubation, 57b
Flaccid, 63
Flail chest, 50, 50f
Flank ecchymosis, 120, 120f, 125b

Flatworms, 258
Fluid imbalance, 182–183
   dehydration and hypovolemia, 182–183, 203b, 204b
   principles, 182
Flutter, atrial, 13, 13f
Focal seizures, 70–71
Foreign bodies
   esophageal, 115, 115t, 128b, 232b
   genitourinary, 143
   gynecological, 137, 158b
   laryngeal, 215, 232b
   otic, 215
   rectal, 115–116
   vegetative, 248b
   wooden, 248b
Forensic evidence collection, 283, 294b
FOUR score, 73
Four Topics Chart, 279, 291b, 293b
Fractures, 238–239, 238f, 249b
   calcaneus, 251b
   knee, 250b
   long bone, 250b
Fragile X syndrome, 100b
Frostbite, 262, 263f, 274b

G

Gallstones, 111, 111f, 130b
Gamma radiation, 259
Gases, toxic, 253
Gastric lavage, 127b
Gastric ulcers, 109–110, 124b
Gastritis, 109, 126b
Gastroenteritis, 116, 126b, 129b
Gastroesophageal reflux disease (GERD), 110–111, 124b, 126b
Gastrointestinal bleeding, 124b
   lower, 108–109, 123b, 124b
   upper, 107–108, 108t, 124b
Gastrointestinal emergencies, 105–121
   abdominal pain, 105, 105f
   abdominal trauma, 119–121, 120f
   acute abdomen, 106–107
   appendicitis, 106, 123b, 124b
   Barrett's esophagus, 110
   bowel obstruction, 118–119, 118t, 129b
   cholecystitis, 111, 111f
   cirrhosis, 111–112, 112f
   diverticulitis, 114, 124b
   esophageal varices, 113–114
   esophagitis, 110–111, 126b
   foreign bodies, esophageal, 115, 115t, 128b
   foreign bodies, rectal, 115–116
   gastritis, 109, 126b
   gastroenteritis, 116, 126b, 129b
   GI bleeding, lower, 108–109, 123b, 124b
   GI bleeding, upper, 107–108, 108t, 124b
   hepatitis, 112–113, 113t, 127b–128b
   hernias, 116
   inflammatory bowel disease, 116–117, 117t, 129b
   intussusception, 117–118
   pancreatitis, 119, 130b
   peritonitis, 106–107, 124b
   ulcers, 109–110, 109b, 110f, 124b
Generalized seizures, 70–71, 86b
Genital herpes, 140t–141t
Genitourinary emergencies, 131–136
   cystitis, 131–132, 162b
   epididymitis, 132, 163b
   foreign bodies, 143
   infection, 131–133
   orchitis, 132–133
   priapism, 87b, 133, 158b
   pyelonephritis, 132
   renal calculi, 133–134, 157b
   testicular torsion, 134, 134f
   trauma, bladder, 135
   trauma, renal, 135, 158b
   trauma, ureters, 135
   trauma, urethral, 136, 161b
   urinary retention, 136
   UTI, 131
Genitourinary infection, 131–133
   cystitis, 131–132, 162b
   epididymitis, 132, 163b
   orchitis, 132–133
   pyelonephritis, 132
   UTI, 131
Geriatrics, respiratory emergencies, 37
Giant cell arteritis, 67
Giardiasis (Giardia infection), 258, 273b
Ginseng, epistaxis, 213–214, 213f, 228b
Glasgow Coma Scale (GCS), 63, 63t, 85b
Glaucoma, 224, 228b
Globe rupture, 225, 230b
Glucose-related endocrine conditions, 186–187, 187t, 205b
Glucose test, CSF, 75, 85b
Gonorrhea, 140t–141t, 158b
Gout, 125b, 239, 251b, 252b
Grasp reflex, 64
Grey Turner sign, 120, 120f, 125b, 135, 158b
Guillain–Barré syndrome (GBS), 66, 80b, 88b
Gynecological emergencies, 136–142
   foreign bodies, 137, 158b
   infection, 138, 157b
   ovarian cyst, 139, 158b
   pelvic inflammatory disease, 138
   sexual assault or battery, 139–142, 159b–160b
   sexually transmitted disease, 139, 140t–141t, 158b
   trauma, 142
   vaginal bleeding, abnormal and dysfunctional, 136
   vaginal discharge, 138
   vaginal hemorrhage, 136–137
Gynecological infection, 138, 157b
   pelvic inflammatory disease, 138
   vaginal discharge, 138

H

Halitosis, 229b
Halo sign (test), CSF, 75, 85b
Handoffs of care, 285–286, 286t
Hazardous material exposure, 259–260
Headaches, 66–67
   cluster, 67, 81b
   migraine, 66–67
   temporal arteritis, 67
   worst, hemorrhagic stroke, 72, 84b
Head injury, blurry vision, 88b
Heart failure, 20–21, 32b. *See also* Cardiogenic shock
   cardiogenic pulmonary edema, 55b
   left-sided, 20, 29b
   vs. non-cardiogenic pulmonary edema, 58b
   right-sided, 20–21
Heat cramps, 260–261
Heat-related emergencies, 260–261, 274b
Heat stroke, 261, 274b
HEELP syndrome, 147–148
Helicobacter pylori, 109b, 126b
Helicobacter pylori ulcers, 109–110, 110f, 126b

Hematemesis, 124b
Hematochezia, 123b, 124b
Hemophilia, 181, 202b
Hemorrhage
   brain and meningeal, 74
   epidural, 74, 80b
   intracerebral, 74
   postpartum, 154
   subdural, 74, 86b
   vaginal, 136–137
Hemorrhagic shock, 96–97
Hemorrhagic stroke, 72, 84b
Hemothorax, 50
   FAST evaluation, 59b
   thoracotomy, emergency, 59b
Hepatitis, 112–113, 113t, 127b–128b
Hernias, 116
Herpes, genital, 140t–141t
Herpes zoster, 197–198, 197f, 209b
Herpes zoster ophthalmicus, 197–198
High altitude pulmonary edema (HAPE), 47
HIPAA, 287–288, 287t, 295b, 296b
HIV, 191, 191f
Homicidal ideation, 168–169, 174b, 176b
Hornet envenomation, 256
Hospital-acquired infection (HAI)
   methicillin-resistant Staphylococcus aureus, 199
   vancomycin-resistant enterococci, 199–200
Hospital Incident Command System (HICS), 289
Human papillomavirus (HPV), 140t–141t
Hydrocephalus, shunt dysfunctions, 68–69, 83b
Hydrofluoric acid, 265, 272b
Hypercalcemia, 185
Hypercoagulation, 100b, 101b
Hyperemesis gravidarum, 144, 161b
Hyperglycemia, 186–187, 187t
Hyperkalemia, 185–186, 204b
Hypernatremia, 184
Hyperosmolar hyperglycemia state (HHS), 186–187, 187t
Hypersplenism, 127b
Hypertension, 21, 33b
Hypertension, portal
   cirrhosis, 111
   esophageal varices, 113–114
   hypersplenism, 127b
Hypertensive crisis (emergency), 21, 34b
Hyperthermia, 260–261
Hyperthyroidism, 188, 188f, 205b, 207b
Hyphema, 225–226, 225f, 230b
Hypocalcemia, 184–185, 204b, 207b
Hypoglycemia, 186–187, 205b
   altered mental status and stroke, 84b, 86b
   stroke mimic, 84b, 85b
Hypokalemia, 185, 202b, 206b
Hyponatremia, 183–184
Hypothermia, 261–262, 262f
   severe, 275b
   submersion injury, 260, 274b
Hypothyroidism, 187–188, 205b
Hypovolemia, 182–183
Hypovolemic shock, 61b, 96–98, 99b, 101b, 103b
   burns, severe, 99b
   damage control resuscitation, 97, 103b
   diabetic ketoacidosis, 103b, 205b
   hemorrhagic, 96–97
   nonhemorrhagic, 97
Hypoxia, tissue, lactate, 102b
Hysterectomy, bowel obstruction, 129b

I

Ibuprofen, nephrotoxicity, 205b
Ibuprofen overdose, 267
Idiopathic thrombocytopenia purpura (ITP), 180–181
Idioventricular rhythm, 16–17, 16f, 32b
Ileus, paralytic, 118–119, 118t
Immunocompromised medical emergencies, 189–191, 206b
Incorporation, radiation, 259b
Inevitable abortion, 163b
Inflammatory bowel disease (IBD), 116–117, 117t, 129b
Influenza, 42
Informed consent, 288
Inhalation injuries, 44
Inhaler, spacer, 55b
INR (international normalized ratio), 102b
Insecticide exposure, 257
Intentional ingestions, 266–268, 275b
Interpretive services, 287
Intracellular fluid (ICF), 182
Intracerebral hemorrhage, 74
Intracranial pressure (ICP), increased, 89b
   Cushing's triad, 68, 83b, 88b
   mannitol, 83b
   shunt dysfunctions, 68–69, 83b
Intraocular pressure, increased, 233b
Intussusception, 117–118
Ipsilateral, 64
Iritis, 224
Ischemic stroke, 72
   transient ischemic attack, 71, 85b
Isolation precautions, 193

J

Jellyfish stings, 256–257, 256f, 276f
Joint effusion, 239
Junctional rhythm, 14, 14f, 32b
J wave, hypothermia, 262, 262f, 275b

K

Kehr's sign, 83b
Keratitis, 224, 230b
Kernig sign, 70
Kidney trauma, 135
Knee fracture, 250b

L

Labor, preterm, 145, 162b
Labyrinthitis, 218–219
Lactate, tissue hypoxia, 102b
Lantus, 205b
Laryngeal foreign body, 215, 232b
Laryngeal trauma, 221
Laryngotracheobronchitis, 40–41, 54b
Learning, lifelong, 280–281, 293b
LeFort fractures, 220–221, 220f, 230b, 233b
Left lower quadrant pain, 105f
Left-sided heart failure, 20, 29b
Left upper quadrant pain, 105f
Leukemia, 181
Level of consciousness, 63, 86b, 89b
Level of Evidence table, 281, 281f
Lifelong learning, 280–281, 293b
Ligament of Treitz, 124b
Listeria, 126b
Liver trauma, 130b
Localizing pain, 63
Long bone fracture, 250b

Loss of consciousness, 89*b*
Low back pain, 239–240
Lower GI bleeding, 108–109, 123*b*, 124*b*
Ludwig's angina, 217, 228*b*, 229*b*, 234*b*
Lumbar puncture, meningitis, 70
Lyme disease, 263–264, 264*f*

M

Malaria, 258
Mandatory reporting, 287–288, 287*t*
Mania, bipolar disorder, 173*b*, 176*b*
Mannitol, 83*b*
Marshall, Barry, 109*b*
Maxillofacial emergencies, 211–221
   abscesses, oral and pharyngeal, 211–212, 211*f*, 228*b*, 231*b*
   dental conditions and abscesses, 212–213, 228*b*, 230*b*
   epistaxis, 213–214, 213*f*, 228*b*
   facial nerve disorders, 55*b*, 214–215, 231*b*, 233*b*
   foreign bodies, 215, 232*b*
   Meniere's disease, 219
   temporomandibular joint dislocation, 219–220
   tympanic membrane rupture, 219, 230*b*
Maxillofacial infection, 215–219
   acute otitis externa, 217
   acute otitis media, 217–218, 230*b*
   epiglottitis, 41–42, 42*f*, 216–217, 216*f*, 233*b*
   labyrinthitis, 218–219
   Ludwig's angina, 217, 228*b*, 229*b*, 234*b*
   necrotizing ulcerative gingivitis, 216, 233*b*
   parotitis, 194–195, 194*f*, 215–216, 233*b*
   sinusitis, 218, 232*b*
Maxillofacial trauma
   laryngeal, 221
   LeFort fractures, 220–221, 220*f*, 230*b*, 233*b*
   zygomatic fractures, 220, 231*b*
McBurney's point, 106, 123*b*
Measles, 193–194, 194*f*, 208*b*
Meconium aspiration, 152
Medical emergencies, 179–192
   allergic reactions and anaphylaxis, 179–180, 179*f*, 202*b*, 209*b*
   blood dyscrasias, 180–181, 180*f*, 202*b*
   disseminated intravascular coagulation, 103*b*, 146, 182, 203*b*
   electrolyte imbalance, 183–186, 202*b*, 204*b*, 206*b*, 207*b*
   endocrine conditions, 186–188, 187*t*, 204*b*, 205*b*
   fever, 188–189, 190*t*, 206*b*
   fluid imbalance, 182–183, 203*b*, 204*b*
   HIV and AIDS, 191, 191*f*
   immunocompromise/oncological, 189–191, 206*b*
   renal failure, 191–192, 205*b*
   sepsis, 192
   sickle cell crisis, 181–182, 182*f*, 203*b*
Medical screening exam (MSE), 282, 285, 289, 294*b*, 296*b*
Melena, 124*b*
Meniere's disease, 219
Meninges, 69*b*
Meningitis, 69–70, 82*b*
   infants, 69, 88*b*
Mental status, altered, 86*b*
   hypoglycemia, 84*b*
Methamphetamine abuse, 260
Methicillin-resistant Staphylococcus aureus (MRSA), 199
Migraine headache, 66–67
Miotic agents, 230*b*, 233*b*
Missed abortion, 163*b*
Missile injuries, 243–244
Mobitz atrioventricular block, 15–16, 15*f*, 27*b*
Monro-Kellie doctrine, 67
Morning sickness, 144, 161*b*

Motor assessment, 63–64
MRSA, 199
Muffled heart tones, 21, 26*b*, 27*b*, 92
   Becks triad, 100*b*, 101*b*, 125*b*
Multi-drug resistant organisms (MDROs), 199–200
   MRSA, 199
   tuberculosis, 200
   vancomycin-resistant enterococci, 199–200
Multiple sclerosis (MS), 65
Mumps, 194–195, 194*f*, 207*b*
   orchitis, 132–133
   parotitis, 194–195, 194*f*, 215–216, 233*b*
Murphy's sign, 111
Myasthenia gravis, 65
Mydriatic agents, 230*b*
Myocardial infarction (MI)
   acute, 28*b*
   inferior wall, 34*b*
Myxedema coma, 187–188, 205*b*, 207*b*

N

Naloxone, 269
Nasal arterial blood supply, 213, 213*f*
National Incident Management System (NIMS), 289
National Institutes of Health Stroke Scale (NIHSS), 72
National Response Framework (NRF), 289
Near-drowning, aspiration pneumonia, 274*b*
Necrotizing ulcerative gingivitis (NUG), 216, 233*b*
Neglect, 165, 174*b*
Neonatal resuscitation, 153–154, 159*b*
Nerve agents, 257
Neurogenic shock, 77, 87*b*, 94, 99*b*, 101*b*
Neurological assessment, 63
Neurological emergencies, 63–89
   AVPU scale, 63
   Alzheimer's disease, 64–65
   blurry vision, after head injury, 88*b*
   chronic neurological disorders, 65–66
   consciousness, level, 63, 86*b*, 89*b*
   cranial nerves and functions, 64, 64*f*, 64*t*, 86*b*, 87*b*
   Glasgow Coma scale, 63, 63*t*, 85*b*
   Guillain–Barré syndrome, 66, 80*b*, 88*b*
   headaches, 66–67
   intracranial pressure, 67–68, 68*t*, 83*b*
   meningitis, 69–70, 82*b*, 88*b*
   motor and sensory assessment, 63–64
   multiple sclerosis, 65
   myasthenia gravis, 65
   Parkinson's disease, 66
   seizure disorders, 70–71, 84*b*, 86*b*
   shunt dysfunctions, 68–69, 83*b*
   spinal cord injuries, 75–78, 87*b*
   stroke, 71–73, 82*b*
   trauma, 73–75, 74*f*
   vascular dementia, 65
Neurologic trauma, 73–75
   assessment/analysis, general, 73
   basilar skull fracture, 74–75, 74*f*
   concussion, 73
   diffuse axonal injury, 73–74
   hemorrhage, 74
Neutropenia, 189, 206*b*
Nitrates, PDE5 inhibitors and, 34*b*
Non-invasive pressure support ventilation (NPPV), 54*b*, 57*b*
Non-rebreather mask, 54*b*
Nonsteroidal anti-inflammatory drugs (NSAIDs), 126*b*
   overdose, 267

Non-ST-segment elevation (NSTEMI) acute coronary syndrome, 5, 6–7, 26b, 31b, 35b
Norovirus, 116

O

Obstetrical emergencies, 143–155
　abruptio placenta, 146–147, 147f, 161b, 162b
　APGAR criteria, 152, 152t
　ectopic pregnancies, 144–145, 144f
　emergent delivery, 148–153
　hyperemesis gravidarum, 144, 161b
　meconium aspiration, 152
　neonatal resuscitation, 153–154
　placenta accreta, 152, 160b
　placenta delivery, 152
　placenta previa, 145–146, 146f, 161b
　postpartum hemorrhage, 154
　postpartum infection, 154–155
　preeclampsia, eclampsia, and HEELP syndrome, 147–148, 162b
　preterm labor, 145, 162b
　threatened/spontaneous abortion, 143–144, 143t, 163b
　trauma, 148, 150t–151t
　umbilical cord prolapse, 152–153
Obstruction. *See specific types*
Obstructive shock, 92–94, 102b
　deep vein thrombosis, 93–94, 102b
　pericardial tamponade, 92, 92f, 99b, 100b
　pulmonary embolus, 47–48, 55b, 58b, 93–94, 100b
　tension pneumothorax, 49–50, 49f, 54b, 58b, 61b, 92–93, 99b, 100b, 102b, 104b
Ocular emergencies, 221–226
　assessment, 221–223, 222f, 223f
　cycloplegics, 230b
　diagnostics and interventions, 223
　evaluation, 223
　extraocular movements, 221, 221f
　eye anatomy, internal, 221f, 228b
　miotic agents, 230b
Ocular medical conditions, 223–225
　central retinal artery occlusion, 224–225, 228b
　conjunctivitis, 223–224
　glaucoma, 224, 228b
　keratitis, 224, 230b
　uveitis/iritis, 224, 229b, 232b
Ocular pressure, preventing, 223
Ocular trauma
　chemical burns, 226, 229b, 234b
　corneal abrasion/laceration, 225
　globe rupture, 225, 230b
　hyphema, 225–226, 225f, 230b
　penetrating injury, 230b
　retinal detachment, 226, 228b
Oculomotor nerve, 64f, 64t, 86b, 87b
Odynophagia, 229b
Olfactory nerve, 231b
Oncological emergencies, 189–191
Open pneumothorax, 50, 56b
Opiate abuse, 269
Optic nerve, 64f, 64t, 86b, 87b, 231b
Oral abscess, 211–212
　peritonsillar, 211, 211f, 228b, 231b
　retropharyngeal, 211–212, 231b
Orchitis, 132–133
Organ donation, 282
Organophosphate exposure, 257, 272b, 273b, 277b
Orthopedic emergencies, 235–241
　Achilles tendon rupture, 241, 241f, 251b, 252b
　amputation, 235–236, 248b, 249b
　bursitis, 239, 252b
　compartment syndrome, 236, 236f, 248b, 252b
　contusions, 236–237, 249b
　costochondritis, 237, 249b
　dislocations, 237–238, 248b, 251b
　fractures, 238–239, 238f, 249b, 250b
　gout and pseudogout, 125b, 239, 251b, 252b
　joint effusion, 239
　low back pain, 239–240
　osteomyelitis, 240
　strains and sprains, 240–241, 249b, 250b
Osborn wave, hypothermia, 262, 262f, 275b
Osler nodes, 20, 20f, 35b
Osteomyelitis, 240
Otalgia, 229b
Otic foreign body, 215
Ovarian cyst, 139, 158b
Overdose, 266–268, 275b

P

Pain
　localizing, 63
　management, 283–284, 295b
Palliative care, 283
Palmar erythema, alcoholic cirrhosis, 112, 112f, 127b
Pancreatitis, 119
　cholelithiasis, 130b
Panic attacks, 166–167, 174b
Paralytic ileus, 118–119, 118t
Parasite infestations, 257–258
Paresis, 64
Parkinson's disease, 66
Parotitis, 194–195, 194f, 215–216, 233b
Patient boarding, 286–287
Patient perception, 293b
Patient safety, 284, 284f
Patient satisfaction, 284–285
Pelvic inflammatory disease (PID), 138
Penetrating injuries, 243–244
Penile fracture, 136
Peptic ulcer disease (PUD), 109–110, 110f, 124b
　Helicobacter pylori, 109
Perception, patient, 293b
Performance improvement, 290
Periapical abscess, 213, 228b
Pericardial effusion, 92
Pericardial tamponade, 92, 92f, 99b, 100b
Pericarditis, 22, 26b, 35b
Pericardium, 92
Periodontal abscess, 213
Periodontitis, 213
Periorbital ecchymosis, 74, 75f, 87b
Peripheral artery disease (PAD), 23
Peripheral vascular disease, 22–24
　acute arterial obstruction, 22–23, 33b
　chronic venous insufficiency, 23–24, 23f, 33b
　peripheral artery disease, 23
　Raynaud's disease, 23, 31b, 33b
　venous thromboembolism, 24, 28b, 33b, 93–94
Peritonitis, 106–107, 124b
　rebound tenderness, 123b
Peritonsillar abscess, 211, 211f, 228b, 231b
Periumbilical ecchymosis, 120, 120f
Personal protective equipment (PPE), 193
Pertussis, 42–43, 55b, 57b, 195–196, 196f
Pharyngeal abscess, 211–212
Phosphodiesterase 5 (PDE5) inhibitors, nitrates and, 34b
Photophobia, 66
Pit vipers, 255–256
Placenta abruptio, 146–147, 147f, 161b, 162b

Placenta accreta, 152, 160b
Placenta delivery, 152
Placenta previa, 145–146, 146f, 161b
Plantar puncture wounds, 244–245, 249b
Plants, toxic, 258–259
Plasmodium falciparum, 258
Plegia, 64
Pleural effusion, 45–46, 46f
Pneumonia, 43, 56b, 57b
Pneumothorax, 46, 61b
  open, 50, 56b
  small, 61b
Pneumothorax, tension, 49–50, 49f, 54b, 58b
  egophony, 55b
  obstructive shock, 49–50, 49f, 54b, 58b, 61b, 92–93, 99b, 100b, 102b, 104b
Portal hypertension
  cirrhosis, 111
  esophageal varices, 113–114
  hypersplenism, 127b
Portuguese man-of-war stings, 256–257
Posterior cord syndrome, 75, 87b
Postictal state, 70–71
Postpartum hemorrhage (PPH), 154
Postpartum infection, 154–155
Post-traumatic stress disorder (PTSD), 171
Posturing
  decerebrate, 63, 64
  decorticate, 63, 64
Potassium hydroxide, 265
Potassium imbalance, 185–186, 202b, 204b, 206b
Preeclampsia, 147–148, 162b
Pregnancy, 37
  ectopic, 144–145, 144f
Preload, 104b
Premature atrial contractions (PACs), 12, 12f
Premature junctional contractions (PJCs), 14
Premature ventricular contractions (PVCs), 17, 17f, 30b
Preparedness, mitigation, response, recovery, 288–289, 289f, 295b
Pressure injuries, 244, 245f, 246f, 251b
Preterm labor, 145, 162b
Priapism, 87b, 133, 158b
Primary hypertension, 21, 33b
Prinzmetal angina, 5, 26b
Privacy, 287–288, 287t, 295b
Procalcitonin, 102b
Procedural sedation, 283–284, 295b
Professional issues, nurse, 279–282
  Critical Incident Stress Management, 279
  ethical dilemmas, 279–280, 291b, 293b
  evidence-based practice, 280, 280f
  Evidence Hierarchy diagram, 281, 282f
  Four Topics Chart, 279, 291b, 293b
  Level of Evidence table, 281, 281f
  lifelong learning, 280–281, 293b
  research, 281, 293b
Professional issues, patient, 282–288
  cultural considerations, 287
  decision making, 288
  discharge planning, 282, 296b
  end-of-life issues, 282–283, 294b
  forensic evidence collection, 283, 294b
  HIPAA, privacy, and mandatory reporting, 287–288, 287t, 295b, 296b
  informed consent, 288
  pain management and procedural sedation, 283–284, 295b
  patient boarding, 286–287
  patient safety, 284, 284f
  patient satisfaction, 284–285
  transfer and stabilization, 285
  transitions of care, 285–286, 286t

Professional issues, system, 288–290
  delegation of tasks, assistive personnel, 288
  disaster management, 288–289, 289f, 295b
  EMTALA, 285, 289–290, 294b, 295b, 296b
  federal regulations, 289–290
  performance improvement, 290
Pruritus, 179–180, 179f, 202b
Pseudogout, 125b, 239, 251b, 252b
Pseudomelena, 124b, 125b
Psychosis, 169, 175b
Psychosocial emergencies, 165–177
  abuse and neglect, 165, 174b
  aggressive violent behavior, 165–166, 173b, 175b
  anxiety, 166–167
  bipolar disorder, 167–168
  bipolar disorder, depression, 168, 177b
  bipolar disorder, mania, 173b, 176b
  depression, 168
  homicidal ideation, 168–169, 174b, 176b
  panic attacks, 166–167, 174b
  post-traumatic stress disorder, 171
  psychosis, 169, 175b
  situational crisis, 169–170, 174b, 175b, 176b
  suicidal ideation and risk, 170–171, 173b, 177b
  telepsychiatry, 171
Pulmonary contusion, 50
Pulmonary edema, 54b, 55b
  cardiogenic vs. non-cardiogenic, 58b
Pulmonary edema, cardiogenic, 54b, 55b, 58b
Pulmonary edema, noncardiogenic, 55b, 58b
  acute respiratory distress syndrome, 47, 48–49, 103b
  high altitude pulmonary edema, 47
Pulmonary embolus, 47–48
  Factor V Leiden, 93, 100b
  obstructive shock, 49–50, 49f, 54b, 58b, 61b, 92–93, 99b, 100b, 102b, 104b
  risk factors, 55b, 58b
Pulpitis, 212
Pulse pressure, widening, Cushing's triad, 68, 83b, 88b
Pulsus alternans, 100b
Pulsus paradoxus, 21, 35b, 38, 39, 56b, 92, 100b
Puncture wounds, 244–245, 249b
  nail-gun, 249b
  plantar, 249b
  tack or screw driver, 249b
Pyelonephritis, 132
Pyridium, on urine color, 162b

Q

qSOFA (QuickSOFA), 96
Quiz, CEN prep, 297–337
  answers, 338

R

Rabies, 264
Raccoon's sign, 74, 75f, 87b
Radiation exposure, 259–260
  alpha, 259, 276b
  beta, 259
  gamma, 259
  time, distance, and shielding, 259, 273b
Rape, 139–142, 159b–160b
Rattlesnake bite, 255–256, 255f, 273b
Raynaud's disease, 23, 31b, 33b
Rebound tenderness, abdomen, 123b, 127b
Receptive aphasia, 71, 80b
Rectal foreign bodies, 115–116
Regulations, federal, 289–290. See also specific types

Renal calculi, 133–134, 157b
Renal colic, 133
Renal failure, 191–192
 ibuprofen-related, 205b
Renal trauma, 135, 158b
Research, nurse, 281, 293b
Respiratory acidosis, 60b
Respiratory alkalosis, 60b
 noncompensated, 54b
Respiratory emergencies, 37–62
 ABG interpretation, 52t, 60b
 acute respiratory distress syndrome (ARDS), 47, 48–49, 103b
 aspiration, 37–38, 55b
 asthma, 38–39, 55b, 60b, 62b
 bi-pap, 40, 40f, 54b, 57b
 capnography, 52, 52f, 61b
 chest wall trauma, 59b
 chronic obstructive pulmonary disease, 39–40, 40f, 56b, 61b
 endotracheal intubation, 54b, 57b, 59b, 60b
 FAST evaluation, 59b
 geriatrics, 37
 infections, 40–44
 inhalation injuries, 44
 obstruction, 45, 45f, 58b
 pediatrics, 37
 pleural effusion, 45–46, 46f
 pneumothorax, 46, 61b
 pneumothorax, open, 50, 56b
 pregnancy, 37
 pulmonary edema, noncardiogenic, 47, 48–49, 55b, 58b, 103b
 pulmonary embolus, 47–48, 55b, 58b, 93–94, 100b
 respiratory alkalosis, 60b
 respiratory alkalosis, noncompensated, 54b
 tension pneumothorax, 49–50, 49f, 54b, 58b, 61b, 92–93, 99b, 100b, 102b, 104b
 thoracotomy, emergency, 59b
 tracheobronchial injuries, 50, 59b
 trauma, 50–51, 50f
Respiratory infections, 40–44
 bronchitis, 41, 56b
 croup (laryngotracheobronchitis), 40–41, 54b
 epiglottitis, 41–42, 42f, 216–217, 216f, 233b
 influenza, 42
 pertussis, 42–43, 55b, 57b
 pneumonia, 43, 56b, 57b
 respiratory syncytial virus, 43–44, 57b
Respiratory obstruction, 45, 45f, 58b
Respiratory syncytial virus (RSV), 43–44, 57b
Resuscitation
 cardiopulmonary, 9–10, 32b
 damage control, 97, 103b
 family presence, 283, 294b
 neonatal, 153–154, 159b
Retinal artery occlusion, central, 224–225, 228b
Retinal detachment, 226, 228b
Retropharyngeal abscess, 211–212, 231b
Rhinosinusitis, 218, 232b
Rib fractures, 50
Right lower quadrant pain, 105f, 128b
 appendicitis, 106
 Crohn's disease, 117t
Right-sided heart failure, 20–21
Right upper quadrant pain, 105f
Rocky Mountain spotted fever, 263
Rosenbaum vision chart, 232b
Rovsing sign, 125b
Rubella, 193–194, 194f
Rubeola, 193–194, 194f
Rule of nines, 272b

S

Safety, patient, 284, 284f
Sarin, 257
Satisfaction, patient, 284–285
Seatbelt sign, 120, 120f, 130b
Secondary hypertension, 21, 33b
Sedation, procedural, 283–284, 295b
Seizure, febrile, 189
Seizure disorders, 70–71, 84b, 86b
Sensory assessment, 63–64
Sepsis, 95–96, 95f, 192
 damage control resuscitation, 97, 103b
 lactate, tissue hypoxia, 102b
 severe, 192
Septic shock, 95–96, 95f, 157b, 192
Seventh cranial nerve, Bell's palsy, 55b, 214, 231b, 233b
Sexual assault or battery, 139–142, 159b–160b
Sexually transmitted disease (STD), 139, 140t–141t, 158b
Shingles, 197–198, 197f, 209b
Shock, anaphylactic, 94–95, 95f, 99b, 179–180, 179f, 202b, 209b
 children, allergic, 101b
 epinephrine, 95, 101b, 102b
Shock, cardiogenic, 61b, 91–92, 101b, 102b
 vasopressors, 91, 99b
Shock, distributive, 94–96
 anaphylactic, 94–95, 95f, 99b, 101b
 neurogenic, 77, 87b, 94, 99b, 101b
 septic, 95–96, 95f, 157b, 192
Shock, hypovolemic, 61b, 96–98, 99b, 101b, 103b
 burns, severe, 99b
 damage control resuscitation, 97, 103b
 diabetic ketoacidosis, 103b, 205b
 hemorrhagic, 96–97
 nonhemorrhagic, 97
Shock, neurogenic, 77, 87b, 94, 99b, 101b
Shock, obstructive, 92–94
 pericardial tamponade, 92, 92f, 99b, 100b
 pulmonary embolus, 47–48, 55b, 58b, 93–94, 100b
 tension pneumothorax, 49–50, 49f, 54b, 58b, 61b, 92–93, 99b, 100b, 102b, 104b
Shock, septic, 95–96, 95f, 157b, 192
Shock, spinal, 77
Shoulder dislocation, 237–238, 248b, 251b
Shunt dysfunctions, 68–69, 83b
Sialolithiasis, 214
Sickle cell crisis, 181–182, 182f, 203b
Sickle cell disease, 181, 182f
Sinus arrhythmia, 11, 11f
Sinus bradycardia, 10, 10f, 31b, 32b
Sinusitis, 218, 232b
Sinus pause/arrest, 12–13, 12f, 28b
Sinus rhythm, normal, 26b, 27b, 30b
Sinus tachycardia, 10–11, 11f, 26b, 33b
Situational crisis, 169–170, 174b, 175b, 176b
Skin layers, burn depth, 253, 253f
Skull fracture, basilar, 74–75, 74f
Slit lamp examination, 223
SLUDGE, 257, 273b, 276b
Smoke exposure and inhalation, 253
 ABG values, 60b
 carbon monoxide, 265–266, 274b
Snellen vision chart, 232b
Sodium imbalance, 183–184
SOFA (sequential [sepsis-related] organ failure assessment) score, 96
Soman, 257
Spacer (inhaler), 55b
Spider angioma, 112, 112f, 127b
Spinal cord, anatomy and function, 76f

Spinal cord injuries, 75–78, 87*b*
    autonomic dysreflexia (hyperreflexia), 77–78, 81*b*
    complete, 75–76
    neurogenic shock, 77, 87*b*, 94, 99*b*, 101*b*
    spinal shock, 77
Spinal shock, 77
Spontaneous abortion, 143–144, 143*t*, 163*b*
Sprains, 240–241, 249*b*, 250*b*
Stabilization, 285
Stable angina, 26*b*, 31*b*
Standard precautions, 193
Stones
    gallstones, 111, 111*f*, 130*b*
    renal, 133–134, 157*b*
Strains, 240–241, 249*b*, 250*b*
Stroke, 71–73
    anisocoria, 82*b*
    assessment scales, 71–72
    Cincinnati Prehospital Stroke Scale, 71, 87*b*
    FAST evaluation, 72
    heat, 261, 274*b*
    hemorrhagic, 72, 84*b*
    hypoglycemia, 84*b*, 86*b*
    ischemic, 72
    ischemic, transient ischemic attack, 71, 85*b*
    National Institutes of Health Stroke Scale, 72
    posterior, 82*b*
    transient ischemic attack, 71, 85*b*
Stroke mimics, 84*b*, 85*b*
ST-segment elevation (STEMI) acute coronary syndrome, 5, 7–8, 7*t*, 26*b*, 31*b*, 34*b*, 35*b*
Study plan, 4*t*
Study tips, 2
Subdural hemorrhage, 74, 86*b*
Submandibular cellulitis, 217
Submersion injury, 260, 274*b*
Substance abuse, 268–271
    alcohol use and abuse, 268–269
    amphetamine abuse, 270
    cocaine abuse, 269–270, 275*b*
    opiate abuse, 269
    synthetic cathinones ("bath salts"), 270–271, 275*b*
Sucking chest wound, 50
Suicidal ideation, 170–171, 173*b*, 177*b*
    carbon monoxide exposure, 274*b*
Supraventricular tachycardia (SVT), 11–12, 11*f*, 26*b*, 28*b*
Surviving Sepsis Campaign (SCC), 96
Sutures, discharge instructions, 251*b*
Swimmer's ear, 217
Swiss Cheese model, 284, 284*f*
Syndrome of inappropriate ADH secretion (SIADH), 183
Synthetic cathinones, 270–271, 275*b*
Syphilis, 140*t*–141*t*
Systemic inflammatory response syndrome (SIRS), 96, 103*b*, 192
Systemic vascular resistance (SVR), 104*b*
Systolic hypertension, 21, 33*b*

T

Tachycardia
    sinus, 10–11, 11*f*, 26*b*, 33*b*
    supraventricular, 11–12, 11*f*, 26*b*, 28*b*
    ventricular, 17–18, 17*f*, 27*b*
Taeniasis, 258
Taenis solium infection, 258, 276*b*
Tampon, retained, 158*b*
Tapeworms, 258
Tdap vaccine, 43, 56*b*

Telepsychiatry, 171
Temperature-related emergencies
    cold-related, 261–262, 262*f*, 263*f*, 274*b*, 275*b*
    heat-related, 260–261, 274*b*
Temporal arteritis, 67
Temporomandibular joint (TMJ) dislocation, 219–220
Tension pneumothorax, 49–50, 49*f*, 54*b*, 58*b*
    egophony, 55*b*
    obstructive shock, 61*b*, 92–93, 99*b*, 100*b*, 102*b*, 104*b*
Testicular torsion, 134, 134*f*
Test preparation, CEN
    prep quiz, 297–337
    prep quiz, answers, 338
Thiamine, post-bariatric surgery, 206*b*
Thoracic trauma, 50–51, 50*f*
Thoracotomy, emergency, 59*b*
Threatened abortion, 143–144, 143*t*, 163*b*
Thrombocytopenia, 180–181, 180*f*
Thromboelastography (TEG), 97, 103*b*
Thromboembolism, venous, 24, 28*b*, 33*b*, 93–94
Thrombophilia, 100*b*
Thrombotic thrombocytopenia purpura, 180–181, 180*f*
Thumb sign, 216, 216*f*
Thyroid disorders, 187–188
    myxedema coma, 187–188, 205*b*, 207*b*
    thyroid storm, 188, 188*f*
Thyroid storm, 188, 188*f*
Thyrotoxic crisis, 188, 188*f*
Tic douloureux, 214–215
Tick-borne illness, 263–264
    Lyme disease, 263–264, 264*f*
    Rocky Mountain spotted fever, 263
Tissue donation, 282
Tissue hypoxia, lactate, 102*b*
Tooth extraction, dental abscess after, 212–213
Total body water (TBW), 182
Total burn surface area (TBSA), 253, 254*f*, 272*b*
Toxic gases, 253
Toxicology emergencies, 265–271
    acids and alkalis, 265, 272*b*
    carbon monoxide, 265–266, 274*b*
    cyanide, 266, 277*b*
    drug interactions, 266
    gases, 253
    insecticides, 257
    organophosphates, 257, 272*b*, 273*b*, 277*b*
    overdose and intentional ingestions, 266–268, 275*b*
    substance abuse, 268–271, 275*b*
    toxic plant exposure, 258–259
Toxic plant exposure, 258–259
Toxic-shock syndrome, 158*b*
Trachea, deviated, 54*b*, 58*b*
Tracheobronchial injuries, 50, 59*b*
Transfer and stabilization, 285
Transient ischemic attack (TIA), 71, 85*b*
Transitions of care, 285–286, 286*t*
Transmission-based precautions, 193
Trauma
    FAST evaluation, 59*b*
Trench mouth, 216, 233*b*
Triage, emergency, 290, 296*b*
Trichomoniasis, 140*t*–141*t*
Tricyclic antidepressant (TCA) overdose, 267–268, 275*b*
Trigeminal nerve, 64*f*, 64*t*, 86*b*
Trigeminal neuralgia, 214–215, 231*b*
Tripod fracture, 220, 231*b*
Trismus, 229*b*
Trochlear nerve, 64*f*, 64*t*, 86*b*, 87*b*
Trousseau sign, 184

Tuberculosis (TB), 200
Tumbling "E" vision chart, 232b
Tympanic membrane rupture, 219, 230b

U

Ulcer, 109–110, 110f
    Helicobacter pylori, 109b
    perforated, 124b
Ulcerative colitis (UC), 116–117, 117t, 129b
Umbilical cord prolapse, 152–153
Unclassified seizures, 70–71
Unstable angina, 5, 26b, 31b
Upper airway, 45, 45f. *See also* Respiratory emergencies
Upper GI bleeding, 107–108, 108t, 124b
Ureter trauma, 135
Urethral trauma, 136, 158b, 161b
Urinary retention, 136
Urinary tract infection (UTI), 131
Urticaria, 179–180, 179f, 202b, 209b
Uveitis, 224, 229b, 232b

V

Vaginal bleeding, abnormal and dysfunctional, 136
Vaginal discharge, 138
Vaginal hemorrhage, 136–137
Vaginal insufflation injuries, 160b
Vagus nerve, 64f, 64t, 86b
Vancomycin-resistant enterococci (VRE), 199–200
Variant angina, 5
Varicella zoster, 196–197, 197f
Varicella-zoster virus (VZV)
    chicken pox, 196–197, 197f, 209b
    herpes zoster, 197–198, 197f, 209b
Varicose veins, 31b
Vascular cognitive impairment (VCI), 65
Vascular dementia, 65
Vasopressors, 99b
    cardiogenic shock, 91, 99b
    neurogenic shock, 94
    septic shock, 95, 96b
Vector-borne illnesses, 263–264
    Lyme disease, 263–264, 264f
    Rocky Mountain spotted fever, 263
    tick-borne illness, 263–264

Venous thromboembolism (VTE), 24, 28b, 33b
    obstructive shock, 93–94
Ventilation, neonatal resuscitation, 153, 159b
Ventricular fibrillation, 18–19, 18f, 26b, 30b
Ventricular tachycardia, 17–18, 17f, 27b
Vestibulocochlear nerve, 64f, 64t, 86b, 231b
Vincent disease, 216, 233b
Violent behavior, aggressive, 165–166, 173b, 175b
Virchow's triad, 93, 101b, 125b
Vision, blurry, after head injury, 88b
Vision chart, 223, 232b
Visual acuity, 222–223, 223f, 232b
Visual field, 222
Volts, 254
Von Willebrand's disease, 100b, 181, 202b
VX, 257

W

Waddell's triad, 101b
Wasp stings, 256
Wenckebach atrioventricular block, 15–16, 15f, 27b, 32b
Wernicke encephalopathy, 206b
Wernicke's aphasia, 71, 80b
Whooping cough, 42–43, 55b, 57b, 195–196, 196f
Withdrawal, 63
Withdrawing care, 283
Withholding care, 283
Wound emergencies, 241–247
    abrasions, 241–242, 242f
    abscess, 243, 250b
    bites, 242–243, 250b
    blast injuries, 247
    debridement, 249b
    foreign body, vegetative, 248b
    foreign body, wooden, 248b
    missile/penetrating injuries, 243–244
    pressure injuries, 244, 245f, 246f, 251b
    puncture wounds, 244–245, 249b
    sutures, discharge instructions, 251b

Z

Zygomatic fractures, 220, 231b

Lightning Source UK Ltd.
Milton Keynes UK
UKHW052044080421
381679UK00005B/66